Emergency
Nursing
Core Curriculum

Emergency Nursing Core Curriculum

Fifth Edition

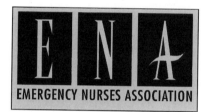

EMERGENCY NURSES ASSOCIATION

SAUNDERS

An Imprint of Elsevier

SAUNDERS
An Imprint of Elsevier

The Curtis Center
Independence Square West
Philadelphia, Pennsylvania 19106

Library of Congress Cataloging-in-Publication Data

Emergency Nurses Association.

Emergency nursing core curriculum / Emergency Nurses Association.—5th ed.

p.   cm.

Includes bibliographical references and index.

ISBN-13: 978-0-7216-8241-9   ISBN-10: 0-7216-8241-3

1. Emergency nursing—Study and teaching.   2. Curriculum
   planning.   I. Title. [DNLM: 1. Emergency Nursing—education
   outlines.   2. Curriculum outlines.   WY 18 E525e 2000]

RT120.E4E45 2000   610.73′61′071—dc21

DNLM/DLC   98–48478

EMERGENCY NURSING CORE CURRICULUM

Permissions may be sought directly from Elsevier's Health Sciences Rights
Department in Philadelphia, PA, USA: phone: (+1) 215 239 3804, fax: (+1) 215 239 3805,
e-mail: healthpermissions@elsevier.com. You may also complete your request on-line
via the Elsevier homepage (http://www.elsevier.com), by selecting 'Customer Support'
and then 'Obtaining Permissions'.

Printed in the United States of America.

ISBN-13: 978-0-7216-8241-9
ISBN-10: 0-7216-8241-3

Last digit is the print number: 9

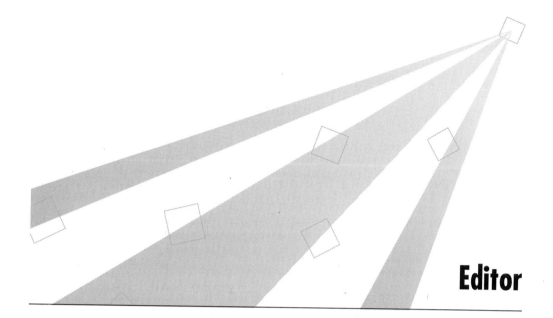

Editor

Kathleen Sanders Jordan, RN, MS, FNP, CCRN, CEN
Family Nurse Practitioner, Emergency Medicine
Mid-Atlantic Emergency Medicine Associates
Charlotte, North Carolina

Contributors

Susan Albrecht, PhD, RN, MPM
Assistant Professor, University of Pittsburgh School of Nursing; Staff
Nurse, South Hills Health System, Pittsburgh, Pennsylvania
Pain Management

Cynthia S. Baxter, RN, BSN, CCRN, CEN
Critical Care Educator, Central Baptist Hospital, Lexington, Kentucky
Genitourinary Emergencies

Lisa Marie Bernardo, RN, PhD
Assistant Professor, Health and Community Systems, University of
Pittsburgh School of Nursing, Pittsburgh, Pennsylvania
Pain Management

Linda Jacobson Bracken, RN, BS, MEd, MPA, CEN
Nurse Manager, Emergency Department, Stanford Healthcare, Stanford,
California
Education

Donna M. Coimbra-Emanuele, RN, MN, CEN, CCRN, FNP
Clinical Preceptor, Family Nurse Practitioner Program, University of
Southern California, Los Angeles, School of Nursing, Los Angeles; Family
Nurse Practitioner, Verdugo Hills Medical Associates, Glendale;
Huntington Memorial Hospital, Pasadena; Emergency Nurse Practitioner,
Long Beach Community Medical Center, Long Beach, California
Dental, Ear, Nose, and Throat Emergencies

Frank L. Cole, PhD, RN, CEN, CS, FNP
Associate Professor of Nursing, Division Head of Emergency Care,

Director of Emergency Nurse Practitioner Education, University of Texas
Health Science Center, School of Nursing, Houston, Texas
Research

Courtney Cosby, MN, MS
Adjunct Faculty, Virginia Commonwealth University/Medical College of
Virginia; Director, Critical Care and Emergency Department, Henrico
Doctors' Hospital, Richmond, Virginia
Organ and Tissue Donation and Post-Transplantation Emergencies

P. Howard Cummings, EdD, RN
Clinical Associate Professor, School of Nursing, University of North
Carolina at Wilmington; Staff Nurse, VitaLink-Mobile Intensive Care
Transport, New Hanover Regional Medical Center, Wilmington, North
Carolina
Abdominal Emergencies

Sally P. Cummings, EdD, RN, FNP
Associate Professor, School of Nursing, University of North Carolina at
Wilmington, Wilmington, North Carolina
Abdominal Emergencies

Kathleen A. Doherty, BS, BSN
Nurse Educator, Emergency, Trauma and Radiology Services Department,
Parkland Health and Hospital System, Dallas, Texas
Cardiovascular Emergencies

Patricia C. Epifanio, RN, MS, CEN
Affiliate Faculty, University of Maryland, Baltimore, Maryland; Partner,
MBA Company, Cape Coral, Florida
Ocular Emergencies

Cynthia A. Horvath, BSN, MSN, CEN
Clinical Nurse Specialist, Emergency Department, UAB Hospital,
University of Alabama at Birmingham, Birmingham, Alabama
Shock Emergencies

Charose James, RN, BSN, CEN
Staff Nurse, Emergency Department, Methodist Hospital, Omaha,
Nebraska
Respiratory Emergencies

Kathleen Sanders Jordan, RN, MS, FNP, CCRN, CEN
Family Nurse Practitioner, Emergency Medicine, Mid-Atlantic Emergency
Medicine Associates, Charlotte, North Carolina
Obstetrical and Gynecological Emergencies

Jorie Klein, RN
Clinical Instructor, Department of Surgery, University of Texas
Southwestern Medical Center; Director, Trauma Services, Parkland Health
and Hospital System, Dallas, Texas
Disaster Preparedness/Disaster Management

Susan Engman Lazear, RN, MN, CEN, CFRN
Director, Specialists in Medical Education, Woodinville, Washington
Emergency Patient Transfer and Transport
Mental Health Emergencies

Genell Lee, JD, MSN, RN
Attorney at Law, Hauth and Lee, LLC, Birmingham, Alabama
Legal Issues

Robin Rosser Martinez, RN, MS
Health Care Consultant, Alexandria, Virginia
Education

Cathy McDeed-Breault, RN, MSN, CEN, CANP
Adult Nurse Practitioner, Veterans Administration Medical Center, La Jolla, California
Toxicological Emergencies

Barbara M. Mitchell, RN, MSN
Senior Quality Specialist, Inova Fairfax Hospital, Falls Church, Virginia
Wound Management Emergencies

Lorene Newberry, RN, MS, CEN
Clinical Nurse Specialist, Emergency Services, WellStar Health System, Marietta, Georgia
General Medical Emergencies: Part II

Sharon Pierce Peabody, MS, CEN, FNP
Affiliate Faculty, University of Alaska-Fairbanks, Fairbanks; Nurse Practitioner, Community Health Aide Program, Alaska Native Medical Center, Anchorage, Alaska
General Medical Emergencies: Part I

Carol Ann Petersen, RN, BSN, MSA
Trauma Program Manager, Nurse Trauma Coordinator, Bryanlgh Medical Center West, Lincoln, Nebraska
Multisystem Trauma and Injury Prevention

Gail E. Polli, RN, MS, CS
Psychiatric Clinical Nurse Specialist and Manager, Psychiatric Service, Emergency Department, South Shore Hospital, South Weymouth, Massachusetts
Mental Health Emergencies

Cherie J. Revere, RN, MSN, CEN, CRNP
Clinical Nurse Specialist, Emergency Department, University of South Alabama Medical Center, Mobile, Alabama
Facial Emergencies

Laura Skidmore Rhodes, BSN, MSN
Executive Secretary, West Virginia Board of Examiners for Registered Professional Nurses, Charleston, West Virginia
Professionalism and Leadership

Reneé Semonin-Holleran, RN, PhD, CEN, CCRN, CFRN
Clinical Faculty, University of Cincinnati College of Nursing and Health,
University of Kentucky, College of Nursing; Chief Flight Nurse,
Emergency Clinical Nurse Specialist, and Sexual Assault Nurse Examiner,
University Hospital, Cincinnati, Ohio
Environmental Emergencies

Diane M. Twedell, MS, BSN, CCRN, CEN
Education Program Coordinator, Department of Emergency Services,
Mayo Clinic and Mayo Foundation, Rochester, Minnesota
Nursing Process: Assessment and Priority Setting

Joan A. Snyder, RN, MS, CEN
Trauma and Emergency Medical Service Systems Consultant, Dahlgren,
Virginia
Neurological Emergencies

Joan Walker, RN, BScN
Orthopaedic Trauma Service Manager, Parkland Health and Hospital
System, Dallas, Texas
Orthopedic Emergencies

Polly Gerber Zimmermann, RN, MS, MBA, CEN
Professor, Harry S. Truman College; Staff Nurse, Swedish Covenant
Hospital; Associate Nurse, American Airlines, O'Hare International
Airport, Chicago, Illinois
Professionalism and Leadership

Reviewers

Susan A. Barnason, PhD, RN-CS, CEN, CCRN
University of Nebraska Medical Center
College of Nursing
Omaha, Nebraska

Dineke M. Boyce, RN, MN, CEN, CFNP
Naval Medical Center, San Diego
San Diego, California

Jonathan L. Burstein, MD, FACEP
Harvard Medical School
Boston, Massachusetts

Col. Edward M. Eitzen, Jr., MD, MPH, FACEP, FAAP
Chief, Operational Medicine Division
U.S. Army Medical Research Institute of Infectious Diseases
Fort Detrick, Maryland

Susan Engman Lazear, RN, MN, CEN, CFRN
Director, Specialists in Medical Education
Woodinville, Washington

Vicki C. Patrick, RN, MS, CS, ACNP, CEN
University of Texas at Arlington
School of Nursing
Arlington, Texas

Preface

In the new millennium, emergency nursing will be faced with tremendous challenges and changes. These will include boundless opportunities for growth and enrichment both for emergency nurses as individuals and for emergency nursing as a specialty organization. Inherent in these opportunities are both intrinsic and extrinsic situations that we must be prepared to successfully manage. The challenges that we now face include the provision of outstanding quality emergency care in the most cost-effective manner, the advancement in technology, the change in overall health care delivery structure and design, and the pressure of remaining competitive in an ever changing health care environment. Emergency care delivery systems have already been greatly affected by the impact of changes in health care restructuring and redesign. It is anticipated that emergency nurses will continue to be challenged by many more changes in the future.

Emergency nursing is an essential component of the health care delivery system, and the Emergency Nurses Association is the world's largest nursing organization devoted entirely to the advancement of emergency nursing practice. The mission of the Emergency Nurses Association is to provide visionary leadership for emergency nursing and emergency care. The Emergency Nurses Association also serves as the expert body to define the future of emergency nursing and emergency care through advocacy, expertise, innovation, and leadership. As a constituent of the association, each individual emergency nurse is an essential component in the evolution of the health care delivery system.

The *Emergency Nursing Core Curriculum, fifth edition,* is designed to articulate the knowledge base required of emergency nurses to meet the challenges that are encountered. The major impetus to prepare a fifth edition of the *Emergency Nursing Core Curriculum* was the need to update as well as expand the depth and breadth of the content contained in the fourth edition, in an effort to increase the core knowledge base of the emergency nurse. There are many similarities in the fifth edition compared with previous editions. The overall organization of clinical content by body systems remains the same. The clinical content is prepared in the framework of the nursing process. The content continues to be presented in outline format in a reader-friendly manner. Each clinical chapter begins with a general strategy approach based on the organ system involved. Discussion outlining specific disease entities follows. There is a major focus in the *fifth edition* to expand upon the pathophysiological basis of each specific disease entity. Chapters have been added to include pain management, multisystem trauma, and injury prevention. A second medical chapter presents content on communicable and infectious diseases. Many other disease entities have been included within specific chapters. The most current research-based diagnostic and treatment modalities have been incorporated throughout the text.

The appendices of the *Emergency Nursing Core Curriculum, fifth edition,* have also been expanded. An appendix is included to present nursing diagnosis–driven patient outcome statements, which incorporate the nursing diagnoses most appropriate to the specialty of emergency nursing. Other new appendices include Rapid Sequence Intubation, Infant Glasgow Coma Scale, ACIP Recommended Schedules of Vaccinations for 1999, Mini-Mental Status Examination, and Advanced Practice.

The *Emergency Nursing Core Curriculum, fifth edition,* is intended to be used by practicing emergency nurses at all levels of expertise for various purposes, including knowledge acquisition, verification, standards development, quality improvement, and education for staff and patients. This text is also designed to be an essential resource in the library of every practicing emergency nurse.

The *Emergency Nursing Core Curriculum, fifth edition,* reflects the expertise and commitment of the contributors and reviewers. Each individual involved in the preparation of this book has made a tremendous contribution and is to be commended. We have attempted in this fifth edition to provide the most current validated knowledge base, outlining both the art and science of emergency nursing. Our goal is still to advance emergency nursing to an even higher level. We welcome your comments and suggestions in this regard.

KATHLEEN SANDERS JORDAN

Acknowledgments

To emergency nurses, physicians, prehospital care providers, and all of the other individuals for their enthusiasm and commitment, which make it possible to provide the high quality of emergency care of which we can all be proud.

To our patients, who provide us with motivation, insight, and wisdom as we strive to improve emergency care.

To our families and friends for their love, encouragement, support, and enthusiasm that help us to keep life in its most important and meaningful perspective.

To the Emergency Nurses Association for their leadership, vision, and endless support:

Patricia Blake, CAE
Executive Director

Claudia Niersbach, RN, JD, CEN, EMT-P
Director, Educational Services

1997 Board of Directors
K. Sue Hoyt, RN, MN, CEN
President

1998 Board of Directors
Anne Manton, RN, PhD, CEN
President

1999 Board of Directors
Jean Proehl, RN, MN, CEN, CCRN
President

Contents

8. General Medical Emergencies: Part II 275
Lorene Newberry, MSN, RN, CEN

9. Genitourinary Emergencies 319
Cynthia S. Baxter, RN, BSN, CCRN, CEN

10. Mental Health Emergencies 343

Gail E. Polli, RN, MS, CS
Susan Engman Lazear, RN, MN, CEN, CFRN

11. Multisystem Trauma and Injury Prevention 371

Carol Ann Petersen, RN, BSN, MSA

26. Education **751**

Linda Jacobson Bracken, RN, BS, MEd, MPA, CEN,
and Robin Rosser Martinez, RN, MS

Diane M. Twedell, MS, BSN, CCRN, CEN

CHAPTER **1**

Nursing Process: Assessment and Priority Setting

MAJOR TOPICS

I. PRIMARY ASSESSMENT

The primary survey is the basis for all emergent interventions delivered in the care of patients. All factors assessed during the primary survey are of such a critical nature that any major deviation from normal requires immediate intervention. The assessment process does not continue until all life-threatening deviations found in the primary survey receive appropriate intervention.

A. Overview of major components

1. **Subjective data collection**
   a. *Content of data*
      1) Brief one-line statement
         a) Chief complaint

        b) Precipitating event/onset of symptoms

        c) Mechanism of injury

    2) Time factor

        a) Chronological sequence of first symptom or injury to initiation of care

  b. *Source of data*

    1) Patient

    2) Family or significant other

    3) Emergency medical services personnel

    4) Bystander

2. Objective data collection

  a. *Airway/cervical spine (C-spine)*

  b. *Breathing*

  c. *Circulation*

  d. *Brief neurological exam*

A mnemonic has been developed to assist in the primary assessment steps.

A = Airway and cervical spine

B = Breathing

C = Circulation

D = Disability (Neurological status)

B. Individual components of primary assessment

  1. Airway and C-spine (any patient whose mechanism of injury, symptoms, or physical findings suggest a spinal injury should have their C-spine stabilized or immobilized)

    a. *Assessment*

      1) Open and clear

        a) Subjective data

          (1) No history related to airway problem

          (2) No dyspnea or dysphagia

        b) Objective data

          (1) Patient able to speak or make sounds appropriate for age

          (2) No foreign material is visible in upper airway (blood, vomitus, loose teeth)

          (3) Chest rises and falls easily with inspired air or positive-pressure ventilation

        c) Action/Intervention

          (1) If patient has mechanism of injury, symptoms, or physical findings to suggest a spinal injury, the C-spine should be stabilized or immobilized

          (2) Verify that airway is established, open, and clear

      2) Partially obstructed or obstructed/unacceptable and requires immediate intervention

        a) Subjective data

          (1) Trauma to face, mouth, pharynx, neck, or chest

          (2) Patient was eating when difficulty began

          (3) Recent vomiting

          (4) Contact with allergen

          (5) Patient was discovered putting objects into mouth

      b) Objective data
- (1) Substernal, intercostal retracting
- (2) Drooling in patient other than infant
- (3) Nasal flaring
- (4) Facial weakness or paralysis
- (5) Violent coughing
- (6) Sitting up and leaning forward; tripod position
- (7) Decreased level of consciousness
- (8) Cyanotic, dusky-gray skin color, especially mucous membranes and nail beds
- (9) Inspiratory and/or expiratory stridor
- (10) Panic behavior, hands on throat
- (11) Patient unable to speak or make sounds appropriate for age
- (12) Absence of breathing

  b. Possible etiologies of airway obstruction
- 1) Tongue falls back, occluding upper airway
- 2) Saliva/sputum
- 3) Vomitus
- 4) Blood
- 5) Teeth/dentures (may be loose or knocked out as a result of facial trauma)
- 6) Food (e.g., hot dogs, hard candy)
- 7) Any item small enough to fit into mouth (e.g., marbles, small toy parts, small parts from pacifier, balloon)
- 8) Airway edema from allergic reactions, inhalation injury, trauma, disease process
- 9) Damaged airway tissue from trauma to face or neck

  c. Nursing diagnoses/collaborative problems
- 1) Anxiety/fear
- 2) Impaired gas exchange
- 3) Ineffective airway clearance

  d. Interventions (see section II. Resuscitation)

  e. Expected outcome/evaluation (see Appendix B)

2. C-spine

  a. Assessment
- 1) Acceptable/stable
  - a) Subjective data
    - (1) No history of trauma; not suspected
    - (2) No history of degenerative bone disease
    - (3) No complaints of pain on movement or palpation of neck
  - b) Objective data
    - (1) Sensation and movement in all extremities without limitation or weakness
    - (2) Breathing not impaired
- 2) Unacceptable or requires immediate intervention/unstable
  - a) Subjective data
    - (1) Direct trauma to head or neck
    - (2) Trauma involving sudden deceleration, as in motor vehicle crash or fall
    - (3) Numbness or tingling of extremities
    - (4) Neck pain may be present or absent
    - (5) Electrical shock
  - b) Objective data: possibility of no objective findings; nondisplaced fractures of C-spine may not compromise neurological system

        (1) Paralysis or paresthesia

        (2) Abdominal breathing indicates possible paralysis of diaphragm

        (3) Decreased or absent sensation or movement below level of injury

        (4) Weakness

        (5) Bowel or bladder incontinence

        (6) Loss of sympathetic motor tone

        (7) Hypotension from vasodilation

        (8) Bradycardia

        (9) Flaccid paralysis

        (10) Loss of sphincter tone

        (11) Cool, dry skin

        (12) Bounding peripheral pulses

        (13) Hypothermia: loss of temperature regulation

        (14) Inability to shiver or sweat

        (15) Poikilothermy: patient assumes temperature of environment

    b. Possible etiologies of cervical spine injury

        1) Trauma

        2) Disease process

    c. Nursing diagnoses

        1) Fluid volume deficit

        2) Impaired gas exchange

        3) Ineffective airway clearance

        4) Ineffective breathing pattern

        5) Ineffective thermoregulation

        6) Risk for aspiration

        7) Risk for injury

    d. Interventions (see section II. Resuscitation)

    e. Expected outcome/evaluation (see Appendix B)

3. Breathing

    a. Assessment

        1) Acceptable

          a) Subjective data

            (1) No distress

            (2) No history of trauma to chest or abdomen

            (3) No deviation from patient's usual breathing pattern

          b) Objective data

            (1) Chest rises and falls spontaneously

            (2) Exhaled air may be felt or heard escaping from nose, mouth, or stoma

            (3) Quality is smooth, even

            (4) Chest expansion equal bilaterally

            (5) Possibly mild degree of retracting, wheezing, and accessory muscle activity

        2) Compromised or absent/unacceptable and requires immediate intervention

          a) Subjective data

            (1) Blunt or penetrating trauma to neck, chest, back, or abdomen

            (2) Severe asthma, emphysema, heart disease

            (3) Dyspnea

            (4) History of respiratory arrest

          b) Objective data

            (1) Apnea

            (2) Agonal breathing less than 10 breaths/min

(3) Shallow, weak, gasping respirations

(4) Marked cyanosis, diaphoresis, and respiratory effort

(5) Absent breath sounds

(6) Unable to converse in phrases or complete sentences

(7) Severe retractions (especially in children)

(8) Pulse oximeter (O_2 saturation) <95%

(9) Arterial blood gas abnormal

    b. Possible etiologies

      1) Disease process

      2) Trauma: blunt or penetrating

      3) Chemical/drug exposure

    c. Nursing diagnoses

      1) Anxiety/fear

      2) Impaired gas exchange

      3) Ineffective breathing pattern

    d. Interventions (see section II. Resuscitation)

    e. Expected outcome/evaluation (see Appendix B)

4. Circulation

    a. Pulse

      1) Assessment

        a) Acceptable

          (1) Subjective data

            (a) No report of prior cardiac arrest

            (b) No report of life-threatening dysrhythmia

          (2) Objective data

            (a) Radial pulse palpable

            (b) Rate >60 (>100 in infants, >80 in small children)

            (c) Rhythm regular

        b) Compromised or absent/unacceptable and requires immediate intervention

          (1) Subjective data

            (a) Unconsciousness

            (b) Reported cardiac arrest

          (2) Objective data

            (a) Heart rate <60 or >100 and weak in adults

            (b) Unresponsive

            (c) Carotid pulse not palpable

            (d) Heart rate <100 in infants, <80 in toddlers

      2) Possible etiologies of pulse abnormalities

        a) Disease process

        b) Trauma: blunt or penetrating

        c) Chemical/drug exposure

        d) Hypothermia

      3) Nursing diagnoses

        a) Tissue perfusion, altered renal, cerebral, cardiopulmonary, gastrointestinal, peripheral

        b) Decreased cardiac output

      4) Interventions (see section II. Resuscitation)

      5) Expected outcomes/evaluation (see Appendix B)

    b. Bleeding

      1) Assessment

        a) Acceptable or adequate for present

          (1) Subjective data

            (a) No history of disease or trauma that would result in bleeding

            (b) Bleeding easily controlled prior to arrival at hospital

        (2) Objective data

            (a) No visible active bleeding

            (b) No visible bleeding but is oozing, low volume, dark red

    b) Unacceptable or requires immediate intervention

        (1) Subjective data

            (a) Extensive blood loss prior to arrival

            (b) Unable to control bleeding en route to hospital

        (2) Objective data

            (a) Uncontrolled, pulsating, or high-flow bleeding

            (b) Marked pallor of sclera and nail beds

            (c) Large clots in emesis, stool, or vaginal discharge

            (d) Gross swelling of extremities (e.g., thigh)

            (e) Systolic blood pressure < 90 mm Hg, rapid heart rate, thready, weak pulse

  2) Possible etiologies

    a) Trauma

    b) Disease process

  3) Nursing diagnoses

    a) Anxiety/fear

    b) Decreased cardiac output

    c) Fluid volume deficit

    d) Impaired gas exchange

  4) Interventions (see section II. Resuscitation)

  5) Expected outcomes/evaluation (see Appendix B)

c. *Perfusion*

  1) Assessment

    a) Acceptable

        (1) Subjective data

            (a) No history that might result in decreased perfusion

        (2) Objective data

            (a) Patient alert and oriented to person, place, time, and event

            (b) Skin warm and dry

            (c) Capillary refill brisk

            (d) Pulse rate within normal limits

    b) Unacceptable/requires immediate intervention

        (1) Subjective data

            (a) Patient weak, lightheaded, nauseated

            (b) Patient verbalizes sense of impending doom

            (c) Patient feels short of breath

        (2) Objective data

            (a) Patient confused, disoriented

            (b) Appears short of breath

            (c) Diaphoretic, cool skin

            (d) Pale, dusky skin color

            (e) Restless

            (f) Peripheral pulses weak, thready, and rapid

            (g) Vomiting, retching

            (h) Capillary refill delayed > 2 seconds

  2) Possible etiologies

    a) Trauma

    b) Disease process

  3) Nursing diagnoses

a) Decreased cardiac output
b) Fear
c) Fluid volume deficit
d) Tissue perfusion, altered cardiopulmonary, renal, gastrointestinal, peripheral
4) Interventions (see section II. Resuscitation)
5) Expected outcome/evaluation (see Appendix B)

5. **Disability (neurological status)**
   a. *Assessment*
      1) Acceptable
         a) Subjective data
            (1) No history of loss of consciousness
            (2) No history of head trauma
            (3) No sudden onset of headache
         b) Objective data
            (1) Determine level of consciousness using "AVPU scale"
               A = Alert, awake; responsive to voice; oriented to person, time, and place
               V = Verbal; responds to voice but not fully oriented to person, time, or place
               P = Pain; does not respond to voice but responds to painful stimuli
               U = Unresponsive; does not respond to voice or pain
            (2) Pupil assessment: pupils equal and reactive to light
            (3) Glasgow Coma Scale (see Appendix C)
            (4) Motor/movement
               (a) Ability to respond to commands and move all four extremities
               (b) Wiggle fingers and toes
               (c) Strength: dorsiflexion, plantar flexion, hand grasp
      2) Unacceptable/requires immediate intervention
         a) Subjective data
            (1) History of loss of consciousness or unconscious
            (2) Head trauma
            (3) Sudden onset of headache
         b) Objective data
            (1) Altered level of consciousness
            (2) Pupillary assessment: unequal, "blown," irregular shape, reaction to light slow or absent
      3) Possible etiologies
         a) Trauma
         b) Disease process
      4) Analysis: differential nursing diagnosis/collaborative problems
         a) Gas exchange impaired
         b) Risk for aspiration
         c) Risk for injury
         d) Tissue perfusion, altered cerebral
      5) Intervention (see section II. Resuscitation)
      6) Expected outcome/evaluation (see Appendix B)

II. RESUSCITATION

The goal of the resuscitation in the primary assessment is to correct all life-threatening deviations from normal. Resuscitation priorities follow the same mnemonic as the primary assessment because they occur simultaneously.

A. Airway

1. **Open airway**
   a. *A jaw-thrust maneuver or chin lift without head tilt should be used in any suspected C-spine injury*
   b. *Remove any loose objects or foreign debris: do not blindly finger sweep the mouth; remove only material that can be visualized*
   c. *Suction gently to clear airway; deep suctioning may stimulate the gag reflex*
   d. *Oropharyngeal airway: use only in unconscious patient; may stimulate vomiting or laryngospasm in conscious patient*
      1) Select proper size airway by measuring from the corner of the mouth to the tip of the ear lobe
      2) Insert the airway with the distal tip of the airway turned toward the roof of the mouth; as the airway passes across the back of the tongue, rotate it 180 degrees; an alternative method of insertion is to use a tongue blade to hold the tongue down and insert into the airway, following the natural curve of the mouth
      3) Reassess airway patency
   e. *If airway is obstructed and it is not possible to ventilate the patient, proceed to back blows, chest thrusts, and abdominal thrusts as indicated*
   f. *Nasopharyngeal airway: use in conscious or semiconscious patient; useful when unable to place oropharyngeal airway (i.e., trismus, massive trauma)*
      1) Select proper size airway by measuring from the tip of nose to ear lobe; use the largest size that will fit in patient's nostril
      2) Lubricate airway with water-soluble lubricant
      3) Insert airway into nare with the bevel facing the nasal septum; direct airway posteriorly until flange rests on nostril
      4) Reassess airway patency
   g. *Endotracheal intubation (see Appendix H: Rapid Sequence Intubation): use to maintain airway patency, reduce risk of aspiration, and provide delivery of high concentrations of oxygen; nasotracheal intubation contraindicated in patients with facial fractures or fractures at base of skull*
      1) Gather all equipment: syringe, laryngoscope, blades, additional ET tubes, different sizes, style and tube ties, tape, suction, tonsil tip, catheter tip, BVM oxygen source, carbon dioxide (CO_2) detector, pulse oximeter, extra batteries
      2) Select appropriate tube size: average adult, 6.5–8.0; pediatric, use Broselow resuscitation tape
      3) Inflate endotracheal (ET) tube to cuff, check for patency of balloon
         a) Term neonates, 3.0–3.5 mm
         b) Infants (6 months to 1 year), 4 mm
         c) Age > 1 year to 8 years of age

$$\text{ET tube size mmID} = \frac{16 + \text{patient's age in years}}{4}$$

      4) Oxygenate patient with bag-valve mask device
         a) Medicate patient (Refer to Appendix H: Medications Used With Rapid-Sequence Intubation)
      5) Obtain proper head position: head extended and neck flexed (i.e., the sniffing position); if C-spine injury is suspected, one person is in charge of maintaining C-spine immobilization
      6) Assist with opening of mouth and insertion of laryngoscope blade
      7) When cords are visualized, insert ET tube into trachea

8) Inflate ET tube cuff with 10–20 mL of air via syringe
9) Confirm tube placement via delivery of manual breath while auscultating breath sounds over both lungs and epigastrium and observing for rise of chest wall
10) If stomach gurgling occurs, the tube is not in the trachea but in the esophagus; tube should be removed and patient oxygenated
11) If the chest wall rises, the lung fields, both at the apexes and anterior bases, should be auscultated and documented
12) Secure the tube via tape, twill ties, or commercial tube holder
13) Obtain chest x-ray film for confirming tube placement
14) End-tidal CO_2 detectors may also be used for determining correct tube placement; once ET tube has been inserted, a disposable end-tidal CO_2 detector can be placed on the end of the tube; color of detector changes based on concentration of CO_2

- Purple: during inspiration when CO_2 is very low
- Yellow: during expiration when CO_2 is very high
- Beige: intermediate concentration of CO_2

If the device is purple during expiration, the tube may be misplaced in the esophagus
h. *Needle cricothyrotomy: indicated when ET intubation is difficult or surgical airways are not available—a needle is passed through the cricothyroid membrane into the trachea*
1) Assemble equipment: antiseptic solution, 10 to 14 gauge over needle catheter, 3-mL syringe, bag-valve device, 3.0 or 3.5 ET tube adaptor, high-flow oxygen source, and suction equipment
2) Position patient in supine position with neck in neutral alignment
3) Cleanse the neck with antiseptic
4) Locate cricothyroid membrane
5) Attach over the needle catheter to 3-mL syringe; insert needle at 90-degree angle through cricothyroid membrane into the trachea, aiming toward patient's feet; air can be aspirated through syringe when trachea is entered
6) Remove syringe and needle, leaving catheter in place
7) Attach catheter to ET tube adaptor
8) Connect bag-valve device to high-flow oxygen and connect to ET tube adaptor
9) Secure catheter with tapes or ties
10) Auscultate chest and observe for chest wall excursion
11) If unable to ventilate with an adult bag-valve mask, try jet insufflation or pediatric bag-valve mask
12) Be prepared for a large amount of subcutaneous emphysema of the face, neck, and chest
i. *Surgical cricothyrotomy: indicated when ET tube cannot be passed through the cords because of edema, trauma, or fracture; this procedure is not recommended in children < 12 years because cricoid cartilage provides the only circumferential support to the upper trachea*
The cricothyroid membrane is opened with a scalpel, and an ET tube or tracheostomy tube is inserted. The emergency department physician will usually perform this procedure.
1) Assemble equipment: sterile gloves, masks, antiseptic solution, gauze dressings, sterile blades, scalpel, hemostat, local anesthetic, tapes or ties to secure tube, tracheostomy or ET tube no. 5

    2) Position patient supine

    3) Cleanse neck with antiseptic solution

    4) Drape neck with sterile towels

    5) Anesthetize area with local anesthetic if patient is conscious

    6) Identify landmarks; stabilize the thyroid cartilage and incise over the cricothyroid membrane

    7) Incise the cricothyroid membrane and open the incision with a hemostat

    8) Insert cuffed ET tube or tracheostomy tube into the trachea

    9) Inflate the cuff and ventilate the patient

    10) Observe respiratory excursion and auscultate lung anteriorly and laterally for breath sounds

    11) Secure tube with ties or tape

    12) Apply dressing around incisional area

    13) Reassess breath sounds and airway patency

  j. Tracheostomy: indicated when unable to perform ET intubation or cricothyrotomy; this procedure is rarely done in an emergency setting because it is a difficult procedure with multiple complications; the emergency department physician will usually perform this procedure

    1) Gather equipment: sterile gloves, masks, goggles, antiseptic solution, scalpel and blades, local anesthetic, tracheostomy tube with obturator (no. 6, 7, or 8 for adults), Metzenbaum scissors, tissue forceps, mosquito forceps, needle holder, tracheal dilator and hook, retractors, adhesive tape, dressings, sterile towels, local anesthetic, suction equipment, bag-valve device, oxygen, suture

    2) Place patient in supine position with neck extended

    3) Cleanse skin with antiseptic from jaw to clavicles

    4) Drape the chest and neck

    5) Infiltrate skin with local anesthetic

    6) Midline incision is made in the trachea to expose pretracheal fascia and thyroid isthmus

    7) Thyroid isthmus is clamped and dissected to expose the trachea; suction should be available

    8) Tracheal rings are incised and the trachea is entered

    9) Insert tracheal tube and obturator; remove obturator and inflate cuff with 5–8 mL of air

    10) Ventilate patient with bag-valve device

    11) Auscultate lung fields and verify tube position with chest x-ray film

    12) Secure tube in place with tape or ties

    13) Dress wound with gauze dressings

  k. Medicated inhalation therapy for bronchospasm

  l. Parenteral epinephrine

    1) Used for allergic reactions with airway compromise

    2) Remain with patient because of possibility of rebound edema to airway

B. Cervical spine (C-spine)

1. Maintain/provide spinal immobilization

  a. Flat on backboard

  b. Stabilize neck with rigid cervical collar

    1) Stabilization includes holding the head in a neutral position or placing bilateral head support devices and using tape to secure the head devices

  c. Immobilize head with locally approved device (e.g., tape with foam blocks or blanket roll).

> 1) Immobilization includes stabilization and application of a backboard and straps
>
> d. *Maintain spinal immobilization until more detailed assessment and radiographs can be completed*
>
> e. *The neck being a joint should be stabilized above and below; top of head and lower legs secured to the board*

2. **Maintain airway**
3. **Monitor/maintain breathing**

C. Breathing

1. **Positive-pressure ventilation**
   a. *Mouth-to-mask ventilation: used for apneic patient*
      1) Gather equipment: pocket mask and one-way valve
      2) Place patient in supine position
      3) Open airway using chin lift and jaw thrust
      4) Assess breathing status
      5) Insert oral or nasal airway if needed
      6) Place mask over patient's nose and mouth with the narrow end of the mask over the nose
      7) Apply pressure to the sides of mask with both hands to seal the air cuff tightly to patient's face
      8) Lift upward on patient's jaw using fingers of both hands to maintain head tilt; if trauma patient, use jaw thrust to maintain C-spine immobilization
      9) Connect oxygen tubing to mask if inlet nipple present
      10) Blow into opening until chest rises
      11) Remove mouth to allow for positive exhalation of air
      12) Ventilate patient 12 times per minute until spontaneous respirations or alternative method of ventilation established
      13) Reassess breathing status frequently
   b. *Bag-valve device ventilation: provides oxygenation and ventilatory support in apneic patient or patient with inadequate respirations*
      1) Gather equipment: oral airway, suction, bag-valve device with oxygen reservoir, oxygen connecting tubing
      2) Open and secure airway
      3) Connect oxygen tubing to oxygen source to attach to oxygen inlet on the bag-valve device
      4) Select appropriate-sized mask and secure to bag
      5) Set mask on patient's face covering the nose, mouth, and tip of chin; narrow end of the mask goes over patient's nose
      6) Hold mask firmly with thumb over patient's nose and fingers grasping the edge of mandible
      7) Squeeze bag to force air into lungs
      8) Assess for symmetrical chest wall excursion
   c. *Mechanical ventilation*
2. **Supplemental oxygen: a variety of devices are available to administer oxygen**
3. **Positioning**
   a. *Semi-Fowler's*
   b. *High Fowler's*
   c. *Arms extended forward and supported*
4. **Needle thoracostomy: indicated when immediate decompression of a**

tension pneumothorax is required because of severe respiratory or cardiac compromise

a. *Gather equipment: antiseptic solution, 20-cc syringe, 14 to 18 gauge over the needle catheter for adults; 20 to 22 gauge for children*

b. *Attach over the needle catheter to a 20-cc syringe*

c. *Determine insertion site; second intercostal space, midclavicular line on the affected side*

d. *Insert needle through skin and direct over top of second rib and into the pleural space, second intercostal space, midclavicular line*

e. *Aspiration of air into the syringe signifies tension pneumothorax*

f. *Remove needle and syringe leaving catheter in place*

g. *Secure catheter with tape and leave open to air*

h. *Prepare for tube thoracostomy as soon as possible; if delay in placement of chest tube, flutter valve or Heimlich valve can be used*

i. *Monitor arterial blood gases*

D. Circulation/bleeding

1. Control of bleeding

a. *Ensure universal blood and body fluid precautions*

b. *Apply direct pressure to source of bleeding*

c. *Elevate source of bleeding (if extremity)*

d. *Use arterial tourniquet as last resort because of nerve damage*

e. *Provide supplemental oxygen*

f. *Obtain venous access: minimum of two large-bore catheters (14–16 gauge for adult; 18–20 gauge for children); if venous access in children is difficult, intraosseous cannulation may be used in children younger than 6 years in a critical situation*

g. *Venous access is used to*

  1) Collect blood samples
     a) Hemoglobin and hematocrit
     b) Type and cross-match
  2) Volume replacement
     a) Crystalloid
     b) Colloid
  3) Deliver medications

h. *Apply pneumatic antishock garment (PASG); use of PASG is controversial, and studies have shown no difference in outcomes for PASG-treated patients versus patients not treated with PASG. Use of PASG may increase peripheral vascular resistance; increase tissue perfusion; help control intra-abdominal, pelvic, and lower extremity hemorrhage; and stabilize fractures of pelvis and lower extremities. Use of PASG is contraindicated in pulmonary edema; abdominal section of PASG should not be used in late pregnancy or abdominal evisceration*

  1) Gather equipment: PASG, foot pump, or inflation device
  2) Examine patient's abdomen, legs, and back because once garment is on, areas will be inaccessible
  3) Remove patient's clothing below the waist if possible; bulky, hard objects may cause skin necrosis if PASG is left on for lengthy duration
  4) Lay PASG open/flat on stretcher and logroll patient onto it; top of abdominal section should lie below lowest rib
  5) Fasten Velcro straps on PASG: first the legs, then the abdominal section

       6) Connect the tubing from the foot pump to the three compartments; many models have color coded tubing

       7) Open stopcocks to leg compartments and close the abdominal compartment stopcock

       8) Inflate the leg compartments until the pressure gauge indicates appropriate amount of pressure; minimum amount of inflation pressure should be used to restore adequate blood pressure; observe for clinical response (improvement of vital signs, capillary refill, skin color, and mental status)

       9) Inflate the abdominal section if systolic BP < 100 mm Hg

      10) Monitor clinical response as noted previously

      11) Monitor respiratory effort

      12) Deflation of the PASG should be monitored closely and done according to strict protocol; patient must be stabilized prior to deflation of garment

    i. Administer blood products

E. Circulation/pulse

1. Interventions for pulselessness

  a. Cardiopulmonary resuscitation

    1) External: assess responsiveness, call for help, appropriately position the victim properly, open airway, assess breathlessness, ventilate patient, confirm pulselessness, and perform closed-chest compressions

    2) Internal

  b. Monitor oxygen saturation by pulse oximetry

  c. Obtain venous access; minimum of two large-bore IV catheters (14–16 gauge for adults; 18–20 gauge for children)

    1) Volume resuscitation

    2) Drug therapy: calculation of IV drip (See Drug Calculation, Appendix I)

  d. Cardioversion

  e. Defibrillation

  f. External cardiac pacing

F. Circulation/perfusion

1. Interventions to increase perfusion

  a. Provide supplemental oxygen

  b. Obtain venous access; minimum of two large-bore needles (14–16 gauge for adults; 18–20 gauge for children), and administer fluids and drugs as indicated; if venous access is difficult in children younger than 6 years, consider intraosseous cannulation

  c. Trendelenburg position

  d. Treat cause of altered perfusion

  e. Monitor vital signs, level of consciousness, urinary output

  f. Remain with patient

G. Disability/neurological

1. Interventions for altered neurologic status

  a. Provide supplemental oxygen

  b. Look for possible causes of decreased level of consciousness: drugs, alcohol, cerebral edema, trauma, underlying disease process

  c. Keep head midline

  d. Administer medications as indicated: steroids, narcotic antagonists, thiamine, dextrose

III. SECONDARY ASSESSMENT

The secondary assessment follows the primary assessment and is brief. The goal of this assessment is to discover all abnormalities or injuries. It is also valuable for discovering occult problems in patients with a poor or confusing history. A useful mnemonic to assist in completion of the secondary survey is

E = *Exposure*
F = *Freezing/Fahrenheit*
G = *Get vitals; gadgets*
H = *Head to toe, history*
I = *Inspect the posterior surface*

A. Subjective data

1. **History of present illness or injury**
   a. *PQRST*
      1) Provocation of current illness, symptoms, precipitating factors
      2) Quality of symptoms
      3) Region/radiation of problem
      4) Severity of symptoms
      5) Time of onset
   b. *Aggravating/relieving factor*
   c. *Effects on other systems and activities*
   d. *Patient's or family's theory or speculation about problem*
   e. *Content and time of most recently ingested food, alcohol/drugs*
   f. *Efforts to treat*
      1) Home remedies
      2) Over-the-counter medications
      3) Body positioning
      4) Physician visits and prescription drugs
      5) Prehospital emergency medical services (EMS) care
   g. *Mechanism of injury/trauma*
      1) Motor vehicle crash
         a) Type of vehicle
         b) Speed of vehicle
         c) Type of vehicle collision
            (1) Moving vehicle hits moving vehicle
            (2) Moving vehicle hits stationary object
            (3) Stationary vehicle hit by moving vehicle
         d) Patient wearing safety belt or helmet
            (1) Type of safety belt (shoulder, lap)
            (2) Vehicle with air bag
         e) Patient remained in vehicle versus being ejected
         f) Position in vehicle prior to crash
         g) Position in vehicle after crash
         h) Direction of forces in collision
            (1) Head-on
            (2) Rear-end
            (3) Broadside
            (4) Corner
      2) Fall

          a) Precipitating event
             (1) Tripped
             (2) Slipped
             (3) Syncope
             (4) Other/unknown
          b) Distance
          c) Position of landing
          d) Surface of landing
       3) Penetrating trauma
          a) Object causing injury
             (1) Knife
             (2) Bullet
             (3) Ice pick
             (4) Screwdriver
             (5) Glass
             (6) Nail
             (7) Other
          b) Force behind object
          c) Estimated depth of penetration
          d) Height and position of assailant/angle of entry
       4) Blunt trauma
          a) Object causing injury
             (1) Steering wheel
             (2) Club, bat, bottle, fist, furniture
             (3) Automobile, truck, train
             (4) Other
          b) Force of impact
          c) Point of body impact
          d) Duration of impact

2. Medical history

   a. General health status
      1) Respiratory disease
      2) Cardiovascular disease
      3) Neurological disease
      4) Endocrine disease
      5) Trauma
      6) Medications or other therapy
      7) Substance use/abuse
      8) Detoxification history
      9) Previous tetanus immunization
      10) Childhood disease immunization
      11) Allergies

   b. Related to present problem or current event
      1) Previous episodes: number, duration, date
      2) Previous injury to same area: number, date
      3) Previous medications or other therapy

3. Social, psychological, and environmental factors

    Although the time constraints of a given situation may make collection of these data difficult, it should be recognized that a complete nursing plan cannot be formulated without them. Incorporating these data into the overall plan may make the critical difference regarding the choice of appropriate treatment and realistic follow-up expectations.

   a. Risk factors

       1) Smoking
       2) Substance abuse
       3) Psychiatric history
    b. *Behavior appropriate for age and developmental stage*
    c. *Occupation/profession*
    d. *Hobbies/vacation*
    e. *Meaning of illness, injury, or event to patient/family*
    f. *Patient's/family's expectations of care*
    g. *Support system*
       1) Family structure
       2) Significant others
       3) Social agencies
       4) Religious affiliation
    h. *Responsibilities*
       1) Self
       2) Family
       3) Business
       4) Community
    i. *Living accommodations*
       1) House
       2) Apartment
       3) Homeless
       4) Stairs
    j. *Ease of access to*
       1) Pharmacy
       2) Market
       3) Transportation
       4) Medical care for follow-up
       5) Assistance with activities of daily living

B. Objective data

1. General survey
    a. *Method of arrival to facility*
    b. *Check for presence of medical information such as medical bracelets*
    c. *Level of consciousness*
    d. *Motor function*
       1) Spontaneous
       2) On command
       3) In response to pain
       4) Purposeful/random
       5) Gait
       6) Speech
       7) Facial expression
       8) Symmetry
       9) Deficit
    e. *Skin/mucous membranes*
       1) Color
          a) Cyanosis
          b) Jaundice
          c) Pallor
          d) Erythema
       2) Moisture/turgor

a) Dry
b) Moist
c) Wet
d) Tenting
e) Edema
f) Pitting
3) Temperature
a) Cool
b) Cold
c) Warm
d) Hot
f. *Odors*
1) Alcohol
2) Acetone, indicative of ketosis
3) Gasoline, indicative of spilled fuel at scene of accident
4) Urine
5) Feces
6) Other
g. *Vital signs*
1) Blood pressure
2) Pulse
a) Apical
b) Radial
c) Femoral
d) Other peripheral pulses, especially distal to injury
e) Rate, rhythm, quality
3) Temperature
a) Oral
b) Axillary
c) Tympanic
d) Rectal
e) Core
4) Respirations
a) Bradypnea
b) Tachypnea
5) Oxygen saturation: pulse oximetry
2. **Head-to-toe assessment: 90 seconds**
a. *Remove clothing (if not already done) as required for inspection; exercise caution for possible sharp objects (e.g., needles) in pockets*
1) If patient is in acute distress or has history indicating potential spine injury, cut off clothing
2) Provide patient with gown and sheet or blanket for privacy and warmth
b. *Rapidly moving from head to toe, assess the following:*
1) Head and face
a) Skin integrity
(1) Lacerations, abrasions, avulsion, puncture
(2) Ecchymosis: "black eyes" may indicate basilar skull fracture
(3) Edema
(4) Presence of pink or gray tissue (brain tissue)
b) Facial features
(1) Asymmetry
(2) Malocclusion of teeth
c) Bony deformities

      (1) Depression
      (2) Angulation
      (3) Open fracture
      (4) Loose teeth
      (5) Tenderness

d) Eyes
      (1) Gross visual acuity
      (2) Pupillary size, equality, reaction to light
      (3) Iris/sclera
         (a) Color
         (b) Bleeding (hyphema)
      (4) Lid edema
      (5) Ptosis
      (6) Excessive blinking (blepharospasm)
      (7) Extraocular movements: able to move eyes in all directions
      (8) Contact lenses (remove if present)

e) Ears
      (1) Blood
         (a) External canal
         (b) Behind tympanic membrane
      (2) Clear fluid: may be cerebrospinal fluid (CSF); do not stop drainage
      (3) Ecchymosis behind ear (Battle's sign); may be indicative of basilar skull fracture (not evident immediately after injury)
      (4) Exposed cartilage
      (5) Purulent drainage/crusting: may be indicative of infection

f) Nose
      (1) Bleeding
      (2) Deformity
      (3) Rhinorrhea (may be CSF)

g) Pain
      (1) Provocation
      (2) Quality
      (3) Region/radiation
      (4) Severity
      (5) Time of onset

2) Neck
a) Skin integrity
      (1) Lacerations, abrasions, avulsion, puncture
      (2) Impaled objects
      (3) Ecchymosis
      (4) Edema: may compromise airway

b) Tracheal deviation
      (1) May be indicative of tension pneumothorax

c) Distended neck veins
      (1) May be indicative of congestive heart failure, tension pneumothorax, or cardiac tamponade
      (2) Palpate/auscultate carotid pulse

d) Subcutaneous emphysema
      (1) May indicate disruption of trachea or bronchial tree

3) Chest and thorax
a) Skin integrity
      (1) Lacerations, abrasions, avulsion, puncture

        (2) Impaled objects

        (3) Ecchymosis

           (a) Round abrasion may indicate steering wheel impact

           (b) Ecchymosis diagonally across chest may indicate seat belt injury

        (4) Edema

        (5) Subcutaneous emphysema: may indicate disruption of trachea or bronchial tree

        (6) Asymmetry: may indicate flail chest

    b) Breathing

        (1) Present

        (2) Wheezes, rales, rhonchi

        (3) Rate

        (4) Depth

        (5) Effort: accessory muscle use

        (6) Pattern

           (a) Kussmaul's respirations: regular, rapid, deep, labored

           (b) Cheyne-Stokes respirations: alternating periods of hyperventilation and apnea

    c) Bony deformities

        (1) Tenderness, crepitus, deformity

    d) Heart sounds

        (1) S_1, S_2: Splitting of S_2 may indicate left bundle branch block

        (2) S_3, S_4

           (a) S_3 indicates left ventricular dysfunction

           (b) S_4 indicates decreased ventricular compliance

        (3) Muffled, distant: may indicate pericardial tamponade

        (4) Murmurs or rubs

           (a) May indicate mitral valve regurgitation

           (b) Friction rub may occur after myocardial infarction (MI) or with pericarditis

    e) Pain

        (1) Provocation

        (2) Quality

        (3) Region/radiation

        (4) Severity

        (5) Time

        (6) Duration

4) Abdomen and flank

    a) Inspection

        (1) Note laceration, abrasion, avulsion, puncture, impaled object, exposed internal organs, scars, contusions, pulsatile masses

        (2) Ecchymosis

           (a) Grey Turner sign—bruising around flank and abdomen—may indicate injury to spleen.

           (b) Cullen sign—bluish discoloration around umbilicus—may indicate hemoperitoneum.

        (3) Contour

           (a) Flat

           (b) Distended

    b) Auscultation

        (1) Bowel sounds

           (a) Absent, indicating paralytic ileus (need to listen at least 1 minute in each quadrant to determine this)

        (b) Hyperactive, indicating increased peristalsis
- c) Percussion
    - (1) Tympany, a hollow sound indicating presence of air or gas
    - (2) Dullness, a heavy sound indicating fluid (e.g., blood) or a mass
- d) Palpation
    - (1) Soft
    - (2) Guarding
    - (3) Rigid, boardlike, indicating peritoneal irritability
- e) Pain
    - (1) Provocation
    - (2) Quality
    - (3) Region/radiation
    - (4) Severity
    - (5) Time
- 5) Pelvis and genitalia
    - a) Surface injuries
        - (1) Laceration, abrasion, avulsion, puncture
        - (2) Ecchymosis: around flank may indicate injury to kidney
        - (3) Edema
    - b) Bone deformities
        - (1) Instability of ischial tuberosities may indicate pelvic fracture
        - (2) Open fracture
    - c) Bleeding
        - (1) Urinary meatus: may indicate injury to bladder, urethra
        - (2) Vagina: may indicate the following:
            - (a) Injury to vagina, cervix, uterus
            - (b) Miscarriage
            - (c) Menstruation
        - (3) Rectum: may indicate injury to anus, rectum, or large bowel
    - d) Altered neurological function
        - (1) Priapism: may indicate spinal cord injury
        - (2) Loss of rectal sphincter tone: may indicate spinal cord injury
    - e) Pain
        - (1) Provocation
        - (2) Quality
        - (3) Region/radiation
        - (4) Severity
        - (5) Time
- 6) Extremities
    - a) Motor function
        - (1) Spontaneous movement
        - (2) Motor strength
        - (3) Symmetry of strength
        - (4) Range of motion
    - b) Sensory function
        - (1) Sharp
        - (2) Dull
    - c) Circulatory status
        - (1) Color, skin temperature
        - (2) Pulses distal to injury
    - d) Surface injuries
        - (1) Laceration, abrasion, avulsion, puncture
        - (2) Ecchymosis

(3) Edema
 e) Deformity
  (1) Closed fracture
  (2) Open fracture
 f) Crepitus
 g) Pain
  (1) Provocation
  (2) Quality
  (3) Region/radiation
  (4) Severity
  (5) Time
7) Posterior
 a) Observe C-spine precautions and splint suspected extremity fractures
 b) Turn patient carefully and assess for ecchymosis, avulsion, laceration or wound, pain
  (1) Back
  (2) Flanks
  (3) Buttocks
  (4) Thighs

IV. FOCUSED ASSESSMENT

The focused assessment is a detailed assessment of any area or system that has an abnormality or injury. Refer to specific chapters for details of focused assessment.

V. DIAGNOSTIC PROCEDURES/DATA

Laboratory studies, radiographs, and electrocardiograms are done in conjunction with findings of the primary, secondary, and focused assessments. When laboratory and diagnostic tests are joined with a thorough history and physical exam, valuable information about a patient's status can be gained. The selection of types of tests for each patient is individualized. Refer to specific chapters for more details. Bedside point of care testing for glucose, hemoglobin, hematocrit, and electrolyte levels are commonly used in the emergency department environment. Daily quality control tests are necessary for accuracy. The results of these tests must be documented daily.

VI. NURSING PROCESS

A. Assessment

Systematic collection of data about patient's actual or risk for health care problems and needs. A general guide is described next; however, the volume of data collected is dependent on several variables, including patient acuity and length of stay.

1. **Subjective data**
 a) *Chief complaint*
 b) *History of present illness*
 c) *Medical/surgical history*
  1) Include allergies, immunizations, and current medications
 d) *Psychosocial history*
  1) Include home situation, significant others, occupation and employment status, and use of alcohol, tobacco, and recreational drugs

> *e) Review of systems*
> **2. Objective data**
> > *a) Vital signs and patient weight (pediatric patients)*
> > *b) Physical examination*

B. Nursing diagnosis (see Appendixes A and B)

Nursing diagnosis is a clinical judgment about the individual, family, or community responses to and risk for actual health problems and life processes. It provides the basis for selection of nursing interventions to achieve outcomes for which the nurse is accountable. A nursing diagnosis made by professional nurses describes actual or potential health problems that nurses, by virtue of their education and experience, are able and licensed to treat.

C. Planning/interventions

This provides a guide for the appropriate nursing activities to manage identified health care problems and needs. These nursing actions include both collaborative and independent interventions. All interventions are patient oriented and goal directed.

D. Expected outcomes/evaluation (see Appendix B)

This is the endpoint determination used to assess whether the desired patient responses to interventions have been achieved. If positive outcomes are not demonstrated, assessment and/or plan of care needs re-evaluation.

E. Recording nursing process

> **1. Format**
> > *a) Subjective data*
> > *b) Objective data*
> > *c) Nursing diagnosis*
> > *d) Plan/intervention*
> > *e) Outcomes/evaluation*

VII. AGE-RELATED CONSIDERATIONS

A. Pediatric: children are not small adults; they have unique anatomical and physiological differences

> **1. Vital signs**
> > *a) Normal ranges change with age; hypotension is a late sign of shock; may not appear until circulating volume is decreased by 50%*
> > *b) Use appropriate-sized cuff for blood pressure*
> > *c) Use brachial or apical site for pulse*
> **2. Airway**
> > *a) Neonates are obligate nose-breathers*
> > *b) Small airway diameter*
> > *c) Greater amounts of soft tissue surrounding airway*
> > *d) Large tongue*
> > *e) Cricoid: narrowest part of airway*
> > *f) Soft laryngeal cartilage*

3. **C-spine**
   a) *Head larger in relation to body; therefore, a greater risk for injury*
4. **Breathing**
   a) *Poorly developed intercostal accessory muscles*
   b) *Thin chest wall*
   c) *Decreased pulmonary reserve*
   d) *Higher oxygen requirements*
5. **Circulation**
   a) *Myocardium: less contractile mass and less compliant*
   b) *Able to maintain cardiac output for long periods of time: strong compensatory mechanisms*
   c) *Less total circulatory blood volume than adults*

6. **Skin temperature**
   a) *May lose heat rapidly; keep covered (especially head in small infants)*

7. **Growth and development**
   a) *Infants*
      1) Trust development
      2) Attachment to parents; minimize separation from parents
      3) Older infants may localize pain
   b) *Toddlers*
      1) Developing autonomy
      2) Increased safety concerns
      3) Fear of pain
   c) *Preschoolers*
      1) Learning to do things for self
      2) Magical thinking
   d) *School-age children*
      1) Able to understand body anatomy and function
      2) Privacy and control important
   e) *Adolescence*
      1) Peer relationship important
      2) Sensitive to being different from peer group
      3) Privacy is critical

8. **"Pearls"**
   a) *Differences in illness in children and adults are anatomical, psychological, and physiological*
   b) *Treat child and parent as one unit; avoid separation*
   c) *Give simple instructions or one choice to increase child's sense of control*
   d) *Use play therapy, if time permits; allow child to have favorite toy for security*
   e) *Avoid threatening behavior such as sudden movement or loud noises*
   f) *Examine painful area last, if possible*
   g) *Be honest with child; if procedure will hurt, say so*
   h) *Protect modesty, respect privacy*
   i) *Explain procedures to the extent possible, according to the child's developmental level*
   j) *Do painful procedures last*

B. Geriatric

1. **Anatomical and physiological changes in the elderly**
   a) *Airway*

1) Diminished airway compliance
2) Increased airway resistance

b) *C-spine*
1) Loss of subcutaneous fat
2) Osteoporosis
3) Degenerative joint changes

c) *Breathing*
1) Loss of thoracic muscle mass
2) Diminished lung compliance
3) Decreased vital capacity
4) Increased anteroposterior chest diameter

d) *Circulation*
1) Decreased cardiac output
2) Decreased blood flow
3) Atherosclerosis

e) *Neurological*
1) Decreased cerebral blood flow
2) Loss of functioning neurons
3) Cerebral atrophy
4) Slowed nerve transmission

f) *Integumentary*
1) Friable, fragile skin
2) Stasis dermatitis and ulcers

2. "Pearls"
a) *Older adults may dismiss significant symptoms as "normal for age": investigate each complaint*
b) *Keep manipulation of body to a minimum to avoid fatigue*
c) *Poor elasticity of skin can mimic dehydration; examine lateral cheeks for turgor*
d) *Do not assume that older patient is hard of hearing; it may offend patient*
e) *Confusion is a common sign of illness in the elderly; do not assume it is dementia*
f) *Elderly are more predisposed to drug toxicities and adverse reactions because of reduced renal excretory function*

VIII. PRIORITIES OF CARE: TRIAGE MODELS

A. Nondisaster triage models

1. Purpose: to provide the best care for each individual patient
2. Sample models for determining priority of care
a) *Models for individual triage*
1) Traffic director
a) Differentiates emergent from nonurgent
b) Sometimes done by nonlicensed personnel
c) Assessment consists of chief complaint
d) No preliminary diagnostics
e) Sent to treatment room or waiting room
f) No further evaluation
g) Little documentation
h) No re-evaluation
2) Spot check
a) Chief complaint: limited subjective and objective data collection

b) Assessment by licensed health care provider (RN or MD)

c) Patient categorized by level or condition: emergent, urgent, delayed

d) May initiate diagnostic procedures

e) Documentation of presenting complaint, objective findings
   (1) No planned re-evaluation: done at patient request

3) Comprehensive

   a) Thorough assessment: subjective and objective data collected; educational needs and primary health needs assessed

   b) Assessment done by RN

   c) Patients placed in categories based on priorities of care
      (1) Immediate: life threatening (cardiac arrest, major trauma)
      (2) Stable but urgent (sickle cell, fractures)
      (3) Stable, nonurgent (small laceration, closed fracture)
      (4) Stable, no distress (rash, "nerves")

   d) Protocol-driven selected diagnostic procedures (extremity radiograph, urinalysis)

   e) Patients who remain in waiting area are reassessed every 15 to 60 minutes, depending on severity of illness or injury

BIBLIOGRAPHY

American Heart Association. (1994). *Advanced cardiac life support.* Dallas, TX: Author.

Bobb, J. (1994). Trauma in the elderly. In S. Veise-Barry (Ed.), *Trauma nursing from resuscitation through rehabilitation* (pp. 721–735). Philadelphia: W. B. Saunders.

Bourn, M. (1993) Pneumatic antishock garment. In J. Proehl (Ed.), *Adult emergency nursing procedures* (pp. 229–232). Boston: Jones and Bartlett.

Bracken, J. (1998) Triage. In L. Newberry (Ed.), *Sheehy's emergency nursing principles and practice* (4th ed., pp. 105–111). St. Louis, MO: Mosby-Year Book.

Chameides, L., & Hazenski, M. F. (Eds.). (1994). *Textbook of pediatric advanced life support.* Dallas, TX: Author.

Echternacht, M. (1993). Tracheostomy. In J. Proehl (Ed.), *Adult emergency nursing procedures* (pp. 129–131). Boston: Jones and Bartlett.

Emergency Nurses Association. (1995). *Trauma nurse core course instructor manual.* Chicago: Author.

Gerardi, M., Saccetti, A., Contor, R., Santamaria, J., Gusche, M., Lucid, W., & Folbin, B. (1996). Rapid sequence intubation of the pediatric patient. *Annals of Emergency Medicine, 28,* 55–73.

Henry, M., & Stapleton, E. (1992). Cardiovascular emergencies. In M. Henry & E. Stapleton (Eds.), *EMT prehospital care* (pp. 207–210). Philadelphia: W. B. Saunders.

Kelly, D. (1993). Surgical cricothyrotomy. In J. Proehl (Ed.), *Adult emergency nursing procedures* (pp. 40–42). Boston: Jones and Bartlett.

Mattox, K. L., Beckell, W., & Pepe, P. E. (1989). Prospective MAST study in 911 patients. *Journal of Trauma, 29,* 1104–1112.

Rogers, J. (1998). Unique characteristics of children. In J. Rogers & T. Soud (Eds.), *Manual of pediatric emergency nursing* (pp. 43–69). St. Louis, MO: Mosby Year Book.

Sellick, B. A. (1996). Cricoid pressure to control regurgitation of stomach contents during induction of anesthesia. *Lancet, 2,* 404–406.

Yamamoto, L. (1991). Rapid sequence anesthesia induction and advanced airway management in pediatric patients. *Emergency Medical Clinics of North America, 9,* 611–637.

Sally P. Cummings, EdD, RN, FNP
P. Howard Cummings, EdD, RN

CHAPTER **2**

Abdominal Emergencies

MAJOR TOPICS

I. GENERAL STRATEGY

A. Assessment

1. **Primary survey/resuscitation** (see Chapter 1)
2. **Secondary survey** (see Chapter 1)
3. **Psychological/social/environmental factors related to abdominal emergencies**
   a. *Stress factors*
      1) Lifestyle
      2) Coping patterns
      3) Precipitating event
   b. *Blunt or penetrating trauma*
      1) Motor vehicle crash
      2) Gunshot wound
      3) Impact on abdomen from object

4. Focused survey
   a. Subjective data collection
      1) History of present illness/chief complaint
         a) Pain
            (1) Provocation
            (2) Quality
            (3) Region/radiation
            (4) Severity of symptoms
            (5) Time of onset
         b) Vomiting
            (1) Pain
            (2) Blood (color)
            (3) Bile
            (4) Feculent matter
            (5) Onset
            (6) Frequency
            (7) Duration
         c) Gastrointestinal (GI) bleeding
         d) Recent changes in weight
         e) Changes in bowel habits
         f) Changes in appetite
         g) Blunt or penetrating trauma
      2) Medical history
         a) Past diseases/surgeries
         b) Current diseases
         c) Current medications
         d) Allergies/immunization status
         e) Alcohol/drug use
         f) Recent foreign travel
   b. Objective data collection
      1) Physical examination
         a) Inspection
            (1) Distention/flatness
            (2) Pulsating mass
            (3) Symmetry
            (4) Contour (flat, rounded, herniation)
            (5) Umbilicus (contour, location, herniation)
            (6) Striae
            (7) Diastasis rectus
            (8) Lesions
            (9) Signs of trauma (e.g., entry/exit wounds, lacerations)
            (10) Scars
            (11) Discolorations
         b) Auscultation
            (1) Bowel sounds (present or absent; character)
            (2) Bruit
         c) Percussion
            (1) Dullness or resonance
            (2) Size of liver
            (3) Borders of any masses
            (4) Fundus of urinary bladder
            (5) Costovertebral angle (CVA) tenderness
         d) Light palpation

         (1) Abdominal tenderness
         (2) Rigidity/guarding
         (3) Masses
         (4) Peritoneal irritation
     e) Deep palpation
         (1) Masses
         (2) Rebound tenderness
         (3) Liver
         (4) Spleen
         (5) Kidneys
         (6) Aorta
     f) Rectal examination: check stool for occult blood
  2) Diagnostic procedures
     a) Laboratory
         (1) Complete blood count with differential
         (2) Calcium, magnesium, and electrolytes
         (3) Liver function tests (aspartate aminotransaminase [AST], alanine aminotransferase [ALT], lactate dehydrogenase [LDH], alkaline phosphatase)
         (4) Serum amylase, lipase
         (5) Sickle cell screen
         (6) Blood for *Helicobacter pylori*
         (7) Type and cross-match blood
         (8) Coagulation studies
         (9) Pregnancy test
        (10) Urinalysis
        (11) Stool for occult blood
        (12) Stool for ova and parasites
        (13) Stool for white blood cell (WBC), mucus, protein
        (14) Stool culture
        (15) Enzyme-linked immunosorbent assay (ELISA) of stool
     b) Radiography
         (1) Flat plate abdomen
         (2) Upright
         (3) Left lateral decubitus
         (4) Cross-table lateral abdomen
         (5) Posteroanterior (PA) chest upright (to detect thoracic involvement)
     c) Other special studies
         (1) Barium enema
         (2) Intravenous urography or cystography
         (3) Intravenous cholangiography
         (4) Upper GI series
         (5) Angiography
         (6) Nuclear scanning
         (7) Gastroscopy or endoscopy
         (8) Sigmoidoscopy/proctoscopy/colonoscopy
         (9) Esophageal manometry
        (10) Abdominal paracentesis
        (11) Peritoneal lavage
        (12) Local wound exploration
        (13) Ultrasonography
        (14) Computed tomography (CT) scan
        (15) Magnetic resonance imaging (MRI)

      d) Preparation of patient and significant others for diagnostic procedures
         (1) Physical preparation
         (2) Emotional support
         (3) Patient and/or family teaching
         (4) Written consents

B. Analysis: differential nursing diagnosis/collaborative problems

1. **Altered nutrition: less than body requirements**
2. **Altered tissue perfusion, gastrointestinal (GI)**
3. **Anxiety/fear**
4. **Body image disturbance**
5. **Constipation**
6. **Diarrhea**
7. **Impaired gas exchange**
8. **Knowledge deficit**
9. **Pain**
10. **Risk for fluid volume deficit**
11. **Risk for infection**

C. Planning/interventions

1. **Determine priorities**
   a. *Control and maintain cardiopulmonary function*
   b. *Prevent complications*
   c. *Control pain*
   d. *Relieve anxiety and/or apprehension*
   e. *Educate patient and/or significant others*
2. **Develop nursing care plan specific to patient's presenting emergency**
3. **Obtain and set up necessary equipment and supplies**
4. **Institute appropriate interventions based on the nursing care plan**
5. **Record data as appropriate**

D. Expected outcome/evaluation (see Appendix B)

1. **Monitor patient responses and outcomes, plans as indicated**
   a. *Specific interventions*
   b. *Disposition/discharge planning*
   c. *If positive outcomes are not demonstrated, assessment and/or plan of care needs re-evaluation.*

E. Age-related considerations for abdominal emergencies

1. **Pediatric**
   a. *Growth or development related*
      1) Higher metabolic rate and lack of kidney reserves (because of immaturity), to properly concentrate, dilute, and excrete waste products
      2) Greater fluid needs related to body surface area make fluid, fluid/electrolyte, and acid-base balance more precarious
      3) Acidosis develops more rapidly in children during dehydration
      4) Hypotension is a late sign of shock and does not appear until 50% of circulating blood volume decreased

5) Diarrhea is a major cause of metabolic acidosis; potassium, glucose, and calcium must be carefully monitored

b. *"Pearls"*

1) Avoid restraining the child as much as possible

2) Use distraction such as television, rhythmic breathing, and imagery for relaxation and pain control

3) Pain medication may be administered in various ways, such as intravenously or in suppositories, cherry syrup elixirs, or pills or capsules in ice cream

4) When obtaining history, use adequate lighting, use face-to-face interviewing, leave enough time for answers, ask specific questions, and use other sources of information too

5) Monitor shock by earlier signs, such as tachycardia, decreased or absent urine output, arterial blood gases, metabolic acidosis, and change in mental status

6) Fluids of choice for oral (PO) replacement include glucose water, apple juice, Gatorade, oral electrolyte solution, broth, carbonated drinks, Jell-O, Kool-Aid, tea, popsicles

7) Intravenous (IV) fluid replacement to correct dehydration should be done with isotonic fluids and fluids containing chloride, glucose, water, sodium, and potassium

2. Geriatric

a. *Age related*

1) About 75% of people older than 65 years have some degree of impaired cognitive function

2) Diminished vision and hearing and slower psychomotor performance may affect responses to health history questions or inquiries

3) Because of older persons' reduced ability to adjust to extremes in environmental temperature, care should be taken to minimize body exposure in the elderly

4) Alterations in GI function with aging include increased gastric secretions and decreased gastric motility

5) Monitor pain and other assessment findings closely, because the elderly tend to under-report symptoms

II. SPECIFIC ABDOMINAL EMERGENCIES

A. Gastritis

Gastritis is inflammation of the stomach that most often originates from dietary indiscretions, such as eating too much or too rapidly, eating food that is noxious to the stomach because of excessive seasoning, and eating foods that are infected. Chronic gastritis may be caused by *H. pylori*, which is present in 30 to 50% of the population with chronic gastritis. Other causes include the ingestion of coffee, NSAIDs, alcohol, salicylates, steroids, and acids or alkalis; uremia; radiotherapy; thermal or mechanical injury; emotional stress; use of tobacco; and diseases that affect the gastric mucosal cells. The gastric mucous membrane becomes edematous and reddened and undergoes superficial erosion, causing excessive secretion of gastric juice containing acid and mucus. Acute episodes may cause nausea, vomiting, colic, diarrhea, anorexia, distress (heartburn), and eructations of gas. Owing to the thinning of the stomach walls and lining as well as gastric atrophy, chronic episodes of gastritis may lead to duodenal and gastric (peptic) ulcers, hemorrhage, pernicious anemia, pyloric obstruction, and perforation.

1. **Assessment**
   a. *Subjective data*
      1) History of present illness
         a) Pain
            (1) Provocation
            (2) Quality: squeezing, burning, dull, gnawing, colicky (relieved by intake of bland foods)
            (3) Region/radiation
            (4) Severity of symptoms
            (5) Time of onset (chronic, intermittent, constant)
         b) Nausea and/or vomiting
            (1) Frequent nausea
            (2) Vomiting (blood, mucus, undigested food)
      2) History of habits and/or occurrences
         a) Allergies
         b) History of ulcer disease, chronic indigestion, malignancy
         c) Irregular eating habits
         d) Hurried eating habits
         e) Consumption of alcohol or tobacco
         f) Unusual or chronic tension or anxiety
         g) Ingestion of an irritant or drugs
         h) Chronic use of antacids (carry antacids with them)
   b. *Objective data*
      1) Physical examination
         a) Vital signs/orthostatic vital signs
         b) Acute epigastric pain on palpation
         c) Hematemesis
         d) Muscular guarding
      2) Diagnostic data and procedures
         a) Electrolyte profile
         b) Complete blood count
         c) Blood for *H. pylori*
         d) Gastric analysis
         e) Stool examination for occult blood
         f) Upper GI series
         g) Endoscopy with gastric biopsy
2. **Analysis: differential nursing diagnosis/collaborative problems**
   a. *Pain related to inflammation*
   b. *Risk for fluid volume deficit related to nausea, decreased intake, and vomiting*
   c. *Knowledge deficit related to diet, habits, and pain*
3. **Planning/interventions**
   a. *Administer pain medication as indicated*
   b. *Monitor vital signs*
   c. *Initiate IV fluids*
   d. *Ensure patient takes nothing by mouth (NPO), initially*
   e. *Insert nasogastric tube, initially*
   f. *Monitor intake and output*
   g. *Monitor urine specific gravity*
   h. *Administer antiemetics as indicated*
   i. *Administer antacids as indicated*
   j. *Administer histamine receptor antagonists as indicated*
   k. *Administer anticholinergics as indicated*
   l. *Provide sodium and potassium supplements as needed*

m. *Monitor gastric emesis/chyme for blood*

n. *Monitor all stools for tarry appearance and/or occult blood*

o. *Minimize environmental stimuli*

p. *Encourage patient to follow prescribed diet and medication regimen*

q. *Instruct patient about importance of avoiding causative factors: stressful events, alcoholic beverages, tobacco products*

r. *Encourage medical follow-up after discharge*

4. **Expected outcome/evaluation** (see Appendix B)

B. Ulcers

An ulcer results from the sloughing of the mucous membrane of the esophagus, stomach, or duodenum. It is often caused by the action of acidic gastric secretions, causing excoriations to form in the mucosal wall of the stomach, pylorus, duodenum, or esophagus. The etiology is poorly understood, but ulcers do commonly occur in the areas of the gastrointestinal tract that are exposed to hydrochloric acid and pepsin. Duodenal ulcers have been observed most frequently in persons between the ages of 20 and 60 years but have also been observed in children and infants. Gastric ulcers are more commonly seen in those aged 55 to 70 years. Ninety to 95% of persons with ulcers also have gastritis associated with *H. pylori*. Ulcers are more common in men, smokers, and persons who take nonsteroidal anti-inflammatory drugs (NSAIDs) regularly.

1. **Assessment**

   a. *Subjective data*

      1) History of present illness

         a) Pain

            (1) Provocation

            (2) Quality: squeezing, burning, dull, gnawing, colicky, feeling of fullness

            (3) Region/radiation: midback, epigastric

            (4) Severity of symptoms: symptoms worsen during day, are worst at night, are exacerbated during spring and fall seasons

            (5) Time of onset: 1 to 3 hours before meals

      2) History of habits and occurrences

         a) Allergies

         b) Medical history of ulcer disease

         c) Bleeding tendencies

         d) Recurring or chronic gastritis

         e) Consumption of alcohol, tobacco, and/or caffeine

         f) Unusual or chronic tension, anxiety, or stress

         g) Chronic ingestion of irritants or drugs

         h) Hurried or irregular eating habits

         i) Change in appetite

   b. *Objective data*

      1) Physical examination

         a) Acute midepigastric pain on palpation

         b) Nausea or vomiting

         c) Hematemesis

         d) Muscular guarding

         e) Decreased or absent bowel sounds

      2) Diagnostic data and procedures

         a) Complete blood count

    b) Serum electrolyte profile

    c) Blood for *H. pylori*

    d) Type and cross-match blood

    e) Liver enzymes

    f) Upper GI barium contrast study

    g) Gastric analysis

    h) Urinalysis

    i) Fiberoptic gastroscopy and duodenoscopy

    j) Stool examination for occult blood

    k) Exfoliative cytology

2. **Analysis: differential nursing diagnosis/collaborative problems**

    a. *Pain related to inflammation, disease process*

    b. *Risk for fluid volume deficit related to nausea, vomiting*

    c. *Anxiety/fear related to discomfort, change in health status*

    d. *Knowledge deficit related to diet, habits, and pain*

3. **Planning/interventions**

    a. *Acute exacerbation*

      1) Give analgesics as indicated

      2) Insert nasogastric tube

      3) Ensure NPO

      4) Initiate IV fluids or blood transfusion

      5) Monitor intake and output

      6) Administer antiemetics as indicated

      7) Administer antacids as indicated

      8) Administer histamine receptor antagonists as indicated

      9) Administer anticholinergics as indicated

     10) Give sodium and potassium supplements as needed

     11) Monitor urine specific gravity

     12) Monitor gastric emesis/chyme for blood

     13) Monitor stool for occult blood

     14) Minimize environmental stimuli

     15) Initiate saline lavages for hemorrhage; note: research indicates that ice water or saline lavage may be ineffective in controlling bleeding and may impede normal coagulation

     16) Prepare patient for surgical intervention as indicated

     17) Calmly explain all procedures in simple terms

     18) Answer patient questions, and address concerns to the extent possible

    b. *Conservative management*

      1) Give pain medication as indicated

      2) Give antacids as indicated

      3) Give histamine receptor antagonists as indicated

      4) Give medications for treatment of *H. pylori* as indicated

      5) Give proton pump inhibitors as indicated

      6) Give anticholinergics as indicated

      7) Limit environmental stimuli

      8) Instruct patient on medications

      9) Instruct patient on importance of adequate rest

     10) Instruct patient in bland diet in six small feedings each day

     11) Instruct patient in avoidance of stressful events, if possible, and alcoholic beverages, smoking, caffeine, and spicy foods

     12) Calmly explain all procedures in simple terms

4. **Expected outcome/evaluation** (see Appendix B)

C. Bowel obstruction

An intestinal obstruction results in the inability of intestinal contents to flow normally along the intestinal tract. Obstruction may be partial, in which the bowel lumen is narrowed, or complete, in which the bowel lumen is closed. Major sites of obstruction include the esophagus, duodenum, small bowel, and large bowel. Causes include cancer, foreign bodies (e.g., fruit stones, parasitic worms), stricture of the bowel, incarcerated hernias, postoperative peritoneal adhesions, volvulus, paralytic ileus, intussusception, congenital defects, stenosis, and neurogenic conditions. A bowel obstruction results in the accumulation of intestinal contents, fluids, and gas proximal to the obstruction. The absorption of fluids is decreased and gastric secretions are increased. Fluids and electrolytes are lost, and increasing pressure within the intestinal lumen causes a decrease in venous and arteriolar capillary pressure. This leads to edema, congestion, necrosis, and eventual rupture or perforation of the intestinal wall.

1. **Assessment**
   a. *Subjective data*
      1) History of present illness
         a) Pain
            (1) Provocation
            (2) Quality: colicky, crampy, intermittent, wavelike
            (3) Region/radiation: localized
            (4) Severity of symptoms: moderate intensity
            (5) Time of onset: gradual onset in large bowel, rapid onset in small bowel
         b) Stool passage
            (1) Small bowel: feces passed for a short time
            (2) Large bowel: absolute constipation; no passage of stool or flatus
         c) Vomiting
      2) Medical history
         a) Allergies
         b) Weight loss
         c) Anorexia
         d) History of abdominal surgery
   b. *Objective data*
      1) Physical examination
         a) Minimal abdominal distention (small bowel)
         b) Maximal abdominal distention (large bowel)
         c) Diffuse abdominal tenderness and rigidity
         d) High-pitched peristaltic rush sounds proximal to the area of obstruction
         e) Reverse peristaltic waves
         f) Audible borborygmi (hyperactive bowel sounds)
         g) Absent bowel sounds: late
         h) Elevated temperature, pulse, and blood pressure
         i) Vomiting: usually small bowel content (frequent and copious, bile, feces)
      2) Diagnostic data and procedures
         a) Serum amylase
         b) Blood urea nitrogen (BUN) and creatinine
         c) Complete blood count: note whether WBC elevated
         d) Electrolyte profile (especially for sodium, potassium, and chloride)
         e) Type and cross-match blood
         f) Urinalysis

g) Stool for mucus and occult blood

h) Barium studies (both upper and lower GI)

i) Radiograph flat and upright of abdomen

2. **Analysis: differential nursing diagnosis/collaborative problems**

   a. *Pain related to abdominal cramping, nausea, vomiting*

   b. *Fluid volume deficit related to nausea and vomiting*

   c. *Altered nutrition: less than body requirements, related to nausea, vomiting, discomfort*

   d. *Anxiety/fear related to vomiting bowel contents, pain, change in health status*

3. **Planning/interventions**

   a. *Administer pain medications/analgesics as indicated*

   b. *Monitor vital signs*

   c. *Initiate nasogastric intubation (nasoenteric intubation with Levin, Cantor, Harris, or Miller-Abbott tube to decompress affected bowel)*

   d. *Ensure NPO*

   e. *Initiate IV therapy*

   f. *Monitor central venous pressure as indicated*

   g. *Monitor intake and output*

   h. *Monitor urine specific gravity*

   i. *Administer potassium supplements as indicated*

   j. *Measure baseline abdominal girth*

   k. *Assess for pitting and dependent edema*

   l. *Administer antibiotic therapy as indicated*

   m. *Prepare for surgical intervention as indicated*

   n. *Ensure minimal environmental stimuli*

   o. *Calmly explain all procedures in simple terms*

4. **Expected outcome/evaluation** (see Appendix B)

D. Gastroenteritis/infectious diarrhea

This is an inflammation of the lining of the stomach and intestines that may be due to viral, protozoan, bacterial, or parasitic causative agents. Gastroenteritis may also be caused by an imbalance in the normal flora of the gut, such as can be caused by antibiotic therapy. Gastroenteritis will usually run an acute course with no sequelae. Caution should be used in infants, children, and the elderly because dehydration may occur sooner in these groups. Infectious diarrhea may be caused by agents that are viral (Rotavirus, Norwalk-type virus, parvovirus), protozoan (amebic dysentery), bacterial (*Salmonella, Shigella dysenteriae, Escherichia coli, Staphylococcus aureus, Clostridium difficile*), or parasitic (trichinosis, hookworm, pinworm, tapeworm). Traveler's diarrhea is an example of an infectious diarrhea. This occurs as a result of consumption of contaminated foods or water. Causative agents may also infect by person-to-person contact, contact with feces such as with diaper changing, or consumption of raw or inadequately prepared shrimp, shellfish, or meat. Some agents cause diarrhea from colonizing the bowel, producing enterotoxins that attach to specific carbohydrate binding sites and adhere to the cell wall mucosa. This overrides the colon's capacity to reabsorb fluid (*C. difficile, Giardia lamblia, E. coli*). Other causative agents such as rotavirus, Norwalk agent, *S. dysenteriae, Salmonella*, enterohemorrhagic *E. coli*, and *Campylobacter jejuni* invade the intestinal mucosa and secrete toxins that destroy the intestinal mucosal epithelial cells. Bacterial toxins causing food poisoning include *S. aureus, Clostridium perfringens*, and *Bacillus cereus*. Food poisoning is characterized by a short (2–6 hour) incubation period, prominent vomiting, and a number of people affected.

1. **Assessment**
   a. *Subjective data*
      1) History of present illness
         a) Pain
            (1) Provocation
            (2) Quality: cramping, colicky
            (3) Region/radiation: epigastric
            (4) Severity of symptoms
            (5) Time of onset
         b) Nausea and/or vomiting and diarrhea
      2) Medical history
         a) Allergies
         b) Stool pattern: cramping diarrhea
         c) Travel to foreign country
         d) Recent dietary change
         e) Emotional upset
         f) Use of antibiotics
         g) Consumption of raw or inadequately cooked shrimp, shellfish, meat
         h) Employed in a day care center or custodial institution
   b. *Objective data*
      1) Physical examination
         a) Hyperactive bowel sounds
         b) Anorexia
         c) Nausea and vomiting
         d) Decreased urine output
         e) Diarrhea/abdominal cramps
         f) Anal excoriation
         g) Weakness, malaise
         h) Fever
         i) Headaches
         j) May have liver tenderness
         k) Mucus in stools
      2) Diagnostic data and procedures
         a) Electrolyte profile
         b) Complete blood count: expect leukocytosis
         c) Stool examination for ova/parasites, WBC, mucus, protein
         d) Stool culture
         e) Stool examination for occult blood
         f) ELISA testing of stool
         g) Lower GI series
2. **Analysis: differential nursing diagnosis/collaborative problems**
   a. *Fluid volume deficit related to nausea, vomiting, diarrhea*
   b. *Diarrhea related to infectious/inflammatory process*
   c. *Pain related to abdominal cramping, diarrhea, vomiting*
3. **Planning/interventions**
   a. *Monitor vital signs*
   b. *Keep NPO until vomiting stops*
   c. *Initiate IV therapy as indicated*
   d. *Give sodium and potassium supplements as indicated*
   e. *Monitor intake and output*
   f. *Give antiemetics as indicated*
   g. *Give analgesics as indicated*
   h. *Give antibiotics as indicated*

      i. Give anticholinergics as indicated

      j. Maintain enteric precautions

      k. Give corticosteroids with parasitic gastroenteritis

      l. Monitor stool for occult blood

     m. Identify causative agent

      n. When taking food PO, give low-residue, bland diet

      o. Give protein and iron supplements as needed

      p. Maintain skin integrity around anal area

      q. Instruct patient to wash all foods well prior to eating/cooking

      r. Instruct patient to cook all foods thoroughly and heat canned foods to greater than 80°C (176°F) for 30 minutes

      s. Instruct patient to refrigerate stored food and use covers on containers and food to protect against insects and rodents

      t. Instruct patient not to eat foods from punctured and swollen cans or jars with defective seals

      u. Instruct patient in use of medications after discharge

      v. Instruct patient to wash hands thoroughly after toileting or after handling diapers

     w. Discuss need for follow-up for some of the causative agents

  4. Expected outcome/evaluation (see Appendix B)

E. Gastroesophageal reflux disorder (GERD)

GERD is the backflow of gastric contents into the esophagus. Approximately 10% of the population has GERD. It is seen more predominantly in obese and elderly people. It can be caused by decreased tone of the lower esophageal sphincter, esophageal irritation from refluxed acidic gastric contents, slowed motility or peristalsis, or slowed gastric emptying. GERD can occur with or without a hiatal hernia, a condition in which muscle weakness causes the sphincter of the stomach to pass or herniate above the diaphragm into the thoracic cavity. Hiatal hernias occur in 5 per 1000 of the population and are more frequent in females. The incidence is especially high in people older than 60 years. Hiatal hernias are usually treated like GERD unless the herniation is severe enough to warrant surgery.

  1. Assessment

    a. Subjective data

      1) History of present illness

        a) Pain

          (1) Provocation

          (2) Quality: burning sensation that moves up and down the esophagus

          (3) Region/radiation: epigastric, may radiate to back, neck, jaw, chest

          (4) Severity of symptoms: variable

          (5) Time of onset: 30 to 60 minutes after meals, with activities that increase intra-abdominal pressure, such as lifting or straining

        b) Reflux

        c) Dysphagia: intermittent when lying or supine

      2) Past history of habits and occurrences

        a) Allergies

        b) Peptic ulcer disease

        c) Obesity or weight gain

        d) Use of tobacco products

        e) Consumption of caffeine, high-fat diet

        f) Taking theophylline, anticholinergic drugs, calcium channel blockers, salicylates

    b. Objective data
      1) Physical examination
        a) Vital signs normal
        b) Slight epigastric tenderness
        c) Hoarseness or laryngitis
      2) Diagnostic data and procedures
        a) Upper GI/barium swallow
        b) Endoscopy with biopsy
        c) Esophageal manometry
        d) Analysis of gastric secretions
        e) Negative response to sublingual nitroglycerin differentiates noncardiac origin of chest pain

2. Analysis: differential nursing diagnosis/collaborative problems
    a. Pain related to chemical irritation and inflammation
    b. Knowledge deficit related to dietary measures, weight loss, eating habits, avoiding anticholinergic drugs, channel blockers, theophyllines

3. Planning/intervention
    a. Administer antacids as indicated
    b. Administer H_2 receptor antagonists as indicated
    c. Administer cholinergic medications as indicated
    d. Administer proton pump inhibitors as indicated
    e. Instruct patient to eat frequent, small meals; avoid caffeine, very hot or cold food, spicy food, alcohol, and high-fat foods
    f. Instruct patient to raise head of bed on 6- to 8-inch blocks
    g. Explain the effect of weight loss in decreasing episodes of reflux
    h. Instruct patient to avoid use of tobacco, salicylates

4. Expected outcome/evaluation (see Appendix B)

F. Intussusception

    Intussusception is a telescoping of a segment of the bowel by peristalsis within itself, causing a mechanical bowel obstruction. It is most commonly found in infants and small children. Intussusception most commonly develops at or near the ileocecal valve or at the point of attachment of a colon tumor, polyp, or Meckel's diverticulum. Without treatment, death can occur within 2 to 4 days because of the compromised blood supply to the bowel and mesentery and the resulting gangrene and sepsis.

1. Assessment
    a. Subjective data
      1) History of present illness
        a) Pain
          (1) Provocation
          (2) Quality: spasmodic with peristalsis
          (3) Region/radiation
          (4) Severity of symptoms
          (5) Time of onset: explosive, sudden onset
        b) States use of cathartics
      2) Medical history
        a) Allergies
        b) Diarrhea
        c) Constipation
    b. Objective data
      1) Physical examination

a) Paroxysms of acute abdominal pain followed by normal activity

b) Knee flexed, then relaxing as pain eases

c) Rectal blood

d) "Currant jelly" mucous stools

e) Progressive lethargy

f) Tender "sausage-shaped" mass at site of intussusception in right lower and middle abdomen

g) Fever

h) Vomiting food, mucus, and/or fecal matter

i) Dehydration, as evidenced by decreased urine output, dry mouth, poor skin turgor

2) Diagnostic data and procedures

a) Barium enema with fluoroscopic examination: may be both diagnostic and therapeutic; there is a high incidence of reduction of intussusception as a result of this test

b) Complete blood count with differential

c) Serum electrolytes

2. **Analysis: differential nursing diagnosis/collaborative problems**

a. *Pain related to bowel ischemia*

b. *Tissue perfusion related to interruption of blood flow*

c. *Anxiety/fear related to pain and change in health status*

3. **Planning/interventions**

a. *Give analgesics as indicated*

b. *Maintain NPO*

c. *Nasogastric intubation and suction*

d. *Begin IV therapy as indicated*

e. *Monitor intake and output*

f. *Catheterize urethral bladder*

g. *Monitor vital signs*

h. *Administer antispasmodics as indicated*

i. *Administer anticholinergic as indicated*

j. *Prepare for surgical interventions as necessary*

k. *Calmly explain all procedures in simple terms*

4. **Expected outcome/evaluation** (see Appendix B)

G. Appendicitis

Appendicitis is an inflammation or obstruction of the appendix, a blind tube that extends from the inferior part of the cecum. This condition can then lead to ischemia of the vermiform appendix, resulting in necrosis, perforation, and subsequent abscess formation or peritonitis. Inflammatory or obstructive edema of the appendix compromises its vascular supply, increasing its permeability and allowing for bacterial invasion of the wall of the appendix by organisms of the normal flora.

1. **Assessment**

a. *Subjective data*

1) History of present illness

a) Pain

(1) Provocation

(2) Quality

(3) Region/radiation: localized to right lower quadrant (RLQ) between umbilicus and right iliac crest (McBurney's point)

(4) Severity of symptoms: mild to severe

              (5) Time of onset
            b) Loss of appetite
          2) Medical history
            a) Allergies
      b. *Objective data*
        1) Physical examination
          a) Nausea and vomiting
          b) Low-grade fever
          c) RLQ tenderness
          d) Muscle rigidity
          e) Rovsing's sign (left lower quadrant [LLQ] pressure will intensify RLQ pain)
          f) Rebound tenderness over McBurney's point
        2) Diagnostic data and procedures
          a) Complete blood count—elevated WBC possible
          b) Abdominal CT scan
  2. **Analysis: differential nursing diagnosis/collaborative problems**
      a. *Pain related to inflammation and infectious process*
      b. *Risk for fluid volume deficit related to vomiting*
      c. *Risk for infection related to inflammation and infection*
      d. *Anxiety related to pain and change in health status*
  3. **Planning/interventions**
      a. *Position comfortably (often in fetal position)*
      b. *Give analgesics as indicated: be aware of masking of symptoms*
      c. *Administer antipyretic as indicated*
      d. *Monitor vital signs*
      e. *Insert nasogastric tube as indicated*
      f. *Start IV fluids as indicated*
      g. *Monitor intake and output*
      h. *Monitor temperature*
      i. *Monitor WBC count*
      j. *Administer antibiotic as indicated*
      k. *Calmly explain procedures in simple terms*
      l. *Prepare for surgical intervention as indicated*
  4. **Expected outcome/evaluation** (see Appendix B)

H. Pancreatitis

   Pancreatitis is an inflammation of the pancreas with release of the digestive enzymes into the interstitium of the gland, leading to autolysis. Acute pancreatitis can arise from many causes, including injury, local infection, and alcoholism, and glucocorticoid, thiazide diuretic, sulfonamide, or acetaminophen toxicity. Approximately 50% of patients with acute pancreatitis have a mechanical obstruction of the biliary tract. Respiratory symptoms, such as atelectasis and pleural effusion, are often seen as complications of acute pancreatitis. Chronic pancreatitis is an inflammatory state that results in irreversible damage to pancreatic structure and function. In chronic pancreatitis, the organ's endocrine functions are preserved until late in the disease course; however, the production of the pancreatic enzymes needed for the digestion of proteins, carbohydrates, and fats is diminished. Hypocalcemia may result as a complication of pancreatitis because the free fatty acids formed by the release of lipase into the soft tissue spaces bind the calcium, causing a decrease in ionized calcium.

1. **Assessment**
   a. *Subjective data*
      1) History of present illness
         a) Pain
            (1) Provocation: eating
            (2) Quality: severe
            (3) Region/radiation: epigastric, back, chest
            (4) Severity of symptoms: more severe after meals and unrelieved by antacids
         b) Loss of appetite
         c) Precipitating event/trauma
      2) Medical history
         a) Allergies
         b) Alcohol intake
         c) Usual medications
   b. *Objective data*
      1) Physical examination
         a) Temperature elevated
         b) Abdomen distended
         c) Hypotension and elevated pulse (caused by acute hemorrhagic state and/or loss of protein-rich fluid into tissues and peritoneal cavity because of increased vascular permeability)
         d) Vomiting, may be bile tinged
         e) Pain on abdominal palpation or when patient supine
         f) Dyspnea with cough from abdominal distention, pleural effusion
         g) Crackles and rhonchi
         h) Malaise
         i) Bulky, fatty, foul-smelling stool
         j) Weight loss
         k) Signs of tetany as a result of hypocalcemia
      2) Diagnostic data and procedures
         a) Elevated serum amylase (peaks at 24 hours)/pancreatic isoamylase
         b) Elevated WBC count
         c) Elevated serum lipase
         d) Elevated serum bilirubin levels
         e) Elevated serum glucose levels
         f) Elevated urine glucose levels
         g) Serum calcium levels reduced to less than 8 mg/100 mL
         h) Elevated serum glutamic-oxaloacetic transaminase (SGOT) levels
         i) Hematocrit reduced
         j) Abdominal flat plate shows epigastric opacities
         k) Chest radiograph shows diaphragmatic elevation caused by fluid accumulation
         l) Ultrasonography
         m) CT scan
         n) MRI
2. **Analysis: differential nursing diagnosis/collaborative problems**
   a. *Fluid volume deficit related to loss of appetite, vomiting, blood loss (in acute hemorrhagic disease)*
   b. *Gas exchange, impaired, related to hypotension, abdominal distention, and pulmonary sequelae*
   c. *Pain related to inflammatory process*

    d. Anxiety/fear related to change in health status and pain

    e. Knowledge deficit related to diet, lifestyle with chronic pancreatitis

3. Planning/interventions

    a. NPO

    b. Insert nasogastric tube

    c. IV fluid administration with normal saline, Ringer's lactate, or whole blood, packed red blood cells, or albumin, as indicated

    d. Monitor intake and output

    e. Monitor vital signs

    f. Monitor serum amylase, calcium, magnesium, electrolytes, BUN, creatinine, glucose as well as urine glucose

    g. Monitor arterial blood gases

    h. Provide oxygen therapy as indicated

    i. Administer analgesics (usually Demerol [meperidine]) as indicated (avoid opiates, such as morphine, which cause biliary pancreatic duct spasms)

    j. Give anticholinergic as indicated to block nerve impulses that would stimulate pancreatic secretions

    k. Monitor calcium, magnesium, electrolytes

    l. Minimize environmental stimuli

    m. Calmly explain all procedures in simple terms

    n. If chronic pancreatitis, instruct patient to avoid alcohol, caffeine, spices

4. Expected outcome/evaluation (see Appendix B)

I. Cholecystitis

Cholecystitis is an inflammation of the gallbladder that is most frequently caused by gallstones. Other causes include typhoid fever and a tumor obstructing the biliary tract. Cholecystitis may also present secondary to a systemic staphylococcal or streptococcal infection. Obstruction or acute inflammation of the bile ducts causes blockage of bile secretion and possible gangrene.

1. Assessment

    a. Subjective data

      1) History of present illness

        a) Pain

          (1) Provocation

          (2) Quality

          (3) Region/radiation: right upper quadrant (RUQ), referred to right scapula and shoulder

          (4) Severity of symptoms: symptoms aggravated by deep breathing; worse after meals

          (5) Time of onset: after meals

        b) Indigestion, nausea, anorexia, vomiting

      2) Medical history

        a) Allergies

        b) Fatty food diet

    b. Objective data

      1) Physical examination

        a) Low-grade fever

        b) Elevated pulse rate

        c) Malaise

        d) Belching and flatulence

        e) Possible jaundice

f) RUQ tenderness and rigidity on palpation

g) Rebound tenderness in RUQ

h) Tenderness over liver on percussion

i) Murphy's sign (inability to take deep breaths during palpation beneath right costal arch below hepatic margin)

  2) Diagnostic data and procedures

a) WBC count elevated

b) Serum and urine bilirubin elevated

c) Serum glutamate pyruvate transaminase (SGPT) elevated

d) Coagulation studies if surgery indicated

e) Cholecystography

f) Ultrasonography

g) Cholangiography

h) Flat and upright radiographs of abdomen

2. **Analysis: differential nursing diagnosis/collaborative problems**

  a. *Pain related to inflammation and/or spasm*

  b. *Fluid volume deficit related to nausea and vomiting, anorexia*

  c. *Knowledge deficit related to low-fat diet and eating habits*

3. **Planning/interventions**

  a. *Administer analgesics as indicated (avoid opiates such as morphine, which cause biliary duct spasms)*

  b. *Monitor vital signs*

  c. *Administer IV fluids as indicated*

  d. *Monitor intake and output*

  e. *Insert nasogastric tube as indicated*

  f. *Administer antiemetics as indicated*

  g. *Administer anticholinergics as indicated*

  h. *Administer antibiotics as indicated*

  i. *Minimize environmental stimuli*

  j. *Instruct patient in low-fat diet regimen*

  k. *Instruct patient to eat several small meals daily*

  l. *Instruct patient to avoid alcohol consumption*

4. **Expected outcome/evaluation** (see Appendix B)

J. Diverticulitis

Diverticulitis is an inflammation of the diverticula of the colon, usually the sigmoid colon. It is caused by weakness of the colon muscles, sometimes produced by constipation, which leads to small, blind pouches in the lining and wall of the colon. These pouches collect bacteria and other irritating substances. In the United States, the occurrence rate is 10%; diverticulitis occurs predominantly in persons older than 50 years.

1. **Assessment**

  a. *Subjective data*

    1) History of present illness

      a) LLQ crampy abdominal pain

      b) Change in bowel habits

      c) Anorexia

    2) Medical history

      a) Allergies

      b) History of diverticulitis

  b. *Objective data*

1) Physical examination
   a) Low-grade fever
   b) Occult blood in stool
   c) Nausea and vomiting
   d) Abdominal tenderness and guarding on palpation
   e) LLQ tenderness on palpation
2) Diagnostic data and procedures
   a) WBC count elevated
   b) Stool for occult blood
   c) Urinalysis
   d) Sigmoidoscopy
   e) Colonoscopy
   f) Barium enema
   g) Abdomen ultrasound: to detect calcifications

2. **Analysis: differential nursing diagnosis/collaborative problems**
   a. *Pain related to bowel inflammation*
   b. *Constipation related to bowel inflammation*
   c. *Knowledge deficit related to diet and medications, avoidance of alcohol*

3. **Planning/interventions**
   a. *Administer analgesics as indicated*
   b. *Administer antispasmodics as indicated to relax smooth muscles*
   c. *Administer antibiotics as indicated*
   d. *Administer stool softeners as indicated, avoid harsh laxatives that irritate the bowel and cause pain*
   e. *Monitor intake and output*
   f. *Encourage fluid intake of at least eight glasses of water daily to facilitate bowel movement*
   g. *Give Fleet or warm water and soap suds enema as needed for acute constipation*
   h. *Instruct patient to avoid straining while defecating*
   i. *Monitor bowel movement pattern*
   j. *Instruct patient in low-fat diet and low-fiber diet during acute phase and high-fiber diet after acute phase to avoid constipation*
   k. *Instruct patient in use of stool softeners (bulk preparations, mineral oil, suppositories) and the need to drink about 8 glasses of water per day to aid in their effectiveness*
   l. *Instruct about antispasmodics*
   m. *Instruct to avoid alcohol consumption, nuts, and popcorn (nuts and popcorn may become trapped in diverticula)*
   n. *Prepare for surgery as indicated*

4. **Expected outcome/evaluation** (see Appendix B)

K. Irritable Bowel Syndrome

Irritable bowel syndrome (IBS), also called spastic colon, is the most common cause of chronic or recurrent abdominal pain not resulting from structural or biochemical factors. It is a disorder of intestinal motility influenced by the number of stimuli and increased sensitivity to abdominal stimuli. Signs and symptoms are first seen in early adulthood and in males more than females. More than half of those with IBS have underlying depression or anxiety.

1. **Assessment**
   a. *Subjective data*

1) History of present illness
   a) Pain
      (1) Provocation
      (2) Quality: intermittent, crampy, relieved somewhat by defecation
      (3) Region/radiation: LLQ
      (4) Severity of symptoms: moderate intensity
      (5) Time of onset: precipitated by meals, fatigue, neurohormonal agents
2) Medical history
   a) Allergies
   b) Anorexia
   c) Anxiety or depression
   d) Bowel pattern: diarrhea or constipation

b. *Objective data*
   1) Physical examination
      a) Tender LLQ
      b) Hyperresonance on abdominal percussion
      c) Abdominal distention and bloating
   2) Diagnostic data and procedures
      a) Complete blood count
      b) Erythrocyte sedimentation count
      c) Serum albumin
      d) Stool for occult blood
      e) Stool for mucus
      f) Stool for ova and parasites
      g) Flexible sigmoidoscopy
      h) Barium enema
      i) Colonoscopy
      j) Test for lactose intolerance

2. **Analysis: differential nursing diagnosis/collaborative problems**
   a. *Pain related to inflammation*
   b. *Fluid volume deficit related to anorexia, diarrhea*
   c. *Constipation related to inflammatory process*
   d. *Diarrhea related to inflammatory process*

3. **Planning/interventions**
   a. *Administer pain medications as indicated*
   b. *Administer anticholinergic medications for spasms as indicated*
   c. *Administer antispasmodic medications 30 to 60 minutes before meals as indicated*
   d. *Administer antidiarrheal medications as indicated only for severe diarrhea*
   e. *Monitor intake and output*
   f. *Ensure minimal environmental stimuli*
   g. *Calmly explain all procedures in simple terms*
   h. *Answer patient's questions, and address concerns to the extent possible*
   i. *Discharge teaching: high-fiber diet, identify spasm stimuli, avoid sorbitol-containing foods, use of bulk agents such as psyllium*

4. **Expected outcome/evaluation** (see Appendix B)

L. Esophagitis

Esophagitis is a nonspecific inflammatory response of the mucosa of the esophagus related to a variety of stimuli, including achalasia, GERD, infection, or medication. The response is of variable severity; the most severe is upper GI bleeding and stricture. Achalasia is impaired motility of the lower 2/3 of the esophagus as a result of alteration in the neurological functioning in the esophagus or lack of lower esophageal sphincter receptors. In GERD, the inflammation is caused by reflux of gastric secretions. Infections such as *Candida*, herpes simplex, and cytomegalovirus can occur in the esophagus, most commonly in immunosuppressed people. Prolonged exposure to drugs such as NSAIDs, potassium chloride, quinidine, and antibiotics can irritate the esophagus, especially if not much fluid was used to swallow the pills or if the person taking the medication was supine immediately after taking medication.

1. **Assessment**
    a. *Subjective data*
        1) History of present illness
            a) Pain
                (1) Provocation
                (2) Quality
                (3) Region/radiation: chest, epigastric, substernal
                (4) Severity of symptoms
                (5) Time of onset
            b) Reflux
            c) Dysphagia
        2) Medical history
            a) Allergies
            b) Currently taking NSAIDs, quinidine, potassium chloride, antibiotics
            c) Possible immunosuppression: AIDS, organ replacement, leukemia, lymphoma
            d) Taking medications influencing achalasia such as anticholinergics, calcium channel blockers
            e) History of GERD
    b. *Objective data*
        1) Physical examination
            a) Vital signs normal
            b) Slight epigastric tenderness
            c) Herpetic mouth or nose lesions if viral cause
        2) Diagnostic data and procedures
            a) Upper GI/barium swallow
            b) Endoscopy with biopsy
            c) Esophageal manometry
2. **Analysis: differential nursing diagnosis/collaborative problems**
    a. *Pain related to reflux and chemical irritation*
    b. *Knowledge deficit related to diet, frequency of eating, medication taking*
3. **Planning/interventions**
    a. *Monitor vital signs*
    b. *Administer antibiotics as indicated*
    c. *Identify causative agent and treat*
    d. *Administer analgesics as indicated*
    e. *Administer proton pump inhibitors as indicated*
    f. *Nutritional support as indicated: percutaneous endoscopic gastrostomy (PEG) tube*
    g. *Instruct patient to remain sitting up 30 minutes after meals, avoid high-fat diet and spicy foods, chew food thoroughly*
    h. *Instruct patient to elevate head of bed on 4- to 6-inch blocks*
    i. *Anticipate esophageal dilatation or surgery for stricture*

4. Expected outcome/evaluation (see Appendix B)

M. Esophageal varices

Esophageal varices are dilated veins found in the submucosa of the lower esophagus that may extend into the upper esophagus and stomach. This condition occurs most often as a result of obstructed portal circulation associated with liver cirrhosis from alcoholism. Hemorrhage from ruptured esophageal varices is frequently the cause of death in patients with cirrhosis of the liver.

1. **Assessment**
   a. *Subjective data*
      1) History of present illness
         a) Pain in chest
         b) Nausea and vomiting
         c) Actions prior to bleeding: lifting heavy objects; straining at stool; sneezing, coughing, or vomiting; swallowing poorly chewed food
         d) Ingesting irritating fluids, salicylates, or drugs that erode mucosa or interfere with cell replication
      2) Medical history
         a) Allergies
         b) Alcoholism, liver disease
         c) Gastritis
         d) Duodenal ulcer
         e) Bleeding disorders
   b. *Objective data*
      1) Physical examination
         a) Hematemesis
         b) Hepatomegaly
         c) Splenomegaly
         d) Ascites/restlessness/drowsiness
         e) Melena
         f) Diaphoresis
         g) Pallor
      2) Diagnostic data and procedures
         a) Hemoglobin, hematocrit (normal or decreased from blood loss)
         b) Liver function tests
         c) BUN, creatinine
         d) Type and cross-match blood
         e) Stool for occult blood
         f) Serum ammonia level
         g) Bleeding panel: prothrombin time (PT), partial thromboplastin time (PTT), clotting time
         h) Upper GI series
         i) Chest radiograph
         j) Liver scan
         k) Esophagoscopy
2. **Analysis: differential nursing diagnosis/collaborative problems**
   a. *Fluid volume deficit related to bleeding*
   b. *Pain related to esophageal bleeding*
   c. *Anxiety/fear related to visible blood loss*
   d. *Knowledge deficit related to dietary restrictions/lifestyle changes*
3. **Planning/interventions**

   a. *Monitor vital signs*
   b. *Monitor central venous pressure*
   c. *Administer intravenous fluids: normal saline, whole blood, or packed red blood cells as indicated*
   d. *Ensure NPO*
   e. *Prepare for insertion of Sengstaken-Blakemore tube or other tubes (e.g., Minnesota tube)*
   f. *Maintain gastric suction*
   g. *Perform gastric lavage as indicated; note: research indicates that this practice may be ineffective in controlling bleeding and may impede the normal coagulation mechanism*
   h. *Maintain oxygen therapy*
   i. *Administer vasopressin as needed to control bleeding*
   j. *Administer vitamin K as needed*
   k. *Monitor serum electrolytes*
   l. *Monitor hemoglobin and hematocrit*
   m. *Monitor arterial blood gases*
   n. *Monitor capillary refill*
   o. *Monitor skin turgor*
   p. *Administer analgesic as indicated*
   q. *Prepare for admission*
   r. *After patient stabilized, instruct patient to*
      1) Avoid taking salicylates such as aspirin
      2) Take small bites and chew food well
      3) Avoid ingesting medication that interferes with cell replication or erodes mucosa, such as aspirin
      4) Avoid irritating foods, fluids, and alcohol
      5) Avoid straining at stool
      6) Avoid lifting heavy objects
   s. *Explain relationship between alcoholism and esophageal varices*
 4. **Expected outcome/evaluation** (see Appendix B)

N. Liver injuries

   Liver injuries are usually caused by motor vehicle crashes and blunt or penetrating trauma and should be suspected if lower right rib fractures are present. The mortality rate, which is 10 to 20%, is affected by associated injuries. Because one fifth of the cardiac output goes to the liver, there is a great potential for significant blood loss with liver injuries. Injury to the liver affects its functions, including blood storage and filtration; secretion of bile; conversion of sugars into glycogen; synthesis and breakdown of fats and temporary storage of fatty acids; and synthesis of serum proteins (globulins, albumin) that help regulate blood volume and essential clotting factors (fibrinogen and prothrombin).
 1. **Assessment**
   a. *Subjective data*
      1) History of present illness
         a) Pain in RUQ, hypochondriac or epigastric region
         b) Mechanism of injury: blunt or penetrating trauma
      2) Medical history
         a) Allergies
         b) Bleeding tendencies
         c) Liver disease or enlarged liver

      b. Objective data
        1) Physical examination
          a) Hypotension
          b) Rapid, thready pulse
          c) Diaphoresis
          d) RUQ spasms and guarding
          e) Possible decreased level of consciousness
          f) Possible increase in abdominal girth
        2) Diagnostic data and procedures
          a) Complete blood count with differential
          b) Type and cross-match blood
          c) Hematocrit/hemoglobin decreases over time
          d) Elevated liver enzymes: alkaline phosphate, SGPT, SGOT
          e) Coagulation studies: PT, PTT
          f) Flat plate of abdomen
          g) MRI
          h) Angiography for possible hepatic vein damage
          i) CT scan

2. Analysis: differential nursing diagnosis/collaborative problems
   a. Fluid volume deficit related to bleeding
   b. Pain related to injury
   c. Anxiety/fear related to trauma/precipitating event and prognosis

3. Planning/interventions
   a. Monitor vital signs
   b. Monitor central venous pressure
   c. Monitor arterial blood gases
   d. Initiate oxygen therapy as indicated
   e. Initiate IV fluid resuscitation with crystalloid fluids, blood, or blood components
   f. Insert urinary bladder catheter
   g. Monitor intake and output
   h. Insert nasogastric tube as indicated
   i. Administer analgesic when permissible
   j. Minimize environmental stimuli
   k. Prepare for surgical intervention as indicated

4. Expected outcome/evaluation (see Appendix B)

O. Splenic injuries

    The spleen is the abdominal organ most frequently injured by blunt trauma. Splenic injuries are suspected if left rib fractures are evident or left pneumothorax is present. Injury to the spleen inhibits its functions, which include collecting reticuloendothelial cells, maintaining a reservoir of blood, containing erythrocytes, helping keep the blood free from unwanted wastes and infecting organisms, and temporarily storing hemoglobin. Of particular concern is the potential for blood loss into the abdomen after splenic trauma. Such loss may go undetected until it is life threatening.

1. Assessment
   a. Subjective data
      1) History of present illness
        a) Left upper quadrant (LUQ) pain

          b) Kehr's sign (pain referred to left shoulder)

          c) Mechanism of injury: blunt or penetrating trauma to the abdomen

       2) Medical history

          a) Allergies

          b) Bleeding tendencies

   b. Objective data

       1) Physical examination

          a) Hypotension, especially when upright

          b) Rapid, thready pulse

          c) Diaphoresis

          d) Possible decreased level of consciousness

          e) Possible increase in abdominal girth

          f) Balance's sign (dullness on percussion, especially when patient changes position)

          g) Possible areas of ecchymosis on LUQ

          h) Left rib fractures (especially lower two to three ribs on left side)

       2) Diagnostic data and procedures

          a) Complete blood count with differential: expect elevation of WBCs and decreasing hematocrit

          b) Type and cross-match blood

          c) Chest radiograph indicates elevated diaphragm, possible pneumothorax, or fractured eighth to tenth ribs

          d) CT scan

          e) Spleen scan

          f) Angiography

          g) Flat plate of abdomen

          h) Ultrasonogram

2. Analysis: differential nursing diagnosis/collaborative problems

   a. Fluid volume deficit related to blood loss

   b. Pain related to intra-abdominal bleeding

   c. Anxiety/fear related to discomfort, procedures, surgery, precipitating events, and prognosis

3. Planning/interventions

   a. Monitor vital signs

   b. Maintain IV fluid resuscitation with crystalloid fluids, blood, or blood components

   c. Monitor central venous pressure

   d. Monitor arterial blood gases

   e. Insert nasogastric tube as indicated

   f. Insert urinary bladder catheter

   g. Monitor intake and output

   h. Initiate oxygen therapy as indicated

   i. Monitor level of consciousness

   j. Monitor peripheral skin perfusion

   k. Administer analgesic as indicated

   l. Minimize environmental stimuli

   m. Prepare for immediate surgical intervention as indicated

   n. Antiembolic stockings to prevent thrombus formation secondary to rebound elevation of thrombocytes

4. Expected outcome/evaluation (see Appendix B)

P. Stomach injuries

Stomach injuries are usually associated with penetrating injuries, such as gunshot wounds, but may be associated with blunt trauma in motor vehicle crashes (e.g., a shearing force by a steering wheel to the abdomen). Most stomach trauma is penetrating and accounts for about 19% of all intra-abdominal injuries. Injury to the stomach interferes with peristalsis and digestion. If the stomach is penetrated, corrosive hydrochloric acid, enzymes, and mucin may leak into the abdominal cavity and cause peritonitis. Injury to the stomach interferes with the action of enzymes that help break down food molecules into smaller parts; mucin, which acts on certain sugars and protects the stomach lining; and hydrochloric acid, which aids in dissolving food before the enzymes begin working on it.

1. **Assessment**
   a. *Subjective data*
      1) History of present illness
         a) Pain in epigastric area or LUQ
         b) May be associated with pancreas or intestinal injuries
         c) Hematemesis
         d) Mechanism of injury: blunt or penetrating trauma to abdomen
      2) Medical history
         a) Allergies
         b) Bleeding tendencies
   b. *Objective data*
      1) Physical examination
         a) Hypotension
         b) Rapid pulse
         c) Abdominal muscle guarding
         d) Rebound tenderness
         e) Diaphoresis
      2) Diagnostic data and procedures
         a) Serum electrolytes
         b) Complete blood count with differential
            (1) Elevated WBC count
            (2) Decreased hemoglobin and hematocrit
         c) CT scan
         d) Abdominal upright radiograph shows free air
         e) Nasogastric lavage positive for blood
         f) Type and cross-match blood
2. **Analysis: differential nursing diagnosis/collaborative problems**
   a. *Fluid volume deficit related to blood loss, diaphoresis*
   b. *Pain related to traumatic injury, bleeding in abdomen*
   c. *Anxiety/fear related to prognosis, precipitating event or trauma, procedures*
3. **Planning/interventions**
   a. *Monitor vital signs*
   b. *Monitor arterial blood gases*
   c. *Initiate oxygen therapy as indicated*
   d. *Initiate IV resuscitation with crystalloid fluids, blood, or blood components*
   e. *Monitor central venous pressure*
   f. *Monitor level of consciousness*
   g. *Monitor capillary refill*
   h. *Insert nasogastric tube as indicated*
   i. *Insert urinary bladder catheter as indicated*
   j. *Monitor intake and output*

> k. *Administer analgesics when permissible*
> l. *Minimize environmental stimuli*
> m. *Calmly explain all procedures in simple terms*
> n. *Answer patient's questions, and address concerns to the extent possible*
> o. *Prepare for surgical intervention as indicated*

4. Expected outcome/evaluation (see Appendix B)

Q. Pancreatic injuries

Pancreatic injuries are often associated with other abdominal injuries. Such an injury can occur as a result of impact with the steering wheel during a motor vehicle crash. Mortality rates are reported as high as 50% for blunt injury, 25% for gunshot wounds, and 8% for stab wounds. The single most important factor influencing morbidity and mortality is a delay in diagnosis, which is why morbidity is so high for blunt trauma. Pancreatic injury alters the secretion of pancreatic juices containing enzymes that break down proteins, fats, and carbohydrates. The bicarbonate ions in pancreatic juice help neutralize chyme that is passed from stomach to duodenum. Altered glucagon and insulin secretion as a result of pancreatic injury is one of the greatest problems and concerns.

1. Assessment
> a. *Subjective data*
>> 1) History of present illness
>>> a) Pain in epigastric area or back
>>> b) May be asymptomatic unless peritoneal irritation present
>>> c) Symptoms may not develop until 12 hours after injury
>>> d) Mechanism of injury: blunt or penetrating trauma to abdomen
>> 2) Medical history
>>> a) Allergies
>>> b) Bleeding tendencies
> b. *Objective data*
>> 1) Physical examination
>>> a) Abdominal guarding and tenderness
>>> b) Absent bowel sounds: ileus
>>> c) Hypotension
>>> d) Rapid pulse with decreased blood pressure
>> 2) Diagnostic data and procedures
>>> a) Elevated serum or urine amylase
>>> b) Elevated serum glucose
>>> c) Elevated serum lipase
>>> d) Peritoneal lavage positive for amylase
>>> e) CT scan
>>> f) Type and cross-match blood

2. Analysis: differential nursing diagnosis/collaborative problems
> a. *Fluid volume deficit related to bleeding, loss of pancreatic fluid into abdomen*
> b. *Pain related to traumatic injury*
> c. *Anxiety/fear related to procedures, precipitating event from trauma, prognosis*

3. Planning/interventions
> a. *Monitor vital signs*
> b. *Monitor arterial blood gases*
> c. *Initiate IV fluid resuscitation with crystalloid fluids, blood, blood components*
> d. *Monitor central venous pressure*
> e. *Initiate oxygen therapy as indicated*

      f. Monitor serum amylase and lipase
      g. Monitor serum and urine glucose
      h. Monitor skin for temperature, capillary refill
      i. Insert nasogastric tube as indicated
      j. Insert urinary bladder catheter as indicated
      k. Monitor intake and output
      l. Administer analgesics when permissible
      m. Minimize environmental stimuli
      n. Prepare for surgical intervention as indicated
   4. Expected outcome/evaluation (see Appendix B)

R. Mesenteric/bowel/colon injuries

    These injuries are often associated with other abdominal injuries. Blunt trauma is usually caused by deceleration or motor vehicle crashes resulting in the shearing force of body contact with the steering wheel. Penetrating wounds are most often caused by gunshot injuries. Injury to the mesentery and intestines inhibits peristalsis, nutrient breakdown and absorption, fluid absorption, and waste excretion.

   1. Assessment
     a. Subjective data
       1) History of present illness
         a) Pain in abdomen
         b) Nausea and vomiting
         c) Mechanism of injury: blunt or penetrating trauma to abdomen
       2) Medical history
         a) Allergies
         b) Bleeding tendencies
     b. Objective data
       1) Physical examination
         a) Absent bowel sounds
         b) Rebound pain tenderness
         c) Abdominal muscle guarding or rigidity
         d) Palpable abdominal mass
         e) Hypotension or shock
       2) Diagnostic data and procedures
         a) Elevated WBC count
         b) Elevated serum amylase
         c) Stool specimen positive for blood
         d) Serum electrolytes
         e) Type and cross-match blood
         f) Arterial blood gases
         g) Flat plate of abdomen shows free air
         h) Peritoneal lavage positive for blood and fecal matter
         i) Chest radiograph
         j) CT scan
   2. Analysis: differential nursing diagnosis/collaborative problems
     a. Fluid volume deficit related to hemorrhage, leaking of bowel contents
     b. Pain related to blunt or penetrating abdominal injury, hemorrhage into abdominal cavity
     c. Anxiety/fear related to prognosis, event precipitating trauma, procedures
     d. Risk for infection related to peritoneal contamination
   3. Planning/interventions
     a. Monitor vital signs

    b. Monitor arterial blood gases

    c. Initiate IV fluid resuscitation with crystalloid fluids, blood, or blood components

    d. Monitor central venous pressure

    e. Insert nasogastric tube as indicated

    f. Insert urinary bladder catheter as indicated

    g. Monitor level of consciousness

    h. Monitor intake and output

    i. Administer analgesic when permissible

    j. Minimize environmental stimuli

    k. Monitor for signs of peritonitis: rebound tenderness, muscle rigidity/spasm, fluid wave, decreased or absent bowel sounds

    l. Administer antibiotics as indicated

    m. Prepare for surgical intervention as indicated

  4. Expected outcome/evaluation (see Appendix B)

S. Greater vessel injuries

    Greater vessel injuries may be associated with other abdominal injuries. The cause of death is exsanguination. Damage to the aorta causes loss of blood supply to the major organs. Loss of blood supply to the lower limbs results from damage to the femoral and iliac vessels. Traumatic rupture of the aorta may be caused by sudden deceleration in a motor vehicle crash or a fall from a height. Mortality rates range from 30 to 60%.

  1. Assessment

    a. Subjective data

      1) History of present illness

        a) Pain in abdomen

        b) Nausea and vomiting

        c) Mechanism of injury: blunt or penetrating trauma to abdomen

      2) Medical history

        a) Allergies

        b) Bleeding tendencies

    b. Objective data

      1) Physical examination

        a) Increased abdominal girth

        b) Ecchymosis of midline of peritoneum

        c) Abdominal tenderness, rigidity, guarding

        d) Femoral pulses diminished or absent

        e) Diminished bowel sounds

        f) Hypotension/shock

      2) Diagnostic data and procedures

        a) Complete blood count

        b) Type and cross-match blood

        c) Coagulation studies

        d) CT scan

        e) Flat plate of abdomen

        f) Angiography shows area of injury

        g) Peritoneal lavage positive for blood

        h) MRI

  2. Analysis: differential nursing diagnosis/collaborative problems

    a) Fluid volume deficit related to blood loss

    b) Pain related to bleeding and injury

    c) Anxiety/fear related to prognosis, surgery

3. **Planning/interventions**

    a) Monitor vital signs

    b) Monitor arterial blood gases

    c) Initiate IV fluid resuscitation with crystalloid fluids, blood, or blood components

    d) Monitor central venous pressure

    e) Monitor level of consciousness

    f) Insert nasogastric tube as indicated

    g) Insert urinary bladder catheter

    h) Administer analgesics when permissible

    i) Prepare for surgical intervention as indicated

4. **Expected outcome/evaluation** (see Appendix B)

BIBLIOGRAPHY

Andreoli, T., Bennett, J., Carpenter, C., & Plum, F. (1997). *Cecil essentials of medicine* (4th ed.). Philadelphia: W. B. Saunders.

Bates, B. (1995). *A guide to physical examination and history taking* (6th ed.). New York: J. B. Lippincott.

Black, J., & Matassarin-Jacobs, E. (1997). *Medical surgical nursing: Clinical management for continuity of care* (5th ed.). Philadelphia: W. B. Saunders.

Butler, K., Moore, E., & Harken, A. (1996). Traumatic rupture of the descending thoracic aorta. *AORN Journal, 63,* 917.

Cardona, V., Hurn, R., Mason, P., Scanlon-Schilpp, A., & Veise-Berry, S. (1992). *Trauma nursing: From resuscitation through rehabilitation*. Philadelphia: W. B. Saunders.

Carlson, E. (1998). Irritable bowel syndrome. *The Nurse Practitioner Journal, 23,* 82–88.

Castiglia, P., & Harbin, R. (1992). *Child health care: Process and practice* (4th ed.). St. Louis, MO: C. V. Mosby.

Clevenger, F., & Tepas, J. (1997). Preoperative management of patients with major trauma injuries. *AORN Journal, 65,* 583–594.

Cummings, P. H. (1993). *Drugs and protocols common to prehospital and emergency care*. Boston: Jones & Bartlett.

Dickerman, R., & Dunn, E. (1981). Splenic, pancreatic, and hepatic injuries. *Surgical Clinics of North America, 61*(1), 3.

Emmick, R., & Peterson, S. (1996). Evaluation of pancreatic injury after blunt abdominal trauma. *Annals of Emergency Medicine, 27,* 658–661.

Fischbach, F. (1998). *A manual of laboratory diagnostic tests* (2nd ed.). Philadelphia: J. B. Lippincott.

Kandel, G. (1990). Management of nonvariceal upper GI hemorrhage. *Hospital Practitioner, 25*(2), 167–184.

Kane, R., Ouslander, J., & Abrass, I. (1994). *Essentials of clinical geriatrics* (3rd ed.). New York: McGraw-Hill.

Lewis, S., Collier, I., & Heitkemper, M. (1996). *Medical surgical nursing: Assessment and management of clinical problems*. St. Louis, MO: C. V. Mosby.

Long, B., Phipps, W., & Cassmeyer, V. (1993). *Medical surgical nursing: A nursing process approach* (3rd ed.). St. Louis, MO: C. V. Mosby.

Middlemiss, C. (1997). Gastroesophageal reflux disease: A common condition in the elderly. *The Nurse Practitioner, 22,* 51–59.

Miller, B., & Keane, C. (1992). *Encyclopedia and dictionary of medicine, nursing, and allied health* (5th ed.). Philadelphia: W. B. Saunders.

Pagana, K., & Pagana, T. (1997). *Diagnostic testing and nursing implications: A case study approach* (3rd ed.). St. Louis, MO: C. V. Mosby.

Price, S., & Wilson, L. (1997). *Pathophysiology: Clinical concepts of disease processes* (5th ed.). New York: Mosby-Year Book.

Richardson, J., & Brewer, M. (1996). Management of upper abdominal solid organ injuries. *AORN Journal, 63,* 907–916.

Rutledge, R., Thomason, M., Oller, D., Meredith, W., Moylan, J., Clancy, T., Cunningham, P., & Baker, M. (1991). The spectrum of abdominal injuries associated with the use of seatbelts. *Journal of Trauma 31*(6), 820–826.

Sheehy, S. (1993). *Manual of emergency care* (4th ed.). St. Louis, MO: C. V. Mosby.

Soud, T., & Rogers, J. (1997). *Manual of pediatric emergency nursing*. St. Louis, MO: C. V. Mosby.

Stobo, J., Hellman, D., Ladenson, P., Petty, B., & Traill, T. (1996). *The principles and practice of medicine* (23rd ed.). Stamford, CT: Appleton & Lange.

Thompson, S. (1990). *Emergency care of children*. Boston: Jones & Bartlett.

Tierney, L., McPhee, S., & Papadikis, M. (Eds.). (1996). *Current medical diagnosis and treatment* (35th ed.). Stamford, CT: Appleton & Lange.

Kathleen A. Doherty, BS, BSN

CHAPTER **3**

Cardiovascular Emergencies

MAJOR TOPICS

General Strategy

Specific Medical Cardiovascular Emergencies

  Angina

  Myocardial Infarction

  Right Ventricular Infarction

  Heart Failure and Cardiogenic Pulmonary Edema

  Cardiac Dysrhythmias

  Hypertensive Emergencies

  Acute Aortic Dissection

  Acute Pericarditis

  Infective Endocarditis

  Acute Arterial Occlusion

  Venous Thrombosis

  Peripheral Vascular Disease

Specific Surgical Cardiovascular Emergencies

  Myocardial Contusion

  Cardiac Tamponade

  Traumatic Aortic Injury

  Arterial Trauma

I. GENERAL CARDIOVASCULAR EMERGENCIES

A. Assessment

    1. Primary survey/resuscitation (see Chapter 1)

    2. Secondary survey (see Chapter 1)

    3. Psychological, social, environmental factors

       a. Unmodifiable

         1) Age (cardiac disease increases with aging)

         2) Sex (male sex predominates)

         3) Heredity

         4) Race

       b. Modifiable

         1) Blood pressure (BP)

         2) Obesity

         3) Dyslipidemia

         4) Smoking

        5) Physical inactivity

        6) Stress

        7) Diabetes

4. Focused survey

  a. Subjective data

      1) Chief complaint

      2) History of present illness

         a) Pain: PQRST

           (1) Provocation

           (2) Quality

           (3) Region/radiation

           (4) Severity

           (5) Time

              (a) Duration

              (b) Development over time

              (c) Periodicity (when it comes and goes)

         b) Dyspnea

           (1) Shortness of breath

              (a) Dyspnea on exertion (DOE)

              (b) Positional dyspnea (trepopnea)

           (2) Paroxysmal nocturnal dyspnea (PND)

           (3) Orthopnea

          c) Cough

           (1) Dry, "cardiac" cough

           (2) Hemoptysis

          d) Syncope

          e) Palpitations

          f) Fatigue

          g) Nausea, vomiting

          h) Headache

          i) Behavioral change

          j) Activity limitations

          k) Injury: mechanism and time

      3) Medical history

         a) Coronary heart disease (CHD)

           (1) Angina

           (2) Previous myocardial infarction (MI)

           (3) Hypertension

           (4) Congestive heart failure (CHF)

         b) Pulmonary disease

         c) Diabetes

         d) Renal disease

         e) Vascular disease

         f) Previous cardiac surgery

         g) Congenital anomalies

         h) Current/past medication use

           (1) Nitrates

           (2) Beta blockers

           (3) Calcium channel blockers

           (4) Antihypertensives

           (5) Digitalis

           (6) Diuretics

           (7) Antidysrhythmics

    (8) Anticoagulants
    (9) Steroids
    (10) Specific pulmonary drugs
    (11) Illicit drugs
    (12) Over-the-counter medications
   i) Allergies
  b. *Objective data*
   1) Physical examination
    a) General survey
     (1) Level of consciousness
     (2) Respiratory status
      (a) Rate
      (b) Regularity
      (c) Effort
      (d) Breath sounds
     (3) Integument
      (a) Color
      (b) Temperature
      (c) Moisture
      (d) Capillary refill time
     (4) Edema
      (a) Dependent: extremities, sacrum
      (b) Cardiac (pitting)
     (5) Cyanosis
      (a) Central: if cardiac output severely decreased
      (b) Peripheral: decrease in blood flow in the periphery
     (6) Clubbing: of the nail beds
     (7) BP measurement
      (a) Both arms
      (b) Orthostatic (supine, sitting, standing)
     (8) Apical heart rate
      (a) Regular rate, tachycardia or bradycardia
      (b) Regular or irregular rhythm
     (9) Peripheral pulses (present, absent, diminished, bounding)
     (10) Pupils
      (a) Size
      (b) Equality
      (c) Reaction to light
    b) Inspection
     (1) Tracheal position (midline or deviated)
     (2) Neck veins
      (a) Internal jugular vein appearance
      (b) Estimate central venous pressure: when sitting at 45-degree angle from horizontal, venous pulses should ascend no more than a few centimeters above clavicle
     (3) Thorax
      (a) Configuration: symmetry; deformities; anteroposterior (A-P) diameter; movement with respirations
      (b) Injuries: penetrating; blunt (ecchymosis, contusions); evidence of previous thoracic injuries and/or surgery
      (c) Abnormal chest wall movements (e.g., asymmetric, paradoxical)
     (4) Precordium
      (a) Apical impulse

        (b) Abnormal precordial movements: heaves; lifts; pulsations; retractions

    (5) Epigastrium (pulsations)

c) Palpation

    (1) Areas of tenderness or crepitus

    (2) Precordial areas

        (a) Point of maximal impulse (PMI): location is normally fifth left intercostal space (ICS), midclavicular line (MCL); size is normally 2 cm; force (amplitude); duration

        (b) Thrills: feels like a purring cat

    (3) Epigastrium

        (a) Direction of pulsation

        (b) Differentiate between abdominal aorta and right ventricular pulsation

d) Auscultation

    (1) Breath sounds

        (a) Depth

        (b) Equality

        (c) Location of bronchial, vesicular, and bronchovesicular sounds

        (d) Adventitious sounds: crackles are fine or coarse; wheezes have musical quality, high pitched; pleural friction rub is grating, harsh

    (2) Heart sounds

        (a) Auscultatory sites: aortic (second right ICS); pulmonic (second left ICS); tricuspid (lower left sternal border [LSB]); mitral (apex); Erb's point (third left ICS); epigastric area (below xiphoid).

        (b) Identify S_1 and S_2 (S_1: mitral, tricuspid valves close; S_2: aortic, pulmonic valves close)

        (c) Identify presence of S_3 and S_4 (S_3 may be normal in children, young adults)

        (d) Murmurs: systolic or diastolic; location

        (e) Variations related to dysrhythmias: premature extra systoles; atrial fibrillation; complete heart block

        (f) Extra cardiac sounds: pericardial friction rubs; venous hum; arterial bruits; clicks

2) Diagnostic procedures

a) Electrocardiogram (ECG): 12 lead, 15 lead

    (1) Rate and rhythm

    (2) Presence of cardiac dysrhythmias

    (3) Evidence of myocardial ischemia, injury

    (4) Presence of intraventricular conduction defect

    (5) Evidence of previous MI

b) Laboratory

    (1) Complete blood count (CBC)

    (2) Serum electrolytes

    (3) Cardiac serum markers (creatinine kinase [CK], treponin, myoglobin, lactic dehydrogenase [LDH])

    (4) Serum glucose

    (5) Coagulation studies

    (6) Digoxin level

    (7) Serum creatinine and blood urea nitrogen (BUN)

    (8) Type and cross-match blood

        (9) Arterial blood gas (ABG)

        (10) Routine urinalysis

    c) Pulse oximetry

    d) Radiography

        (1) Chest radiograph

           (a) Heart size and location

           (b) Presence of interstitial edema, pulmonary infiltrates, pleural effusions

           (c) Air and fluid levels in trauma patients

           (d) Mediastinal width on serial films

           (e) Bony structure integrity

        (2) Cardiac catheterization

        (3) Transesophageal echocardiogram

        (4) Arteriography, aortogram

        (5) Venogram

        (6) Ultrasonography

        (7) Other special procedures

        (8) Preparation of patient and family for diagnostic procedures

           (a) Emotional support

           (b) Physical preparation

           (c) Teaching of patient/family

           (d) Informed consent

B. Analysis: Differential nursing diagnosis/collaborative problems

  1. Anxiety/fear

  2. Cardiac output, decreased

  3. Gas exchange, impaired

  4. Ineffective airway clearance

  5. Knowledge deficit

  6. Pain

  7. Risk for injury

  8. Tissue perfusion, altered (cardiac, cerebral, renal, peripheral)

C. Planning/interventions

  1. Determine priorities

    a. Control and maintain airway, breathing, and circulation

    b. Closely monitor patient; watch for changes in

      1) Airway

      2) Vital signs

      3) Cardiac rhythm

      4) ABG values

      5) Pulse oximetry

    c. Control pain

    d. Relieve anxiety/apprehension

    e. Educate patient/significant others

    f. Prevent complications

  2. Develop nursing care plan specific to patient's cardiac emergency

  3. Obtain and set up emergency equipment and supplies

  4. Institute appropriate interventions based on nursing care plan

  5. Document and record data as appropriate

D. Expected outcomes/evaluation

1. **Monitor patient responses and outcomes and modify nursing care plans as indicated**
   a. *Specific interventions*
   b. *Disposition/discharge planning*
2. **If positive outcomes are not demonstrated, assessment and/or plan of care needs reevaluation**

E. Age-related considerations

1. **Pediatric**
   a. *Growth/development related*
      1) Congenital heart disease (e.g., congenital heart defects)
      2) Acquired heart disease (e.g., rheumatic fever)
      3) Endocrine or metabolic disorders (e.g., diabetes)
      4) Other
         a) Drug ingestion: e.g., tricyclic antidepressants, digoxin
         b) Trauma (e.g., falls, motor vehicle crashes [MVCs])
         c) Suffocation (e.g., plastic bags, drowning, accidental hanging)
   b. *"Pearls"*
      1) Cardiac arrest in the pediatric population usually the result of progressive deterioration in respiratory and circulatory function
      2) Congestive heart failure, cardiogenic shock, and multiple varieties of dysrhythmias are unusual in pediatric patients and often related to congenital anomalies of heart
      3) Immaturity of conduction system and its autonomic innervation may contribute to dysrhythmias

2. **Geriatric**
   a. *Aging-related*
      1) Presence of chronic diseases: may obscure or confound cardiac picture
      2) Altered drug metabolism: slower in the elderly; concurrent medication use may decrease drug metabolism
      3) Multiple physiological differences (e.g., diminished responses to stress and decreased hepatic and renal function) and changes in laboratory values must be taken into account when assessing elderly patients
      4) Psychological and social changes: geriatric patients may have different goals for their treatment plan regarding prolonging life and use of life support; these topics should be discussed with all patients but are particularly important in elderly
      5) Some geriatric patients adapt so well to cardiac disease that signs that would otherwise be remarkable go undetected
      6) Arteriosclerotic changes in the aorta and peripheral pulses may result in difficulty palpating pulse
      7) Rhythm abnormalities are so common that they may be "normal"
   b. *"Pearls"*
      1) "Go slow, stay low" when treating elderly with pharmacotherapeutics
      2) Concurrent use of other medications poses a variety of problems; providing medications that are easy to use (transdermal) and are taken once or twice daily results in improved compliance; frequent evaluation of all medications is essential to preventing complications, which are much more common in geriatric population

II. SPECIFIC MEDICAL CARDIOVASCULAR EMERGENCIES

A. Angina

Angina is the result of an imbalance between myocardial oxygen supply and demand, usually related to atherosclerotic changes in the coronary arteries. There are three types of angina: stable, unstable, and variant (also known as Prinzmetal's angina). When discussing stable and unstable angina, it is important to stress that angina is part of a continuum of a disease process. Stable angina is a symptom of myocardial ischemia described by the patient as pain or discomfort in the chest or adjacent areas, which is poorly localized. It is associated with physical exertion, emotional stress, or exposure to extreme temperatures and is relieved with rest or sublingual nitroglycerin within a few minutes. Variant angina may or may not occur with atherosclerotic changes; instead, it is generally thought to occur as a result of coronary artery spasm. It often occurs in a cyclical fashion, it may occur at the same time each day, almost exclusively at rest, and it is not usually precipitated by physical exertion or emotional stress. Patients with variant angina are usually younger than those with chronic stable angina or unstable angina. The resulting ST-segment elevation seen during the variant anginal episode returns to baseline once the pain is gone. The diagnosis of unstable angina is dependent on one of the following three features: 1) angina at rest as well as with minimal exertion, usually lasting longer than 20 minutes; 2) angina of new onset (within several weeks), which starts with physical exertion and produces marked limitation of ordinary physical activity; 3) previously diagnosed stable angina that has become more severe, prolonged, or frequent.

Pain similar to angina may also accompany esophageal spasm, gastroesophageal reflux disease (GERD), biliary colic, chest wall pain, pericarditis, pulmonary embolism, aortic dissection, and cardiac dysrhythmias. Careful examination and history taking are essential to making the diagnosis.

1. **Assessment**
   a. *Subjective data*
      1) History of present illness
         a) Pain or "discomfort"
            (1) Provocative factors (anything that may increase myocardial oxygen requirements)
               (a) Physical activity/exercise
               (b) Emotional stress
               (c) Cold weather
               (d) After meals
               (e) May occur at rest (variant)
            (2) Palliative factors
               (a) Rest and/or cessation of activity
               (b) Sublingual nitroglycerin
            (3) Quality
               (a) Squeezing
               (b) Clutching
               (c) Crushing
               (d) Pressure: "weight on my chest"
               (e) Burning
               (f) Indigestion
            (4) Region/radiation
               (a) Substernal
               (b) Epigastric

(c) Neck, mandible, lower jaw

(d) Left shoulder, inner surface of arm to ulnar surface of hand

(5) Severity: commonly described as discomfort rather than pain; patient may even deny pain

(a) Stable: unchanged from "normal" angina pain

(b) Unstable: more intense than "normal" angina pain

(c) Variant: extremely severe, referred to as pain

(d) Use of numerical pain scale (e.g., 1–10, 1 = pain free to 10 = severe pain)

(6) Timing

(a) Stable: usually lasts 3 to 5 minutes

(b) Unstable: more prolonged; may last as long as 30 minutes

(c) Variant: may occur at same time each day; attacks tend to cluster at night between midnight and 0800 hours

(d) May awaken patient from sleep

2) Medical history

a) Previous episodes of angina

b) Previous MI

c) Hypertension: increases cardiac workload

d) Diabetes mellitus: may cause vessel damage

e) Medications (e.g., nitroglycerin)

f) Allergies

g) Illicit drug use (e.g., cocaine)

h) Heavy smoker: common with variant-type angina

i) Hypercholesterolemia

j) Physical inactivity

k) Obesity

l) Other

b. *Objective data*

1) Physical examination (following signs may be present):

a) Elevated BP

b) Increased heart rate

c) Rapid, shallow respirations

d) Diaphoresis

e) Third or fourth heart sound

f) Pulsus alternans

g) Transient pulmonary crackles (with pain)

2) Diagnostic procedures

a) ECG

(1) ST depression may accompany pain with stable angina

(2) Transient ST-segment deviations (depression or elevation) and T-wave inversion occur commonly with unstable angina

(3) With variant angina, ST-segment elevation occurs with pain; ST segment returns to baseline when pain subsides

(4) May also see patterns of left ventricular (LV) hypertrophy, old MI, nonspecific ST- and T-wave abnormalities and atrioventricular (AV) defects

b) CBC to assess for anemia-induced angina

c) Cardiac serum markers: no elevation should occur unless myocardial cell damage has occurred

d) Chest radiograph may reflect CHF, cardiomegaly

2. **Analysis: differential nursing diagnosis/collaborative problems**
   a. *Impaired gas exchange related to decreased cardiac output*
   b. *Anxiety/fear related to alteration in health status, inability to control or alter symptoms, and/or fear of death*
   c. *Decreased cardiac output related to conduction disturbances secondary to myocardial oxygen supply-demand imbalance*
   d. *Pain related to myocardial oxygen supply-demand imbalance*
   e. *Risk for injury related to myocardial ischemia*
   f. *Knowledge deficit related to etiology, pathophysiology, interventions, potential complications, and prognosis*

3. **Planning/interventions**
   a. *Continuous cardiac monitoring for potential dysrhythmias*
   b. *Provide supplemental oxygen via nasal cannula or other oxygen delivery device as indicated*
   c. *Obtain intravenous (IV) access, saline lock*
   d. *Obtain blood for laboratory studies (e.g., CBC, electrolytes, cardiac serum markers)*
   e. *Obtain 12- to 15-lead ECG*
   f. *Rest: decrease exertion*
   g. *Decrease anxiety: answer questions, explain procedures*
   h. *Administer sublingual nitroglycerin if patient's systolic BP is at least 90 mm Hg; may follow with intravenous nitroglycerin drip*
      1) Assess patient's BP frequently; peripheral vasodilation may cause hypotension
      2) Assess for headache; may be caused by cerebral vasodilation
      3) Assess for reflex tachycardia
      4) In elderly, venodilatory effect of nitroglycerin is greater and time to onset of action of sublingual nitroglycerin may be prolonged, owing to dry mouth; nitroglycerin spray may be a better choice
   i. *Administer morphine as ordered*
      1) Morphine provides analgesia and sedation, reduces apprehension, decreases preload and afterload
      2) Morphine is used for severe angina when nitroglycerin has not been effective
   j. *Administer beta blockers as ordered*
      1) If clinical situation deteriorates after administration of beta blockers, consider coronary artery spasm as cause of angina
      2) Assess for signs of cardiac failure resulting from negative inotropic effect of beta blockers
      3) Adverse effects of beta blockers are considered more common and severe in the elderly
   k. *Administer calcium antagonists as ordered*
      1) Second-line therapy in patients with continued ischemia despite nitroglycerin and beta blockers
      2) More effective than beta blockers in treating variant-type angina
      3) Assess for CHF resulting from calcium antagonists' negative inotropic effect
      4) Calcium antagonists may increase digoxin levels, and elderly patients are more susceptible to digoxin toxicity

  l. Administer antiplatelet agents
   1) Aspirin or ticlopidine (for those in which acetylsalicylic acid [ASA] is contraindicated) should be administered as soon as possible to decrease platelet activation and thrombus formation
  m. Allow support of significant other if patient's condition permits
  n. Assess patient's knowledge regarding management of anginal episodes
   1) Review identification of anginal pain
   2) Instruct patient to stop activity and sit down
   3) Use of nitroglycerin tablets
    a) Use only sublingually
    b) Should sting, taste bitter
    c) Use one tablet every 3 to 5 minutes
   4) If chest pain not alleviated after using three nitroglycerin tablets over a 15-minute period, call physician or dial 911
   5) Answer questions of patient/significant other regarding pain management
   6) Discuss changes in pain that may indicate worsening of disease
4. Expected outcomes/evaluation (see Appendix B)

B. Myocardial infarction

  Necrosis of the myocardium as a result of prolonged ischemia is referred to as an MI. Almost all MIs occur as a result of coronary artery atherosclerosis complicated by thrombosis formation. Nonatherosclerosis causes of MI include coronary artery spasm, congenital abnormalities, and connective tissue disorders, among others. New understanding of the pathophysiology of MI has lead to the term "acute coronary syndromes," which is used to refer to patients presenting with ischemic chest pain. It is important to realize that this is a continuum of a disease process that includes unstable angina (USA), non-Q-wave MI, and Q-wave MI. MI caused by atherosclerotic disease occurs as a result of the rupture of an unstable atheromatous plaque and subsequent exposure of substances that promote platelet activation and fibrin clot formation. The resultant coronary thrombosis interrupts blood flow and leads to an imbalance of myocardial oxygen supply and demand, which, if severe and/or persistent, leads to myocardial necrosis.

  Physiologically, the ischemia produces irreversible cellular damage. Depending on the amount of ischemia and myocardial tissue involvement, myocardial contractility, stroke volume, and ventricle capability will begin to decline. Peripheral vascular resistance increases secondary to the infarction because of catecholamine release, which increases preload and afterload. The subsequent demands placed on the infarcting myocardium can become overwhelming.

1. Assessment
  a. Subjective data
   1) History of present illness
    a) Pain or "discomfort"
     (1) Provocative factors
      (a) Emotional or physical stressors
      (b) May occur at rest
     (2) Palliative factors: unrelieved by change of position, nitrate use
     (3) Quality: pain may be "different" from usual angina; quality may be described as squeezing, crushing, heaviness, pressure, or "something sitting on my chest"; may also be described as burning or indigestion (especially in the elderly), stabbing, or knifelike
     (4) Radiation/region: chest, substernal, epigastric, neck, intrascapular,

jaw, or ulnar aspect of the left arm or elbow producing tingling in the wrist, hand, and fingers

    (5) Severity: vague, severe, more intense than angina, numerical pain scale

    (6) Timing: continuous or lasting more than 30 minutes; circadian variability, peaks from 6 AM to noon; usually in the first 2 to 3 hours after arising

  b) Nausea and/or vomiting

  c) Dyspnea or orthopnea

  d) Diaphoresis

  e) Weakness and dizziness (especially in elderly patients)

  f) Palpitations

  g) Syncope

  h) Feeling of impending doom

2) Medical history

  a) Angina: variant or atherosclerotic

  b) Previous MI

  c) Hypertension: increased workload for heart

  d) Cerebrovascular accident (CVA): potential for embolus

  e) Diabetes mellitus: increases likelihood of MI, more likely to experience vague symptoms, "silent MI"

  f) Surgery (general or cardiothoracic)

  g) Thromboembolic event: may embolize to the heart

  h) Trauma: to the thoracic area

  i) Medications

  j) Allergies

  k) Dyslipidemia

  l) Tobacco use

  m) Obesity

  n) Physical inactivity

  o) Drug use

b. *Objective data*

1) Physical examination

  a) General appearance

    (1) Anxious and in distress

    (2) Anguished facial expression

    (3) Restless: attempting to get comfortable

    (4) Clenched fist against sternum (Levine sign)

  b) Heart rate

    (1) May be normal

    (2) Tachycardia (most common) or bradycardia

    (3) Regular or irregular: premature ventricular contractions (PVCs) common

  c) Arterial BP

    (1) Majority of patients with uncomplicated MI are normotensive

    (2) May be elevated because of sympathetic stimulation (pain/anxiety)

    (3) Decreased as a result of impaired cardiac function or secondary to administration of nitrates and morphine

  d) Respiratory rate

    (1) Elevates initially

    (2) Should return to normal with pain relief

    (3) In patients with concomitant heart failure, respiratory rate correlates with severity of heart failure

Table 3–1 ECG SIGNS OF MI

ECG	Onset/Appearance	Area of Injury	Indicates
T waves, peaked	Very early sign; tall, peaked T wave	Subendocardial	Ischemia; will disappear if ischemia alleviated
T waves, inverted	T wave inversion: appears deep and symmetrical	Myocardium	Ischemia; will disappear if ischemia alleviated
ST-segment elevation	Indicator of acuteness; ST segment elevates from isoelectric line	Epicardium	Injury returns to isoelectrical line within hours or days
Pathological Q wave	Within first day of infarct, 0.04 second or more in duration or greater than 25% of the R wave in depth, or both	Myocardium	Infarct; may remain permanently

    e) Peripheral (skin) perfusion: alterations will be dependent on the degree of heart failure
      (1) Pallor
      (2) Cyanosis
      (3) Diaphoresis
      (4) Mottled
      (5) Cool
      (6) Peripheral pulses: variable
    f) Temperature
      (1) Often begins to rise 4 to 8 hours after onset of MI
    g) Heart sounds
      (1) Muffled
      (2) Fourth heart sound almost universally present
      (3) Third heart sound indicative of LV dysfunction
      (4) Murmurs: may be transient or permanent
  2) Diagnostic procedures
    a) Continuous cardiac monitoring for dysrhythmias
    b) Twelve-lead, 15-lead ECG
      (1) ECG changes may not be apparent initially; may be completely normal, which does not rule out MI, especially in early hours of occlusion
      (2) ECG signs of MI (Table 3–1)
      (3) Location of infarct (Table 3–2): determined by presence of ECG

Table 3–2 LOCATION OF INFARCT

Location	Lead Changes
Anterior	Leads V_1, V_2, V_3, or V_4 Septal: V_1 and V_2
Lateral	Leads I, aVL, V_5, V_6 Apical infarct: V_5, V_6
Posterior	"Reciprocal" V_1 and V_2 No Q wave, but tall R wave ST depression Upright T wave
Inferior	Leads II, III, aVF
Right ventricular	Leads V_{4R}–V_{6R}

changes in lead sites listed in Table 3–2; infarct may involve more than one surface of LV

 (4) Repeat ECGs are helpful in detecting significant changes

c) Cardiac serum markers: of importance to note, any of these should be serially evaluated for rise and fall

 (1) CK

  (a) Elevated 2 to 4 hours after acute MI peak at 24 to 36 hours, returns to baseline in about 3 days

  (b) Most sensitive and reliable enzyme used in diagnosis of MI

  (c) CK may be elevated by muscle damage caused by trauma, exercise, chronic alcoholism, intramuscular (IM) injections

  (d) Isoenzymes CK-MB most indicative of MI

 (2) Myoglobin

  (a) Elevated 1 to 4 hours after onset of MI, peaks in 6 to 7 hours, and returns to baseline within 24 hours

  (b) Lacks specificity; also found in skeletal muscle

  (c) Should be supplemented by a more cardiac-specific marker

 (3) Cardiac-specific troponins: most recent myocardial cell marker, considered more sensitive and specific for myocardial damage; most commonly measured cardiac troponins are TnT and TnI

  (a) Elevated 3 to 12 hours after onset of MI; peaks in 24 hours with TnI and in 12 to 48 hours with TnT; returns to normal in 5 to 12 days

  (b) TnT may be elevated in patients with renal failure, which is not the case with TnI; therefore, TnI may be more cardiospecific

  (c) Rapid bedside testing of TnT and TnI are available

  (d) Independent diagnostic ability of troponins versus CK-MB is currently under investigation

 (4) Lactate dehydrogenase (LDH)

  (a) Elevated 8 to 48 hours after MI, peaks in 3 to 5 days, returns to baseline in 8 to 10 days

  (b) Concentrated in liver, striated muscles, red blood cells (RBCs), and kidney

  (c) "Flipped" pattern: LDH_1 greater than LDH_2; appears after the CK-MB and indicates myocardial necrosis

  (d) Although sensitive, it is not specific, and it is likely that LDH analysis will be superseded by newer, more specific cardiac markers

2. Analysis: differential nursing diagnosis/collaborative problems

a. Pain related to imbalance between myocardial oxygen supply and demand

b. Tissue perfusion, altered related to decreased cardiac output from dysrhythmias, conduction disturbances, and heart failure

c. Decreased cardiac output related to conduction disturbances secondary to imbalance between myocardial oxygen supply and demand

d. Anxiety/fear related to diagnosis, treatment, and prognosis of acute MI

3. Planning/interventions (See A. Angina, Planning/interventions *h* to *n.*)

a. Maintain airway, breathing, circulation

b. Provide oxygen via nasal cannula or nonrebreather mask

c. Administer IV or sublingual nitrates as ordered if systolic BP greater than 90 mm Hg

d. Obtain and maintain IV access with normal saline solution at keep vein open (KVO) rate

  e. Provide analgesia with morphine or meperidine (Demerol); assess for
   1) Respiratory depression; administer naloxone if necessary
   2) Hypotension
  f. Administer aspirin as ordered
  g. Obtain 12- to 15-lead ECG
  h. Obtain blood samples for laboratory tests
  i. Assist patient in position of comfort
  j. Prepare for thrombolytic therapy if appropriate
   1) Consider guidelines for candidacy
   2) Obtain additional IV access sites; avoid arterial sampling
   3) Prepare thrombolytic agents as specified by package inserts
   4) Follow specific guidelines for administration
   5) Administer nitrates, heparin, antiarrhythmics, beta blockers, angiotensin converting enzyme (ACE) inhibitors as ordered (See A. Angina, Planning / interventions, *h* to *n*.)
   6) Observe patient for
    a) Reperfusion dysrhythmias
    b) Change in neurological status
    c) Bleeding
  k. Continually monitor and assess
   1) Cardiac rhythm for
    a) Ventricular ectopy
    b) AV blocks
   2) Vital signs, including oxygen saturation
   3) Heart and lung sounds
   4) Level of consciousness
   5) Peripheral (skin) perfusion
   6) Intake and output
   7) Level of chest pain or discomfort
  l. Obtain portable chest x-ray film (within 30 minutes)
  m. Be prepared to initiate basic and advanced life support measures
  n. Prepare to transfer for definitive care (e.g., cardiac catheterization lab)
  n. Maintain calm efficient manner; minimize environmental stimuli
  o. Explain all procedures to patient and significant others
  p. Allow significant other at patient's bedside if possible
 4. Expected outcomes/evaluation (see Appendix B)

C. Right ventricular infarction

  Right ventricular infarctions (RVIs) generally occur as a result of occlusion of the proximal right coronary artery. Occasionally, they may result from occlusions in the left circumflex or left anterior descending artery. Isolated RVI is rare; it is generally associated with inferior wall (IW) MI, and occurs in one third to one half of this patient population. RVI with IWMI has a higher mortality than IWMI alone. Injury to the right ventricle produces ventricular dilation and decreased contractility. This inability to pump venous return into the pulmonary vasculature for oxygenation results in a decrease in blood return to the left ventricle, causing decreased cardiac output, which may be profound, producing cardiogenic shock. The symptoms may be mild to severe and life threatening. The clinical triad of hypotension, clear lung sounds, and increased jugular venous pressure is highly sensitive for RVI; however, this occurs only in one quarter of patients presenting with RVI. The clinician must have a high index of suspicion for this condition, based on physical and diagnostic findings. As with all MIs, management revolves around early reperfusion; however, with RVI the clinician must be vigilant to maintain right ventricular preload, usually by the administration of IV fluids, provide inotropic support, and reduce afterload, especially if there is significant concurrent LV injury and failure. The administration of nitrates, diuretics, and morphine sulfate should be avoided because of their preload reducing effects.

1. **Assessment**
    a. *Subjective data*
        1) History of present illness
            a) Pain or "discomfort"
                (1) Provocative factors
                    (a) Emotional or physical stressors
                    (b) May occur at rest
                (2) Palliative factors: unrelieved by change of position, nitrate use
                (3) Quality: pain may be "different" from usual angina; quality may be described as squeezing, crushing, heaviness, pressure, or "something sitting on my chest"; may also be described as burning or indigestion (especially in the elderly), stabbing, or knifelike
                (4) Radiation/region: chest, substernal, epigastric, neck, intrascapular, jaw, or ulnar aspect of left arm or elbow producing tingling in wrist, hand, fingers
                (5) Severity: vague, severe, more intense than angina, use of numerical pain scale
                (6) Timing: continuous or lasting more than 30 minutes; circadian variability, peaks from 6 AM to noon; usually in the first 2 to 3 hours after arising
            b) Nausea and/or vomiting
            c) Dyspnea or orthopnea
            d) Diaphoresis
            e) Weakness and dizziness (especially in elderly patients)
            f) Palpitations
            g) Syncope
            h) Feeling of impending doom
        2) Medical history
            a) Angina: variant or atherosclerotic
            b) Previous MI
            c) Hypertension: increased workload for heart
            d) CVA: potential of embolus
            e) Diabetes mellitus: increases likelihood of MI, more likely to experience vague symptoms
            f) Surgery (general or cardiothoracic)
            g) Thromboembolic event: may embolize to heart
            h) Trauma: to thoracic area
            i) Medications
            j) Allergies
            k) Dyslipidemia
            l) Tobacco use
            m) Obesity
            n) Physical inactivity
    b. *Objective data*
        1) Physical examination
            a) General appearance
                (1) Anxious and in distress

(2) Anguished facial expression

(3) Restless: attempting to get comfortable

(4) Clenched fist against sternum (Levine sign)

b) Heart rate

(1) May be normal

(2) Tachycardia (most common, 100–110 bpm) or bradycardia

(3) Regular or irregular: PVCs common

c) Arterial BP

(1) Majority of patients with uncomplicated MI are normotensive

(2) May be elevated because of sympathetic stimulation (pain/anxiety)

(3) Decreased as a result of impaired cardiac function or secondary to the administration of nitrates and morphine

d) Respiratory rate

(1) Elevates initially

(2) Should return to normal with pain relief

(3) In patients with concomitant heart failure, respiratory rate correlates with severity of heart failure

e) Peripheral (skin) perfusion: alterations will be dependent on degree of heart failure

(1) Pallor

(2) Cyanosis (with profound shock)

(3) Diaphoresis

(4) Mottled

(5) Cool

(6) Peripheral edema

f) Temperature

(1) Nonspecific response to tissue necrosis

(2) Often begins to rise 4 to 8 hours after onset of MI

g) Heart sounds

(1) Tricuspid regurgitation

(2) Right ventricular gallop

2) Diagnostic procedures

a) Continuous cardiac monitoring for dysrhythmias

b) Twelve-lead ECG, 15-lead ECG

(1) ST elevation in leads II, III, and aVF, indicative of IW involvement, is highly suspicious for RVI

(2) Right-sided ECG: ST elevation in V_{4R} considered highly sensitive and specific for RVI

(3) Right bundle branch block and third-degree heart block are common conduction defects; atrial fibrillation may occur with concurrent atrial infarction or dilation

(4) Repeat ECGs are helpful in detecting significant changes

c) Cardiac serum markers: of importance to note, any of these should be serially evaluated for rise and fall

(1) CK

(a) Elevated 2 to 4 hours after acute MI, peaks at 24 to 36 hours, returns to baseline in about 3 days

(b) CK may be elevated by muscle damage caused by trauma, exercise, chronic alcoholism, IM injections

(c) Isoenzymes CK-MB most indicative of MI

(2) Myoglobin

(a) Elevated 1 to 4 hours after onset of MI, peaks in 6 to 7 hours, returns to baseline within 24 hours

(b) Lacks specificity; also found in skeletal muscle

(c) Should be supplemented by a more cardiac-specific marker

(3) Cardiac-specific troponins: most recent myocardial cell marker, considered more sensitive and specific for myocardial damage; most commonly measured cardiac troponins are TnT and TnI

(a) Elevated 3 to 12 hours after onset of MI, peaks in 24 hours with TnI and in 12 to 48 hours with TnT, returns to normal in 5 to 12 days

(b) TnT may be elevated in patients with renal failure, which is not the case with TnI; therefore, TnI may be more cardiac specific

(c) Rapid bedside testing of TnT and TnI are available

(d) Independent diagnostic ability of troponins versus CK-MB is currently under investigation

(4) LDH

(a) Elevated 8 to 48 hours after MI, peaks in 3 to 5 days, returns to baseline in 8 to 10 days

(b) Concentrated in liver, striated muscles, RBCs, and kidney

(c) "Flipped" pattern: LDH_1 greater than LDH_2; appears after the CK-MB and indicates myocardial necrosis

(d) Although sensitive, it is not specific, and it is likely that LDH analysis will be superseded by newer, more specific cardiac markers

d) Echocardiography: may detect right ventricular dilatation, right ventricular wall asynergy

e) Nuclear imaging: the standard for estimating the right ventricular ejection fraction and may display wall abnormalities

2. **Analysis: differential nursing diagnosis/collaborative problems**

a. *Pain related to imbalance between myocardial oxygen supply and demand*

b. *Tissue perfusion, altered related to decreased cardiac output from dysrhythmias, conduction disturbances, heart failure*

c. *Cardiac output decreased related to conduction disturbances secondary to imbalance between myocardial oxygen supply and demand and/or hypotension secondary to decreased cardiac output, decreased preload*

d. *Anxiety/fear related to diagnosis, treatment, and prognosis of acute MI*

3. **Planning/interventions**

a. *Maintain airway, breathing, circulation*

b. *Provide oxygen via nasal cannula*

c. *Obtain and maintain IV access with normal saline, administer fluid bolus as necessary for hypotension*

d. *Provide analgesia with morphine or meperidine (Demerol); assess for*

1) *Respiratory depression; administer naloxone if necessary*

2) *Hypotension*

e. *Administer aspirin as ordered*

f. *Obtain 12- to 15-lead ECG*

g. *Obtain blood samples for laboratory tests*

h. *Assist patient in position of comfort*

i. *Prepare for thrombolytic therapy if appropriate*

1) *Consider guidelines for candidacy*

2) *Obtain additional IV access sites; avoid arterial sampling*

3) *Prepare thrombolytic agents as specified by package inserts*

4) *Follow specific guidelines for administration*

5) *Administer nitrates, heparin, antiarrhythmics, beta blockers, ACE inhibitors as ordered*

      6) Observe patient for
        a) Bleeding
        b) Change in neurological status
        c) Reperfusion dysrhythmias
      7) Thrombolytic therapy is currently under scrutiny in elderly patients (> 75 years) because of increased risk of intracerebral hemorrhage
    j. Continually monitor and assess
      1) Cardiac rhythm for
        a) Bundle branch or AV blocks
        b) Atrial fibrillation
      2) Vital signs, including oxygen saturation
      3) Heart and lung sounds
      4) Level of consciousness
      5) Peripheral (skin) perfusion
      6) Intake and output
      7) Level of chest pain or discomfort
    k. Obtain portable chest x-ray film (within 30 minutes)
    l. Be prepared to initiate basic and advanced life support measures
    m. Maintain calm efficient manner; minimize environmental stimuli
    n. Explain all procedures to patient
    o. Allow significant other at patient's bedside if possible
  4. Expected outcomes/evaluation (see Appendix B)

D. Heart failure and cardiogenic pulmonary edema

    Heart failure is a clinical syndrome that can be a complication of any type of heart disease. In the pediatric population, heart failure is usually the result of congenital heart defects. It is the result of many complex interactions with the various systems of the body, including the renal, pulmonary, and neurohormonal systems. In its essence, heart failure is the heart's inability to pump enough blood to meet the body's metabolic needs. The wide spectrum of clinical symptoms with heart failure ranges from acute and dramatic to chronic and insidious. There are many forms of heart failure: right sided versus left sided, systolic versus diastolic, and low output versus high output. Ultimately, heart failure results in intravascular and interstitial volume overload and decreased tissue perfusion.

    Pulmonary edema is the result of left-sided heart failure. This LV failure may occur as a result of mechanical overload or MI. Subsequently, an abnormal accumulation of fluid in the pulmonary interstitial tissue and the alveoli develops. Commonly, long-standing LV failure will compromise the right ventricle and lead to right-sided failure, which will produce signs of venous congestion.

1. Assessment
    a. Subjective data
      1) History of present illness
        a) Dyspnea on exertion
        b) Fatigue and weakness
        c) Paroxysmal noctural dyspnea
        d) Orthopnea
        e) Weight gain
        f) Extremity swelling
        g) Palpitations
        h) Reduced exercise capacity
        i) Nocturia

   j) Gastrointestinal (GI) symptoms: nausea, anorexia, bloating, and consti-
    pation
  2) Medical history
   a) Chronic heart failure: heart already compromised
   b) MI: decreased ability of LV to function
   c) Hypertension: increase in afterload
   d) Endocrine disorders: may increase cardiac workload (e.g., diabetes,
    thyroid disease)
   e) Cardiomyopathy: increased myocardial stiffness and/or inability of heart
    to relax, may also have conduction deficits
   f) Collagen vascular diseases: may restrict myocardial movement
   g) Toxins, iatrogenic drugs: may have cardiac depressive effects
   h) Medications
   i) Allergies
 b. *Objective data*
  1) Physical examination
   a) General appearance
    (1) Uncomfortable, anxious
    (2) Air hunger
    (3) Malnourished, cachectic: with chronic failure
    (4) Dusky skin color
   b) Physical findings
    (1) Tachycardia
    (2) Decreased pulse pressure
    (3) Diaphoresis/ cool
    (4) Pulmonary crackles or wheezes
    (5) Tachypnea
    (6) Jugular venous distension
    (7) Hepatomegaly
    (8) Hepatojugular reflux
    (9) Increased venous pressure
    (10) Pulsus alternans
    (11) S_3 gallop
    (12) Edema: extremity, anasarca, ascites
    (13) Pleural effusion (hydrothorax)
  2) Diagnostic procedures
   a) Continuous cardiac monitoring for dysrhythmias
   b) Twelve- to 15-lead ECG
    (1) May reveal acute MI or ischemia as a cause
    (2) Evidence of ventricular hypertrophy, atrial enlargement, or conduc-
    tion abnormalities
   c) Laboratory findings
    (1) Proteinuria and high urine specific gravity
    (2) Elevated BUN and creatinine
    (3) Hyponatremia: in severe heart failure
    (4) Hypokalemia: if patient is taking thiazides or loop diuretics
    (5) Abnormal liver function tests
    (6) Anemia: decreased erythrocytes cause increased workload, may be
    precipitating event
   d) Chest radiograph
    (1) Cardiomegaly
    (2) Pulmonary edema
    (3) Pleural effusion

2. **Analysis: differential nursing diagnosis/collaborative problem**
   a. *Impaired gas exchange related to fluid volume overload*
   b. *Ineffective breathing pattern related to fluid volume overload and impaired gas exchange*
   c. *Decreased cardiac output related to ineffective myocardial pump activity*
   d. *Altered tissue perfusion: renal, cerebral, cardiopulmonary, GI, peripheral related to ineffective myocardial pump activity*
   e. *Fluid volume excess related to decreased myocardial pump effectiveness*
   f. *Risk for injury: dysrhythmias related to myocardial stretching, fluid volume overload, or decreased cardiac output*
   g. *Anxiety/fear related to unknown outcomes, difficulty breathing*

3. **Planning/interventions**
   a. *Maintain airway, breathing, circulation*
   b. *Maintain patent airway/effective ventilation*
      1) Provide supplemental oxygen
      2) Anticipate endotracheal intubation
      3) Suction as needed
      4) Provide humidified oxygen
      5) Elevate head of bed semi- to high-Fowler's position
   c. *If the patient is intubated, anticipate need for mechanical ventilation and positive end-expiratory ventilation (PEEP)*
   d. *Obtain IV access with normal saline solution at KVO rate or saline lock*
   e. *Obtain ABG specimens*
   f. *Obtain chest radiograph*
   g. *Administer pharmacological agents as ordered*
      1) Diuretics: furosemide
         (a) Decrease preload secondary to reduction in blood volume, although onset of action may take as long as 30 minutes
         (b) Anticipate need for Foley catheterization
         (c) Maintain accurate intake and output record
         (d) Diuretics are very effective, but geriatric patients are prone to diuretic-induced hypokalemia and hyponatremia
      2) Morphine
         (a) Reduces anxiety and subsequent sympathetic stimulation of the heart, decreasing myocardial workload
         (b) Decreases preload and afterload by causing venous and arterial vasodilatation
         (c) Must use caution when giving a sedative to patients with acute dyspnea
         (d) Should avoid in patients with decreased level of consciousness, inadequate ventilation, or hypercarbia
      3) Vasodilators
         (a) Venodilators: increase venous pooling (e.g., nitroglycerin, isosorbide dinitrate); nitroglycerin is preferred for treatment of pulmonary edema in patients with coronary artery disease (CAD) because it improves coronary artery blood flow; in acute settings, sublingual or IV nitroglycerin is recommended over paste or oral (PO) form secondary to its inconsistent absorption in the latter routes
         (b) Arteriolar dilators (e.g., hydralazine, minoxidil): act on arteries to decrease systemic arterial resistance; these are usually administered concurrently with venodilators; hydralazine will increase renal blood flow; therefore, may be a good choice for patient who cannot tolerate and ACE inhibitor

(c) Combined dilators (e.g., nitroprusside): affect both veins and arteries; reduce both preload and afterload; onset is rapid; nitroprusside can cause cardiac ischemia in setting of CAD, secondary to coronary steal phenomenon

(d) ACE inhibitors (e.g., captopril, enalapril): block formation of angiotensin II and therefore produce vasodilation; inhibits production of aldosterone, which decreases preload and afterload. ACE inhibitors have been shown to reduce mortality and directly improve cardiac function. Avoid overdiuresis before use to prevent hypotension or renal insufficiency. Hypotension can be treated easily with fluid. ACE inhibitors are cleared by the kidneys; therefore, dose requirements may be necessary in patients with renal failure

4) Positive inotropic agents, which include digitalis glycosides, sympathomimetics (dopamine, dobutamine), and phosphodiesterase inhibitors (amrinone, milrinone)

(a) Increased contractility and cardiac output

(b) Decreased myocardial workload

(c) Improve oxygen delivery to tissues

(d) Dobutamine is drug of choice for pulmonary edema in normotensive patient

(e) Dopamine is useful for pulmonary edema in patient with hypotension; at higher infusion rates, produces peripheral vasoconstriction

(f) Digoxin not recommended for the acute management of heart failure; dose must be determined by body size and renal function in geriatric patient

(g) Phosphodiesterase inhibitors are considered inodilators because of their positive inotropic and vasodilator effects; it is currently reserved for refractory acute heart failure

5) Administer bronchodilator if ordered

(a) Assess for side effects, such as nausea, vomiting, and tachyarrhythmias

(b) Assess for pulmonary wheezing

h. *Continually monitor and assess*

1) Cardiac rhythm

2) Vital signs, including pulse oximetry

3) Heart rate, lung sounds, BP, respiratory rate

4) Level of consciousness

5) Peripheral (skin) perfusion

6) Intake and output

7) Side effects of pharmacotherapeutics

i. *Be prepared to institute advanced cardiac life support (ACLS) measures if required*

j. *Explain all procedures*

k. *Maintain calm, efficient manner*

l. *Minimize environmental stimuli*

4. **Expected outcomes/evaluation** (see Appendix B)

E. Cardiogenic shock (see Chapter 19)

F. Cardiac dysrhythmias

A cardiac dysrhythmia is a deviation from the normal sinus rhythm and rate. The pathogenesis of cardiac dysrhythmias can be divided into three categories of

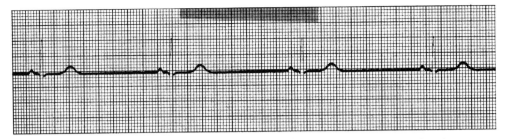

FIGURE 3-1. Sinus bradycardia. From Kitt, S. (1990). Emergency Nursing: A physiologic & clinical perspective. Philadelphia: W. B. Saunders. Used with permission.

disorders: impulse formation, impulse conduction, or a combination of both. The disorder of impulse formation may be due to the abnormal automaticity or, by a triggering activity, may be due to afterdepolarizations (a depolarization that occurs after the action potential of a cardiac cell). Disorders of impulse conduction may be a result of a conduction delay or block, which can lead to bradycardias or tachycardias. These tachycardias are likely due to reentry. Reentry occurs when an impulse reactivates myocardial tissue for a second or multiple times. Reentry occurs as a result of unidirectional block (only allows the impulse to conduct in one direction) and slow conduction (which allows the stimulated tissue to recover).

Contributors to cardiac dysrhythmias are varied and may be the focus of treatment. Examples include metabolic derangements (e.g., hypoxia, acidosis, alkalosis, hypo- and hyperkalemia or hypocalcemia), chronic illness (e.g., CAD, chronic obstructive pulmonary disease [COPD]), cardiac trauma, various medications (e.g., digoxin, bronchodilators), and illicit drugs (e.g., cocaine, amphetamines).

Emergent treatment of cardiac dysrhythmias is dependent on the patient's hemodynamic status. The major consequence of dysrhythmias is inadequate cardiac output; the greater the decrease in the cardiac output, the greater is the urgency of treatment.

1. **Sinus dysrhythmias**
    a. *Sinus bradycardia*
        Sinus bradycardia is characterized by a decrease in the rate of discharge in the sinus node, less than 60 bpm (Fig. 3–1). It may be normal in athletes and while sleeping or may be a response to vagal stimulation. Other causes include inferior wall MI, eye surgery, intracranial tumors, increased intracranial pressure (ICP), myxedema, hypoxia, hypothermia, obstructive jaundice, anorexia nervosa, and medications (digoxin, propranolol, verapamil). In most cases, sinus bradycardia is a benign dysrhythmia and requires treatment only if the patient is symptomatic.
        1) Assessment
            a) Subjective
                (1) History of presenting illness
                    (a) Asymptomatic
                    (b) "Lightheaded" or dizziness
                    (c) Syncope
                    (d) Chest pain/ SOB
                (2) Medical history: as above
            b) Objective
                (1) Physical assessment
                    (a) Heart rate less than 60 bpm
                    (b) Hypotension
                    (c) Decreased level of consciousness

        (d) Cool, clammy skin
     (2) Diagnostic procedures
        (a) Twelve- to 15-lead ECG: rate less than 60 bpm, regular rhythm, P waves consistent and normal, precede every QRS, PR interval, and QRS within normal limits
        (b) Pulse oximetry: decreased arterial oxygen saturation (SaO_2) may reveal hypoxia
        (c) Serum digoxin level
  2) Analysis: differential nursing diagnosis/collaborative problems
    a) Cardiac output decreased related to dysrhythmia
    b) Altered tissue perfusion secondary to decreased cardiac output
    c) Anxiety/fear related to altered health status
  3) Planning/interventions
    a) Monitor airway, breathing, circulation
    b) Establish IV access, saline lock
    c) Continuously monitor
      (1) Level of consciousness
      (2) Heart rate
      (3) BP
      (4) Respiratory rate, rhythm, and depth
      (5) Heart and lung sounds
      (6) Skin/mucous membrane color
      (7) Urine output
    d) Administer atropine as ordered
    e) Treat underlying cause: consider transcutaneous pacemaker, dopamine, epinephrine, isoproterenol
    f) Maintain calm, efficient manner
    g) Minimize environmental stimuli
    h) Explain all procedures
    i) Assess patient/significant other's knowledge of factors that caused dysrhythmia, potential sequelae, reasons for monitoring
    j) Allow family/significant other at bedside
  4) Expected outcomes (see Appendix B)
 b. Sinus tachycardia

     Sinus tachycardia is characterized by an increase in the rate of discharge in the sinus node, which is greater than 100 bpm (Fig. 3–2). It is a normal response to multiple factors, including exercise, anxiety, fever, hypovolemia, anemia, and myocardial ischemia. It is a physiological response to a demand for an increase in cardiac output. Many drugs can also cause sinus tachycardia,

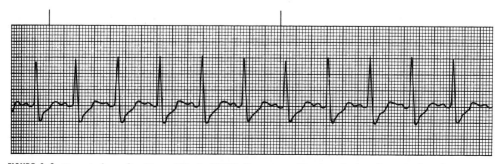

FIGURE 3–2. Sinus tachycardia. From Kitt, S. (1990). Emergency Nursing: A physiologic & clinical perspective. Philadelphia: W. B. Saunders. Used with permission.

including atropine, epinephrine, dopamine, cocaine, and caffeine. The rule of thumb with sinus tachycardia is to treat the underlying cause, not the rhythm.

1) Assessment
    a) Subjective
        (1) History of presenting illness
            (a) Asymptomatic
            (b) Strenuous exercise
            (c) Fever/chills
            (d) Decreased fluid intake
            (e) Chest pain
            (f) Trauma
            (g) Anxiety
        (2) Medical history
            (a) Anemia
            (b) Illicit drug use
            (c) Tobacco use
            (d) Caffeine intake
            (e) Alcohol use/abuse
    b) Objective
        (1) Physical assessment
            (a) Heart rate greater than 100 bpm
            (b) Hypotension
            (c) Temperature greater than 38°F, skin hot
            (d) Diaphoresis
        (2) Diagnostic procedures
            (a) Twelve- to 15-lead ECG: rate greater than 100 bpm (usually 101–150 and rarely exceeds 180); regular rhythm; P waves consistent, normal, and precede every QRS; PR interval usually normal, may be difficult to measure if obscured in preceding T wave; QRS usually normal
            (b) CBC: may reveal anemia
            (c) Toxicology screen: may reveal illicit drug use, particularly stimulants cocaine and amphetamines

2) Analysis: differential nursing diagnosis/collaborative problems
    a) Decreased cardiac output secondary to decreased diastolic filling time
    b) Coronary tissue perfusion, altered related to decreased diastolic time (coronary arteries perfuse during diastole)
    c) Anxiety/fear related to altered health status

3) Planning/interventions
    (a) Monitor airway, breathing, circulation
    (b) Establish IV access, saline lock
    (c) Continuously monitor
        (1) Level of consciousness
        (2) Heart rate, cardiac monitor
        (3) BP
        (4) Respiratory rate, rhythm, and depth
        (5) Heart and lung sounds
        (6) Skin/mucous membrane color
        (7) Urine output
    (d) Treat underlying causes as appropriate; may include
        (1) Administer antipyretics ordered, if febrile
        (2) Administer IV fluids for hypovolemia

(3) Prepare to administer blood, if ordered, for anemia or hypovolemia secondary to blood loss
  (e) Maintain calm, efficient manner
  (f) Minimize environmental stimuli
  (g) Explain all procedures
  (h) Assess patient/significant other's knowledge of factors that caused dysrhythmia, potential sequelae, reasons for monitoring
  (i) Allow family/significant other at bedside
  4) Expected outcomes (see Appendix B)

2. Atrial dysrhythmias

a. Premature atrial contractions (PAC)

A PAC occurs when an ectopic focus in the atria conducts a beat before the next beat was due (Fig. 3–3). The development of PACs is often related to the use of stimulants (e.g., coffee, tea, alcohol, and nicotine) or may be a warning of the development of more serious dysrhythmias. PACs are often seen with atrial enlargement, heart failure, myocardial ischemia or infarction, COPD, fever, infections, and anxiety and with some medications, such as digitalis. PACs indicate atrial irritability and may precipitate the occurrence of a sustained supraventricular tachycardia (SVT) (atrial flutter/fibrillation). Rarely do they produce ventricular dysrhythmias.

1) Assessment
  a) Subjective data
    (1) History of present illness:
      (a) Asymptomatic
      (b) Irregular heart rate
    (2) Medical history: as above
  b) Objective data
    (1) Physical examination:
      (a) Heart rate 60 to 100 bpm
      (b) Heart rhythm irregular
      (c) Pulse deficit
      (d) Fever
    (2) Diagnostic procedures
      (a) Twelve- to 15-lead ECG: irregular rhythm; P waves have different configuration than those originating in the SA node; they may be inverted or concealed in previous T wave; PR interval may be normal or prolonged; QRS complex may be normal, aberrant, or absent; noncompensatory pause is usually present
      (b) Serum digitalis level: may be subtherapeutic
      (c) Serum potassium: hypokalemia; increases susceptibility to digitalis toxicity

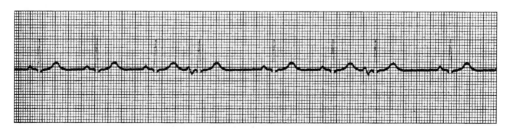

FIGURE 3–3. Premature atrial contractions. From Kitt, S. (1990). Emergency Nursing: A physiologic & clinical perspective. Philadelphia: W. B. Saunders. Used with permission.

2) Analysis: differential nursing diagnosis/collaborative problems
   a) Decreased cardiac output related to dysrhythmia
   b) Anxiety/fear related to need for altered health status
3) Planning/interventions
   a) Monitor airway, breathing, circulation
   b) Establish IV access, saline lock
   c) Continuously monitor
      (1) Level of consciousness
      (2) Heart rate and rhythm
      (3) BP
      (4) Respiratory rate, rhythm, depth
      (5) Heart and lung sounds
      (6) Color of mucous membranes
      (7) Urine output
   d) Administer potassium as ordered if serum potassium is less than 3.5
   e) Administer antipyretics as ordered
   f) Maintain calm, efficient manner
   g) Minimize environmental stimuli
   h) Explain all procedures
   i) Allow family or significant other at bedside if possible
   j) Assess patient's/significant other's knowledge of factors that cause dysrhythmia, potential sequelae, reasons for monitoring
   k) Teach patient/significant other
      (1) How to take pulse and report irregularities
      (2) Name of medicine, dosage, time of doses, purpose, side effects, special considerations
4) Expected outcomes/evaluation (see Appendix B)

b. Atrial tachycardia/paroxysmal atrial tachycardia

Atrial tachycardia occurs when an irritable focus within the atria takes over as the pacemaker. It is a rapid atrial rhythm with a rate of 150 to 250 bpm. When the rhythm starts and ends abruptly, it is termed paroxysmal atrial tachycardia. Causes include emotional stress, fatigue, alcohol, smoking, caffeine, myocardial ischemia, MI, cor pulmonale, and digoxin intoxication. Symptoms are dependent on the rate and underlying cardiovascular disease. Treatment is directed toward determining and eliminating the underlying cause and decreasing the ventricular rate.

1) Assessment
   a) Subjective
      (1) History of presenting illness
         (a) Chest pain
         (b) Dyspnea
         (c) Palpitations
         (d) Anxiety
      (2) Medical history
         (a) Coronary heart disease
         (b) Myocardial infarction
         (c) Digitalis use
         (d) Smoker
         (e) Caffeine use
         (f) Alcohol use
   b) Objective
      (1) Physical assessment
         (a) Heart rate greater than 150 bpm

    (b) Hypotension

    (c) Decreased level of consciousness

    (d) Cool, clammy skin

    (e) Increased intensity of first heart sound

   (2) Diagnostic procedures

    (a) Twelve- to 15-lead, 15-lead ECG: atrial rate, 150 to 250; ventricular rate may be the same or may be less if there is a block in the AV node; rhythm is usually regular, unless there is a variable AV block; P waves are usually different from normal sinus P waves; will precede each QRS except when a block is present, and may be obscured by preceding T waves; QRSs are usually normal

    (b) Serum digitalis level

 2) Analysis: differential nursing diagnosis/collaborative problem

  a) Cardiac output decreased secondary to decreased ventricular filling time

  b) Anxiety/fear related to altered health status

 3) Planning/intervention

  a) Monitor airway, breathing, circulation

  b) Establish IV access, saline lock

  c) Continuously monitor

   (1) Level of consciousness

   (2) Heart rate and rhythm

   (3) BP

   (4) Respiratory rate, rhythm, depth

   (5) Heart and lung sounds

   (6) Color of mucous membranes

   (7) Urine output

  d) Initiate/assist with procedures to decrease heart rate

   (1) Valsalva maneuver

   (2) Head-down tilt with deep inspiration

   (3) Carotid massage

  e) Administer sedatives as ordered to decrease anxiety

  f) Administer medication to slow ventricular response; may include adenosine, digoxin (if patient not already on it), beta blocker, or calcium channel blocker

  g) Prepare for synchronized cardioversion if hemodynamically unstable

   (a) Premedicate if patient is conscious;

   (b) 100 J for initial attempt; may increase gradually to 360 J if necessary

   (c) Pediatric patients: synchronized cardioversion at 0.5 to 1.0 J/kg

  h) Maintain calm, efficient manner

  i) Minimize environmental stimuli

  j) Explain all procedures

  k) Allow family or significant other at bedside if possible

  l) Assess patient's/significant other's knowledge of factors that cause dysrhythmia, potential sequelae, reasons for monitoring

  m) Teach patient/significant other

   (1) How to take pulse and report irregularities

   (2) Name of medicine, dosage, time of doses, purpose, side effects, special considerations

 4) Expected outcomes/evaluation (see Appendix B)

c. *Atrial flutter*

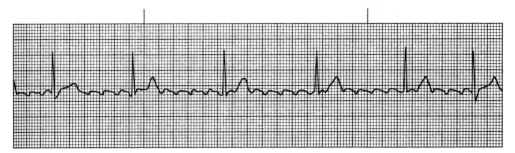

FIGURE 3–4. Atrial flutter. From Kitt, S. (1990). Emergency Nursing: A physiologic & clinical perspective. Philadelphia: W. B. Saunders. Used with permission.

Atrial flutter is demonstrated by the atria depolarizing at a rate of 250 to 350 bpm (Fig. 3–4). It may be due to an extremely irritable focus in the atria, but is more likely the result of impulse reentry in the atria. Ordinarily, in typical atrial flutter, many of the impulses fail to conduct to the ventricles, and the ventricular rate is slower than the atrial rate, usually 2:1. Thus, if the atrial rate is 300, then the ventricular rate would likely be 150. The P waves on the cardiogram are "sawtooth" in appearance and are referred to as flutter waves. Atrial flutter may be associated with valvular heart disease, rheumatic or ischemic heart disease, cardiomyopathy, atrial dilation, CAD, and thyrotoxicosis. It may also occurs following pulmonary embolization and cardiac surgery.

1) Assessment
   a) Subjective data
      (1) History of present illness
         (a) Palpitations
         (b) Dyspnea
         (c) Chest pain
         (d) Sensation of "racing heart"
      (2) Medical history
         (a) Cardiac disease
         (b) Thyrotoxicosis
         (c) COPD
         (d) Recent cardiac surgery
   b) Objective data
      (1) Physical examination
         (a) Tachycardia
         (b) Signs of CHF: S_3 on cardiac auscultation, wheezes/crackles, jugular vein distention (JVD)
         (c) Hypotension
         (d) Cool, clammy skin
         (e) Decreased level of consciousness
      (2) Diagnostic procedures
         (a) ECG: atrial rate has range of 250 to 350 bpm; ventricular rate usually is one half, one third, or one fourth the atrial rate (130–170); regular atrial rhythm; ventricular rate regular, unless variable degree of AV block is present; P waves: flutter waves, "sawtooth" or "picket fence" appearance; PR interval is regular; QRS is usually normal
         (b) Serum digitalis level
2) Analysis: differential nursing diagnosis/collaborative problems

a) Cardiac output decreased related to cardiac rhythm abnormality

b) Anxiety/fear related to alteration in health status

3) Planning/interventions

a) Monitor airway, breathing, circulation

b) Administer oxygen via nasal cannula

c) Establish IV access; infuse normal saline at KVO rate

d) Initiate cardiac monitor, non-invasive blood pressure monitor, pulse oximetry

e) Continuously monitor

(1) Level of consciousness

(2) Heart rate/rhythm

(3) BP

(4) Respiratory rate, rhythm, depth

(5) Skin color

(6) Urine output

f) Obtain 12- to 15-lead ECG

g) Obtain portable chest radiograph

h) Initiate/monitor response to vagal maneuvers; may aid in diagnosis by decreasing ventricular response and allowing better visualization of flutter waves; vagal maneuvers will only temporarily slow the ventricular rate

i) Administer medications as ordered to decrease atrial and ventricular rates

(1) Diltiazem, current drug of choice

(2) Beta blockers

(3) Verapamil

(4) Digoxin

(5) Procainamide

(6) Quinidine

j) If patient is hemodynamically unstable, assist with synchronized cardioversion, initially at 100 J up to 360 J; premedicate patient if time permits

k) Maintain calm, efficient manner

l) Explain all procedures

m) Minimize environmental stimuli

n) Encourage verbalization of concerns/questions

o) Allow significant other at bedside if possible

4) Expected outcomes/evaluation (see Appendix B)

d. *Atrial fibrillation*

Atrial fibrillation (AF) is characterized by a chaotic atrial rhythm and an irregular ventricular rhythm (Fig. 3–5). It may result from multiple irritable

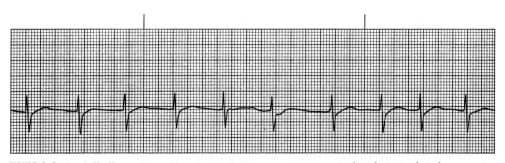

FIGURE 3–5. Atrial fibrillation. From Kitt, S. (1990). Emergency Nursing: A physiologic & clinical perspective. Philadelphia: W. B. Saunders. Used with permission.

foci or from multiple areas of reentry. The electrical activity of the atria is variable and rapid, at a rate of 400 to 700 bpm. This electrical activity produces small waves in the atria but no atrial contractions. Only a small percentage of the stimuli are conducted through the AV node to the ventricles; thus, the ventricular rate is generally between 100 and 180. Atrial fibrillation may be associated with heart failure, atrial enlargement, HTN thyrotoxicosis, and arteriosclerotic or rheumatic heart disease. The clinical significance of atrial fibrillation is (1) a decrease in cardiac output because of the loss of the atrial kick, which normally contributes 20 to 30% to the stroke volume; (2) the atria are unable to completely empty during atrial fibrillation, which results in pooling of blood, thus possibly causing the formation of clot and subsequent emboli release; and (3) if the ventricular response is rapid, the patient may quickly experience heart failure, syncope, or angina.

1) Assessment
  a) Subjective data
    (1) History of present illness
      (a) Palpitations
      (b) Fatigue
      (c) Syncope
      (d) Change in mental status
      (e) May be asymptomatic
    (2) Medical history
      (a) Common in older persons
      (b) Restrictive pericarditis
      (c) Heart failure: geriatric patients often have decreased ventricular compliance; therefore, any tachycardia can precipitate a heart failure event
      (d) Cor pulmonale
      (e) Rheumatic heart disease in childhood
      (f) Some geriatric patients have sinus node dysfunction; when tachydysrhythmia has been treated, sinus node may fail
      (g) Hypertension
  b) Objective data
    (1) Physical examination
      (a) Irregular heart rhythm
      (b) Pulse deficit
      (c) Signs of congestive heart failure: S_3, wheezes or crackles, JVD
      (d) Hypotension
      (e) Decreased level of consciousness
      (f) Cool, clammy skin
    (2) Diagnostic procedures
      (a) ECG: atrial rate 400 to 700 bpm or cannot be counted; undigitalized patient may have a ventricular rate of 160 to 180 bpm; ventricular rhythm is irregular except when there is digitalis intoxication; P waves: nonexistent; chaotic activity, wavy baseline, or F waves may be seen; QRS: ventricular depolarization is usually normal, occasionally QRS complexes are aberrantly conducted
      (b) Cardiac serum markers
      (c) Chest radiograph
2) Analysis: differential nursing diagnosis/collaborative problems
  a) Cardiac output decreased related to cardiac rhythm disturbance
  b) Anxiety/fear related to altered health status

3) Planning/interventions
    a) Monitor airway, breathing, circulation
    b) Administer supplemental oxygen
    c) Establish IV access; infuse normal saline at KVO rate
    d) Initiate cardiac monitor, NIBP, pulse oximetry
    e) Continuously monitor
       (1) Level of consciousness
       (2) Heart rate and rhythm
       (3) Apical-radial pulse volume
       (4) BP
       (5) Respiratory rate, rhythm, depth, pulse oximetry
       (6) Heart and lung sounds
       (7) Skin color
       (8) Urine output
    f) Obtain 12- to 15-lead ECG
    g) Obtain portable chest radiograph
    h) Initiate/monitor response to vagal maneuvers
    i) Administer medications as ordered for rate control
       (1) Diltiazem
       (2) Beta blockers
       (3) Verapamil
       (4) Digoxin
       (5) Procainamide
       (6) Quinidine
    j) Assist with chemical cardioversion
       (1) Administer anticoagulant as ordered
       (2) Procainamide
    k) If patient is hemodynamically unstable, assist with synchronized cardioversion, 50 J to 100 J for the initial attempt; may gradually increase to 360 J; cardioversion is priority for patient who is symptomatic or if atrial fibrillation is of new onset (1–3 days); anticoagulation must be considered
    l) Maintain calm, efficient manner
    m) Minimize environmental stimuli
    n) Explain all procedures
    o) Encourage verbalization of concerns or questions
    p) Allow significant other in treatment area if possible
4) Expected outcomes/evaluation (see Appendix B)

e. *Supraventricular tachycardia*

    Paroxysmal SVT is used to describe a group of tachycardias that originate above the ventricle (Fig. 3–6). SVT may originate in the atria or junction. However, the exact origination cannot be determined. SVT can include atrial tachycardia, atrial flutter, and junctional tachycardia. Causative factors include any of the causes of previously discussed tachycardias. SVT may also be seen in young persons not having organic heart disease. The main consequence of SVT, as with any tachyarrhythmia, is a shortened diastolic filling time and, therefore, a decreased cardiac output. SVT is the most common tachydysrhythmia in the pediatric population.

1) Assessment
    a) Subjective data
       (1) History of present illness
         (a) Chest pain
         (b) Dyspnea

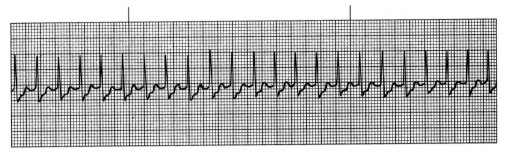

FIGURE 3–6. Supraventricular tachycardia. From Kitt, S. (1990). Emergency Nursing: A physiologic & clinical perspective (1st ed.). Philadelphia: W. B. Saunders. Used with permission.

          (c) Anxiety
       (2) Medical history
          (a) Recent cardiac surgery
          (b) Rheumatic heart disease
          (c) Digitalis use
          (d) Thyroid disease
          (e) Tobacco use
          (f) Caffeine use
          (g) Alcohol use
    b) Objective data
       (1) Physical examination
          (a) Tachycardia: 100 to 240 bpm; pediatric heart rate can be up to 300 bpm
          (b) S_3 on cardiac auscultation
          (c) Tachypnea
          (d) Hypotension
          (e) Cough
          (f) Crackles or wheezes
          (g) Cool, clammy skin
          (h) Decreased level of consciousness
       (2) Diagnostic procedures
          (a) ECG: rate is 100 to 240 bpm; regular rhythm, usually 1:1 AV conduction; P waves are not usually visible; PR interval is usually unmeasurable because of inability to visualize P waves; QRS complex may be normal or prolonged because of bundle branch block or aberrant conduction
          (b) Chest radiograph: pulmonary venous congestion if LV failure has occurred
          (c) Serum digitalis level
          (d) ABGs: possible hypoxemia related to impaired gas exchange
  2) Analysis: differential nursing diagnosis/collaborative problems
    a) Cardiac output decreased related to decreased diastolic filling time
    b) Tissue perfusion altered coronary related to decreased diastolic filling time
    c) Anxiety/fear related to altered health status
    d) Knowledge deficit related to treatment regimen
  3) Planning/interventions
    a) Monitor airway, breathing, circulation
    b) Secure airway if necessary
    c) Administer oxygen via nasal cannula or nonrebreather

    d) Establish IV access with normal saline at KVO rate

    e) Initiate cardiac monitor, NIBP, and pulse oximetry

    f) Obtain 12- to 15-lead ECG

    g) Obtain portable chest radiograph

    h) Initiate/assist with procedures to decrease heart rate

        (1) Valsalva maneuver

        (2) Head-down tilt with deep inspiration

        (3) Carotid massage

        (4) Administer medications as ordered

            (a) Adenosine

            (b) Verapamil: use in infants carries significant risk

            (c) Digitalis (if no toxicity)

        (5) Synchronized cardioversion if hemodynamically unstable

            (a) Premedicate if patient is conscious

            (b) Fifty to 100 J for initial attempt, may increase gradually to 360; check pulse and rhythm after each countershock

            (c) Pediatric patients: synchronized cardioversion at 0.5 to 1.0 J/kg

    i) Continuously monitor

        (1) Level of consciousness

        (2) Heart rate and rhythm

        (3) BP

        (4) Respiratory rate, rhythm, and depth, pulse oximetry

        (5) Heart and lung sounds

        (6) Skin color

        (7) Urine output

    j) Maintain calm, efficient manner

    k) Explain all procedures

    l) Allow significant other at bedside if possible

    m) Assess patient/significant other's knowledge of factors relating to dysrhythmia: potential sequelae, signs and symptoms of dysrhythmia, how to monitor, and follow-up care

    n) Teach patient/significant other

        (1) Factors that cause dysrhythmia, signs and symptoms, potential sequelae

        (2) How to modify risk factors

        (3) How to monitor pulse and report irregularities

        (4) Name of medicine and dose, route, purpose, timing, side effects, and special considerations for medication

        (5) Importance of follow-up care

    o) Provide written discharge instructions tailored to the patient/significant other in terms of intellectual ability, developmental level, and sensory functioning

  4) Expected outcomes/evaluation (see Appendix B)

3. Junctional dysrhythmias

    a. Premature Junctional Complex

        A premature junctional complex (PJC) occurs when an ectopic focus in the AV junction conducts an electrical impulse before the next expected sinus impulse. PJCs result in retrograde atrial depolarization; consequently, the P waves may occur before, during, or after the QRS. Because the conduction to the ventricles is usually normal, the QRS is normal appearing. PJCs can occur in response to vagal tone, irritability resulting from CAD or MI, and use of stimulants (e.g., caffeine, nicotine) and certain drugs, particularly digitalis. Treatment for PJCs is rarely necessary and usually is directed toward removing the offending stimulus.

1) Assessment
  a) Subjective
    (1) History of presenting illness
      (a) Asymptomatic
      (b) Irregular heart/pulse rate
    (2) Medical history
      (a) CAD
      (b) Previous MI
      (c) Cardiac medications
      (d) Nicotine use
  b) Objective
    (1) Physical assessment
      (a) Heart rate 60 to 100 bpm
      (b) Irregular heart rhythm
      (c) Pulse deficit
    (2) Diagnostic procedures
      (a) Twelve- to 15-lead ECG: heart rate 60 to 100 bpm; irregular rhythm; P waves inverted; may occur before, during, or after QRS; PR interval less than 0.12 when P wave precedes QRS; noncompensatory or compensatory pause may occur; QRS is usually normal but may be aberrant
      (b) Serum digitalis level
2) Planning/interventions
  a) Monitor airway, breathing, circulation
  b) Establish IV access, saline lock
  c) Initiate cardiac monitor, NIBP, pulse oximetry
  d) Continuously monitor
    (1) Level of consciousness
    (2) Heart rate and rhythm
    (3) Apical-radial pulse volume
    (4) BP
    (5) Respiratory rate, rhythm, depth
    (6) Heart and lung sounds
    (7) Skin color
    (8) Urine output
  e) Obtain 12- to 15-lead ECG
  f) If patient is on digitalis, hold next dose
  g) Maintain calm, efficient manner
  h) Minimize environmental stimuli
  i) Explain all procedures
  j) Encourage verbalization of concerns or questions
  k) Allow significant other in treatment area if possible
  l) Assess patient/significant other's knowledge of factors relating to dysrhythmia: potential sequelae, signs and symptoms of dysrhythmia, how to monitor, and follow-up care
  m) Teach patient/significant other
    (1) Factors that cause dysrhythmia, signs and symptoms, potential sequelae
    (2) How to modify risk factors
    (3) How to monitor pulse and report irregularities

(4) Name of medicine and dose, route, purpose, timing, side effects, and special considerations for medication

(5) Importance of follow-up care

n) Provide written discharge instructions tailored to patient/significant other in terms of intellectual ability, developmental level, sensory functioning

3) Analysis: differential nursing diagnosis/collaborative problem

a) Anxiety/fear related to altered health status

b) Knowledge deficit related to treatment regimen

4) Expected outcomes/evaluation (see Appendix B)

b. *Junctional rhythm and junctional tachycardia*

Junctional rhythms occur when the junction takes over as the pacemaker (Fig. 3–7). This can occur when the sinus node falls below the intrinsic rate of the junction, which is 40 to 60 bpm. Junctional tachycardia occurs when the junction is acting as the pacemaker but at a rate higher than its intrinsic rate, usually > 70 bpm. Causes include inferior MI, underlying heart disease, hypokalemia, and, most commonly, digitalis toxicity. Symptoms will vary depending on the rate, cause, and underlying cardiovascular disease. Slow rates may compromise cardiac output and may allow for breakthrough ventricular dysrhythmias. Rapid rates can also produce a decrease in cardiac output. Patients with junctional rhythms may experience symptoms related to the loss of atrial contribution. Treatment focuses on the cause and on providing cardiac support if necessary.

1) Assessment

a) Subjective

(1) History of presenting illness

(a) Asymptomatic

(b) "Lightheadedness" or dizziness

(c) Syncope

(d) Chest pain

(e) Dyspnea

(2) Medical history

(a) CAD

(b) Previous MI

(c) Cardiac medications

b) Objective

(1) Physical assessment

(a) Tachycardia or bradycardia

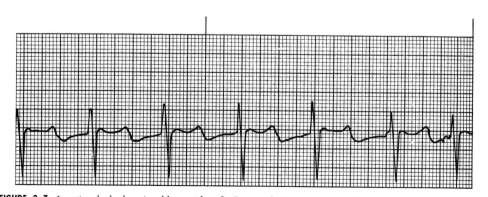

FIGURE 3–7. Junctional rhythm (unable to identify P waves). From Kitt, S. (1990). Emergency Nursing: A physiologic & clinical perspective. Philadelphia: W. B. Saunders. Used with permission.

       (b) Regular rhythm; occasionally it may be irregular, secondary to breakthrough rhythms

       (c) Hypotension

       (d) Diaphoresis

       (e) Cool, clammy skin

       (f) Decreased level of consciousness

   (2) Diagnostic procedures

       (a) Twelve- to 15-lead ECG: rate for junctional rhythm, 40 to 60, for junctional tachycardia, 70 to 130; essentially, regular rhythm may be irregular if escape complexes or ventricular breakthrough occur; P waves usually absent but may seen before or after QRS and are inverted in II, III, and aVF; PR interval is less than 0.12 second if P wave is conducted before the QRS; QRS is usually normal, unless aberrantly conducted

       (b) Serum digitalis level

       (c) Serum potassium

2) Analysis: differential nursing diagnosis/collaborative problems

   a) Decreased cardiac output related to dysrhythmia, loss of atrial kick

   b) Altered tissue perfusion related to decreased cardiac output

3) Planning/interventions

   a) Monitor airway, breathing, circulation

   b) Establish IV access, saline lock

   c) Initiate cardiac monitor, NIBP, pulse oximetry

   d) Continuously monitor

     (1) Level of consciousness

     (2) Heart rate and rhythm

     (3) Apical-radial pulse volume

     (4) BP

     (5) Respiratory rate, rhythm, depth

     (6) Heart and lung sounds

     (7) Skin color

     (8) Urine output

   e) Obtain 12- to 15-lead ECG

   f) If patient is on digitalis, hold next dose

   g) Administer medications as ordered

     (1) Atropine for symptomatic bradydysrhythmia

     (2) Potassium if serum level less than 3.5

     (3) Hold Digoxin and administer Digibind if patient is hemodynamically unstable

     (4) Verapamil, propranolol, or digitalis (if patient not already taking) to slow/terminate tachydysrhythmia

   h) Prepare/assist with synchronized cardioversion if patient is hemodynamically unstable secondary to tachydysrhythmia

     (1) Sedate if possible

     (2) Begin at 100 J and gradually increase to 360 J, as indicated; check pulse and rhythm after each countershock

     (3) Pediatric dose is 0.5 J/kg initially, then increased to 1 J/kg

   i) Maintain calm, efficient manner

   j) Minimize environmental stimuli

   k) Explain all procedures

   l) Encourage verbalization of concerns or questions

   m) Allow significant other in treatment area if possible

   n) Assess patient's/significant other's knowledge of factors relating to dysrhythmia: potential sequelae, signs and symptoms of dysrhythmia, how to monitor, and follow-up care

    o) Teach patient/significant other

        (1) Factors that cause dysrhythmia, signs and symptoms, potential sequelae

        (2) How to modify risk factors

        (3) How to monitor pulse and report irregularities

        (4) Name of medicine and dose, route, purpose, timing, side effects, and special considerations for medication

        (5) Importance of follow-up care

    p) Provide written discharge instructions tailored to the patient/significant other in terms of intellectual ability, developmental level, and sensory functioning

    4) Expected outcomes/evaluation (see Appendix B)

4. AV node conduction disturbances/heart block

Heart blocks occur as a result of a disturbance in the conduction of impulses through the heart. They can be temporary or permanent. Heart blocks can occur at any place there is impulse conduction; however, the most common site is between the atria and the ventricle (AV block; Fig. 3–8). Heart blocks are classified by severity: first degree, second degree (in which there are two types), and third degree.

a. First-degree AV block

First-degree AV block is characterized by a prolonged PR interval in an otherwise normal-appearing cardiac rhythm. A P wave precedes each normal QRS, but the PR interval is longer than 0.20 seconds. This delay usually occurs in the AV node, but can occur in the His-Purkinje system. This dysrhythmia may occur in healthy persons, but pathological conditions such as hypokalemia, myocardial ischemia, inferior MI, rheumatic heart disease, and vagal stimulation may be the cause. Cardiac medications (digitalis, quinidine, and procainamide) may also cause this dysrhythmia. This block does not produce symptoms or have any specific treatment except to treat the underlying cause. It should be carefully monitored in the presence of myocardial ischemia for worsening.

    1) Assessment

        a) Subjective data

            (1) History of present illness

                (a) Most patients are asymptomatic unless the rhythm is severely bradycardic

                (b) Syncope

            (2) Medical history

                (a) Cardiac disease

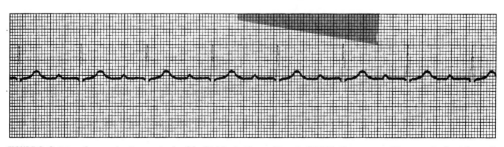

FIGURE 3–8. First-degree (atrioventricular block) block. From Kitt, S. (1990). Emergency Nursing: A physiologic & clinical perspective. Philadelphia: W. B. Saunders. Used with permission.

(b) Use of cardiac medications (as mentioned)

(c) Previous MI

b) Objective data

(1) Physical examination

(a) Bradycardia: heart rate decreases linearly with age and is lower in men; sinus bradycardia is much more common in geriatric population

(b) Chest pain

(c) Hypotension

(2) Diagnostic procedures

(a) ECG: regular rhythm; each P wave is normal, consistent, and followed by a QRS; PR interval is prolonged beyond 0.20 seconds and is usually constant but may vary; QRS morphology is unaffected, unless block occurs in His-Purkinje system

(b) Serum levels of cardiac medications

(c) Serum potassium level

(d) Cardiac enzymes

2) Analysis: differential nursing diagnosis/collaborative problems

a) Knowledge deficit related to dysrhythmia

3) Planning/interventions

a) Monitor airway, breathing, circulation

b) Establish IV access, saline lock

c) Initiate cardiac monitor, NIBP, pulse oximetry

d) Obtain 12- to 15-lead ECG

e) Administer medications as ordered, such as atropine or isoproterenol, if patient is symptomatic

f) Continuously monitor

(1) Level of consciousness

(2) Heart rate and rhythm

(3) BP

(4) Respiratory rate, rhythm, depth

(5) Skin color

(6) Urine output

g) Maintain calm, efficient manner

h) Minimize environmental stimuli

i) Explain all procedures

j) Allow significant other at bedside

k) Assess patient's/significant other's knowledge of cardiac dysrhythmia, potential sequelae, signs and symptoms of sequelae, treatment, and follow-up

l) Teach patient and significant other

(1) Factors that can be related to conduction disturbances

(2) How to take pulse and report irregularities

(3) Medication names, dosages, side effects, purposes, special considerations

m) Provide written instructions specific to the patient's/significant other's ability in terms of reading and comprehension

4) Expected outcomes/evaluation (see Appendix B)

b. *Second-degree AV block: Mobitz type I (Wenckebach)*

Mobitz type I heart block is characterized by a progressive increase of the PR interval with an eventual failure of one impulse to conduct to the ventricle resulting in a "dropped" beat (Fig. 3–9). The pattern is usually repetitive and results in a "grouped-beating" pattern on the ECG. Mobitz I

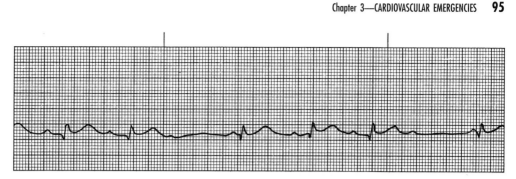

FIGURE 3–9. Mobitz type I. From Kitt, S. (1990). Emergency Nursing: A physiologic & clinical perspective. Philadelphia: W. B. Saunders. Used with permission.

type AV block almost always occurs as a result of a delay in the AV node. It is often associated with increased parasympathetic tone, inferior MI, drug effects (e.g., digitalis, propranolol). If it occurs in the presence of an inferior MI, it is often transient, and it rarely requires temporary pacing.

1) Assessment
    a) Subjective data
        (1) History of present illness
            (a) Palpitations/"missing a beat"
            (b) Chest pain
            (c) Nausea and vomiting
            (d) Diaphoresis
            (e) Symptoms of digitalis toxicity
        (2) Medical history
            (a) Cardiac dysrhythmias
            (b) Use of cardiac medications (verapamil, digitalis, propranolol)
            (c) Heart block, which in the pediatric patient is usually related to congenital abnormalities or overdose of cardiac medication
    b) Objective data
        (1) Physical examination
            (a) Irregular heart rate
            (b) Bradycardia
            (c) Hypotension
        (2) Diagnostic procedures
            (a) ECG: atrial rate unaffected, but ventricular rate will be less than the atrial rate; atrial rhythm usually regular, whereas ventricular rhythm usually irregular with progressive shortening of RR interval before block impulse; P waves will appear normal; progressive increase in PR interval until one P wave is blocked; QRS is usually normal
            (b) Serum potassium level
            (c) Digitalis levels
            (d) Cardiac serum markers
2) Analysis: differential nursing diagnosis/collaborative problems
    a) Cardiac output decreased related to conduction disturbance
    b) Anxiety/fear related to alteration in health status
3) Planning/interventions
    a) Monitor airway, breathing, circulation
    b) Supplemental oxygen
    c) Establish IV access, saline lock

       d) Initiate cardiac monitor, NIBP, pulse oximetry

       e) Obtain 12- to 15-lead ECG

       f) Continuously monitor

         (1) Level of consciousness

         (2) Heart rate and rhythm

         (3) BP

         (4) Respiratory rate, rhythm, depth

         (5) Skin color

         (6) Urine output

       g) If patient is hemodynamically unstable

         (1) Administer medications as ordered to increase heart rate (atropine)

         (2) If medications unsuccessful, apply external cardiac pacer, prepare patient for pacing

         (3) Assist with insertion of temporary transvenous cardiac pacemaker; prepare patient for pacing

       h) Maintain calm, efficient manner

       i) Minimize environmental stimuli

       j) Explain all procedures

       k) Encourage verbalization and questions

       l) Allow significant other at bedside if possible

    4) Expected outcomes/evaluation (see Appendix B)

  c. Second-degree AV block: Mobitz type II

      This dysrhythmia is due to a conduction delay below the level of the AV node, either at the bundle of His or, more commonly, at the bundle branches (Fig. 3–10). Second-degree AV block is differentiated from first-degree AV block in that the PR interval does not lengthen before a dropped beat, and the beats drop unexpectedly and unpredictably. It is associated with a bundle branch block, and the dropped beat is due to a bilateral bundle branch block. Mobitz type II dysrhythmia is usually the result of an organic lesion in the conduction pathway; rarely is it the result of a drug effect. It is less common than a Mobitz type I dysrhythmia but is more serious. In the presence of an MI, it can require pacing (temporary or permanent) and is associated with a higher mortality.

    1) Assessment

      a) Subjective data

        (1) History of present illness

          (a) Syncope

          (b) Angina

          (c) Dyspnea

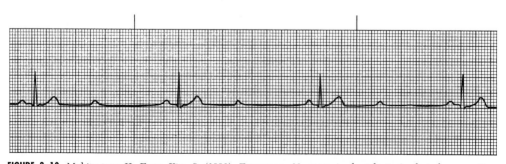

FIGURE 3–10. Mobitz type II. From Kitt, S. (1990). Emergency Nursing: A physiologic & clinical perspective. Philadelphia: W. B. Saunders. Used with permission.

(d) Symptoms of MI, including chest pain, nausea and vomiting, and diaphoresis

(2) Medical history

(a) Cardiac disease

(b) Previous MI

b) Objective data

(1) Physical examination

(a) Irregular heart rate

(b) Hypotension

(c) Diaphoresis

(d) Cool, clammy skin

(2) Diagnostic procedures

(a) Twelve- to 15-lead ECG: atrial rate is unaffected, but ventricular rate is less than atrial rate; atrial rhythm is regular; ventricular rate is irregular; P waves appear normal, followed by normal QRS except when a P wave is blocked; PR interval may be normal or prolonged but will be constant; QRS will be normal if level of block is proximal to bundle of His; QRS will be wide if block is at bundle branch level

(b) Serum potassium

(c) Cardiac enzymes

2) Analysis: differential nursing diagnosis/collaborative problems

a) Cardiac output decreased related to conduction disturbance

b) Myocardial tissue perfusion altered related to decreased cardiac output

c) Anxiety/fear related to change in health status

3) Planning/interventions

a) Monitor airway, breathing, circulation

b) Provide supplemental oxygen

c) Establish IV access; infuse normal saline at KVO rate

d) Initiate cardiac monitor, NIBP, pulse oximetry

e) Obtain 12- to 15-lead ECG

f) If patient is hemodynamically unstable

(1) If medication unsuccessful, apply external cardiac pacer, prepare patient for pacing

(2) Assist with insertion of temporary transvenous cardiac pacemaker; prepare patient for pacing

g) Continuously monitor

(1) Level of consciousness

(2) Heart rate and rhythm

(3) BP

(4) Respiratory rate, rhythm, depth

(5) Skin color

(6) Urine output

h) Provide complete rest for patient

i) Maintain calm, efficient manner

j) Minimize environmental stimuli

k) Explain all procedures

l) Encourage questions and verbalization of fears

m) Allow significant other at bedside if possible

4) Expected outcomes/evaluation (see Appendix B)

d. *Third-degree (complete) AV block*

Third-degree AV block is characterized by a complete absence of conduction between atria and ventricles; both the atria and ventricles are controlled

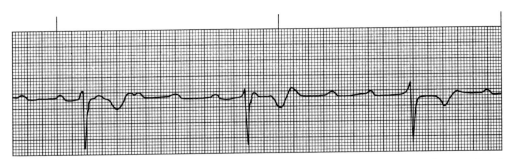

FIGURE 3–11. Third-degree heart block. From Kitt, S. (1990). Emergency Nursing: A physiologic & clinical perspective. Philadelphia: W. B. Saunders. Used with permission.

by independent pacemakers (Fig. 3–11). This may occur at the level of the AV node, the bundle of His, or the bundle branches. With a higher level of block (AV node), the junction will take over as the pacemaker; these types of block are usually transient and carry a good prognosis. With a lower block (bundle branch), the ventricle will take over as the pacemaker; this is very unstable and has a poor prognosis. The pathogenesis includes MI, cardiac disease states, digitalis toxicity, and congenital anomalies.

1) Assessment
   a) Subjective data
      (1) History of present illness
         (a) Syncope
         (b) Angina
         (c) Dyspnea
         (d) Symptoms of MI, including chest pain, nausea, vomiting, and diaphoresis
         (e) Palpitations
         (f) Symptoms of digitalis toxicity, including fatigue, anorexia, nausea and vomiting, blurred vision, and mental confusion
      (2) Medical history
         (a) Cardiac disease
         (b) Use of cardiac medications
         (c) Previous MI
   b) Objective data
      (1) Physical examination
         (a) Slow, regular heart rate
         (b) Hypotension
         (c) Decreasing or loss of consciousness
         (d) Wheezes and crackles if heart failure occurs
         (e) Diaphoresis
         (f) Cool, clammy skin
      (2) Diagnostic procedures
         (a) Twelve- to 15-lead ECG: atrial rate is 60 to 100 bpm; ventricular rate will be less than 40 bpm if activated by ventricular pacemaker or 40 to 60 bpm if activated by junctional pacemaker; atrial rhythm is regular; ventricular rhythm is regular; P wave is normal; PR interval is highly variable; if block occurs at bundle of His, QRS will appear normal; if block occurs at bundle branch level, QRS will be widened
         (b) Serum potassium, digitalis, procainamide, and quinidine levels, if appropriate

(c) Cardiac serum markers

(d) Pulse oximetry, ABGs

2) Analysis: nursing diagnosis/collaborative problems

a) Cardiac output decreased related to conduction disturbance

b) Tissue perfusion, altered related to decreased cardiac output

c) Anxiety/fear related to change in health sttus

3) Planning/interventions

a) Establish and maintain airway, breathing, circulation

b) Administer supplemental oxygen

c) Establish IV access; infuse normal saline at KVO rate

d) Initiate cardiac monitor, NIBP, pulse oximetry

e) Obtain 12- to 15-lead ECG

f) If patient is hemodynamically unstable

(1) Administer medications as ordered to increase heart rate

(2) Apply external cardiac pacer, prepare patient for pacing

(3) Assist with insertion of temporary transvenous cardiac pacemaker; prepare patient for pacing

(4) Prepare catecholamine infusions for continued hypotension despite pacing (e.g., dopamine, epinephrine)

g) Continuously monitor

(1) Level of consciousness

(2) Heart rate and rhythm

(3) BP

(4) Respiratory rate, rhythm, depth

(5) Heart and lung sounds

(6) Peripheral pulses

(7) Skin color

(8) Urine output

h) Maintain calm, efficient manner

i) Minimize environmental stimuli

j) Explain all procedures

k) Encourage questions and verbalization of fears

l) Allow significant other at bedside if possible

4) Expected outcomes/evaluation (see Appendix B)

5. **Ventricular dysrhythmias**

a. *Premature ventricular contractions*

A premature ventricular beat is a complex arising from one of the ventricles before the next expected sinus beat (Fig. 3–12). PVCs are characterized by a QRS complex that is bizarre in shape and has a duration that usually exceeds 0.12 seconds. The causes of PVCs are usually related to conditions that enhance ventricular automaticity, such as anxiety, hypoxia, electrolyte imbalance (e.g., hypokalemia), infection, myocardial ischemia, cardiac disease,

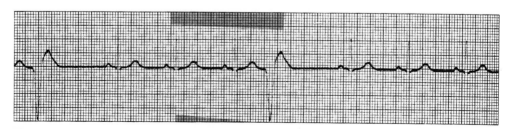

FIGURE 3–12. Uni-formed premature ventricular contraction. From Kitt, S. (1990). Emergency Nursing: A physiologic & clinical perspective. Philadelphia: W. B. Saunders. Used with permission.

a variety of medications (e.g., digitalis, phenothiazines, tricyclic antidepressants) and irritation from pacemaker malfunctions. PVCs are thought to be benign if they are rare and unifocal, occurring in an asymptomatic patient without cardiac disease. However, PVCs may become life threatening when they are multifocal (arise from different areas in the ventricles), occur at a rate of more than six per minute (although this may be a conservative number), occur in couplets (PVCs occurring in pairs), occur close to the preceding T wave, or occur in patients suffering from an acute MI (considered a presage to ventricular fibrillation). Three or more PVCs in a row is considered a run of ventricular tachycardia.

1) Assessment
   a) Subjective data
      (1) History of present illness
         (a) Palpitations
         (b) Feeling lightheaded/dizzy
         (c) Chest pain
         (d) Sensation of "skipped beats"
         (e) Hypotension
         (f) Discomfort in neck/chest (secondary to force of PVC)
         (g) Forceful heartbeat
      (2) Medical history
         (a) Cardiac disease
         (b) Use of cardiac medications
         (c) COPD/asthma/pneumonia
         (d) Prevalence of ventricular ectopy activity increases with age and in males
   b) Objective data
      (1) Physical examination
         (a) Heart rate: 60 to 100 bpm
         (b) Heart/pulse rhythm is irregular
         (c) Decreased intensity of heart sounds, S_1 varies in intensity
         (d) Pulse deficit
         (e) Hypotension
      (2) Diagnostic procedures
         (a) Twelve- to 15-lead ECG: irregular rhythm; P wave usually obscured by PVC but may be seen; retrograde P wave may occur or nonconducted P wave may be seen at expected time; QRS is wide and greater than 0.12 second. The ST segment and T wave are commonly large and often opposite in polarity to QRS; morphology of QRS is bizarre; compensatory pause often seen
         (b) Serum electrolytes, digitalis, aminophylline levels
         (c) ABGs and pulse oximetry
2) Analysis: nursing diagnosis/collaborative problems
   a) Cardiac output decreased related to cardiac rhythm abnormality and/or conduction disturbance
   b) Anxiety/fear related to change in health status
   c) Knowledge deficit related to etiology, pathophysiology, treatments, sequelae, and prognosis of dysrhythmia
3) Planning/interventions
   a) Monitor airway, breathing, circulation
   b) Administer supplemental oxygen via nasal cannula
   c) Establish IV access; infuse normal saline at KVO rate

d) Initiate cardiac monitor, NIBP, pulse oximetry
e) Obtain 12- to 15-lead ECG
f) Continuously monitor
   (1) Level of consciousness
   (2) Heart rate and rhythm
   (3) BP
   (4) Respiratory rate, rhythm, depth
   (5) Heart and lung sounds
   (6) Skin color
   (7) ABG results, pulse oximetry
g) Administer cardiac medications as ordered
   (1) Lidocaine is drug of choice
   (2) Bretylium, procainamide, quinidine, and propranolol may also be used; oral agents include tocainide, mexiletine, and disopyramide
h) Maintain calm, efficient manner
i) Minimize environmental stimuli
j) Encourage questions and verbalization of fears
k) Allow significant other at bedside if possible
l) Explain all procedures
m) Assess patient's/significant other's knowledge of cardiac dysrhythmia: etiology, potential sequelae, signs and symptoms of dysrhythmia and sequelae, how to monitor dysrhythmia, follow-up care
n) Teach patient/significant other
   (1) Factors that can cause dysrhythmia, potential sequelae, signs and symptoms of dysrhythmia, sequelae
   (2) How to monitor pulse and report irregularities
   (3) Medication names, dosages, routes, times for use, purposes, side effects, special considerations
o) Provide written instructions for aftercare and management of subsequent episodes; tailor instructions to patient/significant other in terms of ability to read and comprehend instructions
4) Expected outcomes/evaluation (see Appendix B)

b. *Ventricular tachycardia*

Ventricular tachycardia (VT) is a dysrhythmia characterized by a succession of three or more ventricular beats at a rate greater than 100 bpm (Fig. 3–13). A patient's tolerance of this dysrhythmia will be dependent on the rate and duration of the tachycardia and the underlying cardiovascular disease. The primary cause of VT is acute MI; other causes include cardiomyopathy, primary electrical disease, mitral valve prolapse, valvular heart disease, congenital heart disease, LV hypertrophy, digitalis or quinidine toxicity, hypoxia,

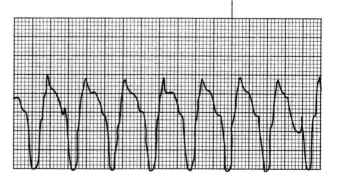

FIGURE 3–13. Ventricular tachycardia. From Kitt, S. (1990). Emergency Nursing: A physiologic & clinical perspective. Philadelphia: W. B. Saunders. Used with permission.

and hypokalemia. In the pediatric population, VT is uncommon. When VT does occur in this age group, the etiologies include underlying structural deficits, prolonged QT interval, hypoxia, acidosis, electrolyte imbalance, and poisoning, such as those caused by tricyclic antidepressant and cardiac medications. VT is labeled sustained when it lasts longer than 30 seconds or requires termination secondary to hemodynamic collapse and is labeled nonsustained if it lasts fewer than 30 seconds and terminates spontaneously.

Torsades de pointes is a form of ventricular tachycardia in which the QRS complexes demonstrate a changing amplitude, which appears to be twisting around the isoelectric line. Its most common causes are factors that may prolong the QT interval, including drug toxicities, reactions to certain antiarrhythmics (particularly type Ia, quinidine and procainamide), hypokalemia, congenital anomalies, and severe bradycardia. Clinical manifestations of torsades de pointes are dependent on rate and duration, just as with any form of VT. This form of VT is more common in women than men. Because it is a precipitated event, treatment involves identifying and treating the offending circumstance.

1) Assessment
   a) Subjective data
      (1) History of present illness
         (a) Altered level of consciousness
         (b) Palpitations
         (c) Chest pain
         (d) Dyspnea
         (e) Syncope/near syncope
         (f) Lightheadedness, weakness, or dizziness
      (2) Medical history
         (a) Hypertension
         (b) Recent MI
         (c) Use of cardiac medications, particularly antiarrhythmics
         (d) Atherosclerotic heart disease
         (e) Congenital anomalies
   b) Objective data
      (1) Physical examination
         (a) Decreased or loss of consciousness
         (b) Hypotension
         (c) Diminished pulses
         (d) Cool, clammy skin
         (e) Pulmonary rales/wheezing
         (f) Cardiac arrest
      (2) Diagnostic procedures
         (a) ECG: rate is greater than 100 bpm, usually less than 220 bpm; usually regular rhythm; in rapid VT, P waves often not discernible; at slower ventricular rates, P wave may be seen as the atria depolarize from the SA node at a rate slower than VT or as they are conducted retrograde from ventricle; for the most part, there is no relationship between atrial and ventricular rates; therefore, PR interval is not measurable; QRS complex is wide, greater than 0.12 second, and may be monomorphic or polymorphic
         (b) Serum electrolytes, procainamide and quinidine levels, as appropriate
         (c) Cardiac serum markers

(d) ABGs and pulse oximetry

2) Analysis: differential nursing diagnosis/collaborative problems

   a) Cardiac output decreased related to cardiac rhythm abnormality and/or conduction disturbance

   b) Decreased tissue perfusion secondary to decreased cardiac output

   c) Anxiety/fear related to change in health status

3) Planning/interventions

   a) Monitor and assist with maintaining airway, breathing, circulation

   b) Determine pulselessness

     (1) If pulse is present

       (a) Administer supplemental oxygen

       (b) Establish IV access with large-bore catheter; infuse normal saline at KVO rate or saline lock

       (c) Initiate cardiac monitor, NIPB, pulse oximetry

       (d) Continuously monitor: level of consciousness; heart rate and rhythm; BP; respiratory rate, rhythm, depth; heart and lung sounds; skin color; peripheral pulses; capillary refill; urine output; ABG results (as available); pulse oximeter

       (e) Obtain 12- to 15-lead ECG

       (f) Obtain portable chest radiograph

       (g) If stable, administer medications as ordered (if unstable go to item h below): start with lidocaine bolus, followed by doses 5 to 10 minutes apart to maximum dose or until VT resolves; if unsuccessful, bretylium; if unsuccessful, procainamide; continuous infusion of drug that converted patient out of VT; if chemical cardioversion unsuccessful, prepare for synchronized cardioversion (see below)

       (h) If unstable or if unsuccessful with antiarrhythmics, initiate/assist with synchronized cardioversion: administer sedation if ordered; put defibrillator in to "synchronized" mode and cardiovert starting at 100 J, gradually increasing up to 360 J; if recurrent, add lidocaine, then bretylium, and, last, procainamide as ordered; pediatric dose 0.5 to 1.0 J/kg with a lidocaine bolus (if readily available) before cardioversion

       (i) Regarding digitalis excess, prepare to administer digoxin immune Fab (Digibind) and a rapid-acting antiarrhythmic (such as lidocaine, magnesium, or phenytoin) as ordered; with unstable VT secondary to digitalis excess, cardioversion should begin at 25 to 50 J, followed 200 J, 300 J, and 360 J

       (j) For patients in torsades de pointes, interventions may include the following: prepare to administer magnesium sulfate as ordered; prepare/assist with overdrive pacing; transcutaneous pacing can be used until a transvenous pacemaker is placed; prepare to administer isoproterenol as ordered (may chemically overdrive ventricle and break VT); avoid any medications that may prolong ventricular repolarization (quinidine, procainamide, phenothiazines)

       (k) Administer potassium if serum level is below 3.5 mEq/L as ordered

       (l) Maintain calm, efficient manner

       (m) Minimize environmental stimuli

       (n) Explain all procedures

       (o) Remain at bedside as much as possible

(2) If pulse is absent

    (a) Begin cardiopulmonary resuscitation (CPR) until defibrillator available; continue as long as patient remains pulseless

    (b) Defibrillate beginning at 200 J, repeat at 300 J and then 360 J, if necessary, for persistent VT

    (c) Assist with intubation, ensure bilateral breath sounds, secure airway

    (d) Obtain IV access

    (e) Administer medications per ACLS protocols

    (f) Once spontaneous pulse returns, obtain and continuously monitor vital signs; support airway and breathing; prepare to administer medications to augment BP, heart rate, and rhythm, as appropriate, as ordered

4) Expected outcomes/evaluation (see Appendix B)

c. *Ventricular fibrillation*

Ventricular fibrillation (VF) is a lethal dysrhythmia characterized by unorganized electrical activity of the ventricles, which produces ineffective quivering of the ventricles (Fig. 3–14). There is no cardiac output or pulse with VF. The terms "coarse" and "fine" are often used to describe the size or amplitude of the waveforms in VF. Generally, coarse VF is considered more recent in onset and may be corrected more readily. Fine VF indicates VF of a longer duration since its onset and is more difficult to reverse. The situation is life threatening and must be treated with prompt defibrillation. The most common cause of VF is acute MI. Other causes include hypoxia, electrical shock, sudden death syndrome, and digitalis or quinidine toxicity. VF is an uncommon event in the pediatric age group and is especially rare in infants.

1) Assessment

    a) Subjective data

        (1) History of present illness

            (a) Unresponsiveness

        (2) Medical history

            (a) Recent MI

            (b) Cardiac disease (advanced)

            (c) Cardiac drug use

    b) Objective data

        (1) Physical examination

            (a) Loss of consciousness

            (b) Pulse absent

            (c) Heart sounds absent

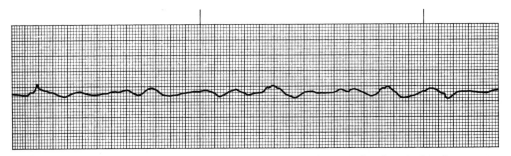

FIGURE 3–14. Ventricular fibrillation. From Kitt, S. (1990). Emergency Nursing: A physiologic & clinical perspective. Philadelphia: W. B. Saunders. Used with permission.

   (d) Apnea
   (e) BP absent
  (2) Diagnostic procedures
   (a) ECG: rate is very rapid, usually too unorganized to count; irregular rhythm; waveforms vary in size and shape; no P wave, QRS, ST segment, or T wave
   (b) ABGs
   (c) Serum electrolytes, digitalis, quinidine levels
   (d) Cardiac serum markers
2) Analysis: nursing diagnosis/collaborative problems
  a) Ineffective airway clearance related to decreased level of consciousness
  b) Gas exchange impaired related to cardiovascular dysrhythmia
  c) Cardiac output decreased related to cardiac dysrhythmia
  d) Tissue perfusion altered related to absent cardiac output
  e) Anxiety/fear (significant other) related to magnitude of physiological problems and potential death of patient
3) Planning/interventions
  a) Establish patent airway
   (1) Jaw-thrust/chin-lift maneuver
   (2) Oropharyngeal or nasopharyngeal suctioning
   (3) Oropharyngeal or nasopharyngeal airways
   (4) Endotracheal tube
  b) Initiate mouth-to-mask ventilation if necessary
  c) Initiate artificial ventilation with bag-valve-mask device using 100% oxygen
  d) Witnessed/monitored VF
   (1) Precordial thump: must be delivered immediately and only if defibrillator is not available
   (2) If rhythm converts, administer IV bolus of lidocaine, followed by continuous lidocaine infusion (proceed to Item g below)
   (3) If VF persists, proceed to Item e (next)
  e) Unmonitored or unwitnessed VF
   (1) Initiate CPR
   (2) Identify VF via ECG monitor or defibrillator monitor
   (3) Defibrillate at 200 J, check rhythm
   (4) If unsuccessful, defibrillate again at 300 J, check rhythm
   (5) If unsuccessful, defibrillate at 360 J, check pulse and rhythm
   (6) If unsuccessful, resume CPR
   (7) If patient not intubated, prepare/assist with intubation at this time
   (8) Establish IV access with large-bore catheter, infuse normal saline at KVO rate
   (9) Administer epinephrine via IV or endotracheal route; allow all drugs given during the resuscitation 30 to 60 seconds to circulate before defibrillating; always check a pulse and rhythm after every intervention; administer epinephrine every 3 to 5 minutes as necessary
   (10) Defibrillate at 360 J, check pulse and rhythm
   (11) If unsuccessful, administer lidocaine via IV or endotracheal route, check pulse and rhythm; repeat as necessary to maximum dose
   (12) If unsuccessful, defibrillate at 360 J; check pulse and rhythm
   (13) Administer bretylium if lidocaine and defibrillation remain unsuccessful; check pulse and rhythm
   (14) If VF persists, defibrillate up to 360 J; check pulse

    (15) Consider administration of sodium bicarbonate if
        (a) Patient has pre-existing hyperkalemia
        (b) Patient has known acidosis
        (c) Known tricyclic antidepressant overdose
        (d) Long arrest interval
    (16) Consider correctable causes of VF in the pediatric population (e.g., metabolic abnormalities, drug intoxication)
    (17) Optimal energy dose has not been established for pediatric patient; it has been suggested that 2 J/kg should be used initially; if unsuccessful, dose is doubled and repeated twice; if VF continues, assess ventilation, oxygenation, and correction of acidosis
  f) Nasogastric tube insertion to protect airway from aspiration
  g) Once spontaneous pulse returns, continuously monitor
    (1) Level of consciousness
    (2) Heart rate and rhythm
    (3) BP
    (4) Respiratory effort/mechanical ventilation
    (5) Peripheral pulses
    (6) Skin and mucous membrane color
    (7) Urine output
  h) Provide ventilatory support
  i) Prepare to administer medications to augment BP, heart rate, and rhythm
  j) Attempt to provide private waiting area for significant others
  k) Provide consistent liaison (chaplain) with same personnel among staff/significant others
  l) Provide significant others with accurate and realistic information regarding patient's status
  m) Maintain calm, empathetic manner
  n) Encourage questions; demonstrate therapeutic emotional response, address denial with gentle, reality-based response
  o) Offer to notify clergy or other support persons
4) Expected outcomes/evaluation (see Appendix B)

d. *Ventricular asystole*

Asystole is a cardiac condition resulting from the complete absence of electrical and mechanical cardiac function. It results from severe end-stage cardiac disease or prolonged cardiac arrest. Asystole has a grim prognosis and usually represents confirmation of death. Treatment is focused on determining the possible cause and aggressively treating it. Asystole is not a shockable rhythm, and countershocks to this rhythm could eliminate any possibility of the return of spontaneous cardiac activity. CPR and ACLS measures must be immediately instituted for any chance of patient survival.

1) Assessment
  a) Subjective data
    (1) History of present illness
        (a) Obtaining history should never delay initiation of resuscitation
        (b) Duration of arrest
        (c) Time interval from occurrence of arrest to initial resuscitation efforts
        (d) Duration of prehospital resuscitation efforts
    (2) Medical history
        (a) Coronary heart disease
        (b) Pulmonary disease and its sequelae

        (c) Traumatic injury

        (d) Electrical: malfunctioning pacemaker, electrocution, lightning

        (e) Cerebrovascular disease

        (f) Drowning

        (g) Overdose/ingestion

        (h) Renal failure

     (3) Risk factors

        (a) Previous cardiac arrest

        (b) Coronary heart disease

        (c) Chronic illness or malignancy

  b) Objective data

     (1) Physical examination

        (a) Unresponsiveness to any stimulus

        (b) Absent heart and lung sounds

        (c) Absent BP, pulses

        (d) Peripheral and central cyanosis

        (e) Pupils unresponsive to light

     (2) Diagnostic procedures

        (a) ECG: absence of electrical activity; must confirm in at least two lead configurations, because fine VF may appear as asystole

        (b) ABGs

        (c) Serum electrolytes

        (d) CBC

        (e) Type and cross-match blood (for trauma)

        (f) Toxicology studies (if suspected overdose/ingestion)

2) Analysis: nursing diagnosis/collaborative problems

  a) Ineffective airway clearance related to cardiopulmonary arrest or unconscious state

  b) Gas exchange impaired related to decreased cardiac output

  c) Cardiac output decreased related to cardiopulmonary arrest

  d) Tissue perfusion altered (systemic) related to cardiopulmonary arrest

  e) Anxiety/fear (family/significant other) related to potential death of patient

3) Planning/interventions

  a) Open airway

     (1) Chin lift or jaw thrust

     (2) Remove any obstruction per basic life support protocol

     (3) Oropharyngeal/nasopharyngeal airway

     (4) Endotracheal/nasotracheal intubation

  b) Intubation, ventilation, and oxygenation always precede drug therapy

     (1) Initiate mouth-to-mask ventilation if necessary; mouth and nose in infants

     (2) Initiate ventilations with bag-valve-mask device using 100% oxygen

     (3) Avoid pressure-cycled automatic breathing devices

     (4) Continuously monitor and assess

        (a) Symmetry of chest wall expansion

        (b) Bilateral breath sounds

        (c) Resistance to artificial ventilation: indication of lung compliance

        (d) ABGs

  c) Begin CPR immediately

  d) Place patient on monitor; check two leads to confirm asystole

  e) If rhythm is unclear and possibly VF, defibrillate as in VF

  f) If asystole, continue CPR

  g) Establish IV access; use large-bore catheter
  h) Administer medications as ordered
    (1) Epinephrine, every 3 to 5 minutes
    (2) Atropine, every 3 to 5 minutes until maximum dose achieved, up to 0.03 to 0.04 mg/kg
    (3) Sodium bicarbonate for
      (a) Known pre-existing hyperkalemia
      (b) Known acidosis
      (c) Known tricyclic antidepressant overdose
    (4) Appropriate antidote for overdose/toxicity
  i) Intubate if patient not already intubated
  j) Prepare/assist with trancutaneous/transvenous pacemaker placement
  k) Pediatric considerations
    (1) Prevent hypothermia in infants and children
    (2) Consider intraosseous cannulation in children younger than 6 years
    (3) CPR begins in the infant when the heart rate is 60 bpm
  l) If hypovolemia is suspected, consider
    (1) Autotransfusion
    (2) Group O, Rh-negative red cells, or group-specific whole blood
    (3) Establish IV access with two large-bore (14-gauge, 16-gauge) catheters and infuse warmed lactated Ringer's or normal saline at "wide open" rate
    (4) Use rapid fluid infusion devices, if available
  m) Insert nasogastric and Foley catheter tubes
  n) Assist family with anticipatory grief and anxiety
    (1) Keep significant others informed of patient's status; same staff member should serve as liaison
    (2) Attempt to prepare significant others for possible death of patient
    (3) Respond to denial with gentle, reality-based statements
    (4) Provide significant others with access to telephone, rest rooms, refreshments, tissues, and privacy
    (5) Notify clergy or support persons
    (6) Allow significant others to view patient body if resuscitation is unsuccessful
    (7) Provide contact name and telephone number for unanticipated questions
4) Expected outcomes/evaluation (see Appendix B)
e. *Pulseless electrical activity*
    Pulseless electrical activity (PEA) describes the presence of electrical activity (other than VT/VF) but no detectable pulse. PEA is a group of dysrhythmias that includes electromechanical dissociation (EMD), pseudo-EMD, idioventricular rhythms, ventricular escape rhythms, and bradyasystolic rhythms. These dysrhythmias are often associated with specific clinical states; therefore, early identification and treatment are paramount in potentially reversing the dysrhythmia. Common etiologies include hypovolemia, hypoxemia, tension pneumothorax, cardiac tamponade, hypothermia, massive pulmonary embolism, hyperkalemia, acidosis, and massive MI. Pediatric PEA is usually related to hypoxemia and acidosis. Prognosis is poor in PEA, unless the underlying cause can be identified and treated quickly.
1) Assessment
  a) Subjective data
    (1) History of present illness

           (a) Unresponsiveness

           (b) Chest pain

           (c) Syncope

           (d) Chest trauma or any other trauma

           (e) Drug overdose

           (f) Prolonged exposure to the cold

        (2) Medical history

           (a) Previous MI

           (b) Shock state

           (c) Recent trauma

           (d) Renal failure

           (e) Previous overdoses

    b) Objective data

        (1) Physical examination

           (a) Loss of consciousness

           (b) Absent pulses

           (c) Absent heart sounds

           (d) Absent BP

           (e) Tracheal deviation (may be present)

           (f) Distended neck veins (may be present)

           (g) Unilateral absent breath sounds

           (h) Obvious signs of trauma

        (2) Diagnostic procedures

           (a) ECG: may appear normal or exhibit any rhythm

           (b) CBC with platelets

           (c) Prothrombin time (PT) and partial thromboplastin time (PTT)

           (d) Serum electrolytes

           (e) ABG analysis

           (f) Serum calcium

           (g) BUN and creatinine

           (h) Urinalysis

           (i) Type and cross-match blood

           (j) Cardiac serum markers

           (k) Urine toxicology screen

           (l) Chest radiograph

          (m) Diagnostic peritoneal lavage

           (n) Pulse oximetry

        (3) Possible therapies and treatments

           (a) Pericardiocentesis

           (b) Needle thoracostomy

           (c) Thoracostomy

           (d) Open thoracotomy

2) Analysis: differential nursing diagnosis/collaborative problems

    a) Airway clearance ineffective related to decreased level of consciousness

    b) Gas exchange impaired related to decreased cardiac output

    c) Cardiac output decreased related to mechanical failure

    d) Tissue perfusion altered related to absence of cardiac output

    e) Anxiety/fear (family/significant other) related to altered health status of patient

3) Planning/interventions

    a) Establish patent airway

        (1) Jaw-thrust/chin-lift maneuver

        (2) Oropharyngeal/nasopharyngeal suctioning

      (3) Mouth sweep

      (4) Oropharyngeal/nasopharyngeal airway

      (5) Endotracheal tube

  b) Initiate mouth-to-mask ventilation if necessary

  c) Initiate ventilation with bag-valve-mask device and 100% oxygen

  d) Continuously monitor and assess

      (1) Bilateral, symmetrical chest wall expansion

      (2) Breath sounds

      (3) Resistance to mechanical ventilation: indication of lung compliance

      (4) ABG results

  e) CPR

  f) Obtain IV access with two large-bore IV catheters; infuse normal saline or Ringer's lactate as ordered

  g) Nasogastric tube to prevent aspiration

  h) In case of severe hypovolemia

      (1) Control obvious hemorrhage

      (2) Infuse warmed IV fluids at bolus/wide-open rate; use rapid fluid infuser device if available

      (3) Increase venous return to the heart by

         (a) Elevating legs

         (b) Putting patient into modified Trendelenburg's position

      (4) Replace blood volume

         (a) Warm, type-specific or type O Rh-negative blood

         (b) If clotting factors depleted, administer fresh frozen plasma (FFP)

         (c) Consider autotransfusion

      (5) Insert Foley catheter

      (6) Prepare patient for transfer to the operating room for definitive management of hemorrhage

  i) If cardiac tamponade is suspected

      (1) Prepare/assist with possible

         (a) Pericardiocentesis

         (b) Open thoracotomy

         (c) Internal cardiac massage

         (d) Internal cardiac defibrillation

      (2) Prepare patient for transfer to operating room suite or to facility with bypass capacity

  j) If tension pneumothorax is suspected

      (1) If open chest wound is covered with occlusive dressing, lift one side of dressing

      (2) Perform or assist with needle thoracostomy

      (3) Assist with tube thoracostomy

  k) Administer medications as ordered

      (1) Epinephrine as soon as peripheral IV or endotracheal access obtained

      (2) Bolus 50 mL of IV fluid after epinephrine administration

      (3) Repeat epinephrine every 5 minutes

      (4) Atropine for

         (a) Absolute or relative bradycardia

         (b) Bolus 50 mL of IV fluid after atropine administration

         (c) Repeat every 3 to 5 minutes as necessary or until maximum dose is reached

      (5) Consider other causes

(a) Hypokalemia

(b) Hypoxemia

(c) Hypothermia

(d) Massive pulmonary embolism

(e) Massive myocardial infarction

(6) Sodium bicarbonate for

(a) Known pre-existing hyperkalemia

(b) Known acidosis

(c) Known tricyclic antidepressant overdose

(7) Appropriate antidotes for overdoses/toxicities

l) Maintain CPR to support ventilation and circulation if interventions unsuccessful

m) Provide quiet waiting area for family if possible

n) Provide consistent liaison (chaplain) between same personnel among staff/significant other

o) Provide significant other with accurate and realistic information regarding patient status

p) Maintain calm, empathetic manner

q) Encourage questions; demonstrate therapeutic emotional response; address denial with a gentle, reality-based response

r) Offer to notify clergy or other support persons

4) Expected outcomes/evaluation (see Appendix B)

G. Hypertensive emergencies

Hypertensive emergency is a rapid decompensation of vital organ function as a result of a sudden onset of markedly increased diastolic BP (DBP), usually greater than 130 mm Hg. True hypertensive emergencies are rare and life threatening, requiring rapid recognition and aggressive treatment to decrease mortality and morbidity (unlike hypertensive urgencies, which can be treated more slowly). Any hypertensive disease can cause a hypertensive emergency, but pheochromocytoma, renovascular hypertension, and use of certain medications, particularly monoamine oxidase (MAO) inhibitors, have the highest incidence.

It is not the absolute BP that determines a hypertensive emergency, but the rapidity of the rise and resulting end-organ dysfunction. The BP that is a hypertensive emergency for one patient may not be for another. An example is the patient with chronic hypertension versus a woman with eclampsia. The woman with eclampsia would likely be symptomatic with a DBP of 90 to 100 mm Hg, whereas the patient with chronic hypertension may not become symptomatic until his or her DBP was greater than 130 mm Hg. This is due to autoregulation. In normotensive patients, autoregulation is the body's ability to maintain adequate cerebral blood flow (CBF) despite changes in BP (usually by maintaining a mean arterial pressure [MAP] of 50–150 mm Hg). In hypertensive patients, this mechanism has adapted by shifting upward (these patients maintain CBF with a MAP of 120–180 mm Hg). When the BP exceeds the upper limits, the brain becomes hyperperfused. If this state is persistent, the vessels in the brain will dilate and eventually begin to leak fluids into the surrounding tissues, producing cerebral edema. This will produce an increase in ICP, which decreases cerebral perfusion pressure and subsequently decreases CBF. It is this decrease in CBF that necessitates rapid therapy to reduce the BP. However, caution must be used not to decrease the BP too low or below the level of autoregulation (which is high in the patient with chronic hypertension), because this can produce hypoperfusion and ischemia. Therefore, it is recommended that the BP be reduced 20 to 30% over 2 to 3 hours. The overall goal of therapy is to reduce target end-organ damage. In addition to the brain, organs at risk are the heart, kidneys, large vessels, and eyes. The pathophysiology of end-organ dysfunction is produced by fibrinoid necrosis and microthrombi of arterioles accompanying the extreme organ strain produced by severely elevated BP.

When treating a hypertensive emergency, a fast-acting potent vasodilator is generally needed to prevent death or end-organ damage. Pharmacology choice will depend on the patient's clinical status, end-organ impairment, fluid status, and comorbidities (e.g., coronary heart disease, end-stage renal disease). These patients will need observation in an intensive care unit (ICU) setting and placement of an arterial catheter for continuous accurate BP monitoring. The use of NIBP monitoring is currently under scrutiny.

1. **Assessment**
   a. *Subjective data*
      1) History of present illness
         a) Headache
         b) Dizziness
         c) Visual complaints
         d) Chest pain
         e) Symptoms of heart failure
         f) Patient may be asymptomatic
      2) Medical history
         a) Hypertension
            (1) Poorly controlled
            (2) Sudden discontinuation/withdrawal of HTN medications
         b) Renal disease
         c) Adrenal disease (particularly pheochromocytoma)
         d) Eclampsia
         e) Hypertension associated with contraceptive pills
   b. *Objective data*
      1) Physical examination
         a) Diastolic BP usually greater than 130 to 140 mm Hg
         b) Retinopathy
            (1) Optic hemorrhages and exudates
            (2) Papilledema (presence of papilledema is termed malignant HTN)
         c) Altered neurological status
            (1) Signs of increased ICP
            (2) Seizures (possible)
            (3) Drowsiness, confusion, lethargy, stupor; may progress to coma
            (4) Hemiparesis
         d) Altered cardiac status
            (1) Prominent apical pulse
            (2) S_3, S_4
            (3) Crackles in lung fields (associated with heart failure)
         e) Oliguria, hematuria
         f) Abdominal bruits
      2) Diagnostic procedures
         a) Serum electrolytes, creatinine, BUN
         b) Urinalysis
         c) CBC

      d) Chest radiograph

      e) Twelve- to 15-lead ECG

         (1) Ischemic changes

         (2) Axis deviation

         (3) Left ventricular hypertrophy

         (4) ST- and T-wave abnormalities

      f) Computed tomography (CT) of brain

2. Analysis: differential nursing diagnosis/collaborative problems

    a. Tissue perfusion, altered cerebral related to decrease of blood flow secondary to increased ICP

    b. Tissue perfusion, altered renal related to pathological changes associated with HTN

    c. Ineffective gas exchange related to pulmonary congestion secondary to acute MI, fluid overload, or heart failure

    d. Anxiety/fear related to altered health status

3. Planning/interventions

    a. Maintain patent airway

      1) Oral or nasal airway

      2) Endotracheal or nasotracheal intubation

    b. Provide supplemental oxygen as needed

    c. Establish IV access and infuse normal saline at KVO rate

    d. Be prepared to administer ACLS measures if necessary

    e. Administer medications as ordered for BP

      1) Nitroprusside

         a) Most common and most effective

         b) Produces arterial and venous dilation, decreasing preload and afterload

         c) Hypotension is a common complication

         d) Observe patient for thiocyanate and cyanide toxicity with long-term therapy

      2) Nitroglycerin

         a) Preferred in patients with CAD or cardiac ischemia due to its ability to dilate coronary arteries

         b) Vasodilator that affects venous vessels more than arterial vessels

         c) May cause tachycardia and occasionally bradycardia

      3) Labetalol

         a) Alpha and beta blocker (noncardioselective)

         b) Onset and cessation of action slower than nitroprusside (Nipride) and nitroglycerin; can be unpredictable

         c) Contraindicated in patients with heart failure, greater than first-degree block, bradycardia, and reactive airway disease

      4) Hydralazine

         a) Vasodilator, mostly arterial

         b) Drug of choice in eclampsia; not for other types of hypertension emergencies

      5) Diazoxide (Hyperstat)

         a) Direct vasodilator that primarily affects arterial vessels

         b) Requires dose adjustment with renal failure

         c) May precipitate hyperglycemia

         d) Contraindicated in setting of angina, MI, aortic dissection

         e) May produce severe hypotension in presence of volume depletion

      6) Nicardipine

         a) Calcium channel blocker

         b) Increases heart rate, may precipitate angina

           c) Increases ICP

           d) Lack of experience in treatment of hypertensive emergencies to date

        7) Phentolamine

           a) Alpha and beta blocker

           b) Used in treatment of catecholamine crisis (pheochromocytoma)

        8) Propranolol or esmolol

           a) Short-acting beta blocker

           b) Not a primary agent in the treatment of hypertensive emergencies; should not be used for cocaine-induced hypertensive emergencies

           c) Propranolol preferred over esmolol for treatment of aortic dissection

        9) Trimethaphan

           a) Vasodilator that dilates resistant and capacitant vessels

           b) Tachyphylaxis tends to occur early

           c) Useful in setting of aortic dissection

           d) Blurred vision, bowel and bladder paresis, orthostatic hypotension common complications

           e) Does not increase ICP; thus, is useful in setting of increased ICP

    f. Be prepared to assist with arterial monitoring

    g. Administer medications to decrease cardiac workload

        1) Diuretics

        2) Morphine

        3) Nitrates

        4) Propranolol

    h. Continuously monitor and assess

        1) Heart and lung sounds

        2) Peripheral perfusion

        3) Cardiac rhythm

        4) Level of consciousness

        5) Glasgow Coma Score (see Appendix C), neurological evaluations

        6) Seizure activity

        7) BP every 5 minutes until stable

        8) Intake and output

        9) Pulse oximetry

        10) Airway, breathing, circulation

    i. Maintain calm, efficient manner

    j. Minimize environmental stimuli

    k. Explain all procedures to patients

    l. Allow significant other at the bedside if possible

  4. Expected outcomes/evaluation (see Appendix B)

H. Acute aortic dissection

    Acute aortic dissection is an uncommon but potentially lethal condition resulting from a tear in the intimal layer of the aorta, which exposes the degenerated medial layer to the forces of blood pressure. These forces cleave, or dissect, the two layers of the arterial wall, creating two lumens within the aorta: the true lumen and the false lumen. The false lumen can extend to unpredictable length, usually anterograde but occasionally retrograde. The blood in the false lumen can clot within the false lumen or may reenter the true lumen, producing a relatively stable patient. However, it may rupture and will quickly lead to death. There are several classifications of aortic dissection, all of which are based on the fact that dissections usually occur in one of two locations: the ascending aorta superior to the aortic valve or the descending aorta at the site of the ligamentum arteriosum. The most common and most lethal of all dissections occur in the ascending aorta, accounting for two thirds of all dissections. The rest occur in the descending aorta, aortic arch, and rarely in the abdominal aorta. Aortic dissections may be acute, present less than 2 weeks, or chronic, present greater 2 weeks. Two thirds of aortic dissections are acute. Hypertension is a major predisposing factor for aortic dissection; others include hereditary defects of connective tissue, most commonly Marfan's syndrome, bicuspid aortic valve, coarctation of the aorta, pregnancy, blunt trauma, and iatrogenic factors (e.g., intra-arterial catheterization). It is more common in the 60- to 70-year age group; men are two times more likely to experience an aortic dissection than women. The initial treatment goals are to reduce the propagation of the dissection by decreasing the blood pressure and velocity of systolic ejection. Prognosis is dependent on the location of the dissection. Left untreated, aortic dissection carries a 1-year mortality rate in excess of 90%.

1. **Assessment**
   a. *Subjective data*
      1) History of present illness
         a) Pain
            (1) Provoked/palliative
                (a) Sudden, abrupt onset, as severe at onset as it will ever be
                (b) Opiates may not relieve pain
            (2) Quality
                (a) Sharp
                (b) Knifelike
                (c) Tearing/ripping
            (3) Region/radiation
                (a) Substernal, neck, throat, jaw, and face associated with ascending aorta
                (b) Interscapula, back, abdomen, flank, and lower extremities associated with descending aorta
                (c) Migratory: from site of origin to other sites as dissection extends down aorta
            (4) Severity
                (a) Excruciating
                (b) Catastrophic
                (c) Unbearable
            (5) Timing: sudden onset; usually unabated until intervention
         b) Symptoms of heart failure
         c) Syncope
         d) Paraplegia
         e) Altered level of consciousness
      2) Medical history
         a) Hypertension
         b) Marfan's syndrome or other connective tissue disease
         c) Congenital heart disease
         d) Pregnancy
         e) Chest trauma
   b. *Objective data*
      1) Physical examination
         a) Variable right- and left-sided BPs
         b) Precordial systolic murmur or diastolic aortic valve murmur, especially heard at right sternal border
         c) Decreased peripheral pulses/pulse deficits
         d) Paresthesia, hemiplegia, paraplegia

        e) Pallor or diaphoresis

        f) Oliguria

        g) Peripheral cyanosis

        h) Hypertension: common with distal dissection

        i) Altered level of consciousness/coma

        j) Hypotension: common with proximal dissection

        k) Patient in extreme pain, attempting to find position of comfort

    2) Diagnostic procedures

        a) Laboratory

           (1) CBC

               (a) Hematocrit tends to fall

               (b) White blood cell count 12,000 to 20,000 cells/mm^3

           (2) Type and cross-match blood

           (3) Serum creatinine and BUN

        b) ECG

           (1) Normal in one third of patients

           (2) LV hypertrophy (if patient previously hypertensive)

           (3) Patient with proximal dissection may demonstrate signs of MI or coronary insufficiency secondary to dissecting flap involving coronary arteries

        c) Chest radiograph

           (1) Widening of aortic silhouette

           (2) Nonspecific widening of superior mediastinum

           (3) "Calcium sign": intimal calcification

           (4) Left-sided pleural effusion

        d) Aortogram

           (1) Visualization of two lumina

           (2) Visualization of intimal tear

           (3) Deformity of aortic lumen

           (4) Thickening of aortic walls

           (5) Aortic valve insufficiency

           (6) Branch vessel abnormalities

        e) CT scan

        f) Magnetic resonance imaging (MRI)

        g) Transesophageal echocardiography

2. Analysis: differential nursing diagnosis/collaborative problems

  a. Pain related to dissection

  b. Altered cerebral, renal, and peripheral tissue perfusion related to decreased blood flow

  c. Anxiety/fear related to altered health status, treatment, and prognosis

3. Planning/interventions

  a. Maintain airway, breathing, circulation

  b. Pain relief indicative of dissection stability: monitor intensity, location, provocation, quality, time

  c. Obtain IV access with a large-bore catheter at two sites

  d. Initiate cardiac monitor, NIBP, and pulse oximetry

  e. Administer pharmacological agents to reduce arterial BP as ordered

    1) Nitroprusside

    2) Labetalol

    3) Trimethaphan: does not require adjunct beta blockers

  f. Administer pharmacological agents to decrease force of myocardial contraction as ordered

    1) Beta blocker: first choice

2) Calcium channel antagonist, if beta blockers contraindicated
g. *Administer morphine as ordered for pain*
h. *Assist patient in finding position of comfort*
i. *Continuously monitor and assess*
1) Level of consciousness
2) Pupillary response
3) Bilateral motor strength, ability
4) Urine output
5) Skin color
6) Skin temperature
7) Skin moisture
8) Capillary refill
9) Pulse quality
10) Peripheral neurological status
a) Paresthesia
b) Paralysis or decreased movement
c) Pain or tingling
11) BP in both arms
j. *Administer IV fluids in setting of hypotension*
k. *Insert Foley catheter*
l. *Anticipate possibility of emergency department thoracotomy*
m. *Anticipate possibility of immediate need for operative intervention and preparation for surgery*
n. *Anticipate/assist with arterial cannulation and BP monitoring*
o. *Anticipate/assist with central venous catheter or pulmonary artery catheter*
p. *Maintain calm, efficient manner*
q. *Explain all procedures to patient*
r. *Allow significant other at bedside if possible*
4. **Expected outcomes/evaluation** (see Appendix B)

I. Acute pericarditis

Acute pericarditis occurs as a result of inflammation of the pericardium. The acute changes seen with pericarditis include infiltration of polymorphonuclear leukocytes into the pericardium, increased pericardial vascularity, and deposition of fibrin. The inflammation may extend to adjacent structures and may produce an exudate. The causes of acute pericarditis include idiopathic, viral, bacterial, and fungal infections; connective tissue diseases (lupus erythematosus, rheumatoid arthritis); renal failure; neoplastic disorders; radiation, and drug-induced myxedema, and ischemia; and tissue injury (MI, cardiac surgery, trauma). It is more common in men than women and in adults than children. Management is dependent on the etiology. Viral, idiopathic, post-MI and postpericardiotomy are usually self-limiting. Complications of pericarditis include recurrence of episodes, which is the most common and most troublesome, and hemodynamic compromise secondary to cardiac compression. Cardiac compression may be due to an effusion, resulting in pericardial tamponade, fibrosis formation, which results in cardiac restriction, or a combination of both.

1. **Assessment**
a. *Subjective data*
1) History of present illness
a) Chest pain
(1) Provocative factors
(a) Deep inspiration

        (b) Recumbency

        (c) Coughing

        (d) Movement

        (e) Swallowing

    (2) Palliative factors

        (a) Sitting forward

        (b) Leaning forward

    (3) Quality

        (a) Severe, sharp

        (b) Dull ache

        (c) Oppressive

    (4) Region/radiation

        (a) Retrosternal

        (b) Left precordial regions

        (c) Radiates to back, neck, or side

        (d) Epigastrium

    (5) Timing

        (a) Sudden in onset

        (b) Persistent for days

  b) General malaise

  c) Fever/chills: maximal on first day

  d) Dyspnea

  e) Cough

  f) Weight loss

2) Medical history

  a) Tuberculosis: may infect the pericardium

  b) Congenital anomalies: congenital pericardial cysts

  c) Immune or collagen disorders: systemic lupus erythematosus, rheumatic fever

  d) MI: Dressler's syndrome

  e) Neoplastic disease: radiation therapy, adenocarcinoma of breast

  f) Drug use (hydralazine, procainamide, and anticoagulants)

  g) Uremia: pericarditis is common in patients receiving hemodialysis

  h) Cardiac surgery: postpericardiotomy syndrome

  i) Cardiac trauma

b. *Objective data*

1) Physical examination

  a) Pericardial friction rub: hallmark of acute pericarditis

    (1) Heard best to left of lower part of sternum with patient leaning forward, end expiration

    (2) Sounds scratchy, superficial; occasionally has a "leathery" quality

    (3) Usually triphasic

        (a) Ventricular systole

        (b) Ventricular diastole

        (c) Atrial systole

    (4) Characteristically transient and may change in quality

  b) Tachycardia

  c) Fever (in pediatric patient, may be very high or low grade)

  d) Tachypnea

2) Diagnostic procedures

  a) ECG

    (1) Four stages

(a) ST-segment elevation (early), with upright T waves, usually present in all leads except aVR and V_1

(b) T waves flatten, ST returns to baseline after several days

(c) T-wave inversion

(d) T waves return to normal, may take weeks to months

(2) Best seen in inferior leads (II, III, and aVF) and sometimes in apical leads (V_5, V_6)

(3) ECG changes occur in approximately 90% of patients with acute pericarditis

b) CBC

c) Creatinine, BUN

d) Serum electrolytes

e) Blood cultures

f) Urinalysis

g) Chest radiographs: are helpful in detecting pericardial effusion and/or underlying etiology (i.e., malignancy, tuberculosis [TB])

h) Echocardiogram: most sensitive and accurate in detecting pericarditis

2. **Analysis: differential nursing diagnosis/collaborative problems**

   a. *Pain related to inflammation*

   b. *Infection risk related to altered immune response*

   c. *Anxiety/fear related to pain, altered health status*

3. **Planning/interventions**

   a. *Provide supplemental oxygen, cardiac monitoring*

   b. *Assist patient in assuming a position of comfort*

   c. *Administer anti-inflammatory agents (e.g., aspirin, ibuprofen, indomethacin) as ordered*

   d. *Prepare patient for pericardiocentesis if necessary*

      1) Gram's stain

      2) Aerobic, anaerobic cultures

   e. *Obtain blood cultures as ordered*

   f. *Administer antipyretics as ordered*

   g. *Administer antibiotics as ordered*

   h. *Monitor vital signs*

   i. *Maintain calm, efficient manner*

   j. *Explain all procedures to patient*

   k. *Allow significant other at bedside if possible*

   l. *Provide reassurance*

4. **Expected outcomes/evaluation** (see Appendix B)

J. Infective endocarditis

Infective endocarditis is an infection of the endocardium and heart valves. The infection may be subacute or acute, depending on the presentation and progression of the disease and the virulence of the pathogen. Subacute bacterial endocarditis (SBE) usually occurs in patients with congenital or acquired valvular heart disease, it evolves over several weeks to months, and patients are generally less toxic. Acute bacterial endocarditis (ABE) is differentiated from SBE by the greatly accelerated pace of days to weeks, it usually affects normal heart valves, and patients present extremely toxic with metastatic infection. *Staphylococcus aureus* is the most common pathogen in ABE and *Streptococcus viridans* the most common in SBE, but many bacteria, fungi, mycobacteria, and a host of other organisms may be the causative pathogen in infective endocarditis. The entry of the pathogen to the system may be from a very minor infection on the skin to major surgery. Most pathogens originate from the upper airway, genitourinary and gastrointestinal tracts, or skin. Risk factors include valvular disease, particularly mitral valve prolapse with systolic murmur, congenital heart defects, rheumatic heart disease, prosthetic heart valves, intravenous drug users, and patients with long-term venous access catheters. The pathophysiology behind the development of infective endocarditis includes an alteration in the normal endothelium to which platelets and fibrin deposit. At this time, circulating organisms adhere to the valvular surface and colonization begins. Further growth of the organism coupled with platelet-fibrin aggregation in a complex process forms a vegetation that can shed microorganisms and embolize fragments into the blood. The embolization of the septic fragments can infarct or infect any distal site. Pulmonary emboli are common with tricuspid involvement; however, any organ/ tissue may be infected, including the brain, kidney, spleen, bone, and joints. The infection of the cardiac tissue can be catastrophic, destroying the valve and extending to adjacent structures, producing rupture of the chordae tendinea and formation of abscesses or fistulas through the cardiac vessels and chambers, all of which can lead to progressive heart failure, conduction disturbances, and dysrhythmias. Endocarditis is uncommon in the pediatric patient and is primarily associated with congenital heart abnormalities, particularly status postsurgical repair.

1. **Assessment**
   a. *Subjective data*
      1) History of present illness
         a) Fever: in SBE usually low grade and remittent; in ABE acute and abrupt, greater than 102°F with chills
         b) Anorexia
         c) Weight loss
         d) Night sweats
         e) Arthralgia/myalgia
         f) Fatigue/malaise
         g) Dyspnea
         h) Cough
         i) Pleuritic chest pain
         j) Hemoptysis
         k) Headache/signs of stroke
         l) Confusion
         m) Abdominal pain
         n) Back pain
      2) Medical history
         a) Cardiac surgery, prosthetic heart valve
         b) Congenital or acquired valve disease
         c) IV drug abuse
         d) Rheumatic heart disease
         e) Cardiac pacemaker
         f) Recent GI or genitourinary disorder
         g) Patient with valve disease or prosthetic valve who underwent recent dental procedure and not treated prophylactically
   b. *Objective data*
      1) Physical examination
         a) Fever: may be absent in elderly, debilitated, those with chronic renal failure
         b) Murmur
         c) Janeway lesions: petechial lesions on hands, feet

  d) Roth's spots: on ophthalmic examination
  e) Splinter hemorrhages of nails: caused by emboli
  f) Osler's nodes: painful lesions to fingertips
  g) Splenomegaly: from emboli in spleen, more common with SBE
  h) Hematuria: from emboli in kidney
  i) Proteinuria: decreased glomerular filtration
  j) Signs of cardiac failure (may be evident)
  k) Petechiae: on conjunctiva, palate, neck upper trunk, extremities
  l) Clubbing: with long-standing SBE
  m) Neurological changes associated with embolic stroke
 2) Diagnostic procedures
  a) Blood cultures: most important in making diagnosis
  b) CBC: anemia common with SBE
  c) Creatinine, BUN
  d) Electrolytes, serum glucose
  e) Sedimentation rate: elevated in both groups
  f) Urinalysis: proteinuria and microscopic hematuria common
  g) Twelve- to 15-lead ECG: conduction abnormalities may be present with septal abscess
  h) Echocardiogram: can visualize mobility and extent of vegetations, valve dysfunction, regurgitation, and myocardial abscesses
  i) Head CT: for patients with neurological signs and symptoms
  j) MRI

2. **Analysis: differential nursing diagnosis/collaborative problems**
  a. *Infection, high risk for related to dissemination of septic emboli*
  b. *Cardiac output decreased related to potential development of heart failure secondary to valve leaflet destruction*
  c. *Anxiety/fear related to altered health status and prognosis*

3. **Planning/interventions**
  a. *Monitor and maintain airway, breathing, circulation*
  b. *Establish IV access and infuse normal saline at KVO rate*
  c. *Obtain four to six specimens for blood culture over 2 to 3 hours; cultures should be aerobic, anaerobic, and fungal*
  d. *Begin antibiotic therapy after blood cultures obtained*
  e. *Administer antipyretic medications as ordered*
  f. *Continuously monitor and assess*
   1) Cardiac rhythm
   2) Vital signs
   3) Heart, lung sounds
   4) Level of consciousness
   5) Peripheral perfusion
   6) Intake and output
   7) Jugular vein distention
  g. *Prepare for/assist with pulmonary artery catheter placement if patient is in heart failure*
  h. *Maintain calm, efficient manner*
  i. *Explain all procedures to patient*
  j. *Attempt to remain with patient if echocardiogram performed in emergency department*
  k. *Encourage questions from patient; allow significant other at bedside, if possible*

4. **Expected outcomes/evaluation** (see Appendix B)

K. Acute arterial occlusion

Acute disruption of arterial blood flow results when an embolism, thrombosis, or trauma occludes the vessel. Embolism is the most common cause of acute arterial occlusion; approximately 80% of emboli originate in the heart. The majority of emboli lodge in the femoral artery, followed by the iliac, aortic, popliteal, mesenteric, branchial, and renal arteries. Occlusion secondary to thrombosis generally occurs at areas of stenosis, which is due to atherosclerosis or is iatrogenic (i.e., intra-arterial catheters). Less common causes include trauma, vasospasm (usually secondary to IV drug use), occlusions of vascular grafts, and dissecting aneurysms. The sudden interruption of blood flow, without collateral circulation, leads to ischemia of the tissues supplied by the affected artery. If untreated, cellular necrosis occurs, which may lead to the development of gangrene and a subsequent loss of the involved extremity. There is no set time when restoration of blood flow will reverse the injury or cellular necrosis; therefore, it is imperative that recognition and treatment be expeditious to maintain limb or organ viability.

1. **Assessment**
   a. *Subjective data*
      1) History of present illness
         a) Pain
            (1) Provocation
               (a) Movement/exercise
               (b) Pain at rest
            (2) Quality
               (a) Discomfort
               (b) Burning
               (c) Throbbing
            (3) Region/radiation: to area distal to occlusion
            (4) Severity: excruciating
            (5) Timing
               (a) Instantaneous
               (b) Relentless
         b) Coldness
         c) Numbness
         d) Paralysis
      2) Medical history
         a) Predisposition for mural thrombi
            (1) History of MI
            (2) Rheumatic heart disease
            (3) Atrial fibrillation
            (4) Previous cardiac surgery
               (a) Mitral commissurotomy
               (b) Prosthetic cardiac valve
            (5) LV aneurysm
            (6) Chronic CHF
            (7) Recent MI
         b) Peripheral atherosclerotic disease
         c) Extremity trauma
         d) Recent placement of intra-atrial catheters
   b. *Objective data*
      1) Physical examination
         a) Pallor, cyanosis, or mottled appearance
         b) Pulselessness (distally)

c) Paresthesia
d) Paralysis
e) Polar coldness
f) Tenderness with muscle palpation
g) Muscle rigor: with prolonged ischemia
h) Petechiae: associated with microemboli
2) Diagnostic procedures
a) Arteriography
b) Doppler ultrasound flow study
c) PT, PTT
d) CBC
e) ECG

2. Analysis: differential nursing diagnosis/collaborative problems
a. *Tissue perfusion, altered related to occlusion*
b. *Pain related to ischemia secondary to occlusion*
c. *Anxiety/fear related to altered health status, treatments, prognosis*

3. Planning/interventions
a. *Elevate head of bed to allow gravitational blood flow to ischemic extremity*
b. *Administer anticoagulants as ordered*
c. *Prepare patient for possibility of one of following procedures:*
1) Thrombolytic infusion
2) Embolectomy
3) Balloon catheter extraction
4) Bypass grafting
d. *Continuously monitor and assess*
1) Pain (presence or absence)
2) Pulses (quality, capillary refill)
3) Pallor (skin color)
4) Paresthesia (sensation)
5) Paralysis (movement)
6) Skin temperature
e. *Assist patient in finding position of comfort*
f. *Administer analgesics as ordered*
g. *Provide warm environment: do not apply heat to area*
h. *Do not elevate ischemic extremity*
i. *Maintain calm, efficient manner*
j. *Explain all procedures to patient*
k. *Allow significant other at bedside if possible*

4. Expected outcomes/evaluation (see Appendix B)

L. Venous thrombosis

Venous thrombosis is the occlusion of a vein by a blood clot, commonly in the lower extremities, often accompanied by inflammation. Signs and symptoms vary depending on the patient's underlying disease and location and extent of the thrombosis. The etiology is related to the integrity of the veins, stasis of blood flow, and hypercoagulability states (Virchow's triad). The major complication associated with venous thrombosis is pulmonary embolism, which occurs when a segment of the thrombosis breaks off and lodges in the pulmonary vasculature. Risk factors for venous thrombosis include age greater than 40 years, cardiac disease, malignancy, history of hypercoagulability, and use of estrogens and oral contraceptives. Elderly patients are particularly at risk related to the venous changes associated with aging.

1. Assessment

a. *Subjective data*
   1) History of present illness
      a) Pain
         (1) Provocation: walking
         (2) Quality: aching, throbbing
         (3) Region: localized at point of occlusion
         (4) Severity: aching, throbbing
         (5) Timing: constant
      b) Swelling
      c) Deep muscle tenderness
      d) Fever
   2) Medical history
      a) Recent surgery and anesthesia
      b) Recent traumatic event (injury)
      c) Postpartum
      d) Recent prolonged bed rest
      e) Heart failure
      f) Hematological disorders
      g) Malignancy
      h) Obesity
      i) Oral contraceptive use
      j) Venous disorders
      k) Recent MI
      l) Thrombotic disease
b. *Objective data*
   1) Physical examination
      a) Erythema
      b) Swelling/induration
      c) Warmth
      d) Deep muscle tenderness on palpation/at rest
      e) Asymmetry between extremities
      f) Fever
      g) Positive Homans's sign
   2) Diagnostic procedures
      a) CBC
      b) Sedimentation rate
      c) PT, PTT
      d) Radioactive fibrinogen scintigraphy
      e) Doppler ultrasonic flow study
      f) Impedance plethysmography
      g) Venography: gold standard

2. **Analysis: differential nursing diagnosis/collaborative problems**
   a. *Pain related to inflammation and obstructed venous output*
   b. *Risk for injury related to risk of pulmonary embolus*
3. **Planning/interventions**
   a. *Assist patient in finding position of comfort*
   b. *Elevate affected extremity*
   c. *Administer analgesia as ordered*
   d. *Provide warm, moist compresses to area*
   e. *Administer anticoagulants for thrombosis, as ordered*
   f. *Administer thrombolytics, as ordered*
   g. *Apply elastic stockings or Ace bandages as ordered*
   h. *Assist patient in maintaining bed rest*

     i. Monitor intake/output; provide fluids
     j. Continuously monitor and assess
       1) Vital signs
       2) Heart and lung sounds
       3) Cardiac rhythm
       4) Presence of chest or abdominal pain, dyspnea, or cough
       5) Peripheral pulses
       6) Skin temperature and color
4. Expected outcomes/evaluation (see Appendix B)

M. Peripheral vascular disease

    Peripheral circulation is usually defined as the circulation outside of the heart. Arteriosclerosis is a major cause of peripheral vascular disease (PVD). Arteriosclerosis is a hardening of the arteries. Atherosclerosis is a form of arteriosclerosis, in which intimal fatty lesions are produced and narrow the vessel's lumen. Atherosclerosis affects the large and medium-sized arteries. It is an insidious process that begins in very young persons (usually in their 20s), but does not begin to manifest clinically until 20 to 40 years later (at 40–60 years of age). Symptoms are due to the narrowing of the vessel lumen, to which blood flow is directly related. Symptoms become increasingly severe with disease progression. The etiology remains unclear; however, many risk factors have been identified, including heredity, male sex, increasing age, cigarette smoking, HTN, and hyperlipidemia. Diabetes, obesity, and inactivity are considered associated risk factors.

    Two other conditions of PVD are Raynaud's disease and thromboangiitis obliterans (Buerger's disease). Raynaud's disease is characterized by episodic intense vasospasm of the digits, particularly the fingers, in response to the cold or stress. Women are more prone to Raynaud's disease. The ischemia produced by the vasospasm produces pallor followed by cyanosis, coldness, and numbness of the affected digit. There may also be decreased mobility. As the vasospasm and ischemia resolve, hyperemia produces intense rubor and throbbing pain, after which there is a return to normal color. Raynaud's disease is divided into two types: primary, or Raynaud's disease, for which there is no known cause; and secondary, or Raynaud's phenomenon, which is associated with previous vessel injury. The former tends to be less severe. Chronic and frequent attacks may lead to ischemic changes, including thickening of the fingertips and nails, ulceration, and the development of gangrene. The treatment is aimed at decreasing or eliminating the vasospasm and reducing the ischemic injury.

    Thromboangiitis obliterans is an inflammatory disorder characterized by thrombus formation, usually affecting the medium-sized arteries in the lower leg and foot. The etiology is unknown, but it predominately affects males between the ages of 25 and 40 years who are heavy smokers. The disease produces decreased blood flow to the affected limb, which results in ischemia, pain, intermittent claudication, decreased or absent peripheral pulses, and changes in skin color (from cyanotic to reddish blue). Because of the decreased blood flow, the skin becomes thin and shiny, with decreased hair growth and nail thickening; eventually ulcerations and gangrene may develop. The treatment priorities are to increase blood flow to the affected extremity and prevent further injury. Smoking cessation is mandatory for these patients.

1. Assessment
    a. Subjective
      1) Pain
        a) Palliative/provocative

(1) Cold environment

(2) Stress

(3) Exercise

(4) Relieved by removal/discontinuation of agonist

b) Quality

(1) Severe

(2) Throbbing

c) Radiation/region

(1) Fingers, toes

(2) Calf, foot

d) Timing

(1) After exercise

(2) During stressful situations

(3) Exposure to cold environment

2) Numbness

3) Tingling

b. *Objective*

1) Physical assessment

a) Coldness to touch

b) Decreased/absent pulses

c) Pallor

d) Cyanosis

e) Rubor

f) Thin, shiny skin

g) Thickened fingertips and nails

h) Ulcerations/necrosis

2) Diagnostics

a) Antinuclear antibody (ANA), CBC

b) Doppler studies

c) Angiography

d) MRI

e) Impedance plethysmography

f) Thermography

2. Analysis: differential nursing diagnosis/collaborative problems

a. *Altered tissue perfusion related to vasospasm, narrowing of vessel lumen*

b. *Pain related to ischemia secondary to vasospasm*

c. *Anxiety/fear related to altered health status, treatments, prognosis*

3. Planning/interventions

a. *Discontinue precipitating factors (e.g., stress, cold)*

b. *Prepare to administer vasodilators, as ordered*

1) Calcium channel blockers

2) Adrenergic blocking agents

c. *Continuously monitor and assess*

1) Pain (presence or absence)

2) Pulses (quality, capillary refill)

3) Pallor (skin color)

4) Paresthesia (sensation)

5) Paralysis (movement)

6) Skin temperature

d. *Assist patient in finding position of comfort*

e. *Administer analgesics as ordered*

f. *Provide warm environment*

g. *Do not elevate ischemic extremity*

h. Maintain calm, efficient manner
i. Explain all procedures to patient
j. Allow significant other at bedside if possible
4. Expected outcomes/evaluation (see Appendix B)

III. SPECIFIC SURGICAL CARDIOVASCULAR EMERGENCIES

A. Myocardial contusion

Myocardial contusion is usually the result of blunt trauma from vehicular, industrial, or sports injuries. The most common mechanism is the direct impact of the chest into the steering wheel in motor vehicle collisions (MVCs). Blunt injury to the heart may range from subepicardial petechiae to full-thickness contusions with fragmentation and necrosis to actual rupture of the heart. The pathological lesions of cardiac contusion are similar to those of acute MI resulting from coronary artery occlusion. The difference lies in the amount of hemorrhage, which may be marked in cardiac contusion. The areas most frequently injured include the right anteroapical wall, the anterior interventricular septum, and the left anteroapical wall. The sequelae of myocardial contusion is rarely fatal; however, patients are at risk for sudden dysrhythmias and very rarely, if there is a significant transmural injury, a ventricular aneurysm may develop. MVCs are the usual mechanism of injury among children, whereas pedestrian-auto crashes and falls are the common mechanism among the elderly.

1. Assessment
  a. Subjective data
   1) History of present illness
    a) Recent blunt trauma to chest
    b) Chest pain
     (1) Character, location, and radiation similar to MI
     (2) Usually unaffected by coronary vasodilatory drugs
    c) Pain with inspiration usually secondary to sternal fracture
    d) Patient may be asymptomatic
   2) Medical history
    a) Angina
    b) Previous MI
    c) HTN
    d) Chronic heart failure
    e) Alcohol or drug use
    f) Previous cardiovascular surgery
  b. Objective data
   1) Physical examination
    a) May be normal without physical signs of trauma
    b) May be associated with severe multisystem injuries
    c) Contusion, ecchymosis on chest wall
    d) Tachycardia
    e) Rapid, shallow respirations
    f) Elevated or low BP
    g) Signs of LV failure
     (1) Pulmonary crackles
     (2) S_3 gallop
   2) Diagnostic procedures
    a) ECG
     (1) Sinus tachycardia

      (2) Conduction and rhythm disturbances

         (a) Premature atrial or ventricular contractions

         (b) Atrial fibrillation

         (c) SA block, nodal rhythm, AV block

         (d) VF and VT

      (3) Nonspecific ST- and T-wave abnormalities

      (4) Pattern of pericarditis

      (5) Bundle branch block: usually right

      (6) Infarct pattern

   b) Cardiac serum markers

   c) Echocardiography

   d) Chest radiograph

   e) Central venous pressure (CVP): may indicate right ventricular dysfunction

   f) Multiple gated acquisition (MUGA) scan

  2. Analysis: differential nursing diagnosis/collaborative problems

   a. Risk for decreased cardiac output related to myocardial dysfunction secondary to myocardial contusion

   b. Pain related to chest wall and cardiac injury

   c. Anxiety/fear related to need for medical intervention for sudden alteration in health status, treatments, and prognosis

  3. Planning/interventions

   a. Maintain airway, breathing, circulation

   b. Provide supplemental oxygen

   c. Obtain IV access with two large-bore catheters; replace fluid volume as needed

   d. Initiate cardiac monitor, NIBP, and pulse oximetry

   e. Provide analgesia as necessary; avoid nitrates

   f. Treat dysrhythmias if necessary

   g. Continuously monitor and assess

      1) Vital signs

      2) Heart and lung sounds

      3) Level of consciousness

      4) Peripheral perfusion

      5) Intake and output

   h. Assist patient in finding position of comfort

   i. Administer analgesics if ordered

   j. Maintain calm, efficient manner

   k. Explain all procedures to patient

   l. Allow significant other at bedside if possible

   m. Eliminate unnecessary stressors to decrease myocardial workload

  4. Expected outcomes/evaluation (see Appendix B)

B. Cardiac tamponade

    Cardiac tamponade occurs when fluid accumulates in the pericardial space. This results in an elevation in the intracardiac pressure, a decrease in diastolic filling, which is progressive, and, subsequently, reduction in stroke volume and cardiac output. The etiology of cardiac tamponade is diverse; the most common causes are malignancies, pericarditis, uremia, and trauma. The condition may be acute, as with trauma, or chronic, as with malignancies. Clinical manifestations will be dependent on the onset. Acute tamponade produces a patient who is in extremis, whereas with chronic tamponade the patient is ill but not in extremis. The classic clinical presentation for cardiac tamponade is known as Beck's triad, in which the patient demonstrates hypotension, an increase in CVP (jugular venous distention), and muffled heart tones. In the acute setting, it may take less than 100 cc of fluid to produce significant and life-threatening symptoms, whereas in the chronic environment, it may take 1 to 2 L. Prognosis is dependent on the etiology and timeliness of intervention. It is important to remember that cardiac tamponade is both an injury and a symptom; identification and treatment of the underlying cause are paramount in preventing recurrence.

1. **Assessment**
    a. *Subjective data*
        1) History of present illness
            a) Penetrating or blunt injury of chest, neck, back, or abdomen
            b) Weapon
                (1) Knife
                (2) Gun
                (3) Other missile
            c) Recent repair of cardiac lesions
            d) Dyspnea
            e) Anxious
            f) Chest pain
            g) Fatigue/malaise
        2) Medical history
            a) Cardiac disease
            b) Infectious or neoplastic disease
            c) Renal failure: dependent on hemodialysis
    b. *Objective data*
        1) Physical examination
            a) Penetrating wound to neck, anterior or posterior thorax, upper abdomen
            b) Beck's triad
                (1) Venous pressure elevation
                (2) Decline in arterial pressure
                (3) Muffled heart tones
            c) Tachypnea/rales
            d) Kussmaul's sign: rise in venous pressure with inspiration when breathing spontaneously
            e) Jugular venous distention from elevated venous pressure; may be absent in hypovolemia
            f) Pulsus paradoxus: systolic BP decreases with inspiration 10 mm Hg or more
            g) Narrow pulse pressure
            h) Tachycardia
            i) Cold, moist skin
            j) Lips, digits cyanotic
            k) Decreased urinary output
            l) Decreasing level of consciousness: coma
            m) Hepatomegaly
        2) Diagnostic procedures
            a) Chest radiograph
            b) Pericardiocentesis
                (1) Hematocrit will be lower in blood aspirated from pericardial sac than in simultaneously determined venous sample
                (2) Pericardial blood may or may not clot; if the blood has clotted, aspiration will not benefit patient, and open pericardiotomy will

be necessary; generally, pericardial blood does not clot and is diagnostic
- c) Echocardiogram
- d) Type and cross-match blood
- e) CBC
- f) ECG: only if time permits; do not delay treatment to obtain an ECG; may see electrical alternans, ST- and T-wave abnormalities, pattern of pericarditis, low voltage with limb leads
- g) CVP

2. **Analysis: differential nursing diagnosis/collaborative problems**
    a. *Cardiac output decreased related to impaired cardiac filling and contractility and decreased venous return secondary to increased intrathoracic pressure*

3. **Planning/interventions**
    a. *Maintain airway, breathing, circulation*
    b. *Obtain IV access: two large-bore catheters 14-gauge, 16-gauge; replace volume as indicated*
    c. *Initiate cardiac monitoring, NIBP, and pulse oximetry*
    d. *Prepare for and assist with following procedures as indicated:*
       1) Pericardiocentesis
       2) Thoracotomy
       3) Internal cardiac massage
       4) Internal defibrillation
    e. *Continuously monitor and assess*
       1) Vital signs
       2) Heart and lung sounds
       3) Level of consciousness
       4) Peripheral perfusion
       5) Intake and output
       6) Cardiac rhythm
    f. *Insert urinary catheter and nasogastric tube*
    g. *Prepare patient for immediate surgical intervention*

4. **Expected outcomes/evaluation** (see Appendix B)

C. Traumatic aortic injury

Aortic injury can be the result of blunt or penetrating trauma. MVCs are the most common cause of aortic injury. Aortic injury may result in complete rupture, which often leads to in sudden death at the scene of the accident (approximately 90%). When the aorta is subjected to traumatic forces, it may tear, usually at points of attachment, or it may be pinched between the spinal column and the manubrium. If the injury/tear does not involve the adventitial layer (the outermost layer), the patient may survive. As a result of the intact adventitia, an aneurysm can form. Rupture may occur at any time. Diagnosis is suspected by chest radiograph and confirmed by arteriography, transesophageal echocardiogram, or CT scan. Surgical intervention is indicated.

1. **Assessment**
    a. *Subjective data*
       1) History of present illness
          a) Blunt trauma to chest or abdomen, deceleration mechanism (frontal or lateral impact)
          b) Pain
             (1) Chest, midscapular, back
             (2) Generally severe

           (3) Unrelenting
     2) Medical history
        a) Atherosclerotic heart disease
        b) Prior thoracic injuries or surgery
  b. Objective data
     1) Physical examination
        a) Dyspnea, tachypnea
        b) Tachycardia
        c) Dysphagia/hoarseness
        d) Discrepancy in BP between right and left arms
        e) Possible harsh systolic murmur over precordium
        f) Varying degrees of shock
        g) Chest wall ecchymosis
        h) Paraplegia
        i) Decreased quality of femoral pulses versus radial pulses
     2) Diagnostic procedures
        a) Chest radiograph
           (1) Widened mediastinum
           (2) Obliteration of the aortic knob
           (3) Tracheal deviation to the right
           (4) Presence of pleural cap
           (5) Fractures of first and second ribs
           (6) Depression of left main stem bronchus
           (7) Deviation of esophagus (nasogastric tube) to right
           (8) Shift of right main stem bronchus up and to right
        b) Aortogram: extravasation of dye
        c) CT scan
        d) Transesophageal echocardiography (TEE)
        e) ECG
        f) Type and cross-match blood
        g) CBC

2. **Analysis: differential nursing diagnosis/collaborative problems**
  a. Fluid volume deficit related to hemorrhage secondary to aortic rupture
  b. Cardiac output decreased related to decreased circulating blood volume secondary to hemorrhage

3. **Planning/interventions**
  a. Maintain airway, breathing, circulation
  b. Obtain venous access with two large-bore catheters; fluid resuscitate, as necessary
  c. Administer type-specific or fully cross-matched blood as ordered
  d. Prepare for autotransfusion
  e. Insert Foley catheter and nasogastric tube
  f. Continuously monitor and assess
     1) Vital signs
     2) Heart, lung sounds
     3) Level of consciousness
     4) Peripheral perfusion
     5) Intake and output
     6) Cardiac rhythm
     7) Skin color
     8) Skin temperature, moisture
     9) Capillary refill
     10) Quality of pulses

    g. *Periodically monitor arterial pH*

    h. *Prepare patient for immediate surgical intervention or transfer to surgical facility*

    i. *Administer medications as ordered (if treatment delay for surgical repair)*

       1) Antihypertensives

       2) Beta blockers

    j. *Attempt to minimize patient's anxiety to reduce sympathetic stimulation*

  4. Expected outcomes/evaluation (see Appendix B)

D. Arterial trauma

    Arterial injuries are the result of blunt or penetrating trauma. Penetrating trauma is a more common and obvious cause of injury; however, blunt trauma can be more dangerous because it is not so obvious and occurs in combination with more obvious injuries. Blunt trauma is commonly associated with MVCs and crush injuries, and penetrating trauma is most commonly due to gunshot wounds and stab wounds. Vessel injury can be direct, as when the vessel is lacerated by a knife, or indirect, as in secondary to a displaced fracture or dislocation or a result of the concussive effects associated with gunshot wounds. Injuries to vessels may include lacerations, hematomas, and pseudoaneurysms. Neurological signs often accompany vessel injuries because of the close proximity of nerves to vessels. The major consequence of arterial injuries is ischemia distally, which requires immediate surgical repair

  1. Assessment

    a. *Subjective data*

       1) History of present illness

         a) Shotgun wound or injury

         b) Stabbing

         c) Blast injury

         d) Crush injury with fracture

         e) Numbness/tingling

         f) Pain

         g) Paralysis

       2) Medical history

         a) Diabetes

         b) Peripheral vascular disease

    b. *Objective data*

       1) Physical examination

         a) Hemorrhage from open wound

         b) Signs of shock from blood loss

         c) Signs of pulsatile or expanding hematoma

         d) Difference in BP between extremities

         e) Prolonged capillary refill

         f) Diminished or absent distal pulse

         g) Pallor

         h) Paresthesia

         i) Coolness

         j) Paralysis

       2) Diagnostic procedures

         a) Arteriogram: only in stable patient

         b) Digital subtraction angiography

         c) Doppler study

        d) CBC

        e) Type and cross-match blood

  2. Analysis: differential nursing diagnosis/collaborative problems

     a. Tissue perfusion altered peripheral related to arterial injury

     b. Risk for fluid volume deficit related to continued blood loss

     c. Anxiety/fear related to lack of knowledge regarding treatment and concerns about altered health status

  3. Planning/interventions

     a. Maintain and monitor airway, breathing, circulation

     b. Control bleeding

     c. Supplemental oxygen

     d. Obtain IV access; replace intravascular fluid volume as needed

     e. Prepare patient for surgical intervention

     f. Continuously monitor and assess

        1) Vital signs, pulse oximetry

        2) Arterial pulses

        3) Capillary refill

        4) Skin color, temperature

        5) Sensation

        6) Motor ability

        7) Intake and output

     g. Insert Foley catheter as indicated

     h. Maintain calm, efficient manner

     i. Explain all procedures to patient

     j. If possible, allow significant other to see patient before surgery

  4. Expected outcomes/evaluation (see Appendix B)

BIBLIOGRAPHY

Abolnik, I. Z., & Corer, G. R. (1995). Pinning down infective endocarditis. *Emergency Medicine, 27*(8), 85–90.

American College of Surgeons. (1997). *Advanced trauma life support course.* Chicago, IL: Author.

American Heart Association. (1997–1999). *Advanced cardiac life support.* Dallas, TX: Author.

American Heart Association, American Academy of Pediatrics. (1994). *Textbook of pediatric advanced life support.* Dallas, TX: Author.

Bennett, K. A., & Grines, C. L. (1990). Current controversies in patient selection for thrombolytic therapy. *Journal of Emergency Nursing, 16*(3), 191–194.

Bernardo, L. M., Conway, A., & Bove, M. (1990). The ABC method of emotional assessment and intervention: A new approach in pediatric emergency care. *Journal of Emergency Nursing, 16*(2), 70–76.

Braunwald, E. (Ed.). (1997). *Heart disease* (Vols. 1–2). Philadelphia: W. B. Saunders.

Butler, K. L., Moore, E. E., & Harken, A. H. (1996). Traumatic rupture of the descending thoracic aorta. *AORN Journal, 63,* 917–925.

Calhoun, D. A., & Oparil, S. (1990). Treatment of hypertensive crisis. *New England Journal of Medicine, 323*(17), 1177–1183.

Cardona, V. D., Hurn, P. D., Bastnagal Mason, P. J., Scanlon, A. M., & Veise-Berry, S. W. (Eds.). (1994). *Trauma nursing: From resuscitation through rehabilitation* (2nd ed.). Philadelphia: W. B. Saunders.

Carpenito, L. J. (1989). *Nursing diagnosis: Application to clinical practice.* Philadelphia: J. B. Lippincott.

Colletti, R. C. (1990). Diagnosis of acute myocardial infarction in the emergency department. *Journal of Emergency Nursing, 16*(3), 187–190.

Cunha, B. A., Gill, M. V., & Lazar, J. M. (1996). Acute infective endocarditis: Diagnostic and therapeutic approach. *Infectious Disease Clinics of North America, 10,* 811–833.

Daily, E. K. (1991). Clinical management of patients receiving thrombolytic therapy. *Heart & Lung, 20*(2), 552–565.

Emergency Nurses Association. (1995). *Trauma nursing core course* (4th ed.). Park Ridge, IL: Author.

Fabian, T. C., Richardson, J. D., Croce, M. A., et al (1997). Prospective study of blunt aortic injury: Multicenter trial of the American Association for the Surgery of Trauma. *Journal of Trauma: Injury, Infection, and Critical Care, 42,* 374–380.

Franchello, A., Olivero, G., Summa, M. D., Memore, L., Scavarda, B., & Bertoldo, V. (1997). Rupture of thoracic aorta resulting from blunt trauma. *International Surgery, 82,* 79–84.

Francis, G. S. (1991). Heart failure in 1991. *Cardiology, 78,* 81–94.

Goldberger, E. (1990). *Treatment of cardiac emergencies* (5th ed.). St. Louis, MO: C. V. Mosby.

Hamm, C. W., Goldman, B. U., Heeschen, C., Kreymann, G., Berger, J., & Meinertz, T. (1997). Emergency room triage of patients with acute chest pain by means of rapid testing for cardiac troponin T or troponin I. *New England Journal of Medicine, 337,* 1648–1653.

Hammond, B. B., & Capasso, V. C. (1987). Cardiovascular emergencies. In R. Rea, P. Bourg, J. G. Parker, & D. Rushing (Eds.), *Emergency nursing care curriculum* (pp. 74–168). Philadelphia: W. B. Saunders.

Herlitz, J. (1990). Chest pain in acute myocardial infarction. *Cardiology, 77,* 421–423.

Howell, E., Widra, L., & Hill, M. G. (Eds.). (1988). *Comprehensive trauma nursing: Theory and practice.* Glenview, IL: Scott, Foresman.

Huang, S. H., Kessler, C. A., McCulloch, C. D., & Dasher, L. A. (Eds.). (1989). *Coronary care nursing.* Philadelphia: W. B. Saunders.

Jenkins, J. L., & Loscalzo, J. (1990). *Manual of emergency medicine: Diagnosis and treatment* (2nd ed.). Boston: Little, Brown.

Joy, C. L. (Ed.). (1989). *Pediatric trauma nursing.* Rockville, MD: Aspen.

Katyal, D., McLellen, B. A., Brenneman, F. D., Boulanger, B. R., Sharkey, P. W., & Waddell, J. P. (1997). Lateral impact motor vehicle collisions: Significant cause of blunt traumatic rupture of the thoracic aorta. *Journal of Trauma: Injury, Infection, and Critical Care, 42,* 769–772.

Kelley, S. J. (Ed.). (1988). *Pediatric emergency nursing.* Norwalk, CT: Appleton & Lange.

Kinch, J. W., & Ryan, T. J. (1994). Right ventricular infarction. *New England Journal of Medicine, 330,* 1211–1216.

Kinney, M. R., Packa, D. R., & Dunbar, S. B. (Eds.). (1988). *AACN's clinical reference for critical care nursing* (2nd ed.). New York: McGraw-Hill.

Kitt, S., Selfridge-Thomas, J., Proehl, J. A., & Kaiser, J. (Eds.). (1995). *Emergency nursing: A physiologic and clinical perspective.* (2nd ed.) Philadelphia: W. B. Saunders.

Kohr, L. M., & O'Brien, P. (1995). Current management of congestive heart failure in infants and children. *Nursing Clinics of North America, 30(2),* 261–289.

Kreis, D. J., & Gomez, G. A. (Eds.). (1989). *Trauma management.* Boston: Little, Brown.

Krisanda, T. J. (1990). Atrial fibrillation with cardiac tamponade as the initial manifestation of malignant pericarditis. *American Journal of Emergency Medicine, 8(6),* 531–533.

Madias, J. E., Mahjoub, M., & Wijetilaka, R. (1997). Standard 12-lead ECG versus special chest leads in the diagnosis of right myocardial infarction. *American Journal of Emergency Medicine, 15,* 89–90.

Majorowicz, K., & Hayes-Christiansen, H. (1989). *Cardiovascular nursing.* Springhouse, PA: Springhouse.

Martin, R. E., & Teberian, G. (1990). Multiple trauma and the elderly patient. *Emergency Medicine Clinics of North America, 8(2),* 411–420.

Martin, S., Chesnick, P. A., & Young, J. B. (1990). Invasive cardiac procedures after myocardial infarction: Which procedure when and its relationship to thrombolysis. *Journal of Emergency Nursing, 16,* 202–207.

Mattox, K. L. (1997). Red river anthology. *Journal of Trauma: Injury, Infection, and Critical Care, 42,* 353–368.

Messerli, F. H. (Ed.). (1988). *Cardiovascular disease in the elderly* (2nd ed.). Boston: Martinus Nijhoff.

McGrath, A. (1997). Raynaud's syndrome: Preventing peripheral ischemic injury. *American Journal of Nursing, 97,* 34–35.

Murphy, C. (1995). Hypertensive emergencies. *Emergency Medicine Clinics of North America, 13,* 973–1005.

Navarro, F., & Bacharach, J. M. (1996). Treatment of peripheral arterial and venous disease. *Coronary Artery Disease, 7,* 649–655.

Newbern, V. B. (1991). Cautionary tales on using beta-blockers. *Geriatric Nursing, 3,* 119–122.

Pervaiz, S., Anderson, F. P., Lohmann, T. P., Lawson, C. J., Feng, Y., Waskiewicz, D., Contois, J. H., & Wu, A. H. B. (1997). Comparative analysis of cardiac troponin I and creatine-MB as markers of acute myocardial infarction. *Clinical Cardiology, 20,* 269–271.

Porth, C. M. (Ed.). (1986). *Pathophysiology: Concepts of altered health states* (2nd ed.). Philadelphia: J. B. Lippincott.

Robiolio, P. A. (1996). Right ventricular infarction: Reversing the short-term prognosis. *Emergency Medicine, 28(9),* 16–26.

Ryan, T. J. (1997). Management of acute myocardial infarction: Synopsis of ACC/AHA practice guidelines. *Postgraduate Medicine, 102,* 84–93.

Ryan, T. J., Anderson, J. L., Antman, E. M., Braniff, B. A., Brooks, N. H., Califf, R. M., Hillis, L. D., Hiraatzka, L. F., Rappaport, E., Riegel, B. J., Russell, R. O., Smith, E. E., III, & Weaver, W. D. (1996). ACC/AHA guidelines for the management of patients with acute myocardial infarction: A report of the American College of Cardiology/American Heart Association Task Force on Practice Guidelines (Committee on Management of Acute Myocardial Infarction). *Journal of the American College of Cardiology, 28,* 1328–1428.

Schreiber, W. E. (1997). Laboratory assessment of myocardial damage: Which test is best? *American Journal of Clinical Pathology, 107,* 383–384.

Schron, E. B., & Friedman, L. M. (1990). Cardiovascular options for the 1990s. *Geriatric Nursing, 4,* 187–190.

Symbas, P. (1989). *Cardiothoracic trauma.* Philadelphia: W. B. Saunders.

Tintinalli, J. E., Ruiz, E., & Krome, R. L. (Eds.). (1996). *Emergency medicine: A comprehensive study guide.* New York: McGraw-Hill.

Todd, B. (1989). Diuretics' dangers. *Geriatric Nursing, 4,* 212–214.

Trunkey, D. D., & Lewis, F. R. (Eds.). (1986). *Current therapy of trauma* (2nd ed.). Toronto: B. C. Decker.

Underhill, S. L., Woods, S. L., Froelicher, E. S., & Halpenny, C. J. (Eds.). (1989). *Cardiac nursing* (2nd ed.). Philadelphia: J. B. Lippincott.

Varon, J., & Fromm, R. E., Jr. (1996). Hypertensive crisis: The need for urgent management. *Postgraduate Medicine, 99,* 189–201.

Wallerand, A. H., & Delgin, J. H. (Eds.). (1991). *Drug guide for critical care and emergency nursing.* Philadelphia: F. A. Davis.

Wilkins, E. W. (Ed.). (1989). *Emergency medicine: Scientific foundations and current practice* (3rd ed.). Baltimore: Williams & Wilkins.

Willerson, J. T., & Cohn, J. N. (Eds.). (1995). *Cardiovascular medicine.* New York: Churchill Livingstone.

Wilson, J. M., Kalife, G., Rogers, M., Strickman, N. E., & Massumi, A. (1996). Unusual electrocardiographic presentation of right ventricular infarction. *Texas Heart Institute Journal, 23,* 305–309.

Woods, S. L., Sivarajan Froelicher, E. S., Halpenny, C. J., & Underhill Motzer, S. (Eds.). (1995). *Cardiac nursing* (3rd ed.). Philadelphia: J. B. Lippincott.

Yager, M. (1996). Right ventricular infarction in the emergency department: A review of pathophysiology, assessment, diagnosis, treatment, and nursing care. *Journal of Emergency Nursing, 22,* 288–292.

Donna M. Coimbra-Emanuele, RN, MN, CEN, CCRN, FNP

CHAPTER **4**

Dental, Ear, Nose, and Throat Emergencies

MAJOR TOPICS

I. GENERAL STRATEGY

A. Assessment

1. **Primary survey/resuscitation** (see Chapter 1)
2. **Secondary survey** (see Chapter 1)
3. **Psychological, social, and environmental factors**
   a. *Infrequent dental care or lack of maintenance (e.g., flossing and brushing)*
   b. *Poor nutrition*

      c. Contact sports without correct mouth protectors

      d. Swimming in contaminated water

      e. Trauma resulting from attempts to clean or scratch an itching ear

      f. Blast injuries

      g. Air travel with upper respiratory tract infection without premedication

      h. Domestic violence

      i. Unsanitary living conditions

      j. Sick contacts

      k. Cigarette, cigar, or pipe smoking

      l. Occupational exposures

4. Focused survey

  a. Subjective data

    1) Chief complaint

    2) History of present illness

      a) Pain: PQRST

        (1) Provocation

        (2) Quality

        (3) Region or radiation

        (4) Severity

        (5) Time

      b) Bleeding or hemorrhage: estimated blood loss, syncope, or dizziness

      c) Shortness of breath or obstructed airway

      d) Swelling or edema

      e) Lymphadenopathy

      f) Foreign body

      g) Asymmetry or dislocation

      h) Fever, chills

      i) Nausea, vomiting

      j) Paresthesia, facial numbness

      k) Dysphasia, dysphagia

      l) Foul odor or bad taste in mouth

      m) Loss of hearing

      n) Tinnitus or vertigo

      o) Trismus: spasm of masticatory muscles resulting in difficulty opening mouth

      p) Injury: mechanism and time

      q) Discharge or drainage: ears, nose, or mouth

      r) Itching

      s) Neck pain

      t) Drooling

      u) Bleeding gums

      v) Excessive or decreased salivation

      w) Headache

      x) Dyspnea

    3) Medical history

      a) Hypertension: implications for epistaxis

      b) Cardiopulmonary disease: may result in decreased oxygenation

      c) Atherosclerosis: of particular concern in epistaxis

      d) Neurological disease: dental, ear, nose, and throat (ENT) emergencies may result in neurological deficits owing to cranial nerve involvement

      e) Dental or ENT surgery

      f) Previous trauma or fractures

      g) Previous dental or ENT infections

h) Cancer of head and neck
i) Blood dyscrasia: especially important if bleeding is present
j) Exposure to noxious agents (e.g., chemicals, nicotine, alcohol, and drugs)
k) Allergies or current medications
l) Smoking, alcohol or illicit drug use
m) Diabetes
n) Denture use

b. *Objective data*

1) Physical examination

   a) General survey

     (1) General appearance: dress, gait, behavior, and nutritional status

     (2) Neurological status

     (3) Vital signs: include orthostatic vital signs if bleeding is present

     (4) Skin assessment: color, temperature, moisture, and turgor

   b) Inspection, palpation

     (1) External ear and canal: position, size, and symmetry; skin color; drainage; and abnormalities such as swelling or redness

     (2) Tympanic membrane (necessitates use of otoscope): color (pearl gray); identification of landmarks (cone of light); position, size, and symmetry; mobility (use pneumatic otoscope/insufflator); and abnormalities

     (3) External nose: position, shape, and symmetry; drainage; and abnormalities

     (4) Internal nose: nasal septum (color, integrity, and abnormalities); inferior and middle turbinates and middle meatus (color, size, and abnormalities); nasal mucosa (color, integrity) and abnormalities

     (5) Mouth and pharynx: temporomandibular joint (mobility); teeth (number, color, form, occlusion,); lips (color, symmetry, moisture, surface characteristics); oral buccal mucosa/oropharynx (color, landmarks, surface characteristics, and structures); gingiva (color, surface characteristics); tongue (symmetry, movement, color, surface characteristics, ventral surface); hard and soft palates (color, surface characteristics, landmarks); abnormalities

     (6) Paranasal sinuses: soft tissue over sinus area for erythema or swelling

     (7) Neck: symmetry of structures and abnormalities

2) Diagnostic procedures

   a) Radiology

     (1) Dental emergencies: Panorex radiograph of teeth; chest radiograph to rule out aspiration of foreign body in lungs if teeth are missing; facial radiographic series to detect fractures

     (2) ENT emergencies: radiographs of nasal/facial bones (although sometimes ordered, diagnosis usually made with clinical presentation); Waters' view of orbits, skull, and cervical spine (C-spine) and odontoid view with neck trauma; computed tomography (CT) scan; chest radiograph; possibly other special procedures (e.g., magnetic resonance imaging [MRI])

   b) Laboratory

     (1) Aerobic and anaerobic cultures if infection suspected

     (2) Complete blood count

     (3) Erythrocyte sedimentation rate

     (4) Coagulation studies

(5) *Streptococcus* screen/culture
(6) Arterial blood gas (ABG) values
c) Foreign body removal procedures
(1) McGill forceps
(2) Rigid esophagoscopy
(3) Balloon-tipped Foley catheter
(4) Bougienage
(5) Flexible fiberoptic endoscopy
(6) Pharmacological agents

B. Analysis: differential nursing diagnosis/collaborative problems

1. **Pain**
2. **Anxiety/fear**
3. **Infection**
4. **Risk for fluid volume problem**
5. **Alteration in tissue perfusion**
6. **Knowledge deficit**
7. **Risk for ineffective airway clearance**
8. **Risk for ineffective breathing pattern**

C. Planning/interventions

1. **Determine priorities**
   a. *Control and maintain airway, breathing, and circulation (ABCs)*
   b. *Control bleeding and hemorrhage*
   c. *Maintain fluid volume*
   d. *Control pain*
   e. *Relieve anxiety or apprehension*
   f. *Provide definitive treatment of emergency*
   g. *Prevent complications*
   h. *Educate patient and/or significant other*
   i. *Administer medications*
2. **Develop nursing care plan specific to patient's presenting emergency**
3. **Obtain and prepare necessary equipment and supplies**
4. **Institute appropriate interventions on basis of nursing care plan**
5. **Document and record data as appropriate**

D. Expected outcomes/evaluation

1. **Monitor patient responses and outcomes, adjusting nursing care plan as indicated**
   a. *Specific interventions*
   b. *Disposition or discharge planning*
2. **If positive outcomes are not demonstrated, assessment or plan of care needs re-evaluation**
3. **Record data as appropriate**

E. Age-related considerations

1. **Pediatric**
   a. *Growth and development related*
      1) Eighty-five percent of foreign body (FB) **aspirations** are in children

younger than 3 years. Boys are twice as likely to aspirate an FB than girls; peak incidence occurs between the ages of 1 and 2 years; FB **ingestions** occur equally in boys and girls between ages 6 months to 6 years; those children with neurological disorders, with developmental delays, or who have had esophageal surgery are at higher risk of injury as a result of problems that impair their protective reflexes. In 20 to 38% of children with esophageal FB ingestions, there are no symptoms.

2) Irritability and lack of feeding in infants should not be overlooked as they may be potential signs of ENT and dental emergencies

b. *"Pearls"*

1) Persistent cough or chronic wheezing may be indicative of aspirated FB
2) Difficulty with feeding may be indicative of significant ENT emergency
3) Abrupt onset of upper respiratory and pulmonary symptoms suggest FB ingestion

2. Geriatric

a. *Aging related*

1) Difficulty in mastication and loss of sensation in mouth should be considered
2) Progressive hearing loss occurs as part of aging process and may be difficult to assess in emergency department

b. *"Pearls"*

1) Malignant external otitis media and cholesteatoma should be considered in elderly diabetic with earache or recurrent ear infections
2) Most dental and ENT trauma in elderly is related to falls, visual changes occurring with age, motor vehicle crashes, and assaults
3) Poor eyesight contributes to FBs in pharynx

II. SPECIFIC DENTAL EMERGENCIES

A. Odontalgia

Odontalgia, or toothache, is associated with a carious lesion involving a portion of pulp tissue within the tooth. Pulpal inflammation (pulpitis) invades the soft tissue, producing pain that is provoked by eating sweets and changes in temperature, especially cold. Pain may begin suddenly or gradually, creating sharp to throbbing sensations. Pain may be localized or radiate to the ear, jaw, temple, or neck. If left untreated, the pulpal inflammation extends into the dentin and root apex, producing necrosis. This necrosis increases the risk for periapical and alveolar abscess, facial cellulitis, and tooth extraction. Treatment measures are aimed at prevention of tooth decay from dental caries. Good oral hygiene is essential to prevent oral microbes generated by diet which invade tooth enamel causing decay. When disease is present, it is important to rule out secondary complications that may be associated with abscessed teeth; if required, tooth extraction, root canal, or incision and drainage may be performed. Antibiotics and analgesics can be administered until definitive treatment by a dentist is provided.

1. Assessment

a. *Subjective data*

1) History of present illness

a) Pain

(1) In diseased tooth: dental caries
(2) Referred to gum line, jaw, temple, ear, and neck
(3) Sharp, shooting pain in early phase that progresses to intense,

persistent, throbbing with tooth exquisitely sensitive to touch during later phase (pulp damage)

(4) More intense nocturnal pain from affected tooth

(5) Begins with heat or cold stimulus and occurs spontaneously with continued worsening

(6) Not relieved by analgesics; irreversible pain indicates necessity for root canal or extraction

  2) Medical history

    a) Previous dental caries, injuries, and gum disease

    b) Allergies to medications

    c) Current medications

  b. *Objective data*

    1) Physical examination

      a) Presence of tooth discoloration or obvious decay

      b) Foul odor in mouth

      c) Tenderness/pain on percussion

    2) Diagnostic procedures: dental radiograph

2. Analysis: differential nursing diagnosis/collaborative problems

  a. *Pain related to tooth decay and inflammation/infection*

  b. *Anxiety/fear related to pain*

  c. *Risk for infection related to tooth decay*

3. Planning/interventions

  a. *Topical anesthetic*

  b. *Antibiotics as indicated*

  c. *Administration of analgesic with instructions regarding side effects*

  d. *Appropriate reassurance*

  e. *Explanation of disease process*

  f. *Discussion, explanation, and demonstration of discharge and follow-up instructions*

  g. *Dental nerve blocks*

4. Expected outcomes/evaluation (see Appendix B)

B. Tooth eruption

Odontogenic pain is commonly experienced when the primary teeth in infants and children are erupting from the gums. This can also be experienced when the third molars (wisdom teeth) evolve during the second decade. Low-grade temperature, diarrhea, and refusal to eat or drink may occur in infants and children during tooth eruption. Management is supportive and directed toward pain control, adequate hydration, and control of diarrhea if present. Analgesia (both oral and topical) and nonsteroidal anti-inflammatory drugs (NSAIDs) are used to alleviate discomfort.

1. Assessment

  a. *Subjective data*

    1) History of present illness

      a) Pressure or tenderness

      b) Irritability

      c) Disrupted sleep

      d) Decreased fluid intake

      e) Associated symptoms: cold, diarrhea

      f) Agitation

      g) Nasal discharge

       h) Crying

       i) Fever (low grade)

    2) Medical history

       a) Similar occurrences

       b) Allergies

  b. Objective data

    1) Physical examination

       a) Drooling

       b) Circumoral rash around mouth

       c) Reddened, edematous tissues over erupting tooth

       d) Tenderness on palpation of affected gum area

       e) Reddened nasal mucosa and rhinorrhea

       f) Fever (low grade)

    2) Diagnostic procedures: none indicated

2. Analysis: differential nursing diagnosis/collaborative problems

  a. Pain related to inflammation

  b. Anxiety/fear related to pain

3. Planning/interventions

  a. Gentle massage to overlying gingival tissue with finger or teething ring

  b. Ice chips in cloth placed over gingival tissue

  c. Topical anesthetic: benzocaine (e.g., Orajel or Numzit)

  d. Mild systemic analgesic to decrease pain and overall discomfort and fever

  e. Referral to dentist if eruption site remains soft or swollen (probable eruption cyst, which may rupture and bleed)

  f. Warm saline mouth rinses

  g. Soft solid diet

4. Expected outcomes/evaluation (see Appendix B)

C. Pericoronitis

    Erupting or impacted molar teeth are referred to as pericoronitis. Acute inflammation surrounds the gingival tissue or occurs on the crown of the partially erupted tooth. The space between the crown, overlying tooth, and gingival flap has a tendency to accumulate food and bacteria, causing increased inflammation. This is commonly seen in adults entering their third decade of life but can be found in teenagers as well. Pain is the primary symptom described that may radiate to the ear, throat, and floor of the mouth. General treatment measures consist of saline irrigations, warm mouth rinses, and pain control with analgesic medications. Occasionally, systemic symptoms occur with lymphadenopathy, fever, and fatigue. Antibiotics, debridement, excision of the gingival flap, or extraction of the molar may be necessary. Cellulitis, peritonsillar abscess, and Ludwig's angina are rare complications that should be considered when systemic symptoms are present.

1. Assessment

  a. Subjective data

    1) History of present illness

       a) Nonspecific diffuse extraoral pain or pain on opening mouth

       b) Earache on affected side

       c) Sore throat, neck and jaw pain

    2) Medical history

       a) Unerupted third molar tooth in area of discomfort or pain

       b) Allergies to medications

  b. Objective data

1) Physical examination
   a) Submandibular lymphadenopathy
   b) Red, inflamed soft tissues around crown of partially erupted tooth
   c) Trismus if infection has spread
   d) Temperature greater than 100°F (37.7°C)
2) Diagnostic procedures: dental radiographs

2. Analysis: differential nursing diagnosis/collaborative problems
   a. *Pain related to soft tissue inflammation*
   b. *Risk for infection related to bacterial invasion of soft tissue*

3. Planning/interventions
   a. *Irrigate under pericoronal flap with warm normal saline to remove debris*
   b. *Administer prescribed antibiotic therapy if infection present*
   c. *Assist with draining of abscess, if present*
   d. *Administer antipyretics if elevated temperature*
   e. *Refer to dentist for debridement of pericoronal flap or tooth extraction and follow-up therapy*
   f. *Administer analgesic as prescribed*

4. Expected outcomes/evaluation (see Appendix B)

D. Fractured tooth

Dentoalveolar trauma can cause fractures or injury to the teeth and supporting structures. Traumatic injuries are associated with falls, motor vehicle accidents, physical abuse, sports-related activities, and FBs that strike the oral structures. Seizures may also be responsible for intraoral injury. The Ellis system is commonly used to describe the fracture anatomy of teeth. **Ellis Class I** includes fractures that involve only the enamel portion of the tooth. These fractures are generally minor, involving the maxillary central incisors and producing a "rough" appearance of the tooth that later may be smoothed or cosmetically repaired by a dentist. **Ellis Class II** includes fractures that involve the enamel portion and part of the dentin. These fractures frequently produce pain sensitivities to heat, cold, and air. Treatment is age dependent. Children younger than 12 years usually have less dentin present, which can expose the pulp to bacteria more readily. Therefore, treatment with calcium hydroxide on the exposed dentin using dry gauze is important to delay contaminants from invading the pulp. These patients are referred to a dentist within 24 hours for definitive treatment. **Ellis Class III** includes fractures that involve the enamel portion, dentin, and pulp of the tooth. These fractures are dental emergencies that require immediate referral and attention by an endodontist because of the increased risk of infection from exposed pulp and disruption of neurovascular supply. A piece of tin foil or dry gauze may be placed temporarily to avoid pulpal irritation and minimize pain.

1. Assessment
   a. *Subjective data*
      1) History of present illness
         a) Injury to tooth or related structures
         b) Disfigurement of tooth
         c) Pain from affected tooth (dentin or pulp injury)
            (1) Spontaneous
            (2) From hot or cold agents
            (3) On inspiration of air
            (4) Not relieved by analgesics
            (5) Tooth sore to touch or while eating

       d) Headache

       e) Nausea or vomiting

       f) Loss of consciousness or amnesia: assess for concomitant head injury

       g) Treatment since injury

     2) Medical history

       a) Previous dental injury, disease, surgery, or cosmetic repair (e.g., crowns)

       b) Allergies to medications

       c) Tetanus immunization history

  b. *Objective data*

     1) Physical examination

       a) Primary or permanent teeth: number involved

       b) Involvement of enamel, dentin, pulp, or root

       c) Change in color of affected tooth

       d) Tenderness of tooth to touch

       e) Pieces of fractured tooth in oral cavity

       f) Malocclusion

       g) Intraoral or extraoral wounds

       h) Bleeding

     2) Diagnostic procedures

       a) Dental radiographs

       b) Radiographs of facial bones

2. Analysis: differential nursing diagnosis/collaborative problems

  a. *Pain related to injury and possible exposed nerve*

  b. *Anxiety/fear related to injury and pain*

3. Planning/interventions

  a. *Treat fracture involving enamel and dentin*

     1) Apply calcium hydroxide (if available) to protect tooth from further injury or contamination from exposure to saliva and air, which may lead to pulpitis

     2) May use clear nail polish as substitute protective covering

     3) Administer mild oral analgesic

     4) Provide dental referral within 24 hours for definitive treatment

     5) Administer antibiotics

  b. *Treat fracture involving pulp*

     1) Apply calcium hydroxide to exposed crown surface

     2) Administer oral analgesic

     3) Provide dental referral for pulpectomy

     4) Explore soft tissue for possible tooth fragments

     5) Administer antibiotics

  c. *Permit calm significant other to remain in examination room if patient stable*

  d. *Discuss, explain, and demonstrate discharge and follow-up instructions*

4. Expected outcomes/evaluation (see Appendix B)

E. Subluxed/avulsed teeth

Similar forces that result in fractured teeth are also responsible for causing subluxed and avulsed teeth. This "loosening of teeth" occurs in all age groups but is most prevalent in children aged 7 to 10 years. Examining the gingival crevice of the tooth may identify subluxation. Blood is usually visualized. Gentle finger pressure applied to the affected tooth reveals varying degrees of mobility within the socket. Minimal mobility will usually heal within 2 weeks, and patients are placed on a soft diet. Referral to a dentist or maxillofacial surgeon is indicated when the pulp is exposed and the tooth is grossly mobile. When applicable, partially avulsed teeth should be repositioned for stability. Complete tooth avulsion is a dental emergency, and measures should be taken to preserve the tooth for successful replantation. Permanent retention of avulsed teeth should occur within 30 minutes. Each minute the tooth is absent from the socket reduces successful replantation. Minimal handling of avulsed teeth should be encouraged. Only saline should be used if debris is found. The tooth should be immediately placed in the tooth socket to preserve and increase viability. When replantation is delayed, the tooth should be placed in a moist saline gauze or milk during transport for definitive treatment.

1. **Assessment**
   a. *Subjective data*
      1) History of present illness
         a) Injury resulting in displacement of tooth from alveolar socket
         b) Pain at site of avulsion
         c) Bleeding at site of avulsion
         d) Loss of consciousness
         e) Other injuries
         f) Dyspnea
         g) Neck pain
      2) Medical history
         a) Dental injuries or disease
         b) Allergies to medications
         c) Tetanus immunization history
   b. *Objective data*
      1) Physical examination
         a) Primary or permanent tooth involved
         b) Number of teeth involved
         c) Oral cavity for presence of FBs and other injuries
         d) Level of consciousness
         e) Extraoral wounds
         f) Respiratory status
      2) Diagnostic procedures
         a) Dental radiographs
         b) Chest radiograph (if tooth cannot be located) to rule out aspiration
2. **Analysis: differential nursing diagnosis/collaborative problems**
   a. *Pain related to injury and disrupted tissue*
   b. *Anxiety/fear related to injury and pain*
   c. *Risk for infection related to impaired integrity of skin/mucous membrane*
3. **Planning/interventions**
   a. *Administer local anesthesia as ordered*
   b. *Replant avulsed tooth*
      1) Clean by rinsing with normal saline or cold water (do not scrub tooth)
      2) Suction blood from socket
      3) Replant within 30 minutes after injury for best results or up to 6 hours maximum
   c. *Administer analgesic and antibiotics as prescribed*
   d. *Instruct patient not to bite into anything with affected tooth and to avoid hot and cold substances*
   e. *Refer to dentist or oral surgeon for further treatment and follow-up care*
4. **Expected outcomes/evaluation** (see Appendix B)

F. Dental abscess

A dental abscess occurs from the localized accumulation of pus in a cavity of a tooth. Gingival swelling results as plaque and debris collect in the space between the tooth and gingiva. Periodontal disease results when infections extend into the surrounding tissues, gingival epithelium, periodontal ligament, or alveolar bone. Periapical (alveolar) abscess (infection has spread beyond the bone) and periodontal abscess (bony destruction at the periodontal membrane) result when bacterial, viral, or mycotic pathogens are able to colonize. Treatment measures are aimed at managing infection with antibiotics. In some cases, incision and drainage of the soft tissue is necessary to prevent involvement to the extending fascial areas of the head and neck.

1. **Assessment**
   a. *Subjective data*
      1) History of present illness
         a) Pain
            (1) Affected tooth and surrounding tissue radiating to jaw, ear, and neck
            (2) Mild to severe depending on extent of abscess
            (3) Not relieved by analgesics
         b) Swelling of face or neck on affected side
         c) Fever or chills
         d) Malaise
         e) Foul breath
         f) Unpleasant taste in mouth
         g) Sore gums
      2) Medical history
         a) Previous dental abscess
         b) Previous dental space caries or gum disease
         c) Infrequent dental care or lack of maintenance
         d) Diabetes
         e) Alcohol use
         f) Allergies to medications
   b. *Objective data*
      1) Physical examination
         a) Temperature greater than 99°F (37.2°C)
         b) Edematous face (if minor and localized abscess)
         c) Edematous face and neck (if major and extending abscess)
         d) Possible edema of pharynx and surrounding structure on affected side
         e) Tender affected tooth
         f) Agitation or restlessness
      2) Diagnostic procedures
         a) Dental radiograph of affected tooth
         b) Soft tissue radiograph of neck
         c) White blood cell count to determine presence of leukocytosis, a sign of systemic toxicity
         d) Culture and sensitivity testing of any drainage: aerobic and anaerobic
2. **Analysis: differential nursing diagnosis/collaborative problems**
   a. *Pain related to infectious process*
   b. *Infection related to invasion of tissues by bacteria*
   c. *Anxiety/fear related to infection and pain*
3. **Planning/interventions**
   a. *Administer systemic analgesic*
   b. *Administer antipyretic for fever or discomfort*

     c. Assist with incision and drainage of abscess if fluctuance is present, leaving drain in place

     d. Obtain culture and sensitivity testing of exudate

     e. Use warm normal saline mouth rinses every 1 to 2 hours (when patient is awake)

     f. Discuss, explain, and demonstrate discharge and follow-up instructions

     g. Refer to dentist or endodontist for follow-up care

4. Expected outcomes/evaluation (see Appendix B)

G. Ludwig's angina

Ludwig's angina usually results from a secondary dental infection involving the lower second and third molars. Bilateral diffuse swelling and extending cellulitis involving the submandibular, submental, and sublingual areas occurs. The neck and face are swollen with protrusion and elevation of the tongue, which cause difficulty talking and swallowing. Breathing becomes compromised as oropharynx swelling evolves and descends toward the mediastinum. In addition, fever, chills, and trismus are commonly present. Aerobes and anaerobes are responsible for the vast majority of infections that are caused by the proliferation of hemolytic streptococci and *Bacteroides melaninogenicus*. Treatment of infection includes the use of penicillin, clindamycin, or third-generation cephalosporins. Third-generation cephalosporins are preferred because they are more responsive to aerobic gram-negative organisms and penicillin-resistant pathogens. Incision and drainage is performed to provide relief from swelling and infection and to protect the airway further.

1. Assessment

    a. Subjective data

      1) History of present illness

        a) Pain and swelling of jaw and neck

        b) Fever or chills

        c) Malaise

        d) Difficulty swallowing (dysphagia)

        e) Difficulty talking (dysphasia)

      2) Medical history

        a) Dental infection and treatment

        b) Allergies to medications

    b. Objective data

      1) Physical examination

        a) Marked bilateral swelling of jaw and neck

        b) Marked elevation of tongue and floor of mouth toward palate

        c) Dyspnea with tachypnea

        d) Temperature greater than 101°F (38.3°C)

        e) Diaphoresis

        f) Pallor or cyanosis

        g) Possible poor dental hygiene

        h) Agitation

      2) Diagnostic procedures

        a) Complete blood count with differential leukocyte count

        b) Erythrocyte sedimentation rate

        c) Soft tissue radiograph of neck

        d) Culture and sensitivity testing of exudate

        e) ABG values if cyanosis or difficulty in breathing

2. Analysis: differential nursing diagnosis/collaborative problems

     a. Impaired gas exchange related to edema of airways secondary to inflammation

     b. Pain related to inflammatory process

     c. Infection related to invasion of tissues by bacteria

     d. Anxiety/fear related to pain and airway compromise

     e. Risk for ineffective airway clearance related to edema

  3. Planning/interventions

     a. Maintain airway, breathing, circulation

     b. Assist patient to Fowler's position

     c. Provide supplemental oxygen

     d. Continuously monitor and assess

       1) Respiratory rate and depth

       2) Lung sounds

       3) Use of accessory breathing muscles

       4) Tissue perfusion

       5) Level of consciousness or mental status

     e. Assist with intraoral incision and drainage of infected area

     f. Start peripheral intravenous (IV) infusion catheter

     g. Administer systemic analgesic as ordered

     h. Administer IV antibiotic as ordered but perform pharyngeal culture prior to IV

     i. Anticipate possible need for cricothyrotomy if acute airway compromise occurs

     j. Instruct patient to rinse mouth with warm normal saline two or three times every hour while awake

     k. Apply hot, moist compress to jaw and neck every hour while patient is awake

  4. Expected outcomes/evaluation (see Appendix B)

H. Postextraction Pain and Bleeding

     Pain and swelling are generally present up to 24 hours after a tooth extraction. This is known as periostitis and usually responds well to analgesics, NSAIDs, or narcotic analgesics. However, pain lasting more than 2 to 3 days may be caused by alveolitis, commonly referred to as "dry socket." Pain may radiate to the ear and may last from days to weeks. This is most commonly found in patients who have had removal of the mandibular posterior teeth. This is due to a loss of the healing blood clot and localized infection. Alveolitis is best treated with irrigation of the clot and topical analgesic medication or gauze moistened with eugenol that is changed daily. The patient should be monitored for the subsequent development of osteomyelitis. Fever or swelling should be reported. Antibiotic therapy should be initiated, and the patient should be referred to a dentist within 24 hours for definitive management.

     Postextraction bleeding may occur from small vessels that continue to bleed after a tooth extraction. After the clot is removed, a pressure dressing using cotton wrapped in gauze may be applied directly to the extraction site for approximately 30 minutes. This may be repeated until the bleeding resolves. If bleeding continues, the site may be anesthetized using lidocaine with epinephrine and sutured. In addition, oxidized cellulose, topical thrombin in a gelatin sponge, or microfibrillar collagen can be placed in the socket to act as a hemostatic agent and tamponade bleeding. A patient with prolonged bleeding should be referred to the oral surgeon for definitive treatment.

  1. Assessment

     a. Subjective data

    1) History of present illness
        a) Tooth extraction usually within previous 24 hours if there is bleeding
        b) Severe pain several days after tooth extraction (dry socket)
    2) Medical history
        a) Previous difficult extractions
        b) Bleeding disorders
        c) Allergies to medications
  b. *Objective data*
    1) Physical examination
        a) Bleeding from socket
        b) Socket healing (may not be healing in dry socket)
    2) Diagnostic procedures
        a) Clot removal from socket
2. **Analysis: differential nursing diagnosis/collaborative problems**
  a. *Risk for fluid volume deficit related to bleeding or hemorrhage*
  b. *Pain related to tooth extraction*
  c. *Anxiety/fear related to pain, bleeding, and need to seek medical attention*
  d. *Risk for infection related to impaired tissue integrity*
3. **Planning/interventions**
  a. *Bleeding*
    1) Have patient bite on gauze over extraction site for 30 minutes
    2) Instruct patient to avoid hard or hot foods
  b. *Pain*
    1) Administer acetaminophen
    2) Pack with oil of wintergreen or other local anesthetic
  c. *Refer to dentist for follow-up*
4. **Expected outcomes/evaluation** (see Appendix B)

I. Acute Necrotizing Ulcerative Gingivitis (Trench Mouth)

Acute necrotizing ulcerative gingivitis (ANUG) is a noncontagious infection commonly referred to as trench mouth or Vincent's infection. ANUG is associated with debilitating illnesses, emotional stressors, nutritional deficiencies, and smoking. It is often found in patients following an upper respiratory tract infection. It is commonly seen in adolescents and young adults but occurs in all age groups. Both spirochete and fusiform bacilli that affect gingival tissue cause ANUG. Inflammation, painful bleeding gums, fever, cervical lymphadenopathy, and fetid breath may result. Ulcerations may develop within the gingival tissue, forming a gray membrane that bleeds with pressure or when removed. Treatment measures include local debridement, good oral hygiene with one-half strength hydrogen peroxide (H_2O_2) rinses, antibiotics, and adequate nutrition. Efforts to avoid irritation should be encouraged and analgesics provided after initial debridement to minimize pain. Recovery usually occurs within 24 hours. Patients may require gingival curettage.

1. **Assessment**
  a. *Subjective data*
    1) History of present illness
        a) Gingival tissue pain
        b) Fever, chills, and malaise
        c) Bleeding gums
        d) Halitosis
    2) Medical history
        a) Previous dental injury, gum disease, or pharyngeal infection

          b) Poor nutrition and dental habits

          c) Chronic debilitating disease

          d) Immunocompromise

          e) Allergies to medications

     b. *Objective data*

       1) Physical exam

          a) Spontaneous gingival bleeding

          b) Dental papillae ulceration

          c) Edematous gums

          d) Poor oral hygiene

          e) Fetid breath

          f) Fever greater than 101°F (38.3°C)

          g) Lymphadenopathy

          h) Gray pseudomembranous ulcers on pharyngeal structures

2. Analysis: differential nursing diagnosis/collaborative problems

     a. *Pain related to inflammation/infection*

     b. *Infection related to bacterial invasion of tissue*

3. Planning/interventions

     a. *Administer topical or local anesthetics for pain control*

     b. *Administer prescribed antibiotics to treat underlying infections*

     c. *Administer systemic analgesics and antipyretic medications to reduce fever and relieve pain*

     d. *Refer to dentist for definitive management of illness*

     e. *Instruct the patient how to care for gums and teeth on discharge*

4. Expected outcomes/evaluation (see Appendix B)

III. SPECIFIC EAR EMERGENCIES

A. Acute otitis externa

Acute otitis externa (AOE), commonly referred to as "swimmer's ear," is an inflammatory condition of the external auditory canal and auricle of the ear. This inflammatory reaction promotes swelling and maceration of the stratum corneum of the skin, causing pruritus, swollen lymph nodes, and pain in the involved area. Exudate may or may not be present initially. Movement of the external ear and auricle and pressing on the tragus, mastoid, parotid area and upper neck further aggravate the pain response. The etiological agents include infection (viral, fungal, or bacterial), perforation, FB, or dermatosis. Gram-negative bacteria (e.g., *Pseudomonas*) that produce a green exudate visualized in the external canal may cause infections. Yellow exudate or crusting may represent *Staphylococcus aureus*. Other infections associated with fungal pathogens, including *Aspergillus* or *Candida*, produce a fluffy white to black material similar to that of "bread mold." Dermatological chronic skin disorders, such as eczema, can lead to cellulitis in the affected ear canal. General principles for treatment of AOE consist of cleaning debris of the external auditory canal with a cotton-tipped applicator, suctioning, and applying or instilling an antibiotic-steroid solution or powder for bacterial and fungal infections for approximately 1 week. An ear wick (Otowick) saturated with antibiotic solution may be placed in the external canal of some patients in which the swelling is too significant to allow for adequate instillation of the topical antibiotic. The ear wick is generally removed in 2 to 3 days after insertion. The majority of episodes of AOE resolve within 7 days after treatment. When persistent infections occur, cultures of the ear should be taken to identify the underlying pathogen(s). Additional treatment includes protecting the external ear canal from excessive moisture when bathing.

Swimming and frequent cleansing of the ear canal using cotton-tipped applicators should be avoided until the infection has resolved. Persisting infections should be referred to an otolaryngologist.

1. **Assessment**
   a. *Subjective data*
      1) History of present illness
         a) Pain
            (1) Localized to the outer ear and external canal
            (2) Radiation to affected side of head, jaw, and neck
            (3) Moderate to severe pain with movement of external ear (pinna and tragus)
            (4) Poor response to over-the-counter analgesics and NSAIDs
         b) Impaired or diminished hearing (conductive hearing loss)
         c) Swelling, redness, discharge, or debris in external and outer ear
         d) Tender, enlarged lymph nodes over cervical pre- and postauricular areas
         e) Pruritus (1–3 days of progressive ear itch)
         f) Low-grade fever
         g) Malaise
         h) Pressure or sensation of fullness in ear
      2) Medical history
         a) Prior ear infection
         b) Use of medications
         c) Recent upper respiratory tract infection
         d) Recent swimming or water submersion
         e) Recent use of objects to clean or irrigate ears
         f) Allergies
         g) History of diabetes or debilitated patient condition
   b. *Objective data*
      1) Physical examination
         a) Pain with movement of auricle, tragus, and pinna; tympanic membrane (TM) is usually normal appearing
         b) Purulent drainage from external ear canal
         c) Edema, tenderness, and erythema of ear canal
         d) Periauricular, cervical lymphadenopathy
         e) Cellulitis
         f) Decreased hearing: distinguish between sensorineural and conductive loss
         g) Temperature at or greater than 99°F (37.2°C)
      2) Diagnostic procedures
         a) Whisper voice test to determine hearing loss
         b) Tuning fork tests (Rinne's or Weber's) to differentiate conductive from sensorineural hearing loss
2. **Analysis: differential nursing diagnosis/collaborative problems**
   a. *Pain related to inflammation and infection*
   b. *Infection related to bacterial invasion of tissue*
3. **Planning/interventions**
   a. *Administer prescribed medications: analgesic, topical antibiotic, steroid solution (suspension), and antipyretics; insert ear wick when ear canal is too acutely swollen to distribute medication evenly in canal*
   b. *Apply hot, moist compress to affected ear*
   c. *Speak slowly and clearly toward healthy ear while directly facing patient*
   d. *Use visual cues or gestures*

     e. Discuss, explain, and demonstrate discharge and follow-up instructions

     f. Instruct patient to keep ear canal dry in future with use of ear plugs or Burow's solution via ear wick or dropper

  4. Expected outcomes/evaluation (see Appendix B)

B. Acute otitis media

     Acute otitis media (AOM) is a disease of the middle ear that results from a bacterial infection. Common pathogens include *Streptococcus pneumoniae, Haemophilus influenzae, Streptococcus pyogenes,* and *Moraxella catarrhalis.* Barotrauma, eustachian tube dysfunction, and serous otitis media can precipitate AOM. Most cases of AOM occur with an upper respiratory tract infection. As the auditory tube swells, fluid accumulates, preventing effective drainage and allowing bacteria to proliferate. Although AOM is commonly seen in infants and children, all age groups may be affected. Patients with AOM complain of severe earache, ear pressure, and decreased hearing and may present with fever. Infants and children with AOM are observed "tugging" at their ears. Physical exam reveals an erythematous and dull TM with poorly visualized landmarks or dull light reflex. The TM has decreased mobility and may appear as a bulge as a result of pressure, and fluid accumulates within the middle ear. In these cases, rupture of the TM may occur. TM ruptures produce a significant decrease in pain, and discharge within the external canal may be found. Healing of the TM is usually spontaneous, and scar tissue may later be found on visual exam. Treatment of AOM consists of antibiotics and adequate hydration. Analgesics and NSAIDs should be given for pain and fever control. In patients who are immunocompetent or with chronic recurrent AOM, tympanocentesis may be performed to identify the source of infection and obtain fluid for culture. Surgical drainage of the middle ear (myringotomy) with the insertion of ear ventilating tubes may be considered when complications result from AOM such as meningitis, mastoiditis, osteomyelitis, facial paralysis and intracranial abscess or from chronic recurrent episodes of AOM.

  1. Assessment

    a. Subjective data

      1) History of present illness

        a) Otalgia (earache) that increases with prone position

          (1) Pulling at ear (infant or toddler)

          (2) Verbal complaints (older child)

        b) Sensation of fullness in ear

        c) Decreased hearing

        d) Upper respiratory tract infection

        e) Irritability or malaise

        f) Fever or chills

        g) Anorexia or vomiting

        h) Diarrhea

        i) Vertigo/dizziness

        j) Recent air travel

      2) Medical history

        a) Previous ear infections

        b) Use of medications

        c) Allergies

    b. Objective data

      1) Physical examination

        a) Elevated temperature

      b) Purulent nasal discharge
      c) Erythema of pharynx
      d) Erythema of TM
      e) Retracted or bulging TM
      f) Blebs on eardrum surface (bullous myringitis)
      g) White or yellow discoloration of TM
      h) Excessive purulent drainage from ear if TM has ruptured
      i) Conductive hearing loss
      j) Restlessness or agitation
      k) Uncooperativeness
    2) Diagnostic procedures
      a) Pneumatic otoscopy
      b) Hearing tests
      c) Blood cultures as indicated
      d) Tympanocentesis (aspiration of middle ear for effusion)
      e) Myringotomy if TM bulging

2. Analysis: differential nursing diagnosis/collaborative problems
  a. Pain related to infectious process and fluid accumulation
  b. Infection related to invasion of tissues by bacteria
  c. Anxiety/fear related to pain

3. Planning/interventions
  a. Administer prescribed medication (analgesic, antibiotic, and antipyretic)
  b. Speak slowly and clearly toward healthy ear while directly facing patient
  c. Follow-up within 2 weeks

4. Expected outcomes/evaluation (see Appendix B)

C. Ruptured tympanic membrane

    Although the majority of TM perforations are caused primarily by infection, some cases may result from trauma, including impact injury and explosive acoustic trauma. Hearing may be reduced until healing occurs. Healing is usually spontaneous, and during this time efforts to avoid getting the ear wet are advised to avoid secondary complications. When blunt or barotrauma caused a hemotympanum (blood behind an intact TM), resolution of symptoms may take up to several weeks. If hearing loss persists, surgical intervention may be indicated to improve symptoms.

  1. Assessment
    a. Subjective data
      1) History of present illness
        a) Pain in ear
        b) Discharge from ear: bloody or purulent
        c) Vertigo that is transient at time of injury
        d) Tinnitus
        e) Hearing loss
        f) Fever or chills
        g) Nausea or vomiting
        h) Recent injury to ear
        i) Barotrauma: seen with air travel with an upper respiratory tract infection (rupture occurs most commonly on descent), submersion injuries associated with quick water descent or scuba diving
      2) Medical history
        a) Previous ear infections and treatment
        b) Allergies to medications
    b. Objective data

   1) Physical examination
    a) Tear or perforation of TM: slit-shaped or irregular defect
    b) Discharge from ear: purulent or bloody
    c) Decreased hearing in affected ear
    d) Nystagmus: may or may not be present
    e) Other signs of trauma to head or ear
    f) Temperature at or greater than 100°F (37.7°C) possible
    g) Disequilibrium
   2) Diagnostic procedures
    a) Otoscopic examination
    b) Hearing tests (tuning fork and voice tests)
    c) Radiographs of skull, temporal bone, and cervical spine, as indicated

 2. Analysis: differential nursing diagnosis/collaborative problems
  a. Pain related to infection or trauma
  b. Infection related to bacterial invasion of middle ear

 3. Planning/interventions
  a. Administer prescribed medications (analgesic, antibiotic, and antipyretic)
  b. Assist physician in removing blood and debris from ear canal
  c. Speak slowly and clearly toward healthy ear while directly facing patient
  d. Discuss, explain, and demonstrate discharge and follow-up instructions

 4. Expected outcomes/evaluation (see Appendix B)

D. Foreign body in ear

  FBs in the ear are commonly seen in children but are found in adults as well. Foreign objects and material are inserted or introduced into the external canal, where they become lodged and produce local irritation and tissue inflammation. FBs are removed with instruments, including forceps, hooks, and loops, or with syringe irrigation. In some cases, microscopic guidance to remove an FB is required when the object is directed medially toward the TM or displaced deeper into the meatus. Irrigation of vegetable FBs, including peas and beans, should be avoided because they have a tendency to swell with water and absorb moisture, obliterating the canal and making removal difficult. Attempts to remove insects should involve filling the canal with mineral oil or instilling 2% lidocaine to kill and immobilize the insect. This will facilitate easier removal of the foreign object. If maggots are visualized, calomel powder is an effective treatment for removal.

 1. Assessment
  a. Subjective data
   1) History of present illness
    a) Discharge from ear: purulent or bloody
    b) Discomfort or pain in ear
    c) Decreased hearing in ear
    d) Swelling of external ear
    e) Foul odor in ear
    f) Insect buzzing in ear
    g) Sensation of something in ear
    h) Fullness in ear
    i) If present for extended period, inflammatory response
    j) Agitation
   2) Medical history
    a) Allergies to medications
    b) Socioenvironmental conditions
  b. Objective data

      1) Physical examination

        a) Visible foreign body in ear: animal, mineral, or vegetable

        b) Edema and erythema of ear canal

        c) Purulent drainage or bleeding in affected ear canal

        d) Foul odor from affected ear

      2) Diagnostic procedures: otoscopic examination

2. Analysis: differential nursing diagnosis/collaborative problems

    a. Pain related to foreign body and inflammation

    b. Anxiety/fear related to onset of symptoms and need to seek medical attention

3. Planning/interventions

    a. Assist with removal of FB

      1) Irrigation

        a) Normal saline or water at body temperature

        b) Mixture of alcohol and water for organic material (less swelling)

        c) Insect: mineral oil or 2% lidocaine solution

      2) Suction

      3) Direct instrumentation: syringe irrigation or microscope guided removal

      4) Insect: use flashlight to attract live insect out of canal

        a. Administer prescribed medication (analgesic or antibiotic)

        b. Discuss, explain, and demonstrate discharge and follow-up instructions

4. Expected outcomes/evaluation (see Appendix B)

E. Meniere's disease

Meniere's disease or syndrome is a disorder of the vestibular system in the inner ear, termed *endolymphatic hydrops*. Although the cause is unknown, it may occur in any age group but is commonly seen in individuals in their fourth to sixth decade of life. Abnormal fluctuations in the fluid or endolymph accumulate in the hearing balance structure of the ear (cochlea and labyrinth), causing severe rotary vertigo, nausea, vomiting, and tinnitus. This may occur from a blow to the head, infection, allergies, or degeneration of the inner ear. An attack may last for several hours; recurrent symptoms last for weeks to months. The triad of characteristics of Meniere's disease includes unilateral sensorineural loss, tinnitus, and episodic vertigo. Physical examination during an attack may reveal spontaneous nystagmus unaffected by positional changes. When vertigo is present, dizziness, nausea, imbalance, and vomiting are common because of the vagal and vestibular impulses involved. Additional vagal system involvement may produce abdominal pain, diaphoresis, bradycardia, and pallor. Differential diagnoses that produce similar symptoms must be considered and include acoustic neuroma, viral labyrinthitis, multiple sclerosis, syphilitic vertigo, labyrinthine fistula, vestibular granuloma, and temporal bone fracture. Medical treatment involves symptom management using labyrinthine sedatives/antiemetic to control nausea and antihistamines that may assist with increasing blood flow to the inner ear and minimize vertigo. Diuretics may also be prescribed to stabilize body fluid levels and avoid secondary fluctuations in the endolymph. In addition, maintaining an adequate diet that balances sugar and salt intake and avoiding caffeine, alcohol, and smoking can also reduce symptoms. Hydration is important to minimize symptoms. Losses during exercise or excessive heat should be replenished. Surgery may be considered when Meniere's disease is severe and refractory to medical treatment. An endolymphatic shunt to decompress and relieve the fluid pressure in the inner ear, labyrinthectomy to destroy the inner ear, or a vestibular neurectomy to section the vestibular nerve and disconnect it from the brain are options that may be considered.

1. Assessment

   a. *Subjective data*
      1) History of present illness
         a) Rotational vertigo with inability to ambulate without falling (feelings of person spinning or objects spinning around person)
         b) Nausea or vomiting
         c) Diaphoresis
         d) Tinnitus (roaring sensation or ringing in ears)
         e) Mild to severe hearing loss
         f) Feeling of pressure or fullness in affected ear
         g) Heightened sensitivity to loud sounds
         h) Headache
         i) Blurred vision
      2) Medical history
         a) Otitis media
         b) Arteriosclerosis
         c) Leukemia
         d) Smoking or alcohol use
         e) Allergies to medications
   b. *Objective data*
      1) Physical examination
         a) Disequilibrium: falls toward affected ear
         b) Decreased hearing in affected ear
         c) Moist, pale skin
         d) Nystagmus
      2) Diagnostic procedures: caloric tests to differentiate from intracranial lesion are considered but may not be initially performed

2. Analysis: differential nursing diagnosis/collaborative problems
   a. *Risk for injury related to dizziness*
   b. *Risk for fluid volume deficit related to nausea and vomiting*

3. Planning/interventions
   a. *Administer prescribed medication (vasodilator, antihistamine, diuretics, and oral sedative/antiemetic)*
   b. *Maintain bed rest or quiet environment*
   c. *Explain importance of safety in relation to this condition (e.g., vertigo, falling, and medication)*
   d. *Instruct patient to make position changes or other movements slowly and to limit activity*
   e. *Discuss, explain, and demonstrate discharge and follow-up instructions*
   f. *Instruct patient to avoid alcohol and caffeine*

4. Expected outcomes/evaluation (see Appendix B)

F. Labyrinthitis

    Labyrinthitis is an inflammatory response of the inner ear that can occur at any age and may involve the nerves connecting the inner ear to the brain. This is commonly referred to as neuronitis. Both bacterial and viral infections can cause this inflammation, producing disturbances within the cochlea that result in tinnitus and dizziness. When the vestibular system is affected, the symptoms include disturbances in balance and vision that may vary from mild to severe depending on the severity of infection. Bacterial labyrinthitis may damage the labyrinth by infecting the middle ear or surrounding bone of the inner ear. Bacteria may invade the cochlea or vestibular system, resulting in inflammation. More serious symptoms are usually from chronic or untreated middle ear infections and/or inner ear trauma.

Treatment measures are aimed at eliminating the bacteria with appropriate antibiotics. Surgery may be indicated to prevent further disease and complications when the middle or inner ear membranes are involved or have ruptured.

Viruses may also invade the inner ear and cause inflammation to the labyrinth. The symptoms are sudden in onset, with symptoms of severe spontaneous vertigo. These viruses invade the inner ear via the blood stream, causing both local and systemic responses. Influenza, measles, mumps, rubella, polio, hepatitis, herpes, and Epstein-Barr virus have been associated with this disorder. Symptoms of this condition create hearing abnormalities, balance/gait instability, nausea, vomiting, and dizziness. Dizziness and the sensation of spinning (vertigo) are the most common symptoms described. The initial symptoms persist for several days but may continue in varying severity for up to 6 weeks or longer. Diagnosis is contingent on ruling out neurological and cardiovascular disease, trauma, illicit drug or alcohol use, anxiety, allergies, and use of pharmacological agents. Treatment of symptoms is otherwise supportive with the use of antihistamines and antiemetics to manage dizziness and nausea.

1. **Assessment**
   a. *Subjective data*
      1) History of present illness.
         a) Vertigo/peripheral vertigo: patient feels he/she is moving; feelings of unsteadiness; undulating motions; rocking without spatial disorientation; tendency to fall when attempting to walk
         b) Nausea/vomiting
         c) Hearing abnormalities: ringing sensation in ears and sensitivity to loud noises; there is seldom hearing loss
         d) Ear pressure
         e) Headache
      2) Medical history
         a) Ear infection
         b) Meningitis
         c) Smoking and excessive caffeine use
         d) Head or ear trauma
         e) Recent upper respiratory tract infection
         f) Viral illness: measles, mumps, rubella (MMR), Epstein-Barr virus (EBV), hepatitis, polio, herpes or influenza
         g) Hypertension or arteriosclerosis
         h) Illicit drug or alcohol use
         i) Allergies
         j) Anxiety
         k) Systemic lupus erythematosus (SLE) or vasculitis
         l) Neurological disorders
         m) Migraine
         n) Meniere's syndrome
         o) Secondary or tertiary syphilis
         p) Prescription or nonprescription drug use
   b. *Objective data*
      1) Physical exam
         a) Disequilibrium
         b) Spontaneous horizontal nystagmus with peripheral features, away from side of disease; suppression of nystagmus with fixation
         c) Decreased hearing but usually no loss
         d) Caloric testing indicated if symptoms persist; should show absent or decreased response on affected side

e) Normal neurological and neurovascular exam

f) Orthostasis

2. **Analysis: differential nursing diagnosis/collaborative problems**

a. *Risk for physical injury related to dizziness*

b. *Risk for fluid volume deficit related to nausea/vomiting*

c. *Anxiety/fear related to alteration in health status*

3. **Planning/interventions**

a. *Administer labyrinthine suppressant as ordered: antihistamines*

b. *Antiemetics*

c. *Sedatives/anxiolytics*

d. *Intravenous fluids as indicated*

e. *Antibiotics as indicated*

4. **Expected outcomes/evaluation** (see Appendix B)

IV. SPECIFIC NOSE EMERGENCIES

A. Rhinitis

Rhinitis is an inflammatory condition of the nasal mucosa characterized by nasal membrane edema, vasodilation, discharge, and obstruction. It is most frequently seen in patients with viral or bacterial upper respiratory tract infections. Other causes include allergies and vasomotor and atrophic changes. Rhinitis affects all age groups and is spread by direct droplet contact from viruses and bacteria that invade the respiratory system. Symptoms include nasal congestion, runny nose, sneezing, headache, malaise, and scratchy throat. Ocular irritations such as itching and swelling as well as a loss of smell and taste can also occur. Physical exam reveals a swollen, erythematous nasal mucosa and nasal discharge. Symptom management is generally all that is needed to minimize discomfort. Oral decongestants, antihistamines, and topical corticosteroid nasal sprays are administered, and symptoms usually resolve within 7 days. If secondary bacterial infections result, as evident by a change in color of the nasal discharge, antibiotics may be prescribed. Bacterial invasion may occur from *S. pneumoniae*, *S. aureus*, *H. influenzae*, or *M. cattarrhalis*. When conventional treatment methods fail, referral to the otolaryngologist or allergist should be considered.

1. **Assessment**

a. *Subjective data*

1) History of present illness

a) Sneezing

b) Postnasal drip

c) Copious nasal discharge: thin, purulent, mucoid

d) Nasal obstruction

e) Muscle aches

f) Malaise

g) Headache

h) Watery or itchy eyes

i) Sore throat

j) Mild fever or chills

2) Medical history

a) Previous rhinitis

b) Nasal surgery or procedures

c) Allergies

b. *Objective data*

1) Physical examination

  a) Inflammation of throat and sinuses
  b) Nasal mucosa erythematous, edematous, and congested
  c) Injected sclera
  d) Clear drainage from eyes (watery eyes)
  e) Thickened nasal mucous membrane (chronic rhinitis)
  f) Pale turbinates (allergic rhinitis)
  g) Possible nasal polyps
  h) Restlessness
  2) Diagnostic procedures
  a) Nasal speculum examination
  b) Possible sinus radiographs
2. **Analysis: differential nursing diagnosis/collaborative problems**
  a. *Risk for ineffective breathing pattern (infants) related to nasal obstruction*
3. **Planning/interventions**
  a. *Administer prescribed medication: analgesics, antipyretics, decongestant, or antihistamine, nasal corticosteroid*
  b. *Discuss, explain, and demonstrate discharge and follow-up instructions*
  1) Maintain adequate humidification in home environment
  2) Use topical decongestants for only a few days (owing to rebound nasal congestion)
  3) Increase fluid intake
4. **Expected outcomes/evaluation** (see Appendix B)

B. Epistaxis

Spontaneous erosion of the superficial blood vessels originating from the anterior and inferior portions of the nasal septum (Kiesselbach's parea) through the internal and external carotid arteries accounts for the majority of cases of epistaxis. Less commonly, epistaxis originates from the ethmoidal arteries involving the roof of the nasal chamber or posterior septum and the sphenopalatine arteries that cause postnasal and lateral wall bleeding. Factors associated with bleeding result from localized nasal trauma including nose picking, forceful nose blowing, and FB. Rhinitis, excessive dryness of the nasal mucosa, systemic disease, antiplatelet medication, and nasal septum deviation can contribute to nasal bleeding and hemorrhage. Anterior epistaxis may be treated and resolve quickly by applying firm pressure at the bleeding site. This can be achieved by pinching the nasal alae together for approximately 10 minutes. When this fails, attempts to locate the bleeding site are necessary. A mixture of topical anesthetics and vasoconstrictors such as lidocaine, cocaine, and tetracaine (Pontocaine) may be used with a cotton pledget to provide better visualization in locating the bleeding site. When the bleeding site is identified, it may be cauterized using a silver nitrate stick, diathermy, or electrocautery. Nasal packing is then followed by the use of Surgicel strips, petroleum gauze, or Gelfoam and reassessed within 24 hours. Posterior epistaxis most always requires the insertion of nasal packing to control bleeding. The risk of hemorrhage in posterior epistaxis is more likely, and hospitalization is required to monitor patients for sequelae. Emergency measures to manage posterior epistaxis include placing balloon-tipped Foley catheters in the nasopharynx, posterior gauze packs, or Nasostat to tamponade bleeding until the otolaryngologist can perform definitive treatment.

1. **Assessment**
  a. *Subjective data*
  1) History of present illness
  a) Duration, frequency, and amount of bleeding

b) Previous epistaxis alone versus epistaxis and spitting blood (draining out front of nose: anterior; draining down throat: posterior)
c) Possibility of nasal FB
d) Recent nasal trauma or surgery
e) Nausea or vomiting (blood or blood clots)
2) Medical history
a) Use of aspirin or anticoagulants
b) Hypertension
c) Atherosclerosis
d) Previous epistaxis
e) Known bleeding disorders
f) Liver disease or alcohol abuse
g) Allergies to medications
b. *Objective data*
1) Physical examination
a) Bleeding from nostril(s)
b) Fresh blood in oropharynx
c) Active bleeding points on nasal mucosa
d) Erythema and swelling of nasal mucosa and turbinates
e) Blood in auditory canal (blood passing up eustachian tube and through perforated TM) or blood in corners of eyes (passed through lacrimal ducts)
f) Anxiety
g) Elevated or normal blood pressure
h) Tachycardia
i) Fear of dying or sense of impending doom
2) Diagnostic procedures
a) Complete blood count to determine degree of blood loss
b) Coagulation profile
c) Nasal examination to find source of bleeding

2. **Analysis: differential nursing diagnosis/collaborative problems**
a. *Risk for fluid volume deficit related to hemorrhage*
b. *Anxiety/fear related to hemorrhage, treatment, and outcome*
c. *Risk for ineffective airway clearance related to obstruction secondary to bleeding*

3. **Planning/interventions**
a. *Maintain airway, breathing, circulation*
b. *Monitor blood pressure, pulse, and respiration*
c. *Assist in control of hemorrhage*
1) Apply direct pressure to nose
2) Assist with anterior or posterior nasal pack, Nasostat
3) Establish IV catheter
4) Have suction equipment available
5) Assist with cauterization
a) Silver nitrate
b) Electrocautery or diathermy
6) Hemostatic material: oxidized regenerated cellulose (Surgicel), absorbable gelatin sponge (Gelfoam), or petroleum gauze
d. *Administer prescribed medications*
1) Anesthetic
2) Topical vasoconstrictors
3) Decongestant
4) Vasoconstrictor

5) Antihypertensive medications to control elevated blood pressure
    e. Administer blood products if required
4. Expected outcomes/evaluation (see Appendix B)

C. Nasal fracture

The nasal bones are fractured more frequently than any other facial bone; the nasal pyramid is the most fractured bone in the body. Nasal fractures result from direct trauma to the nose and can cause epistaxis, soft tissue swelling, nasal hematoma, periorbital ecchymosis, and subconjunctival hemorrhage. Signs of deformity, asymmetry, and inflammation are present; crepitus is noted on palpation of the nose. Radiological assessment to determine the identification of nasal fractures is important to determine the extent of injury. Three major categories are used to classify nasal fractures: 1) depressed, 2) lateral angulated, and 3) comminuted. Treatment measures include maintaining airway patency, reducing fractures, and controlling bleeding and pain. Applying ice and providing analgesic medications reduce pain and swelling. Intranasal examination is performed to rule out septal hematoma. When this exists, efforts to evacuate the clot immediately are undertaken to avoid secondary complications associated with septal necrosis and nasal deformity. Antibiotics are administered to prevent infection. Cosmetic repair of nasal deformities can be done when the condition permits.

1. **Assessment**
    a. *Subjective data*
        1) History of present illness
            a) Blunt or penetrating trauma to nose
            b) Visual deformity of nasal bone or cartilage
            c) Swelling
            d) Nasal bleeding
            e) Nasal obstruction
            f) Loss of consciousness
        2) Medical history
            a) Nasal surgery or defects
            b) Other pertinent medical conditions
            c) Allergies
            d) Tetanus immunization history if open wounds are present
    b. *Objective data*
        1) Physical examination
            a) Nasal deformity, asymmetry, or depression
            b) Nasal swelling
            c) Crepitus or false motion of nasal bone
            d) Epistaxis
            e) Obstruction of nasal cavity on fractured side
            f) Nasal and periorbital ecchymosis with possible subconjunctival hemorrhage
            g) Pain or tenderness on palpation of nose
            h) Septal fracture or hematoma or submucosal hemorrhage
            i) Mental status and neurological examination: confusion, lethargy, depressed responses
        2) Diagnostic procedures
            a) Radiographic assessment of the nasal/facial bones
2. **Analysis: differential nursing diagnosis/collaborative problems**
    a. *Pain related to fracture/soft tissue swelling*
    b. *Anxiety/fear related to pain and treatment outcome*

3. Planning/interventions
   a. Assess C-spine and maintain airway, breathing, circulation
   b. Assist in control of hemorrhage and evacuation of clot in septum as indicated
      1) Apply direct pressure to nose
      2) Establish IV catheter
      3) Use anterior or posterior nasal pack if necessary
   c. Administer prescribed medications
      1) Anesthetic
      2) Decongestant
      3) Vasoconstrictor
      4) Analgesic
      5) Antibiotics
   d. Apply cold pack to bridge of nose
4. Expected outcomes/evaluation (see Appendix B)

D. Foreign body in nose

Nasal FBs are most commonly seen in children, resulting from play with buttons, beans, pebbles, beads, and small toy parts. Presenting features usually reveal unilateral nasal obstruction. Foul-smelling rhinorrhea may result from the FB remaining in the nose for an extended period of time. The nose may be sore or bleeding from previous attempts at removal. The nose may appear swollen or tender when palpated. Difficulty breathing, stridor, lethargy, and failure to eat may be indicators of FB aspiration and should be managed immediately. Attempts to remove a foreign body or object once it is located can be achieved by several methods. Having the parent gently blow into the child's mouth while obliterating the unaffected nostril, simple nose blowing or suctioning may cause enough pressure to release the foreign body. Forceps and hooked or looped instruments may also be used. In some cases, 1% phenylephrine is applied topically to minimize swelling of the nasal mucosa before retrieving a nasal foreign object. When retrieval is difficult, a 6- or 8-French Foley catheter may be passed beyond the obstruction. When the balloon is inflated and pressure is released, the FB may be easily removed.

1. Assessment
   a. Subjective data
      1) History of present illness
         a) Verbal report of FB in nose
         b) Nose pain or swelling
         c) Purulent nasal discharge
         d) Foul smell from nose
      2) Medical history
         a) Allergies to medications
         b) Previous FB
   b. Objective data
      1) Physical examination
         a) Unilateral purulent nasal discharge
         b) Foul-smelling rhinorrhea
         c) Visualization of FB (usually lodges between middle turbinate and septum)
         d) Edema of nasal mucosa
         e) Unilateral bleeding from nose
         f) Agitation
      2) Diagnostic procedure: nasal examination with speculum
2. Analysis: differential nursing diagnosis/collaborative problems

 a. *Pain related to pressure and edema*
 b. *Anxiety/fear related to need to seek medical attention*
 3. **Planning/interventions**
 a. *Instruct patient to blow nose in attempt to dislodge and remove foreign object*
 b. *Apply topical vasoconstrictive agent (1% phenylephrine) and/or topical anesthetic to involved nostril before manual removal to minimize swelling*
 c. *Assist in removal of foreign object (with suction, forceps, or Foley catheter)*
 d. *Discuss, explain, and demonstrate discharge and follow-up instructions*
 4. **Expected outcomes/evaluation** (see Appendix B)

V. SPECIFIC THROAT EMERGENCIES

A. Pharyngitis

Pharyngitis is commonly described as a "sore throat" and is a frequent cause of emergency department visits. Pharyngitis is usually associated with viral upper respiratory tract infections that cause inflammation in the pharynx. Most cases resolve with symptom management. Bacterial infections caused by group A *beta-hemolytic streptococci* may result in more serious complications such as peritonsillar abscess, retropharyngeal abscess, rheumatic fever, and glomerulonephritis. Pharyngitis affects all age groups, and transmission is by droplet of infected secretions. It is most commonly seen during late fall, winter, and early spring. Clinical symptoms include a sore throat, fever, pain on swallowing, and cervical adenopathy. Physical exam commonly reveals a red and edematous pharynx, palatine petechiae, and tonsils with or without purulent exudate. Some patients may have a scarlatiniform erythematous rash that looks like a sunburn with fine red papules and a sandpaper texture. It will blanch with pressure and resolve within 2 to 5 days. Frequently, there is facial flushing. The tongue may have a characteristic "strawberry" appearance as a result of enlarged papillae. Treatment involves obtaining a throat culture and beginning antimicrobial therapy when clinical suspicion of strep throat is high. Differential diagnosis must be considered and includes adenovirus, mononucleosis, and diphtheria, among others. Chronic or recurrent pharyngitis requires further evaluation to determine whether pathology exists and whether alternative therapy is indicated.

 1. **Assessment**
 a. *Subjective data*
 1) History of present illness
 a) Mild to severe sore throat
 b) Difficulty in swallowing or talking
 c) Pain referred to ears, neck, and jaw
 d) Fever or chills
 e) Harsh cough
 f) Anorexia
 g) Fatigue
 h) Body aches: muscle and joint pain
 i) Feeling of fullness in head or headache
 2) Medical history
 a) Use of medications
 b) Smoking or inhaled illicit drug use
 c) Allergies to medications
 d) Immunization status
 b. *Objective data*
 1) Physical examination

        a) Enlarged tonsils

        b) Cervical lymphadenopathy

        c) Erythema or exudate of pharynx or tonsils

        d) Foul breath odor

        e) Nasal speech

        f) Malaise

        g) Flushed face or hot skin

    2) Diagnostic procedures

        a) Rapid *Streptococcus* screen if available

        b) Throat culture and sensitivity testing

2. Analysis: differential nursing diagnosis/collaborative problems

  a. Pain related to inflammatory process

  b. Infection related to invasion of tissue by bacteria

3. Planning/interventions

  a. Administer prescribed medications

    1) Antipyretic

    2) Analgesic

    3) Topical anesthetic agent

    4) Steroids

    5) Antibiotics

  b. Provide warm saline throat irrigation

  c. Instruct patient on importance of adequate rest and fluid intake

  d. Discuss, explain, and demonstrate discharge and follow-up instructions

4. Expected outcomes/evaluation (see Appendix B)

B. Tonsillitis

Similar organisms that are responsible for pharyngitis can also affect the tonsils and cause infection. As a part of the lymphatic system, tonsils are considered a "filter" for circulating bacteria, lymph, or other foreign material to aid in fighting infections. As bacteria invade the nose and mouth, inflammation and enlargement can occur within the palatine, lingual, and pharyngeal tonsils, causing acute tonsillitis. Infection can sometimes be trapped within these structures and result in sore throat, difficulty swallowing, fever, chills, cervical lymphadenopathy, and fetid breath. Treatment measures include the use of antibiotics, analgesics, and warm salt-water gargles. Chronic tonsillitis may occur in some patients, necessitating surgical removal of the tonsils to avoid recurrent or relapsing infection from sore throat.

1. Assessment

  a. Subjective data

    1) History of present illness

        a) Mild to severe throat pain

        b) Recent upper respiratory tract infection

        c) Pain or difficulty in swallowing

        d) Referred pain to ear and neck

        e) Fever or chills

        f) Fatigue

        g) Headache

        h) Muscle or joint pain

    2) Medical history

        a) Previous infections of pharynx or tonsils

        b) Related surgery

        c) Medication therapy

        d) Allergies to medications

          e) Immunization status
    b. *Objective data*
       1) Physical examination
          a) Tachycardia
          b) Elevated temperature
          c) Red and swollen tonsils
          d) Purulent exudate on tonsillar crypts
          e) Erythematous oropharynx
          f) Enlarged and tender cervical and submandibular lymph nodes
          g) Flushed face
          h) Inflammation and enlargement of pharyngeal or lingual tonsils
       2) Diagnostic procedures
          a) Rapid *Streptococcus* screen as indicated
          b) Culture and sensitivity testing of exudate
  2. **Analysis: differential nursing diagnosis/collaborative problems**
    a. *Pain related to inflammatory/infectious process*
    b. *Infection related to invasion of tissue by bacteria*
  3. **Planning/interventions**
    a. *Maintain airway, breathing, circulation*
    b. *Provide warm saline throat irrigations*
    c. *Instruct patient on importance of adequate diet and rest*
    d. *Administer prescribed medications (antibiotic and antitussive) and steroids to suppress acute inflammation*
    e. *Discuss, explain, and demonstrate discharge and follow-up procedures*
  4. **Expected outcomes/evaluation** (see Appendix B)

C. Laryngitis

Viral infection is the most frequent cause of hoarseness, more commonly referred to as laryngitis. Excessive use of voice, irritating inhaled or ingested substances, bacterial infections, and allergies can produce similar symptoms affecting the larynx and vocal cords. The constant urge to clear the throat and tickling sensations in the pharynx are often described. As inflammation of the mucous membranes increases, the symptoms worsen. The voice sounds harsh and raspy. When significant edema is present, there is stridor or airway impairment, and emergency measures should be taken to prevent further airway obstruction. Differential diagnosis such as polyps, lesions, or tumors must be considered and further examination by direct laryngoscopy performed to rule out pathology. Treatment involves voice rest and use of corticosteroids to suppress inflammation, expectorants to liquefy secretions, and antibiotics to treat suspected bacterial infections.

  1. **Assessment**
    a. *Subjective data*
       1) History of present illness
          a) Dry, tickling sensation in throat
          b) Partial or complete loss of voice, hoarseness
          c) Fever or chills
          d) Sore throat
          e) Dyspnea: increasing dyspnea may be a sign of edematous laryngitis or croup
          f) Difficulty in swallowing
          g) Dry cough
          h) Minor discomfort

       i) Anorexia
   2) Medical history
      a) Recent infections, illness, or injury
      b) Allergies
      c) Immunization status
  b. *Objective data*
   1) Physical examination
      a) Reddened larynx and vocal cords
      b) Swelling of larynx and epiglottis
      c) Dyspnea
      d) Respiratory stridor
      e) Granulation of mucous membrane lining larynx (chronic)
      f) Dysphonia or aphonia
      g) Temperature greater than 99°F(37.2°C)
      h) Restlessness
      i) Postnasal drip and rhinorrhea
   2) Diagnostic procedures
      a) Throat culture and sensitivity testing as indicated
      b) Complete blood count with differential

2. Analysis: differential nursing diagnosis/collaborative problems
  a. *Pain related to inflammatory process*
  b. *Infection related to invasion of tissue by microorganisms*

3. Planning/interventions
  a. *Provide adequately warm room that is adequately humidified*
  b. *Instruct patient to maintain voice rest*
  c. *Administer prescribed medication*
   1) Antibiotic, sometimes in combination with oral or inhaled steroids
   2) Antitussive agents
   3) Oral analgesics
   4) Topical anesthetic agent: viscous lidocaine 2% or chloroseptic spray
   5) Antipyretic
   6) Zinc throat lozenges
  d. *Apply ice bag to anterior aspect of patient's throat*

4. Expected outcomes/evaluation (see Appendix B)

D. Fractured larynx

Direct trauma to the neck resulting from blunt penetration as seen in motor vehicle crashes can cause vascular injuries or larynx fracture of the neck. Penetrating trauma may also occur but is less common. Presenting symptoms may include hoarseness when speaking, pain with swallowing, cough, or hemoptysis. The neck area may appear ecchymotic, with presence of abrasions, subcutaneous emphysema, and loss of thyroid prominence. Because of the danger of spinal cord injury, trauma to the neck must be carefully evaluated to rule out C-spine injury. Efforts to maintain adequate airway, ventilation, and perfusion are essential because they are frequently compromised with this injury. Cricothyrotomy and tracheotomy may be necessary if the extent of trauma prevents nasal or endotracheal intubation. Common causes associated with larynx fracture include motor vehicle crashes, strangulation (both self-inflicted and accidental), and physical trauma associated with sport activities.

1. Assessment
  a. *Subjective data*
   1) History of present illness

   a) Blunt trauma to neck
   b) Hoarseness
   c) Change in voice characteristics
   d) Odynophagia: pain on swallowing
   e) Cough or dyspnea
   f) Hemoptysis
  2) Medical history
   a) Recent surgery in neck area
   b) Allergies to medications
 b. Objective data
  1) Physical examination
   a) Ecchymosis
   b) Abrasions
   c) Loss of normal prominence of thyroid cartilage
   d) Subcutaneous emphysema
   e) Inspiratory stridor
   f) Suprasternal or intercostal retractions
  2) Diagnostic procedures
   a) Fiberoptic laryngoscopy: presence of edema and hematomas indicate need for tracheotomy
   b) Indirect laryngoscopy
   c) CT scan to assess for fractures, hematomas, and dislocations; soft tissue films of the neck are not sensitive to laryngeal injury

2. Analysis: differential nursing diagnosis/collaborative problems
 a. Ineffective airway clearance related to edema, hemorrhage, and fracture
 b. Ineffective breathing pattern related to airway obstruction
 c. Anxiety/fear related to airway obstruction and pain

3. Planning/interventions
 a. Assess C-spine and maintain airway, breathing, circulation
 b. Prepare to assist with cricothyrotomy or tracheotomy as indicated
 c. Administer high-humidity oxygen
 d. Prepare to assist with fiberoptic intubation
 e. Monitor ABG values
 f. Treat concomitant injuries

4. Expected outcomes/evaluation (see Appendix B)

E. Peritonsillar abscess

  Peritonsillar abscess arises through an infection penetrating the tonsillar capsule and superior constrictor muscle into the surrounding areolar tissue. Severe sore throat, odynophagia, trismus, and uvular deviation are common features found in peritonsillar abscess. Streptococci bacteria are generally the pathogens responsible for this infection. Physical exam reveals the tonsil displaced medially. Patients frequently demonstrate a "hot potato" voice and may be unable to swallow their own saliva. Drainage may produce immediate relief by aspirating pus from the peritonsillar fold located superior and medial to the upper pole of the tonsil. An otolaryngologist or oral surgeon should perform the drainage to avoid complications to the retropharyngeal, deep neck, and posterior mediastinal spaces. Antibiotics and warm saline irrigation aid in reducing infection and promoting comfort. Tonsillectomy is performed when infections are relapsing and peritonsillar abscess is recurrent.

1. Assessment

    a. *Subjective data*
      1) History of present illness
        a) Sore throat
        b) Pain on swallowing
        c) Ipsilateral ear fullness, otalgia
        d) Fever or chills
        e) Pus on tonsils
        f) Difficulty in opening mouth or eating
        g) Drooling or inability to swallow
        h) Muffled "hot potato" voice
        i) Difficulty breathing
      2) Medical history
        a) Recent tonsillitis
        b) Present medication
        c) Allergies to medications
    b. *Objective data*
      1) Physical examination
        a) Enlarged affected tonsil
        b) Displacement of uvula toward nonaffected side
        c) Edema and erythema of soft palate
        d) Profuse salivation
        e) Trismus
        f) Torticollis: contracted state of cervical muscles, resulting in twisting of neck in abnormal position
        g) Exudate on tonsil
        h) Increased respiratory rate
        i) Shortness of breath
        j) Elevated temperature
      2) Diagnostic procedures
        a) Needle aspiration of suspected abscess
        b) Culture and sensitivity testing of exudate from abscess

2. **Analysis: differential nursing diagnosis/collaborative problems**
    a. *Risk for ineffective airway clearance related to edema and inflammatory process*
    b) *Pain related to infection*
    c) *Infection related to invasion of tissue by organisms*

3. **Planning/interventions**
    a. *Maintain airway, breathing, circulation*
    b. *Monitor vital signs and respiratory status closely*
    c. *Administer oxygen*
    d. *Elevate head of bed 60 to 90 degrees*
    e. *Initiate IV catheter for hydration and medication*
    f. *Provide warm saline throat irrigations*
    g. *Administer prescribed medications*
      1) Antibiotics
      2) Topical anesthetic throat spray
      3) Local anesthetic injection
      4) Narcotic analgesic
      5) Antipyretic
    h. *Apply ice collar to throat*
    i. *Assist with incision and drainage if ordered*
    j. *Pulse oximetry as indicated*

4. Expected outcomes/evaluation (see Appendix B)

F. Foreign body in throat

FB aspiration is a common cause of accidental death in the United States among children 6 years of age and younger. FBs or objects such as, for example, peanuts, hotdogs, grapes, vegetables, seeds, and metal or plastic objects can obstruct the main stem bronchi or distal trachea near the carina and esophagus. A variety of symptoms may present after ingestion of a FB or object with varying degrees of obstruction observed, such as wheezing, stridor, coughing, failure to eat or drink, or apnea. With any suspected FB, airway management is the priority until location of the FB is confirmed. Treatment and removal of the FB are dependent on its location. Radiographs are used to locate the FB and assist in determining the type of treatment necessary. Emergency department management may include direct laryngoscopy to visualize the FB and facilitate removal with the use of McGill forceps. Tracheal and bronchial FBs are usually removed under general anesthesia, and esophageal FBs that do not pass into the stomach within 12 hours should be removed to avoid secondary complications. When indicated removal of an FB can be achieved with a variety of methods, including rigid esophagoscopy, balloon-tipped Foley catheter, bougienage, flexible endoscopy, and pharmacological agents. The use of the Heimlich maneuver, or chest and abdominal thrusts, can prevent unnecessary deaths associated with FB ingestion and aspiration.

1. **Assessment**
   a. *Subjective data*
      1) History of present illness
         a) Pain or sore throat
         b) Vocal changes
         c) Drooling
         d) Coughing
         e) Difficulty in swallowing or breathing
         f) Difficulty in talking or inability to talk
         g) Recent ingestion of foreign object or food
         h) Diminished ability or inability to take oral fluids/food
      2) Medical history
         a) Current medications
         b) Allergies to medications
   b. *Objective data*
      1) Physical examination
         a) FB visible in pharynx or larynx
         b) Dyspnea or stridor
         c) Respiratory rate greater than 12 breaths/min
         d) Tachycardia
         e) Cyanosis
         f) Excessive salivation or dysphasia
         g) Skin cool and moist
         h) Dysphagia
         i) Hemoptysis or hematemesis
         j) Agitation
         k) Chest pain
      2) Diagnostic procedures
         a) Indirect laryngoscopy

       b) Anteroposterior and lateral chest radiographs with end-inspiratory and end-expiratory views; decubitus views as indicated

       c) Soft tissue radiograph of neck

       d) Examination with radiopaque contrast material

2. Analysis: differential nursing diagnosis/collaborative problems

    a. Ineffective airway clearance related to ingestion of FB

    b. Anxiety/fear related to ineffective airway clearance

3. Planning/interventions

    a. Maintain airway, breathing, circulation

      1) Finger sweep of mouth (age dependent)

      2) Heimlich maneuver or abdominal chest thrust as indicated

    b. Provide supplemental oxygen and pulse oximetry

    c. Initiate IV catheter

    d. Elevate head of bed 60 to 90 degrees

    e. Continuously monitor and assess

      1) Vital signs

      2) Cardiac rhythm

      3) Tissue perfusion

      4) Level of consciousness

      5) ABG values

    f. Prepare for potential emergency medical interventions as indicated

      1) Indirect laryngoscopy

      2) Cricothyrotomy/tracheotomy

    g. Minimize environmental stimuli

    h. Assist with FB removal procedures

      1) Rigid esophagoscopy

      2) Balloon-tipped Foley catheter:

      3) Bougienage: pushes esophageal coin ingestions into the stomach

      4) Flexible endoscopy

      5) Pharmacological agents: diazepam (Valium), meperidine (Demerol), glucagon

4. Expected outcomes/evaluation (see Appendix B)

BIBLIOGRAPHY

Amundson, L. H. (1990). Disorders of the external ear. *Primary Care, 2,* 213–231.

Ballenger, J. J. (1991). *Diseases of the nose, throat, ear, head, and neck* (14th ed.). Philadelphia: Lea & Febiger.

Bluestone, C. D. (1989). Modern management of otitis media. *Pediatric Clinics of North America, 6,* 1371–1386.

Drezner, D. A., Schaffer, S. R., & Finkelstein, J. M. (1991). Nonvascular injuries of the mouth and neck. *Topics in Emergency Medicine, 4,* 48–59.

Finkelstein, J. M., Schaffer, S. R., & Drezner, D. A. (1991). Otologic injuries. *Topics in Emergency Medicine, 4,* 60–66.

Fritz, S., Kelen, G. D., & Sivertson, K. T. (1987). Foreign bodies of the external auditory canal. *Emergency Medicine Clinics of North America, 2,* 183–192.

Giebink, G. S., Canafax, D. M., & Kempthorne, J. (1991). Antimicrobial treatment of acute otitis media. *Journal of Pediatrics, 119,* 495–500.

Hall, S. F. (1990). Peritonsillar abscess: The treatment options. *Journal of Otolaryngology, 3,* 226–229.

Hedges, J. R., & Lowe, R. A. (1987). Approach to acute pharyngitis. *Emergency Medicine Clinics of North America, 2,* 335–350.

Hess, G. P. (1987). An approach to throat complaints. *Emergency Medicine Clinics of North America, 2,* 313–334.

Josell, S. D., & Abrams, R. G. (1991). Managing common dental problems and emergencies. *Pediatric Clinics of North America, 5,* 1325–1342.

Kemp, E. D. (1990). Otitis media. *Primary Care, 2,* 267–286.

Lanzi, G. L. (1991). Mandibular and dental injuries. *Topics in Emergency Medicine, 4,* 27–38.

Lusk, R. P., Lazar, R. H., & Muntz, H. R. (1989). The diagnosis and treatment of recurrent and chronic sinusitis in children. *Pediatric Clinics of North America, 6,* 1411–1429.

McKay, J. I. (1987). Dental, ear, nose, and throat emergencies. In R. E. Rea, P. W. Bourg, J. G. Parker, & D. Rushing (Eds.), *Emergency nursing core curriculum* (3rd ed.). Philadelphia: W. B. Saunders.

Randall, D. A., & Freeman, S. B. (1991). Management of anterior and posterior epistaxis. *American Family Physician, 6,* 2007–2015.

Reich, J. J. (1987). Ear infections. *Emergency Medicine Clinics of North America, 2,* 227–242.

Riley, M. A. K. (1987). *Nursing care of the client with ear, nose, and throat disorders.* Berlin: Springer.

Sweeney, R. L., & Doolin, E. J. (1991). Head and neck trauma: Special considerations in children. *Topics in Emergency Medicine, 4,* 78–86.

Vogt, H. B. (1990). Rhinitis. *Primary Care, 2,* 309–322.

Reneé Semonin-Holleran RN, PhD, CEN, CCRN, CFRN

CHAPTER **5**

Environmental Emergencies

MAJOR TOPICS

General Strategy

Specific Environmental Emergencies

  Heat-Related Emergencies

  Cold-Related Emergencies

Submersion Injuries

Thermal Injuries

Lightning Injury

Bites and Stings

I. GENERAL STRATEGY

A. Assessment

1. **Primary assessment/resuscitation** (see Chapter 1)
2. **Secondary assessment** (see Chapter 1)
3. **Psychological, social, and environmental risk factors**
    a. *Alterations in ability to perceive environmental threats*
        1) Age of the patient
            a) Pediatric: decision making limited to developmental level
            b) Elderly: disease process altering ability for decision making/self-care
        2) Psychiatric illness
        3) Use of any substance that alters patient's ability to react to environment
    b. *Physical factors*
        1) Obesity
        2) Malnutrition
        3) Lack of psychological and physical preparation
    c. *Social risk factors*
        1) Homelessness or lack of appropriate shelter
        2) Lack of appropriate clothing
        3) Maltreatment/neglect
    d. *Occupational risk factors*
        1) Firefighters, emergency medical service (EMS), and rescue personnel

      2) Outside laborers

      3) Occupation that involves exposure to excessive heat or cold

      4) Hazardous material workers

      5) Military recruits

  e. *Recreational risk factors*

      1) Amateur athletes

      2) Marathon running

      3) Vigorous exercise

      4) Heavy exertion

      5) Winter sports

      6) Hiking/walking in unfamiliar areas

  f. *Environmental risk factors*

      1) Weather conditions

         a) Ambient temperature: above 100°F (38°C) or below 32° F (0°C)

         b) Prolonged heat wave

      2) Wind

         a) Chill factor

         b) Still air

      3) Humidity

      4) Contact with metal or water

      5) Enclosed area

         a) Temperature

         b) Ventilation

      6) Animals, insects, spiders, aquatic animals, reptiles indigenous to the specific environment

      7) Raising or working with exotic pets

4. Focused survey

  a. *Subjective data*

      1) History of present illness/injury

         a) Mechanism of environmental exposure/injury

         b) Environmental factors

            (1) Ambient temperature

            (2) Enclosed space

            (3) Type and temperature of the water

            (4) Type of insect, animal, reptile that lives in environment in which patient was found

            (5) Type of clothing/prevention used by the patient

         c) Exposure

            (1) Time of exposure/injury occurred

            (2) Length of time in the environment or since the incident occurred (e.g., time of submersion)

            (3) Underlying factors predisposing patient to exposure/injury: mental status; use of alcohol or mind-altering substances; lack of available shelter or appropriate clothing; activity before exposure/injury

         d) Presence of pain

            (1) Location of injury and severity of pain

            (2) Radiation of injury or toxicity, especially with envenomation

      2) Past medical history

         a) Allergies

         b) Medications

            (1) Alcohol

            (2) Phenothiazines

            (3) Anticholinergics

            (4) Antihistamines

(5) Tricyclic antidepressants

(6) Amphetamines

(7) Lysergic acid diethylamide (LSD)

(8) Cocaine

(9) Monoamine oxidase (MAO) inhibitors

(10) Beta blockers

(11) Sympatholytic antihypertensives

(12) Steroids

(13) Immunosuppressive drugs

(14) Anticoagulants

c) Tetanus immunization history

d) History of rabies immunization

e) History of antivenom therapy

f) Medical problems

(1) Anaphylaxis

(2) Alcoholism

(3) Spinal cord injury

(4) Central nervous system disorders (e.g., cerebrovascular accident [CVA], seizures)

(5) Asthma

(6) Diabetes

(7) Cardiovascular disease

(8) Hepatic disease

(9) Hypoadrenalism

(10) Parkinsonism

(11) Hyperthyroidism

(12) Raynaud's disease

(13) Prior environmental injury (hypothermia, hyperthermia)

(14) Extensive burns

(15) Cystic fibrosis

(16) Scleroderma

(17) Ectodermal dysplasia

(18) Miliaria

b. *Objective data*

1) Physical examination

a) General survey

(1) Inspection

(a) Scene safety: unlike other emergencies, health care provider needs to ensure that it is safe to render care to the patient (e.g., animal contained? Fire under control?)

(b) Airway: patent, maintainable, not maintainable; carbonaceous sputum, singed nasal hairs/eyebrows, conjunctivitis, rhinitis, erythema of the face, palate; facial swelling

(c) Respiratory status

(d) Pupillary function

(e) Motor/sensory function

(f) Signs of other injuries

(2) Auscultation

(a) Breath sounds

(b) Heart tones

(c) Bowel sounds

(3) Palpation

(a) Peripheral and central pulses

          (b) Blood pressure
          (c) Skin temperature
          (d) Pain
          (e) Deformities

      (4) Skin appearance

          (a) Hyperemia   (f) Hives
          (b) Blistering   (g) Ticks
          (c) Edema   (h) Fang/bite marks
          (d) Ulceration   (i) Stingers
          (e) Rash

      (5) Bites/wounds

          (a) Size
          (b) Shape
          (c) Depth
          (d) Visible skin structures: muscle, subcutaneous tissues
          (e) Debris

B. Analysis: differential nursing diagnosis/collaborative problems

1. **Anxiety/fear**
2. **Breathing pattern ineffective**
3. **Fluid volume deficit**
4. **Impaired gas exchange**
5. **Impaired skin integrity**
6. **Ineffective airway clearance**
7. **Ineffective thermoregulation**
8. **Hypothermia**
9. **Knowledge deficit**
10. **Pain**
11. **Risk for infection**
12. **Risk for injury**

C. Planning/interventions

1. **Determine priorities**
   a. *Manage and maintain patient's airway, breathing, and circulation (ABCs); provide cervical spine immobilization as indicated by the patient's specific environmental emergency*
   b. *Obtain information related to the specific environmental emergency, patient's medical history, and interventions initiated before arrival in the emergency department*
   c. *Obtain and monitor patient's vital signs, particularly temperature*
   d. *Prepare patient for particular interventions related to environmental emergency*
   e. *Manage patient's pain*
   f. *Prevent complications*
   g. *Notify appropriate authorities as indicated (i.e., local health department for animal bites)*
   h. *Consult experts as needed to provide patient care for specific environmental emergencies (e.g., envenomation)*
2. **Develop nursing care plan to patient's presenting emergency**
3. **Obtain and prepare necessary equipment and supplies**
4. **Institute appropriate interventions on basis of nursing care plan**
5. **Document and record data as appropriate**

D. Expected outcomes/evaluation

1. **Monitor patient responses and outcomes, adjusting nursing care plans as indicated**
   a. *Specific interventions*
   b. *Disposition and discharge planning*
2. **Record all pertinent data**
3. **If positive outcomes are not demonstrated, assessment and/or plan of care needs to be re-evaluated**

E. Age-related considerations

1. **Pediatric**
   a. *Growth or development related*
      1) Deaths from burns and drowning are among the leading causes of death in children
      2) Infants and small children have small airways, which are more easily obstructed by edema from anaphylaxis or inhalation injury
      3) Children have a large ratio of body surface area to weight and lose body heat more easily
      4) Children have less adipose tissue to maintain body heat and provide insulation
      5) Young and premature infants do not have the ability to shiver to maintain warmth; they use nonshivering thermogenesis for heat generation; when there is a drop in skin temperature, the thermal receptors transmit impulses to the central nervous system (CNS), which stimulates heat production in the brown fat tissue
      6) Children are dependent on caregivers to educate and protect them about the environment in which they live
      7) The potential for maltreatment should be considered (e. g., burns may be inflicted as a form of punishment; drowning may occur as a result of a lack of supervision)
      8) Child's immunization status should be assessed
      9) Children's healing responses are more rapid than those of adults
   b. *"Pearls"*
      1) Children are curious and want to explore their environment and may be exposed to danger from the environment with little fear of the consequences of their actions (e.g., young children may not be afraid of a dog they do not know and may approach the animal without fear)
      2) Adolescents may take more risks because of peer pressure (potential consequences of this behavior include drowning that results from swimming while intoxicated)
      3) Children are at a greater risk for injury from heat and cold emergencies because of their immature nervous system and dependency on caregivers to maintain the environment around them
      4) Children are at greater risk for complications from envenomation because of their smaller size and lower weight
2. **Geriatric**
   a. *Age related*
      1) A decrease in elasticity of lung tissue and a decrease in amount of alveoli may contribute to a limited ability to respond to toxic inhalation exposures
      2) Cardiovascular changes that occur with aging cause decreased distensibility

of blood vessels, increased systemic resistance, decreased cardiac output, and decreased response to stress

3) Increased risk for hyper- or hypothermia because of inability to vasodilate or vasoconstrict blood vessels; decreased cardiac output; and decreased subcutaneous tissue

4) Delayed and diminished sweat response

5) Thirst mechanism becomes less efficient with aging, as does the kidney's ability to concentrate urine, increasing risk of heat-related dehydration

6) Inactivity and immobility increase susceptibility to hypothermia by suppressing shivering and reducing heat-generating muscle activity

b. *"Pearls"*

1) Elderly have thinner skin and may sustain more serious injury from bites

2) Fluid overload during resuscitation could cause serious consequences

3) Elderly patients with an altered mental status are dependent on caregivers to protect them from danger in the surrounding environment

II. SPECIFIC ENVIRONMENTAL EMERGENCIES

A. Heat-related emergencies

Heat-related emergencies occur when the body is no longer able to regulate its body temperature through normal physiologic mechanisms. Thermoregulation occurs through the preoptic anterior hypothalamus. Information about body temperature is sent to the brain by peripheral and central thermoreceptors located in the skin, limb muscles, and spinal cord. The hypothalamus then initiates methods that will help the body maintain a normal or tolerable body temperature. The body attempts to keep itself at a temperature of 98.6°F or 37.1°C. When the body is exposed to excessive heat, it will attempt to dissipate the heat by convection, radiation, or evaporation. Drugs, strenuous activity, and high ambient temperatures can increase internal heat production. Factors such as lack of acclimation, restrictive clothing, and high humidity affect the body's ability to manage excessive heat. As the body's temperature increases, there is stimulation of the sweat response to initiate evaporative heat loss. This is the body's primary mechanism of cooling. Sweating not only assists in cooling the body, but it may also cause loss of body weight, sodium, and potassium. If fluids and electrolytes are not replaced, dehydration can occur. The body will also attempt to dissipate heat by shunting blood to the skin. There is an increase in heart rate, stroke volume, and cardiac output. Additionally, the kidneys conserve fluid for evaporation by retaining salt and water. Under normal circumstances, with time to acclimate, these compensatory mechanisms will assist the body in sustaining a normal temperature. However, if there are additional factors contributing to the heat stress, these mechanisms will fail and will result in a heat-related emergency. People at risk for heat-related emergencies include the young, the elderly, and individuals not acclimated to hot weather.

Heat-related emergencies include heat cramps, heat exhaustion, and heat stroke.

1. Heat cramps

Heat cramps result from depletion of fluids and electrolytes in exerted muscles. The patient is usually in good health, but has not adequately replaced the fluids and electrolytes lost while sweating. The patient complains of pain in the exerted muscles and thirst. Treatment includes cessation of the exertional activity, resting in a cool place, massage of the painful areas, and replacement of fluids with a balanced solution such as a commercially prepared sports drink (e.g., Gatorade).

2. Heat exhaustion

Heat exhaustion is precipitated by major exertion in hot weather. Peripheral vasodilatation occurs to dissipate heat, and fluids and electrolytes are lost through perfuse sweating. The patient's core body temperature may be high-normal or as high as 104°F (39°C). On physical examination, the patient is pale, ashen, and sweating profusely. The patient may complain of weakness or present with an altered mental status. Additional symptoms include hypotension, tachycardia, and severe thirst. Treatment includes placing the patient in a cool environment, managing ABCs, and monitoring for cardiac dysrhythmias, including ventricular aberrance and peaked T waves secondary to electrolyte imbalances. Muscle damage may occur at high temperature, so the patient must be monitored for rhabdomyolysis (e.g., dark urine, muscle cramps).

3. Heat stroke

Heat stroke is a medical emergency. The patient is no longer able to dissipate heat because of failure of the central thermoregulation mechanisms. Morbidity is directly related to the amount of time the patient's body temperature remains elevated. There is a history of extreme exertion in a hot environment, lack of acclimation, and the presence of risk factors such as use of phenothiazines or a CNS disorder. The core body temperature is greater than 106°F (41°C). The patient's mental status ranges from confusion to coma, and the skin is hot and dry. Because of fluid loss, the patient is hypotensive and tachycardic. Treatment includes stabilization of the patient's ABCs along with rapid cooling. There continues to be controversy about which method is best. Cooling methods include removal of clothing, covering with wet sheets, and placing him or her in front of a large fan (evaporative cooling); providing an ice water bath (conductive cooling); and administering cool fluids. Whatever cooling method is chosen, the patient's temperature must be closely monitored and shivering controlled. Fluid and electrolyte imbalances must be corrected and the patient monitored for rhabdomyolysis. Clotting studies should be obtained to monitor the patient for the development of disseminated intravascular coagulation (DIC), a potential complication of heat stroke.

a. Assessment

  1) Subjective data

    a) History of present illness

      (1) Temperature of patient when found

      (2) Relative humidity

      (3) Type of activity in which patient was engaged

      (4) Length of time in environment

      (5) Risk factors for heat-related emergency

        (a) Age (young or elderly)

        (b) Exertion during hot weather

        (c) Lack of acclimation

        (d) Obesity

        (e) Physical conditioning

    b) Medical history

      (1) Medications

        (a) Phenothiazines

        (b) Tricyclic antidepressants

        (c) Cocaine

        (d) Antihistamines

        (e) Ethanol

        (f) Diuretics

      (2) Disease states

(a) Alcoholism

(b) Diabetes

(c) Spinal cord injuries

(d) CNS disorders

(e) Cardiovascular disease

2) Objective data

a) Physical examination

(1) General survey

(2) Pain in exerted muscles

(3) Thirst

(4) Diaphoresis/profuse sweating

(5) Pale, ashen skin

(6) Hot/dry skin (heat stroke)

(7) Altered mental status (confusion to coma)

(8) Weakness

(9) Hypotension

(10) Tachycardia

(11) Tachypnea

(12) Core body temperature greater than 104°F (39°C)

b) Diagnostic procedures

(1) Complete blood count (CBC)

(2) Prothrombin time (PT), partial thromboplastin time (PTT)

(3) Platelets, fibrin split products

(4) Electrolytes

(5) Hepatic and renal profiles

(6) Arterial blood gases (ABGs)

(7) Drug screen

(8) Urinalysis, myoglobin

(9) Chest x-ray film

(10) Computed tomography (CT) of the head

(11) Electrocardiography (ECG)

b. *Analysis: differential nursing diagnosis/collaborative problems*

1) Impaired gas exchange related to ineffective temperature regulation, altered level of consciousness

2) Fluid volume deficit related to fluid and electrolyte loss from sweating and inability to replace volume loss

3) Ineffective thermoregulation related to the development of hyperthermia

4) Knowledge deficit related to lack of identification of risk factors for the development of a heat-related illness

c. *Planning/interventions*

1) Manage and maintain patient's ABCs

2) Establish intravenous (IV) access for fluid resuscitation

3) Place patient in a cool environment

4) For patient with heat stroke, initiate rapid cooling interventions

a) Remove clothing and spray the patient with tepid water; place in front of large fan

b) Immerse in ice water

c) Administer cool intravenous fluids or lavage with cool fluids

5) Monitor patient's core body temperature closely, and manage any shivering

6) Monitor patient's cardiac rhythm for dysrhythmias or signs of electrolyte imbalance such as peaked T waves

7) Monitor patient for rhabdomyolysis

a) Dark urine

      b) Blood in urine

      c) Muscle cramps

      d) Hyperkalemia

   8) Monitor patient for fluid overload and development of pulmonary or cerebral edema

   9) Allow family to remain with patient and participate in care as appropriate

   10) Provide patient and family with information about risk factors for heat-related illnesses

  d. Expected outcomes/evaluation (see Appendix B)

B. Cold-related emergencies

In a cool environment, the body will attempt to maintain a comfortable temperature. Heat is conserved by the body by vasoconstriction and is produced by shivering. Risk factors for the development of a cold-related emergency include extremes of age, ambient temperature, inappropriate clothing, wet clothing, water/metal contact, wind, and length of exposure.

Alcohol, drugs such as phenothiazines, trauma, and illnesses such as diabetes pose additional risks for the development of cold-related emergencies. Two cold-related emergencies include frostbite and hypothermia.

1. Frostbite

Frostbite is "true tissue freezing," which causes the formation of ice crystals in the tissue. Frostbite usually occurs when an individual is not dressed for cold weather. Alcoholism and homelessness are also contributing factors. The initial response to cold stress is peripheral vasoconstriction. Vascular stasis and decreased blood flow contribute to the development of tissue damage. Cooling increases blood viscosity, decreases capillary perfusion, and results in sludging and thrombosis of the vessels. Subsequently, alterations in vascular permeability lead to edema.

Frostbite has been classified into first-, second-, and third-degree injuries or superficial and deep injuries. Tissue appearance will range from pale to blue and mottled.

Any patient with frostbite must always be evaluated for hypothermia. Treatment includes rewarming of the affected area, pain management, and wound care.

 a. Assessment

  1) Subjective data

   a) History of present illness

    (1) Patient age

    (2) Cold ambient temperature

    (3) Improper clothing; constricting clothing or clothing that does not cover high-risk areas, such as ears, nose, hands, fingers

    (4) Alcohol or drug intoxication

    (5) Pain in affected extremity

   b) Medical history

    (1) History of cold injury

    (2) History of cardiovascular disease

    (3) History of diabetes

    (4) Tetanus status

    (5) Present medications

    (6) Allergies to medications

  2) Objective data

   a) Physical examination

    (1) General survey

    (2) First-degree frostbite

(a) Pale skin
(b) Skin may be cyanotic
(c) Edema
(d) Decreased sensation to the injured area
(3) Superficial second-degree frostbite
(a) Skin is cyanotic
(b) Edema
(c) Blisters
(d) Decreased sensation at the injured site
(4) Deep second-degree frostbite
(a) Skin is pale with significant cyanosis
(b) Edema
(c) Anesthesia at the injured site
(d) Skin nonpliable
(5) Third-degree frostbite
(a) Pale skin, cyanosis, necrosis, gangrene
(b) Edema
(c) Anesthesia
(6) Core body temperature
(7) Peripheral pulses
(8) Motor function of the affected area
(9) Sensation to the affected area
b) Diagnostic procedures
(1) CBC
(2) PT, PTT
(3) Electrolytes
(4) Hepatic and renal profiles
(5) Drug screen
(6) Urinalysis
(7) Chest x-ray film
(8) Radiograph of affected extremity
(9) Technetium-99 studies
(10) Pressure monitoring of affected site
b. *Analysis: differential nursing diagnosis/collaborative problems*
1) Impaired skin integrity related to tissue freezing
2) Risk for infection related to impaired skin integrity
3) Hypothermia related to exposure to cold environment
4) Pain related to tissue damage
5) Anxiety/fear related to possible loss of affected extremity, and pain
c. *Planning/interventions*
1) Manage and maintain patient's ABCs
2) Obtain core temperature to rule out hypothermia
3) Begin rewarming of the injured area
a) Remove wet clothing
b) Rapidly rewarm affected extremity in warm water at 104 to 108°F (40–42°C) usually for 15 to 30 minutes
c) Debride blisters and apply topical antimicrobial ointment every 6 hours
d) Leave hemorrhagic blisters intact
e) Elevate affected part
f) Apply loose-fitting dressing to avoid further injury
4) Administer pharmacological therapy as prescribed
a) Pain medications (e.g., morphine)
b) Ibuprofen

c) Antibiotics

d) Tetanus immunization

e) Low-molecular-weight dextran

5) Allow patient's family to remain with patient and participate in care as appropriate

6) Instruct patient and family on hazards of cold exposure, including

a) Need for protective clothing

b) Effects of exposure

c) Early signs and symptoms of frostbite

d) Avoidance of tobacco, caffeine, alcohol

e) Wound care

7) Increased risk of recurrence

d. *Expected outcomes/evaluation* (see Appendix B)

2. Hypothermia

Hypothermia has been defined as a core body temperature of less than 95°F (35°C). Hypothermia results when the body cannot maintain an adequate temperature. The body produces heat through cellular metabolism, muscle activity, and shivering. Heat is lost through conduction, convection, evaporation, and radiation. It is important to note that the ambient temperature does not have to be very low to cause hypothermia. Hypothermia needs to be rapidly recognized and treated for life-threatening complications such as apnea, ventricular fibrillation, and acidosis.

There are multiple risk factors for hypothermia, including age (pediatric patients because of their inability to shiver and decreased body fat, and the elderly because of the high incidence of cardiovascular disease and decreased body fat); medications, such as phenothiazines and neuromuscular blocking agents, which interfere with the patient's ability to shiver; alcohol; traumatic injury; shock; and diseases such as diabetes.

a. *Assessment*

1) Subjective data

a) History of present illness

(1) Ambient temperature

(2) Length of exposure

(3) Patient's clothing

(4) Exposure to water/metal

(5) Traumatic injury

(6) Administration of neuromuscular blocking agents

(7) Patient age

b) Medical history

(1) Alcoholism

(2) Hypothyroidism

(3) Malnutrition

(4) Medications

(a) Phenothiazines

(b) Barbiturates

2) Objective data

a) Physical examination

(1) General survey

(2) Core body temperature

(a) Mild hypothermia: 93 to 95°F (35–36°C)

(b) Moderate hypothermia: 86 to 93°F (30–34°C)

(c) Severe hypothermia: less than 86°F (30°C)

(3) Hypoventilation

(4) Hypotension: difficult to detect blood pressure

(5) Cardiac dysrhythmias: bradycardia, atrial fibrillation, presence of an Osborn ("hump" between QRS and ST segments) or J wave, ventricular fibrillation

(6) Altered mental status (confusion to coma)

(7) Paradoxical undressing: patient removes all clothing even though cold

(8) Shivering diminished or absent at core body temperatures of 86°F (30°C)

(9) Absence of reflexes

(10) Fixed, dilated pupils

(11) Pale, cyanotic skin

b) Diagnostic procedures

(1) CBC

(2) PT, PTT

(3) Platelets, fibrin split products

(4) Electrolytes

(5) Hepatic and renal profiles

(6) Drug screen

(7) ABGs

(8) Urinalysis

(9) Chest radiograph

(10) Arterial catheter

(11) Pulmonary catheter

(12) ECG

b. *Analysis/differential diagnosis/collaborative problems*

1) Ineffective airway clearance related to decrease in level of consciousness

2) Impaired gas exchange related to decrease in core body temperature

3) Ineffective thermoregulation related to the development of hypothermia

4) Knowledge deficit related to risk factors and prevention of hypothermia

c. *Planning/interventions*

1) Manage and maintain patient's airway, breathing, circulation

2) Rewarm patient

a) Passive rewarming: removing wet clothing; applying dry clothing, warm blankets; administering warm fluids

b) Active external: body-to-body contact; application of heating devices such as fluid- or air-filled warming blankets or radiant lights (this must be done with caution because peripheral vasoconstriction will place patient at risk for integument injury); rewarming of extremities may place patient at risk for "afterdrop."

c) Active core warming: administration of warmed IV fluids; heated, humidified oxygen; peritoneal, gastric, or colonic lavage with warmed fluids

d) Hemodialysis or cardiopulmonary bypass to raise the core body temperature

3) Monitor patient for afterdrop, which occurs when cold blood from the periphery reaches the core after warming; can cause hypotension and dysrhythmias; may be avoided by warming the trunk and vascular areas first and then proceeding to extremities

4) Continuously monitor

a) Respiratory status

b) Hemodynamic status

c) Glucose, electrolytes, metabolic status

5) Insert gastric tube to prevent aspiration

6) Allow family to remain with patient and participate in care when appropriate

7) Discuss with patient/family risk factors related to development of hypothermia
   a) Medical illness, medications, age
   b) Early signs and symptoms of hypothermia
   c) Prevention of hypothermia (e.g., proper clothing, when to seek shelter)

d. *Expected outcomes/evaluation* (see Appendix B)

3. Submersion injuries

A submersion emergency results when a person becomes hypoxic from submersion in a substance. The most common substance is water, but people have been submerged in dry chemicals and in grain. Each year in the United States, about 8000 people die from submersion injuries; 40% of these victims are younger than 4 years. The population at greatest risk for a submersion injury are children younger than 5 years and boys between the ages of 15 and 19 years. The primary risk factors related to submersion injuries include inability to swim, intoxication, seizures, trauma, hyperventilation before deep-water swimming, hypothermia, CVAs, myocardial infarctions (MIs), and child maltreatment and neglect.

When a human is submerged, there is initial panic followed by breath holding and hyperventilation, which results in aspiration and swallowing of fluid. It takes a very small amount of substance (e.g., water) to trigger this response. Swallowed water may cause vomiting and additional aspiration. Hypoxia develops, and aspiration may lead to pulmonary injury. The injured lungs may begin shunting blood, causing further hypoxia. Subsequently, hypoxia contributes to cerebral injury, edema, and eventually brain death.

a. *Assessment*
   1) Subjective data
      a) History of present illness
         (1) Presence of risk factors
         (2) Substance in which patient was found
         (3) Length of time submerged in substance
         (4) Temperature of substance
         (5) Potential for child maltreatment
      b) Medical history
         (1) Cardiovascular disease
         (2) CNS disease (e. g., seizures, CVAs)
         (3) Physical conditioning
   2) Objective data
      a) Physical examination
         (1) General survey
         (2) Airway patency
         (3) Ventilatory effort
         (4) Level of consciousness
         (5) Core body temperature
         (6) Cool, clammy, pale, cyanotic skin
         (7) Gastric distention
         (8) Presence of other injuries (e. g., spinal cord injury)
         (9) Signs of maltreatment (e. g., bruising, rope burns)
      b) Diagnostic data
         (1) CBC
         (2) PT, PTT
         (3) Platelets, fibrin split products
         (4) Electrolytes
         (5) Renal and hepatic profiles

        (6) Airway, breathing, circulation

        (7) Chest x-ray film

        (8) Head CT/magnetic resonance imaging (MRI) scan

        (9) ECG

        (10) Pulse oximetry

  b. *Analysis: differential nursing diagnosis/collaborative problems*

    1) Ineffective airway clearance related to decreased level of consciousness, irritation of the respiratory tract, or laryngeal spasm

    2) Impaired gas exchange related to alveolar injury

    3) Ineffective breathing pattern related to altered level of consciousness, spinal cord injury

    4) Ineffective thermoregulation related to loss of heat based on water temperature and length of time in water

    5) Knowledge deficit related to risk factors and prevention of submersion emergencies

  c. *Planning/interventions*

    1) Manage and maintain patient's airway, breathing, circulation

    2) Immobilize patient's cervical spine if trauma is suspected

    3) Supply supplemental oxygen (warm oxygen before administration if patient is hypothermic)

    4) Establish IV access for fluid resuscitation and administer warm fluids if patient is hypothermic

    5) Continuously monitor

      a) Respiratory status

      b) Hemodynamic status

      c) Signs and symptoms of hypoxia

    6) Maintain normothermia with appropriate rewarming as indicated by patient's core body temperature (see section II. B.2. Hypothermia)

    7) Insert gastric tube to decompress the abdomen

    8) Treat complications: respiratory distress syndrome and aspiration; increased intracranial pressure (ICP); seizures (see appropriate chapters for further management)

    9) Allow family to remain with patient and provide care when appropriate

    10) Provide patient/family with information related to risk factors for submersion injuries

    11) Notify appropriate authorities if child maltreatment suspected

  d. *Expected outcomes/evaluation* (see Appendix B)

C. Thermal injuries

    A burn injury is defined as tissue injury that results from exposure to flames, hot liquids, hot objects, caustic chemicals or radiation, or electric current.

1. Thermal burn

    Thermal burns result from contact with a heat source such as a flame or hot substance. Scald burns are a common source of burn injury in children and older adults.

2. Chemical burn

    A chemical burn results from contact with three types of chemicals: acids, alkali, and organic compounds. Acids are found in cleaning products such as drain cleaners. Alkalis are found in such products as rust removers and swimming pool cleaners. Organic compounds include phenols and petroleum products such as gasoline and creosote.

3. Electrical burn

An electrical burn causes injury as a result of heat generated by an electrical current passing through human tissue. Electrical current can either be alternating (most household current) or direct (car battery). One of the major concerns with electrical injuries is the development of cardiac dysrhythmias.

4. Inhalation burn

An inhalation burn results from the inhalation of toxic substances, such as carbon monoxide, that cause cellular hypoxia or superheated air or steam that causes thermal injury to the airway, resulting in upper or lower airway edema and obstruction.

Each year in the United States, more than 2 million people are burned, approximately 60,000 of whom require hospitalization. Deaths from burns have been estimated at between 5000 to 12,000 either directly from the injury or from its complications. Burn injury causes serious pathophysiological responses in all systems of the body. Burn injury initiates an inflammatory response, which includes heat, redness, pain, and localized and systemic edema formation. The amount of edema is related to the extent and depth of the burn injury and the amount of fluid administered during fluid resuscitation. The combinations of fluid shift, edema formation, and evaporative water loss from the burn wound can lead to hypovolemia ("burn shock"). Loss of plasma is greatest during the first 4 to 6 hours after the burn injury. The decreased circulating blood volume becomes thickened and sluggish, which diminishes tissue oxygenation, causing injury to organs such as the kidneys. Hypovolemia reduces cardiac output, and the sympathetic nervous system responds by releasing catecholamines, leading to increased peripheral vascular resistance, increased afterload, and increased heart rate. Fluid resuscitation can stabilize cardiac output during the resuscitative phase of burn injury. Because of the tissue damage that occurs with major burn injuries, hemolysis may occur. Hemolysis results in hemoconcentration, thrombocytopenia, decreased platelets, and potential clotting abnormalities. Burn injuries are classified according to the depth and extent of the injury. Populations at risk for burn injury include children, the elderly, alcoholics, smokers, and people with suicidal ideation.

a. *Assessment*
   1) Subjective data
      a) History of present illness
         (1) Mechanism of injury or exposure: thermal, chemical, electrical, inhalation
         (2) Related injuries: cervical spine, spine, leg or arm fractures, evidence of maltreatment
         (3) Length of time exposed to burn source
         (4) Level of consciousness
         (5) Environment in which patient was found: enclosed space, industrial setting, presence of combustible substances, such as wood, petroleum products, plastics
         (6) Electrical injury: amount of voltage, alternating or direct current, resistance, path of current
         (7) Chemical injury: type of chemical, concentration, chemical's mechanism of action, extent of tissue penetration, duration of contact
         (8) Pain
      b) Medical history
         (1) Cardiovascular disease
         (2) Diabetes
         (3) Alcohol or drug abuse
         (4) Smoking
         (5) Medications

(6) Allergies

(7) Tetanus immunization status

(8) History of suicidal behavior

(9) History of maltreatment

2) Objective data

  a) Physical examination

    (1) General survey

    (2) Airway

      (a) Burns of face

      (b) Singed hair or eyebrows

      (c) Blistering around or in mouth

      (d) Soot or carbonaceous sputum

      (e) Cyanosis

    (3) Ventilation

      (a) Coughing

      (b) Stridor

      (c) Wheezing

      (d) Sternal retractions

      (e) Circumferential chest wall burns

    (4) Hypotension

    (5) Tachycardia

    (6) Absence of peripheral pulses

    (7) Altered level of consciousness: confusion, coma

    (8) Depth of the burn injury (Table 5–1)

      (a) First degree (superficial epidermal burn): involves epidermis; erythematous; blanches with pressure, pain

      (b) Second degree (partial-thickness burn): involves epidermis and extends into dermal layer; moist appearance; blisters; deep red hue; pain

      (c) Third degree (full-thickness burn): involves full thickness of epidermis and dermis; dry, leathery appearance; inelasticity; absence of blanching, pain

Table 5–1 DEPTH OF BURN INJURY

Description	Depth	Characteristics	Healing Period
Superficial epidermal (first degree)	Epidermis	Erythema, dry, blanches, tender, painful	3 to 5 days
Partial thickness Superficial (first degree to second degree)	Epidermis Upper dermis	Deep red to pink, blistering, moist, blanches, painful	10 days to 3 weeks
Deep (second degree)	Epidermis Deep dermis	Mottled, dry or moist, may have blistering, usually intermixed with full thickness, extremely painful	Several weeks to months
Full thickness (third degree)	Epidermis Dermis Subcutaneous tissue	Dry, pearly white to charred, little to no pain or sensation, leathery, inelastic	Skin grafting required

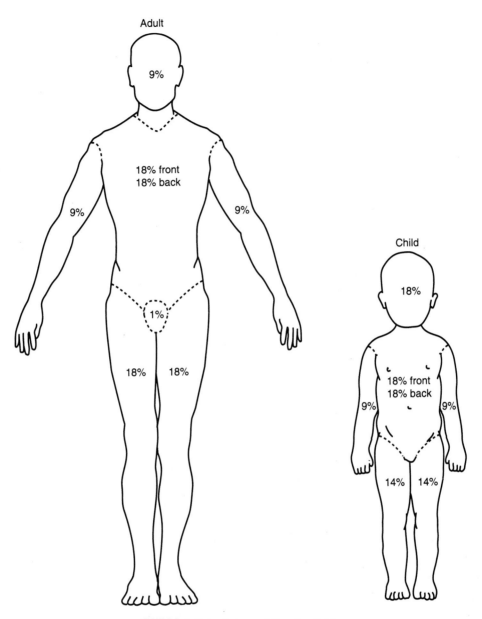

FIGURE 5–1. Rule of nines, adult and pediatric.

(9) Extent of burn: determined by estimation of total body surface area (TBSA) involved

- Rule of nines (Fig. 5–1)
- Lund and Browder chart (Fig. 5–2)

(a) Circumferential burns: burn injury that encompasses an entire extremity or area (e.g., thorax); skin inelasticity and edema cause tissue ischemia and death

(b) Muscle involvement: charred or mummified appearance, absent peripheral pulses, edema, increased in compartment pressure; myoglobinuria

(c) Location of burn: face, hands, feet, genitalia, perineum, areas overlying major joints

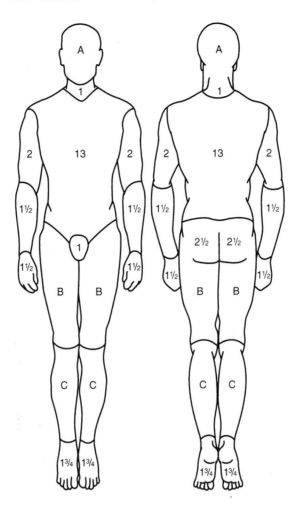

RELATIVE PERCENTAGE OF BODY SURFACE AREA AFFECTED BY GROWTH

AREA	AGE 0	1	5	10	15	ADULT
A = ½ of head	9 ½	8 ½	6 ½	5 ½	4 ½	3 ½
B = ½ of one thigh	2 ¾	3 ¼	4	4 ½	4 ½	4 ¾
C = ½ of one leg	2 ½	2 ½	2 ¾	3	3 ¼	3 ½

FIGURE 5–2. Lund and Browder chart.

b) Diagnostic procedures
   (1) CBC
   (2) Electrolytes
   (3) Blood urea nitrogen (BUN)
   (4) ABGs
   (5) PT, PTT
   (6) Drug screen
   (7) Urinalysis
   (8) Chest radiograph
   (9) Cervical spine radiograph
   (10) CT scan
   (11) Extremity radiographs

(12) Pulse oximetry: use with caution when carbon monoxide (CO) poisoning may be suspected (reading will be falsely elevated)

b. *Analysis: differential nursing diagnosis/collaborative problems*
1) Ineffective airway clearance related to airway edema, altered level of consciousness secondary to hypoxia, pain
2) Impaired gas exchange related to alveolar damage, fluid shifts, CO toxicity, hypovolemia, circumferential burns
3) Ineffective breathing pattern related to pain, circumferential burns
4) Fluid volume deficit related to abnormal fluid losses secondary to increased capillary permeability, fluid shifts, inflammatory response
5) Risk for hypothermia related to injury to the integument, fluid resuscitation, and exposure
6) Risk for infection related to injury to the integument and resuscitative procedures
7) Pain related to tissue injury from exposure to a thermal, chemical, radiation, or electrical current source

c. *Planning/interventions*
1) Stop burning process
   a) Remove all of patient's clothing
   b) Remove all jewelry
   c) Decontaminate patient as indicated
2) Ensure a patent airway, and immobilize the cervical spine when indicated
   a) Administer high-flow oxygen
   b) Intubate when patient's condition indicates: signs of inhalation injury, hypoxemia, oropharyngeal burns
3) Establish IV access for fluid resuscitation
   a) Infuse a crystalloid solution such as Ringer's lactate
   b) Adults: 2 to 4 mL × kg body weight x percent burn
   c) Children: 3 to 4 mL × kg body weight x percent burn
   d) Administer one half of fluid in the first 8 hours from time of burn injury
   e) Remaining fluid is administered over the next 16 hours
   f) Inhalation injury, high-voltage injury, or delayed fluid resuscitation may require more fluid than predicted
4) Insert urinary catheter, and monitor urinary output hourly
   a) Adults: 30 to 50 mL/hour
   b) Children weighing less than 30 kg: 1 mL/kg/hour
   c) Monitor color of urine (rhabdomyolysis)
5) Continuously monitor
   a) Respiratory status
   b) Hemodynamic status: dehydration, fluid overload
   c) Patient's level of pain
6) Prepare for/assist with additional interventions
   a) Escharotomy for circumferential burns
   b) Insertion of invasive monitoring catheters
   c) Compartment pressure monitoring
7) Insert gastric tube to decompress the abdomen
8) Administer pharmacological therapy as prescribed
   a) Analgesia
   b) Sedation
   c) Antibiotics
   d) Tetanus immunization
   e) Topical burn wound medications
9) Apply cool, moistened dressings to burns less than 10% TBSA

a) Do not use ice
b) Do not use antibiotic or chemical solutions
c) Keep patient warm

10) Maintain normothermia by keeping patient covered with clean sheets/blankets

11) Provide burn wound care: may not be initiated in emergency department for severely burned patient
   a) Administer pain medication before beginning treatment
   b) Clean wound gently with soap solution
   c) Debride nonviable epidermis
   d) Treat blisters as prescribed by burn surgeon
   e) Apply topical antimicrobial agent as prescribed; for example,
      (1) Silver sulfadiazine (Silvadene)
      (2) Mafenide acetate (Sulfamylon)
      (3) Water-based ointment to face, ears, neck, and perineum (e.g., bacitracin)

12) Allow family to remain with patient and to participate in care as appropriate

13) Prepare patient for transfer to burn facility
   a) Second-degree burns greater than 10% TBSA
   b) Burns that involve face, hands, feet, genitalia, perineum, and major joints
   c) Third-degree burns in any age group
   d) Electrical burns, including lightning injury
   e) Chemical burns
   f) Inhalation injury
   g) Burn injury in patients with pre-existing illness that will complicate recovery
   h) Patients with burns and concomitant trauma
   i) Pediatric burn patients
   j) Patients who require special social, emotional and/or long-term rehabilitative support, suspected child maltreatment

14) Provide the following discharge instructions
   a) Wound care
   b) Signs and symptoms of infection
   c) Medications
   d) Nutrition
   e) When to return for follow-up care

d. *Expected outcomes/evaluation* (see Appendix B)

5. Lightning injury

Lightning injuries occur as the result of contact with lightning. A person may be injured by a direct hit, splash effect, step voltage, or concussive injury. A bolt of lightning is an electrical current that may reach 200 million volts and 500,000 amperes (A) with a temperature of 8000°C. The path of the bolt and the amount of resistance determine the type of injury that may result. Cardiac dysrhythmias are a potential lethal complication of a lightning strike. Those at risk for lightning strike include hikers, campers, farmers, and golfers. Areas of highest risk for lightning strike in the United States are the South, Gulf Coast, and Rocky Mountains and along the Ohio, Mississippi, and Hudson rivers.

a. *Assessment*
   1) Subjective data
      a) History of present illness

            (1) Patient found down after a storm
            (2) Witnessed strike
            (3) Cardiac arrest during a storm
            (4) Chest pain
            (5) Muscle aches
       b) Medical history
            (1) History of being struck by lightning
            (2) Lack of preparation for outside activity
    2) Objective data
       a) Physical examination
            (1) General survey
            (2) Respiratory arrest
            (3) Ventricular fibrillation
            (4) Seizures
            (5) Deafness
            (6) Confusion
            (7) Amnesia
            (8) Blindness
            (9) Contusions from shock wave
            (10) Tympanic membrane rupture
            (11) Cutaneous burns
            (12) Cataracts
            (13) Myoglobinuria
       b) Diagnostic data
            (1) CBC
            (2) Electrolytes
            (3) Hepatic and renal profiles
            (4) Cardiac enzymes
            (5) ECG
            (6) Radiographs as indicated by injury
  b. Analysis: differential nursing diagnosis/collaborative problems
    1) Ineffective breathing pattern related to injury from lightning strike
    2) Fluid volume deficit related to tissue damage from burn injury
    3) Pain from injuries related to lightning strike
  c. Planning/interventions
    1) Remove patient and rescuers to a safe place
    2) Manage and maintain patient's airway, breathing, circulation; immobilize cervical spine
    3) Establish IV access for fluid resuscitation
    4) Place patient on continuous cardiac monitoring
    5) Obtain 12- to 15-lead ECG
    6) Administer pharmacological therapy as prescribed
      a) Analgesia
      b) Sedation
      c) Tetanus immunization
    7) Perform burn wound care when indicated
    8) Allow family members to remain with patient and participate in care as appropriate
    9) Provide patient and family with information about potential risk for lightning injury
  d. Expected outcomes/evaluation (see Appendix B)

D. Bites and stings

A bite or a sting may produce a puncture wound or laceration and may cause serious complications, including anaphylaxis, envenomation, tissue damage, wound infection, and transmission of illnesses such as rabies or Lyme disease. Each year thousands of patients are treated for bites and stings in the emergency department. There are multiple sources of bites and stings, including mammals, reptiles, marine animals, insects, and spiders. Common sources of bites and stings in the United States are summarized in Table 5–2.

Occasionally, patients will present to the emergency department after having been bitten or stung by an exotic insect or animal. People at greatest risk of being bitten or stung include young children, people working outside, and people unfamiliar with the insect or animal they are handling.

1. **Human bites**

Human bites cause puncture wounds or lacerations and are generally the consequence of a fight or sexual activity. Human bites are dangerous because of the organisms that may contaminate the bite wound, including *Staphylococcus aureus*, *Streptococcus*, and hepatitis virus. Common sites of human bites involve the metacarpophalangeal joint, ears, nose, vagina, and penis.

   a. *Assessment*
   1) Subjective data
       a) History of present illness
           (1) Description of the incident
           (2) Amount of time since injury
           (3) Location of bite
           (4) Amount of bleeding
           (5) Presence of pain
       b) Medical history
           (1) Cardiovascular disease
           (2) Diabetes
           (3) Allergies
           (4) Medications
   2) Objective data
       a) Physical examination
           (1) General survey
           (2) Size of wound
           (3) Depth of wound
           (4) Presence of necrotic tissue

Table 5–2   COMMON SOURCES OF BITES IN THE UNITED STATES

Bites	Stings
Dogs	Bees
Cats	Wasps
Humans	Ants
Rodents	Scorpions
Horses	Some marine animals
Reptiles	
Bats	
Raccoons	
Skunks	
Spiders	

(5) Neuromuscular function of injured area
b) Diagnostic data
(1) CBC
(2) Radiograph of injured area as indicated
(3) Culture of wound
(4) Forensic evidence collection when indicated
b. *Analysis: differential nursing diagnosis/collaborative problems*
1) Impaired skin integrity related to bite injury
2) Risk for infection related to wound contamination
3) Pain related to tissue destruction and inflammatory response
4) Knowledge deficit related to care of the injury
c. *Planning/interventions*
1) Manage and maintain patient's airway, breathing, circulation
2) Consider taking pictures of injury before cleansing if injury associated with a crime
3) Perform wound care
a) Cleanse with a mild antiseptic soap
b) Irrigate with copious amounts of normal saline
c) Anesthetize the wound as needed
d) Assist with or perform tissue debridement
e) Assist with or perform wound closure if indicated; delayed closure is usually preferred in human bites, but is determined by location and age of wound
f) Apply appropriate dressing
4) Administer pharmacological therapy as prescribed
a) Analgesia
b) Antibiotics
c) Immunizations
5) Assist in admission of patient to the hospital if more extensive treatment is required
6) Allow family member to remain with patient and participate in care as appropriate
7) Provide patient/family with discharge instructions, including wound care, signs and symptoms of infections, medication administration, and follow-up care appointment
d. *Expected outcomes* (see Appendix B)

2. **Animal bites**

Animal bites can inflict lacerations and deep puncture wounds and have the potential for infection and the transmission of diseases such as rabies. Animals, particularly dogs, can also produce crush injuries by the power of their jaws closing onto an extremity or other exposed body part. Bite injuries may result in damage to the face, hands, and feet, which may cause long-term scarring and loss of function. Dog bites account for 90% of the bite injuries that are treated in the emergency department. Dog bites are also responsible for the majority of deaths reported from nonvenomous animals. Cats are another source of animal bites. Complications from cat bites may result in deep penetration leading to infection and cellulitis from the organism *Pasteurella*, which is carried in the cat's mouth.

Wild animal bites also pose a risk to humans. The most common animals inflicting these wounds are bats. Those at risk for bat bites are individuals who work with bats, chimney sweeps, and individuals who explore caves, which are bat habitats. Rabies-related deaths have occurred secondary to bat bites.

Children are at greatest risk of being bitten by animals, particularly dogs. Dogs are bred to protect their territory, and when they are approached by someone unfamiliar they feel threatened and will bite in defense. A curious young child may not associate danger with a dog. Animal bites must be reported to health authorities based on local and state regulations.

a. *Assessment*
  1) Subjective data
    a) History of present illness
      (1) Type of animal that inflicted injury
      (2) Animal known to victim
      (3) Provocation of animal
      (4) Rabies status if a domestic animal
      (5) Time of injury
      (6) Location of injury
      (7) Extent of bleeding
      (8) Presence of pain
    b) Medical history
      (1) Cardiovascular disease
      (2) Diabetes
      (3) Medications
      (4) Allergies
      (5) Immunization status
  2) Objective data
    a) Physical examination
      (1) General survey
      (2) Location of wound
      (3) Size of wound
      (4) Depth of wound
      (5) Visible structures such as subcutaneous fat, bones, tendons, muscles
      (6) Neurovascular status
      (7) Function of injured area
    b) Diagnostic procedures
      (1) CBC if indicated
      (2) Wound culture
      (3) Radiograph of injured area
b. *Analysis: differential nursing diagnosis/collaborative problems*
  1) Ineffective airway clearance related to bite wounds on face or neck
  2) Impaired skin integrity related to bite wound
  3) Risk for infection related to wound contamination
  4) Pain related to bite wound
  5) Knowledge deficit related to care of bite wound
c. *Planning/interventions*
  1) Manage and maintain patient's airway, breathing, circulation
  2) Assess and manage wound
    a) Control active bleeding
    b) Assess vascular integrity
    c) Monitor neuromuscular function
  3) Perform wound care
    a) Cleanse with mild aseptic soap
    b) Irrigate with copious amounts of normal saline
    c) Anesthetize wound as needed for patient comfort
    d) Assist with or perform tissue debridement
    e) Assist with or perform wound closure if indicated; delayed closure may be indicated to decrease risk of infection, but is determined by location and age of the wound

4) Administer pharmacological therapy as prescribed
   a) Analgesia
   b) Sedation
   c) Antibiotics
   d) Immunizations
   e) Rabies prophylaxis (generally administered for wild animal bites)
      (1) Rabies immune globulin (RIG)
      (2) Human diploid cell vaccine (HDCV)
      (3) Rabies vaccine absorbed (RVA)
5) Assist in admission of patient to the hospital if more extensive treatment required
6) Allow family member to remain with patient and participate in care as appropriate
7) Provide patient with discharge instructions, including wound care, signs and symptoms of infection, medication administration, rabies prophylaxis schedule, and follow-up care appointment
8) Provide patient and family with information about bite injury prevention, including the following: be familiar with local animal behaviors; remain motionless when approached by an unfamiliar dog; if knocked down by a dog, roll into a ball and lie still; do not keep dangerous animals where children can easily be exposed to them

d. *Expected outcomes* (see Appendix B)

3. Snake bites

Snake bites usually cause either a laceration or a puncture wound. Snake bites may become infected, but the major complication is envenomation. Several thousand snake bites occur in the United States each year. Deaths from venomous snake bites account for 10 to 15 deaths each year. There are five venomous families of snakes. In the United States, the *Crotalidae*, or pit vipers, are responsible for the majority of bites. Pit vipers include rattlesnakes *(Crotalus)*, massasauga rattlesnakes *(Sistrurus)*, and copperheads and cottonmouths, or water moccasin *(Agkistrodon)*. The other family of venomous snakes in the United States are the *Elapidae*, or coral snakes. Occasionally, a patient is bitten by a snake not native to this country, whether it occurs at a zoo or in one's home where the reptile is kept as a pet.

Snake bites generally occur in the lower extremities, but also may occur to the hands and the face.

Envenomation is animal poisoning. Venom contains many enzymes and proteins that can cause local tissue damage, massive tissue edema, hypotension, coagulopathy, shock, and death. The first sign of envenomation is burning at the bite site. Swelling and edema may involve the entire area where the bite is located. Depending on the amount of venom dispensed, extensive tissue destruction can occur. Envenomation can also have systemic manifestations, including a metallic taste, fasciculations, weakness, nausea, vomiting, numbness, and tingling around the mouth. People at risk for snake bite include snake handlers, hikers, campers, and intoxicated individuals.

a. *Assessment*
   1) Subjective data
      a) History of present illness
         (1) Description of incident
         (2) Description and identification of the snake
            (a) Pit vipers have a pit between eye and nostril, catlike elliptical pupils, triangular head, two fangs
            (b) Coral snakes have black, red, and yellow bands (black and

yellow wider than red); black head; slender body; small, fixed fangs; round, black eyes

    (3) Location of bite

    (4) Size and weight of victim

    (5) Prehospital care provided

    (6) Signs and symptoms before arrival

    (7) Time of incident

  b) Medical history

    (1) Cardiovascular disease

    (2) Diabetes

    (3) Previous bite injury

    (4) Previous administration of antivenom

    (5) Medications

    (6) Allergies

2) Objective data

  a) Physical examination

    (1) General survey

    (2) Appearance of wound

      (a) Pit viper: fang marks, semicircle teeth marks

      (b) Coral snake: scratch marks or tiny puncture marks

      (c) Nonvenomous: scratch marks, teeth marks

    (3) Burning pain at site of bite

    (4) Numbness and tingling in mouth

    (5) Ecchymosis

    (6) Vesicles at or around bite site

    (7) Weakness

    (8) Sweating

    (9) Nausea and vomiting

    (10) Dyspnea

    (11) Bleeding

    (12) Seizures

    (13) Flaccid paralysis

    (14) Euphoria

  b) Diagnostic data

    (1) CBC

    (2) Type and cross-match

    (3) Platelets, fibrin split products

    (4) Wound culture

    (5) Radiographs of injured area as indicated

b. *Analysis: differential nursing diagnosis/collaborative problems*

  1) Ineffective airway clearance related to envenomation, anaphylaxis

  2) Fluid volume deficit related to blood loss/hemorrhage from envenomation

  3) Impaired skin integrity related to bite injury

  4) Risk for infection related to contaminated bite wound

  5) Pain from bite wound and envenomation

  6) Anxiety/fear related to source of injury

  7) Knowledge deficit related to treatment and prevention of snake bites

c. *Planning/interventions*

  1) Manage and maintain patient's airway, breathing, circulation

  2) Establish IV access for administration of fluids, blood, blood products, and antivenom

  3) Continuously monitor

    a) Respiratory status

      b) Hemodynamic status

      c) Edema progression

    4) Prepare for/assist with specific interventions

      a) Immobilization of affected part

      b) Fasciotomy for severe tissue injury (an expert should always be consulted before this procedure is considered)

    5) Administer pharmacological therapy

      a) Analgesia

      b) Sedation

      c) Antibiotics

      d) Antivenom

      e) Immunizations

    6) Perform wound care

    7) Allow family to remain with patient and participate in care as appropriate

    8) If antivenom is to be administered:

      a) Perform skin or conjunctival testing for horse serum sensitivity

      b) Monitor patient closely for anaphylaxis

    9) Assist in admission of patient to hospital for further treatment

    10) Provide patient with discharge instructions, including wound care, signs and symptoms of infection, medication administration, follow-up care, and prevention (wear boots or high-top shoes when hiking, do not attempt to pick up or provoke a snake, be familiar with venomous species in areas where camping or hiking, carry first aid for snake bite such as a Sawyer's extractor)

  d. Expected outcomes/evaluation (see Appendix B)

4. Insect stings

    An insect sting causes a break in the skin and the deposit of a stinger, which contains an apparatus that injects venom into its victim. Bees, wasps, and ants are the most common sources of stings. Venom is used for defense and to subdue the insect's prey. A serious complication of stings is anaphylaxis. Each year about 150 people die from an anaphylactic reaction.

    Anaphylaxis is an acute allergic reaction that results from an exposure to a foreign protein to which the patient has already been sensitized. Signs and symptoms of anaphylaxis include facial or oral edema; respiratory distress (stridor, wheezing, sternal retractions); and a rash or hives. People at risk for insect stings include anyone who works outside, hikers, and campers.

  a. Assessment

    1) Subjective data

      a) History of present illness

        (1) Type of insect

        (2) Description of sting

        (3) Location of sting

        (4) Time incident occurred

        (5) Symptoms experienced after sting

        (6) Prehospital treatment

      b) Medical history

        (1) Allergy to stings

        (2) Allergies

        (3) Asthma

        (4) Medications

        (5) Immunizations

    2) Objective data

      a) Physical examination

        (1) General survey
        (2) Appearance of skin site: redness, warmth, wheal formation, blisters
        (3) Presence of stinger
        (4) Pain
        (5) Pruritus
        (6) Shortness of breath
        (7) Stridor
        (8) Wheezing
        (9) Altered mental status
        (10) Hypotension
        (11) Cardiac dysrhythmia
        (12) Vascular collapse
    b) Diagnostic procedures
        (1) CBC if indicated
        (2) Wound culture if indicated
        (3) Chest radiograph
        (4) Pulse oximeter

b. *Analysis: differential nursing diagnosis/collaborative problems*
  1) Ineffective airway clearance related to airway edema
  2) Altered tissue perfusion related to loss of peripheral vascular resistance
  3) Pain related to sting and envenomation
  4) Knowledge deficit related to treatment and prevention

c. *Planning/interventions*
  1) Manage and maintain patient's airway, breathing, circulation
  2) Establish IV access for fluid resuscitation
  3) Treat anaphylaxis
    a) Establish patent airway
    b) Administer high-flow oxygen
    c) Administer medications as prescribed
        (1) Epinephrine, 0.1 to 0.5 mL of 1:10,000 solution
        (2) B_2-selective inhaled agents
        (3) Diphenhydramine
        (4) H_2 blockers
        (5) Steroids IV and orally (PO)
  4) Continuously monitor:
    a) Respiratory status
    b) Hemodynamic status
    c) Edema progression
  5) Administer pharmacologic therapy as prescribed
    a) Analgesia
    b) Antibiotics
    c) Antihistamines
    d) Immunizations
  6) Remove stinger and perform wound care
    a) Scrape off stinger with hard surface such as a credit card
    b) Clean area with mild antiseptic soap
    c) Apply ice, baking soda paste, aloe vera for comfort
  7) Allow family member to remain with patient and participate in care as appropriate
  8) Provide patient/family with discharge instructions, including wound care, signs and symptoms of infection, signs and symptoms of anaphylaxis, follow-up care, and prevention (e.g., wear light-colored clothing, use appropriate insect repellent, carry EpiPen if there is potential for anaphylaxis)

d. Expected outcomes (see Appendix B)
5. **Tick bites**

Ticks are species of arthropods that attach to the host, secreting a cement-like material and burrowing into the skin to feed on blood. Victims are frequently unaware of the presence of the insects because they are small and flat when not engorged with blood and may be in such places as one's head, covered by hair. Some ticks transmit diseases such as Rocky Mountain spotted fever and Lyme disease. Some ticks can inject neurotoxins, which may cause paralysis. People at risk of tick bites are children, outside workers (particularly in high-grass or wooded areas), hikers, and campers.

a. Assessment
1) Subjective data
   a) History of present illness
      (1) Walking in an area where ticks may be present
      (2) Location of bite or where the tick was found
      (3) Report of any signs and symptoms such as weakness, progressing ascending paralysis, fever, chills
   b) Medical history
      (1) Allergies
      (2) Medications
      (3) Immunization status
2) Objective data
   a) Physical examination
      (1) General survey
      (2) Tick attached to body
      (3) Paresthesia in the legs
      (4) Symmetrical ascending paralysis
      (5) Bulbar paralysis and respiratory failure
      (6) Fever
      (7) Chills
      (8) Headache
      (9) Photophobia
      (10) Muscle and joint pain
      (11) Skin rash initially on ankle and wrists, spreading to trunk, palms of hands, soles of feet, and later to axillae, trunk, and face
      (12) Signs of Lyme disease
         (a) First stage (4–20 days after tick bite): expanding skin rash (erythema chronicum migrans); rash starts with small, red spot and often develops into reddish circle 2 to 3 inches in diameter; nonspecific flulike symptoms such as a headache, stiff neck, fatigue, joint and muscle aches. Symptoms will disappear in 2 weeks if not treated
         (b) Second stage (4 days to 22 weeks after initial symptoms), systemic dissemination: monoarticular arthritis, multiple skin lesions, neurological complications such as memory loss, meningitis, poor motor coordination, atrioventricular (AV) block
         (c) Third stage (several months to 2 years after initial skin lesion): meningoencephalitis; myocarditis; recurrent attacks of arthritis
   b) Diagnostic procedures
      (1) CBC
      (2) Electrolytes
      (3) Glucose
      (4) BUN

(5) Creatinine

(6) Calcium

(7) PT, PTT

(8) Urinalysis

(9) Pulse oximetry

(10) ECG

(11) Lyme antibody titers

b. *Analysis: differential diagnosis/collaborative problems*

1) Ineffective airway clearance related to paralysis from tick bite

2) Pain related to inflammatory response from tick bite

3) Knowledge deficit related to treatment for tick bite and prevention

c. *Planning/interventions*

1) Manage and maintain patient's airway, breathing, circulation

a) Patients with Stage 3 Lyme disease may require pacemaker insertion for cardiac rhythm control

2) Continuously monitor

a) Respiratory status

b) Hemodynamic status

c) Pain and discomfort

3) Remove tick

a) Take care not to crush or squeeze tick

b) Coat with nail polish, petroleum jelly (Vaseline), or mineral oil, and wait for disengagement

c) Apply forceps as close to skin and mouth parts of tick as possible, pull straight back gently but firmly, counter to direction in which mouth parts entered patient's skin

d) If head becomes disengaged or mouth parts remain, remove just as though these pieces were a splinter

e) Save tick for species identification

4) Clean site with mild antiseptic soap

5) Administer pharmacological therapy as ordered

a) Analgesia

b) Antibiotics

c) Immunizations

6) Allow family member to remain with patient and participate in care as appropriate

7) Provide patient/family with discharge instructions, including wound care, medication administration, signs and symptoms of infection, follow-up care, and prevention

a) Wear protective clothing, long sleeves, and light colors

b) Tuck pant legs into socks or boots

c) Use tick repellents when outdoors in a known tick area

d) Lyme disease vaccine

d. *Expected outcomes* (see Appendix B)

6. Spider bites

Two particular species of spiders in the United States can cause significant problems with envenomation. These are the black widow (*Latrodectus mactans*) and the brown recluse (*Loxosceles reclusa*) spiders. Black widow spiders are found in all states except Alaska. They live in the ground in secluded, dark areas such as garages, barns, sheds, and outhouses. The venom of the black widow is a neurotoxin. When bitten by a black widow spider, patients will feel a pinprick-like sensation. Twenty minutes later they will experience a dull ache. Systemic symptoms generally occur 30 minutes after envenomation. These include abdominal cramping, hypertension, nausea, vomiting, and tachycardia.

The brown recluse spider is found throughout the southern United States. It is shy and generally found in wood piles or storage areas. The bite is usually insignificant until 24 hours after its occurrence. A painful purple purpura develops, which progresses to a necrotic ulcerating wound. This wound can extend deeper into the tissue and take a long time to heal. Occasionally, a patient may suffer systemic signs and symptoms of brown recluse envenomation, including fever, chills, nausea, and vomiting. People at risk for spider bites include outside workers, anyone working in such areas as wood piles, and curious children.

a. *Assessment*
    1) Subjective data
        a) History of present illness
            (1) History of spider bite or working in area where a spider may be
            (2) Black widow: complaint of sharp pinprick, then dull ache
            (3) Brown recluse: based on location
            (4) Spider identification
                (a) Black widow: shiny, black body with red hourglass or irregular markings on abdomen
                (b) Brown recluse: small, brown or tan color, with dark band shaped like violin on cephalothorax
            (5) Location of bite
            (6) Time of bite
            (7) Presence of pain
        b) Medical history
            (1) Cardiovascular disease
            (2) Diabetes
            (3) Medications
            (4) Allergies
            (5) Immunizations
    2) Objective data
        a) Physical examination
            (1) General survey
            (2) Black widow bite: swelling, presence of tiny fang marks; severe pain 15 to 60 minutes after bite, increasing for 12 to 48 hours; pain in abdomen and back, dyspnea, nausea and vomiting, hypertension, paresthesias
            (3) Brown recluse bite: local reaction beginning in 2 to 8 hours, pain, redness, blister formation and ischemia, dark firm center in 2 to 4 days, ulcer formation in 7 to 14 days, systemic symptoms (e.g., fever, chills, malaise, nausea and vomiting, joint pain)
        b) Diagnostic procedures
            (1) CBC
            (2) Electrolytes
            (3) Renal function
            (4) Urinalysis
            (5) ECG
b. *Analysis: differential diagnosis/collaborative problems*
    1) Pain related to spider envenomation
    2) Impaired skin integrity related to tissue damage in bite area
    3) Risk for infection related to the wound from spider envenomation
    4) Knowledge deficit related to treatment and prevention

   c. Planning/interventions
     1) Manage and maintain patient's airway, breathing, circulation
     2) Continuously monitor
       a) Respiratory status
       b) Hemodynamic status
       c) Wound
     3) Provide care for black widow envenomation
       a) Apply ice to decrease venom absorption
       b) Establish IV access
       c) Administer oxygen as needed
       d) Administer pain medication and muscle relaxants
       e) Administer antivenom after appropriate skin testing
       f) Administer tetanus immunization
     4) Provide care for brown recluse envenomation
       a) Clean area of bite with mild antiseptic soap
       b) Perform wound care: remove necrotic tissue
       c) Administer medication as prescribed: dapsone, antivenom, steroids, antibiotics
       d) Prepare patient for hyperbaric oxygen treatment
       e) Administer tetanus immunization
     5) Allow family member to remain with patient and perform care when appropriate
     6) Provide patient/family with discharge instructions, including wound care, medication administration, signs and symptoms of infection, follow-up care, and prevention (wear gloves when working in wood piles, storage areas; shake out shoes or clothing when outside)
   d. Expected outcomes (see Appendix B)
  7. Bites and stings by aquatic organisms
     Aquatic organisms usually do not prey on people but will inflict injury when they are disturbed. When disturbed, these creatures may bite or sting, causing mechanical injury and/or envenomation. Some of the most toxic substances to humans are found in marine organisms. These wounds may also become infected from contaminated water. There are three types of aquatic organisms: creatures that bite and may cause envenomation such as sharks, barracudas, moray eels, octopi, sea snakes, and sea lions; creatures that sting (coelenterates) by means of nematocysts or stinging capsules and produce a wound and envenomation such as jellyfish, hydrozoans (Portuguese man-of-war), anemones, and corals; and creatures that have spines, which produce traumatic puncture wounds and release toxins from venom sacs such as stingrays, scorpion fish, sea urchin, and cat fish. Envenomation from aquatic organisms can result in a variety of symptoms ranging from localized tissue irritation to death. In addition to envenomation, some stings and bites may cause an anaphylactic reaction. People at risk include snorkelers, unprotected divers, and people walking along the beach. It is important to remember that even dead organisms may be able to inflict an injury, and health care providers and rescuers are at risk of being bitten or stung if appropriate precautions are not taken.
   a. Assessment
     1) Subjective data
       a) History of present illness
         (1) Description of incident
         (2) Unexplained collapse while in water
         (3) Geographical area of incident
         (4) Description of aquatic organism

(5) Location of injury

(6) Extent of bleeding

(7) Subjective complaints of discomfort

(8) Time lapsed since injury

(9) Prehospital care

b) Medical history

(1) Cardiovascular disease

(2) Diabetes

(3) Allergies

(4) Medications

(5) Immunization status

2) Objective data

a) Physical examination

(1) General survey

(2) Location of wound

(3) Signs and symptoms of anaphylaxis: shortness of breath, airway edema, hives, hypotension, vascular collapse

(4) Bites: size of wound, depth of tissues involved, visible structures, presence of teeth, function of involved part

(5) Stings: extent of body affected, urticarial lesions, adhered tentacles, barbs, swelling, redness, pain

(6) Spines: extent of wound, spines, welts, streaks, redness, swelling

(7) Nausea, vomiting

(8) Muscle weakness, stiffness

(9) Paralysis

(10) Seizures

(11) Pain

b) Diagnostic procedures

(1) CBC if indicated

(2) ECG

(3) Radiological examination of affected area if retained parts are suspected

(4) Press transparent tape against affected area to obtain nematocysts for species identification

b. *Analysis: differential diagnosis/collaborative problems*

1) Ineffective airway clearance related to airway edema from an allergic reaction to envenomation

2) Ineffective breathing pattern related to envenomation

3) Pain related to tissue envenomation

4) Impaired skin integrity related to bite or sting

5) Infection related to impaired skin integrity or wound contaminants

6) Knowledge deficit related to treatment and prevention

c. *Planning/interventions*

1) Manage and maintain patient's airway, breathing, circulation

2) Treat anaphylaxis (see section II. D.4. Insect stings)

3) Continuously monitor

a) Respiratory status

b) Hemodynamic status

c) Patient's level of pain

4) Perform wound care: bites

a) Cleanse wound with mild antiseptic soap

b) Irrigate with copious amounts of normal saline

c) Assist or administer local anesthetic

d) Assist or perform wound debridement and closure as indicated by the location and type of wound

e) Apply appropriate dressing

5) Perform wound care: stings

a) Immediately rinse wound with sea water

b) Do not rub area or use fresh water because this will stimulate the nematocysts that have not already fired

c) Remove tentacles with gloved hand or forceps

d) Apply acetic acid 5% (vinegar) to inactivate the toxin

e) Isopropyl alcohol 40 to 70% may be used as an alternative, but not for box-jellyfish stings

f) After soaking wound in vinegar or alcohol, remove remaining nematocysts by applying shaving cream or a paste of baking soda, flour, or talc and shave the area

g) Local anesthetic ointments may be applied after nematocyst removal to decrease pain

6) Administer pharmacological therapy as prescribed

a) Analgesia

b) Sedation

c) Antibiotics

d) Local anesthetics

e) Tetanus immunization

7) Allow family to remain with patient and perform care when appropriate

8) Provide patient with discharge instructions, including wound care, signs and symptoms of infection, medication administration, follow-up care and prevention (remain far away from aquatic organisms that can inflict injury, wear protective clothing such as "stinger suits" and gloves, and leave dead aquatic organisms alone)

  d. *Expected outcomes* (see Appendix B)

BIBLIOGRAPHY

American Burn Association. (1994). *Prehospital burn life support.* Lincoln, NE: American Burn Association.

Anderson, K., Roy, T., & Danzl, D. (1992). Submersion incidents: A review of 39 cases and the development of the submersion outcome score. *Journal of Wilderness Medicine, 3,* 27–36.

Auerbach, P. (1997). Envenomations from jellyfish and related species. *Journal of Emergency Nursing, 23,* 555–568.

Braun R., & Krishel, S. (1997). Environmental emergencies. *Emergency Medicine Clinics of North America, 15,* 451–477.

Callaham, M., & French, S. (1995). Bites and injuries inflicted by mammals. In P. Auerbach (Ed.), *Wilderness medicine* (pp. 927–993). St. Louis, MO: Mosby Year Book.

Chapman, C. (1998). Shock emergencies. In L. Newberry (Ed.), *Sheehy's emergency nursing principles and practice* (4th ed., pp. 515–523). St. Louis, MO: Mosby Year Book.

Danzl, D., Pozos, R., & Hamler, M. (1995). Accidental hypothermia. In P. Auerbach (Ed.), *Wilderness medicine* (pp. 51–103). St. Louis, MO: Mosby Year Book.

Dog-bite related fatalities in the United States, 1995–

1996. (1997). *Morbidity and Mortality Weekly Report, 46,* 463–467.

Electricity related deaths in Oklahoma. (1996). Morbidity and Mortality Weekly Report, *2,* 440–442.

Emergency Nurses Association. (1995). *Trauma nursing core course.* Park Ridge, IL: Author.

Gillenwater, J., Quan, L., & Feldman, K. (1996). Inflicted submersion in childhood. *Archives of Pediatric and Adolescent Medicine, 150,* 298–303.

Haddad, L., & Lee, R. (1998). Toxic marine life. In L. Haddad, M. Shannon, & J. Winchester III (Eds.), *Poisoning and drug overdose* (pp. 386–398). Philadelphia: W. B. Saunders.

Hassan, L., & McNally, J. (1995). Spider bites. In P. Auerbach (Ed.), *Wilderness medicine* (pp. 769–786). St. Louis, MO: Mosby Year Book.

Henry, M., & Stapleton, E. (1992). *EMT prehospital care.* Philadelphia: W. B. Saunders.

Herman, L., & Newberry, L. (1998). Wound management. In L. Newberry (Ed.), *Sheehy's emergency nursing principles and practice* (4th ed., pp. 183–198). St. Louis, MO: Mosby Year Book.

Hubbard, R., Gaffin, S., & Squire, D. (1995). Heat-related illness. In P. Auerbach (Ed.), *Wilderness medicine* (pp. 167–212). St. Louis, MO: Mosby Year Book.

Jolly, B., & Ghezzi, K. (1992). Accidental hypothermia. *Emergency Medicine Clinics of North America, 10,* 311–327.

Kelsey, J., Erlich, M., & Henderson, S. (1995). Exotic reptile bites. *American Journal of Emergency Medicine, 5,* 536–537.

Langley, R., & Morrow, W. (1997). Death resulting from animal attacks in the United States. *Wilderness and Environmental Medicine, 5,* 536–537.

McCauley, R., Smith, D., Robson, M., & Heggers, J. (1995). Frostbite and other cold-induced injuries. In P. Auerbach (Ed.), *Wilderness medicine* (pp. 129–145). St. Louis, MO: Mosby Year Book.

Mills, W. (1991). Frostbite. In J. Vallotton & F. Dubas (Eds.), *Mountain medicine* (pp. 78–91). St. Louis, MO: Mosby Year Book.

Minton, S. (1996). Bites by non-venomous snakes in the United States. *Wilderness and Environmental Medicine, 4,* 297–303.

Minton, S., & Bechtel, H. (1995). Arthropod envenomation and parasitism. In P. Auerbach (Ed.), *Wilderness medicine.* St. Louis, MO: Mosby Year Book.

Neumann, K. (1997). Strategies for outwitting insects. *Wilderness Medicine Letter, 14,* 6–7.

Newman, A. (1995). Submersion incidents. In P. Auerbach (Ed.), *Wilderness medicine* (pp. 1209–1233). St. Louis, MO: Mosby Year Book.

Nieves, J., Buttacavoli, M., Fuller, L., Clarke, T., & Schimpf, P. (1996). Childhood drowning: Review of the literature and clinical implications. *Pediatric Nurse, 22,* 206–210.

Olshaker, J. (1992). Near drowning. *Emergency Medicine Clinics of North America, 10,* 339–350.

Orlowski, J. (1979). Prognostic factors in pediatric cases of drowning and near-drowning. *Journal of the American College of Emergency Physicians, 8,* 176–179.

Patton, B. (1991). Hypothermia. In J. Vallotton & F. Dubas (Eds.), *Mountain medicine* (pp. 92–97). St. Louis, MO: Mosby Year Book.

Tek, D., & Olshaker, J. (1992). Heat illness. *Emergency Medicine Clinics of North America, 10,* 299–310.

Tilton, B., & Hubbell, F. (1994). *Medicine for the backcountry.* Merrillville, IN: ICS Books, Inc.

Tomaszewski, C. (1998). Spiders. In L. Haddad, M. Shannon, & J. Winchester (Eds.), *Poisoning and drug overdose* (3rd ed., pp. 353–357). Philadelphia: W. B. Saunders.

Tunney, F. (1998). Stinging insects. In L. Haddad, M. Shannon, & J. Winchester (Eds.), *Poisoning and drug overdose* (3rd ed., pp. 359–364). Philadelphia: W. B. Saunders.

Weiss, H., Friedman, D., & Coben, J. (1998). Incidence of dog bites injuries treated in emergency departments. *Journal of the American Medical Association, 7,* 51–53.

Cherie J. Revere, RN, MSN, CEN, CRNP

CHAPTER **6**

Facial Emergencies

MAJOR TOPICS

General Strategy

Specific Facial Emergencies

Sinusitis

Temporomandibular Joint
Dislocation

Bell's Palsy

Trigeminal Neuralgia

Facial Lacerations and Soft Tissue
Injuries

Mandibular Fractures

Maxillary Fractures

Zygomatic Fractures

I. GENERAL STRATEGY

A. Assessment

1. **Primary survey/resuscitation** (see Chapter 1)
2. **Secondary survey** (see Chapter 1)
3. **Psychological, social, and environmental factors**
   a. *Lack of restraint devices*
   b. *Lifestyles prone to violence*
   c. *Injuries intentional or unintentional*
4. **Focused survey**
   a. *Subjective data*
      1) Chief complaint
      2) History of present illness
         a) Pain: PQRST
            (1) *Provocation*
            (2) *Quality*
            (3) *Region/radiation*
            (4) *Severity*
            (5) *Timing*
         b) Nature of injury (when applicable)
            (1) *Cause*

(2) Speed and force

(3) Date and time

(4) Blunt or penetrating trauma

(5) Seat belt or restraint device use, airbag deployment

(6) Position in which patient found at injury scene

c) Bleeding/hemorrhage

d) Respiratory distress/shortness of breath

e) Head trauma/loss of consciousness

f) Motor deficits/changes

g) Sensory deficits/changes

(1) Auditory: hearing loss or ringing in ears

(2) Visual: partial or complete blindness, visual field defects, and decreased light perception

(3) Tactile/kinesthetic: decreased sensation, numbness, tingling, and paresthesias

(4) Gustatory: loss of taste or metallic taste

(5) Olfactory: unilateral or bilateral loss of smell

h) Malocclusion or trismus (inability to open mouth)

i) Asymmetry/dislocation

j) Swelling/edema

k) Fever/chills

l) Nausea/vomiting

m) Dizziness/vertigo

n) Dysphagia

o) Excessive salivation

p) Foreign body sensation

q) Exposure to and/or ingestion of noxious agents

(1) Illicit agents (e.g., street drugs)

(2) Other agents (e.g., nicotine, alcohol, contact substances, inhalants)

r) Consistency of patient's presentation with mechanism of injury

s) Other

3) Medical/surgical history

a) Neurological disorders or diseases: neurological assessment, including cranial nerves, may show deficits not related to present illness or injury

b) Hypertension: may be secondary cause of epistaxis

c) Blood dyscrasias: especially important if bleeding is noted in present injury

d) Previous dental; ear, nose, and throat (ENT); or facial trauma, fractures, or surgeries

e) Current medication history

(1) Analgesics: may affect neurological assessment (e.g., slurred speech and altered level of consciousness)

(2) Antibiotics: past/recent regimen may worsen present illness

(3) Anticoagulants: increase bleeding tendencies

(4) Psychotropic drugs: phenothiazine reaction may cause inability to close mouth

f) Compliance with current medication regimen

g) Allergies

(1) Contact substances

(2) Inhalants

(3) Foods

(4) Drugs

h) Immunization history

b. *Objective data*
  1) Physical examination
    a) Assessment for life-threatening emergencies
      (1) Patent airway: facial trauma predisposes to potential airway compromise
      (2) Effective breathing
      (3) Adequate circulation
      (4) Hemorrhage (external and/or internal)
      (5) Signs and symptoms of shock
      (6) Vital signs
    b) General survey
      (1) Mental status or level of consciousness
      (2) General appearance
      (3) Skin assessment
        (a) Color (mucous membrane assessment necessary in dark-pigmented skin)
        (b) Moisture
        (c) Temperature
        (d) Turgor
      (4) Obvious bleeding or swelling
      (5) Obvious deformities/asymmetry (e.g., dislocations, open fractures, lacerations, abrasions)
    c) Assessment for central nervous system (CNS) injury
      (1) Mental status or level of consciousness
      (2) Sensory deficits or changes
      (3) Motor deficits or changes
      (4) Cranial nerve function
      (5) Deep tendon reflexes
      (6) Head/scalp injuries
    d) Inspection
      (1) Face
        (a) Symmetry of structures in size, position, and movement to include palpebral fissures and nasolabial folds
        (b) Color and condition of skin
        (c) Size and depth of facial wounds
        (d) Presence of foreign bodies
        (e) Bleeding
        (f) Swelling or edema
        (g) Facial muscle function
        (h) Facial sensation
        (i) Malocclusion or trismus
      (2) Head
        (a) Symmetry and contour of skull
        (b) Size and depth of facial wounds
        (c) Presence of foreign bodies
        (d) Bleeding
        (e) Swelling, edema, lumps, and hematomas
      (3) Eyes (see Chapter 14)
      (4) Ears (see Chapter 4)
      (5) Nose (see Chapter 4)
      (6) Oral structures and cavity contents (see Chapter 4)
      (7) Neck: symmetry of movement or range of motion
      (8) Spinal processes: symmetry or alignment

e) Palpation
  (1) Face
    (a) Facial bones for stability, crepitus, false motion, bony defects, step defects, pain or tenderness
    (b) Frontal and maxillary sinuses for swelling and pain or tenderness
  (2) Head
    (a) For pain or tenderness
    (b) For lumps, bumps, and deformities
  (3) Eyes (see Chapter 14)
    (a) Lacrimal gland and sac for swelling and pain or tenderness
    (b) Orbital rims for bony defects
  (4) Ears (see Chapter 4)
  (5) Nose (see Chapter 4)
  (6) Oral structures and cavity contents (see Chapter 4)
  (7) Neck and spinal column
    (a) Spinal processes for pain or tenderness
    (b) Symmetry or alignment
    (c) Muscle tenseness
f) Percussion
  (1) Soft tissues over frontal sinuses
  (2) Soft tissues over maxillary sinuses
g) Psychosocial responses of patient or significant others
  (1) Stress factors
    (a) Loss of life
    (b) Disfigurement (temporary vs. permanent)
    (c) Loss of functioning (sensory, motor, occupational, sexual, recreational)
    (d) Financial burden or strain
    (e) Guilt toward self or toward other victims of traumatic event
  (2) Behavioral responses
    (a) Anxiety/fear
    (b) Anger/hostility
    (c) Avoidance, isolation, or withdrawal
    (d) Depression
    (e) Self-pity
    (f) Manipulative or attention-seeking behavior
    (g) Panic
    (h) Embarrassment
2) Diagnostic procedures
  a) Radiology
    (1) Radiographs of facial bones: maxilla, mandible, zygoma, orbits, nasal bone
    (2) Waters' view of facial bones and sinuses
    (3) Skull radiographic series
    (4) Cervical spine or other spinal radiographs
    (5) Chest radiograph if foreign body aspiration suspected
    (6) Panorex radiograph of teeth
    (7) Computed tomography (CT) scan: head, sinuses, and larynx
    (8) Other special procedures (e.g., contrast studies)
  b) Laboratory
    (1) Anaerobic or aerobic cultures of wounds
    (2) Complete blood count (CBC) with differential leukocyte count

(3) Urinalysis

(4) Coagulation studies with platelets

(5) Arterial blood gas (ABG) values

(6) Type and cross-match of blood

(7) Drug or toxicology screen: blood and urine

(8) Pregnancy test

(9) Other

c) Electrocardiography

d) Preparation of patient and significant others for diagnostic procedures

(1) Physical preparation

(2) Emotional support

(3) Teaching of patient/significant others

(4) Written consent for treatment, if possible

B. Analysis: differential nursing diagnosis/collaborative problems

1. **Ineffective airway clearance**
2. **Pain**
3. **Infection**
4. **Anxiety/fear**
5. **Knowledge deficit**
6. **Impaired skin integrity**
7. **Kinesthetic, gustatory, and tactile sensory/perceptual alteration**

C. Planning/interventions

1. **Determine priorities**
   a. *Control and maintain airway, breathing, and circulation (ABC)*
   b. *Control bleeding or hemorrhage*
   c. *Maintain fluid and electrolyte balance*
   d. *Prevent potential CNS complications*
   e. *Control pain*
   f. *Relieve anxiety/apprehension*
   g. *Prevent complications*
   h. *Educate patient/significant others*
2. **Develop nursing care plan specific to patient's presenting emergency**
3. **Obtain and set up necessary equipment and supplies**
4. **Institute appropriate interventions on basis of nursing care plan**

D. Expected outcomes/evaluation (see Appendix B)

1. **Monitor patient's responses and outcomes, adjusting nursing care plan as indicated**

E. Age-related considerations

1. **Pediatric**
   a. *Growth/development related*
      1) During the sixth and seventh years, maximal enlargement of the face occurs. Primarily the eruption of teeth and the development of the midface influence facial proportions at that time.
      2) Circulating blood volume per unit of body weight is greater in children (80 mL/kg) than in adults

3) Children achieve vasoconstriction effectively; therefore, if pediatric patient becomes hypotensive from trauma, major blood loss has usually occurred

4) Child's head is larger proportionately than adult's, and neck muscles are relatively weak for large head mass

5) Height and body mass of child produce less momentum than that of adult

b. *"Pearls"*

1) Infants and young children are prone to hypothermia because of large surface area, especially if unclothed: keep warm

2) Always explain to children what is going to be done to them and be honest

3) Limitation in verbal expressions is disadvantage in evaluation of child and complicates assessment

4) Facial bone fractures in pediatric patients tend to be less severe; most common are comminuted and undisplaced fractures because facial bones in children are softer and more pliable than those in adults

2. Geriatric

a. *Aging related*

1) Changes associated with aging

a) Ventilation

(1) Decreased arterial oxygen tension

(2) Diminished ability to cough

(3) Decreased vital capacity

b) Perception

(1) Visual acuity loss

(2) Diminished hearing

(3) Decreased sense of taste

(4) Decreased sensitivity to touch

c) Consciousness

(1) Loss of short-term memory

(2) Slower thought processing

(3) Increased pain threshold

d) Musculoskeletal

(1) Muscle atrophy

(2) Decreased flexibility

2) Elderly tend to have deterioration in special senses

3) Chronic diseases add further limitations to aged

4) Delayed response to stressors and alterations in perception may contribute to injury

5) Medication use can also contribute to increased injury rates

II. SPECIFIC FACIAL EMERGENCIES

A. Sinusitis

Sinusitis is an inflammatory condition of the mucous membranes that line the paranasal sinuses. Symptoms can range from mild congestion to a severe, progressive infection with lethal complications. The maxillary sinus is most frequently affected. Acute sinusitis frequently follows upper respiratory tract infections. Other causes include allergy, dental infections, trauma, and anatomical obstructions such as polyps. The signs and symptoms of acute sinusitis are related to the location of the involved sinuses; however, true infection of the sinus cavities is not always correlated with the signs and symptoms. Complications of acute sinusitis include chronic sinusitis, orbital cellulitis, orbital abscess, epidural abscess, subdural empyema, meningitis, brain abscess, cavernous sinus thrombosis, and osteomyelitis of the frontal or maxillary bone. Risk factors that may cause sinus drainage or obstruction, and ultimately sinusitis, include a deviated septum, nasal polyps, an adenoid mass, a foreign body, and enlarged turbinates.

1. **Assessment**
    a. *Subjective data*
        1) History of present illness
            a) Pain over area of involved sinus
                (1) Frontal: pain over forehead or around orbit, exacerbated when bending forward
                (2) Maxillary: pain below eyes; pain over cheekbones, upper teeth, or upper jaw; ear pain; pain on chewing; and numbness over middle third of face; major site of infection in children
                (3) Ethmoidal: pain at bridge of nose and behind eyes (retro-ocular) and mastoid pain; seen more frequently in children and associated with puffy eyes; may occur with maxillary sinusitis
                (4) Sphenoidal: pain referred to the top of head and occipital area
            b) Fever: may or may not be present
            c) Headache: usually frontal and worsens with bending over or coughing
            d) Facial pain that is described as achy and dull
            e) Nasal quality to voice
            f) Decreased appetite
            g) Nausea
            h) Nasal congestion/obstruction
            i) Cough
            j) Sore throat: may occur secondary to mouth breathing or postnasal drainage
            k) Pressure sensation over involved sinuses
        2) Medical history
            a) Chronic or acute upper respiratory tract symptoms
            b) Recent cold that is not improving
            c) Recent molar extraction
            d) Recurrent otitis media in children
            e) Fetid breath in young children
    b. *Objective data*
        1) Physical examination
            a) Red, swollen nasal mucosa
            b) Purulent nasal drainage, possibly blood tinged
            c) Conjunctivitis
            d) Tenderness to palpation over area of involved sinuses
            e) Opacification of sinuses to transillumination
            f) Puffy eyes in children
        2) Diagnostic procedures
            a) Sinus cultures: aerobic and anaerobic (e.g., via needle aspiration and/or cannulation of ostia)
            b) Radiographs to include Waters', Caldwell's, submentovertical, and lateral views; three findings show evidence of active infection: presence of radiological opacity, air-fluid level, and mucosal thickening
            c) CT scan: used for patients with suspected complication
2. **Analysis: differential nursing diagnosis/collaborative problems**
    a. *Pain related to congestion and inflammatory changes in sinuses*
    b. *Infection related to bacterial invasion of sinus mucosa*
    c. *Knowledge deficit related to management of sinusitis*
3. **Planning/interventions**

    a. Treatment of acute uncomplicated sinusitis
      1) Relieve obstruction
        a) Nasal or systemic decongestants
        b) Nasal steroids
      2) Control infection with antibiotics
      3) Promote sinus drainage by keeping head of bed (HOB) elevated
      4) Apply heat to face to relieve pressure
      5) Administer analgesic, as indicated
      6) Use room vaporizer
    b. Treatment of acute complicated sinusitis
      1) Admit to hospital
      2) Obtain consultation
      3) Administer intravenous (IV) antibiotics
      4) Prepare for possible surgical intervention
    c. Instruct patient/significant others to return immediately if condition worsens or does not improve in 3 to 4 days
    d. Explain importance of use of vaporizer, steam bath, or hot shower in helping to liquefy and mobilize nasal mucus and exudate
    e. If applicable, instruct parents on use of saline nose drops in children
    f. Prepare patient for discharge; include medication instructions regarding dose, frequency and route of administration, and side effects
      1) Local decongestants should be sprayed into each nostril as directed
      2) Local decongestants should not be used for more than 3 or 4 days to avoid mucosal rebound effect
    g. Instruct patient to increase fluids
    h. Instruct patient to avoid smoking cigarettes or smoke exposure
  4. Expected outcomes/evaluation (see Appendix B)

B. Temporomandibular joint (TMJ) dislocation

TMJ dislocation is an anterior and superior displacement of the jaw in which spasms and muscle contractions of the jaw muscles prevent the condyles from returning to their normal position. TMJ dislocation may be unilateral or bilateral and result from trauma or simply opening one's mouth too widely (e.g., during yawning and when undergoing dental work). TMJ dislocations may accompany mandibular fractures. Risk factors associated with TMJ dislocation include malocclusion, poorly fitted dentures, grinding or clenching of the teeth (bruxism), and emotional stress, which may alter muscular balance.

1. Assessment
    a. Subjective data
      1) History of present illness
        a) Accident/injury to mouth area
        b) Wide and/or prolonged opening of mouth just before dislocation
        c) Inability to close mouth
        d) Malocclusion
        e) Headache
        f) Earache
        g) Discomfort: pain usually worsens with jaw movement
        h) Neck pain
      2) Medical history
        a) Arthritis
        b) Myofascial pain dysfunction syndrome
    b. Objective data

1) Physical examination
    a) Malocclusion
    b) Open mouth with inability to close
    c) Limited range of motion
    d) Pain on palpating masseter muscle
2) Diagnostic procedures
    a) Radiographs of TMJ to include Panorex, transcranial, and Towne's techniques
    b) Postreduction radiograph of TMJ

2. Analysis: differential nursing diagnosis/collaborative problems
   a. *Pain related to dislocated joint*
   b. *Knowledge deficit related to management of TMJ dislocation*
   c. *Anxiety/fear related to inability to close mouth, pain, and knowledge deficit*

3. Planning/interventions
   a. *Reassure patient/significant others that reduction of jaw is possible*
   b. *Explain rationale for all diagnostic tests, procedures, and treatments to patient/ significant others*
      1) Radiographs to rule out mandibular fractures
      2) Manual reduction of jaw
      3) Conscious sedation administration to facilitate reduction, as needed
      4) Postreduction radiographs
      5) Hospital admission if severe pain or spasm after reduction (rare)
   c. *Have pen and paper readily available so patient can communicate via writing*
   d. *Prepare patient for discharge*
      1) Soft diet for 3 to 4 days to reduce chewing
      2) Avoidance of stress on TMJ
      3) Medication instructions (e.g., analgesics and muscle relaxants as needed)
   e. *Instruct patient to become aware of any habits of teeth clenching or grinding and relax the jaw*
   f. *Instruct patient to avoid wide, uncontrolled opening such as "yawning"*

4. Expected outcomes/evaluation (see Appendix B)

C. Bell's palsy

Bell's palsy is the paralysis of all facial muscles on one side of the face, its etiology is unknown, and it occurs without evidence of cerebral pathological changes. Pain in the postauricular region and ear may accompany or precede the paralysis. Bell's palsy is a diagnosis of exclusion. Bell's palsy is presumed to be caused by swelling of the facial nerve as a result of viral or immunodeficiency disease. In the narrow course through the temporal bone, the nerve becomes compressed and ischemic. The syndrome is thought to occur as the result of polyneuritis. Emotional stress, herpes simplex virus infection, and prolonged exposure to drafts or cold have also been implicated as causative agents. Bell's palsy is usually unilateral but may be bilateral. It can occur in children but is more common in adults. The majority of cases occur in people older than 40 years of age and are distributed equally between the sexes. The symptoms of Bell's palsy are usually self-limiting, and complete resolution occurs in 80 to 90% of cases.

1. Assessment
   a. *Subjective data*
      1) History of present illness
         a) Rapid, acute onset of symptoms
         b) Viral prodrome

  c) Sudden, unilateral facial weakness/paralysis (bilateral facial paralysis may occur but is rare)

  d) Retroauricular and/or facial discomfort

  e) Drooling and/or difficulty swallowing

  f) Increased sensitivity to noise on involved side

  g) Loss of taste; difficult to tell whether it is unilateral

 2) Medical history

  a) Diabetes

  b) Sarcoidosis

  c) Lyme disease

  d) Trauma

 b. *Objective data*

  1) Physical examination

   a) Upward movement of eyeball on affected side when attempting to close eye (Bell's phenomenon)

   b) Facial paralysis can be complete or partial

   c) Lag on affected side when closing eyes

   d) Widening of palpebral fissure and inability to close eye on affected side

   e) Decreased lacrimation on affected side

   f) Drooping of mouth on affected side

   g) Flattening of nasolabial fold on affected side

   h) Positive corneal sensation but no blink

   i) Speech difficulties from facial paralysis

   j) Inability to wrinkle forehead on affected side

   k) Drooling

  2) Diagnostic procedures

   Diagnostic tests are performed in facial paralysis to aid in the exclusion of other diagnoses that may be confused with Bell's palsy (e.g., middle ear disease, middle ear tumor, eighth cranial nerve tumor, and CNS disturbances). Tests are also performed when it is necessary to determine the site of the lesion causing facial paralysis. These tests include the following:

   a) Audiogram

   b) Mastoid radiographs to rule out temporal bone fractures

   c) Schirmer's test to evaluate lacrimation

   d) Acoustic reflex testing

   e) Salivary flow testing

   f) Nerve excitability testing

   g) Electronystagmography

   h) Tests of cranial nerve function

2. Analysis: differential nursing diagnosis/collaborative problems

 a. *Anxiety/fear related to physical symptoms*

 b. *Risk for injury related to corneal abrasion secondary to inability to close eyelid on affected side*

 c. *Knowledge deficit related to management of Bell's palsy*

3. Planning/interventions

 a. *Explain Bell's palsy to patient/significant others*

 b. *Reassure patient/significant others that stroke has not occurred*

 c. *Inform patient/significant others that spontaneous recovery occurs in majority of cases within 3 weeks*

 d. *Administer 1% methylcellulose (artificial tears) to affected eye*

 e. *Apply gentle manual closure of eyelid periodically to reduce amount of ocular exposure*

 f. *Offer sunglasses*

g. *Apply eye patch after closing affected eyelid manually*
h. *Inform patient/significant others that Bell's palsy is not contagious*
i. *Inform patient/significant others of usual and likely outcome or prognosis of Bell's palsy*
j. *Encourage patient to keep face warm and avoid drafts*
k. *Administer analgesics and steroids as per physician's orders*
l. *Prepare patient for discharge*
    1) Patient participation in recovery
        a) Moist heat and facial massage
        b) Passive facial muscle exercise
        c) Active facial muscle exercise
    2) Support of sagging facial muscles
        a) Wound closures (Steri-Strips)
        b) Facial sling
    3) Corneal protection: reinforce eye care
    4) Medication instructions
        a) Analgesics
        b) Steroids
        c) Artificial tears
    5) Notification of physician of changes in condition
    6) Follow-up appointment with physician
4. **Expected outcome/evaluation** (see Appendix B)

D. Trigeminal neuralgia

Trigeminal neuralgia is a neurological disorder of the fifth cranial nerve of unknown etiology. Any of the three nerve divisions can be affected. The second and third divisions, which innervate the maxillary and mandibular areas of the face, are more commonly affected. It is characterized by brief, recurrent paroxysms of excruciating facial pain. Structural lesions are believed to be the cause leading to a type of short circuit that allows repetitive firing in the nerve and its divisions. Attacks may be brought on by exposure to the cold and eating, drinking, and washing the face. Females and persons 40 years of age or older are more prone to experience this condition.

1. **Assessment**
    a. *Subjective data*
        1) History of present illness
            a) Pain similar to that from electrical shock that occurs in distribution of one or more branches of trigeminal nerve (lower cheek, jaw, and, less commonly, forehead)
            b) Pain-free interval of minutes, hours, days, or longer; however, recurrences become more frequent and severe
            c) Unilateral pain during any single episode
            d) Minimal to no sensory loss in distribution of trigeminal nerve
            e) Right side affected more than left side
        2) Medical history: noncontributory
    b. *Objective data*
        1) Physical examination
            a) Normal neurological examination results, with minimal or absent sensory loss along distribution of trigeminal nerve
            b) Painful paroxysm precipitated by touching of trigger zone on ipsilateral anterior aspect of face
        2) Diagnostic procedures

a) Diagnosis may be made on basis of history and physical examination alone

b) Medical treatment and response and/or lack of response to treatment may act as therapeutic challenge to diagnosis

c) No further diagnostic tests are required unless intracranial lesion or other neurological disorders are suspected

2. **Analysis: differential nursing diagnosis/collaborative problems**

a. *Pain related to pathophysiologic process of disease*

b. *Knowledge deficit related to management of trigeminal nerve stimulation*

3. **Planning/interventions**

a. *Determine definitive diagnosis of trigeminal neuralgia*

b. *Provide medical pharmacological treatment as prescribed by physician*

1) Carbamazepine

2) Phenytoin

3) Narcotics and analgesics, which are minimally effective

c. *Prepare for surgical intervention if adequate pain relief not achieved pharmacologically*

1) Percutaneous radiofrequency neurolysis

2) Microvascular decompression of trigeminal nerve

3) Trigeminal glycerol chemoneurolysis: injecting glycerol into trigeminal cistern, causing chemical dissolution of nerve

4) Surgical release of scar tissue, vessels, or dural structures surrounding semilunar ganglion in middle cranial fossa

5) Blocking or transection of peripheral branches of trigeminal nerve

d. *Reinforce with patient/significant others goals of treatment, prognosis, and so forth after physician's explanation*

1) Majority of patients with trigeminal neuralgia respond to medical therapy within 48 hours

2) Of these patients, 25 to 50% eventually fail to respond to drug therapy and require surgical intervention

e. *If exposing the affected cheek to sudden cold triggers neuralgia, instruct patient to avoid iced drinks, cold wind, swimming in cold water, and so forth*

f. *Prepare patient for discharge*

1) Medication instructions regarding dose, frequency and route of administration, and side effects

2) Recognition of signs and symptoms and when to call physician

3) Follow-up appointment

4. **Expected outcomes/evaluation** (see Appendix B)

E. Facial lacerations and soft tissue injuries

There are multiple causes of facial lacerations and soft tissue injuries; the most common are vehicular crashes, interpersonal altercations, violent crimes, and animal and human bites. Common types of soft tissue injuries include lacerations, abrasions, puncture wounds, contusions, and avulsion injuries. Presentations may range from simple isolated facial lacerations to those accompanied by airway obstruction, edema, hemorrhage, massive facial trauma, fractures, and multisystem injuries. As a result, it is imperative that a complete review of systems and physical assessment be done for all individuals with facial trauma.

1. **Assessment**

a. *Subjective data*

1) History of present illness

a) Time/date of occurrence

          b) Facial wounds

          c) Facial asymmetry/swelling

          d) Bleeding

          e) Motor deficits

             (1) Systemic

             (2) Local

          f) Sensory deficits

             (1) Systemic

             (2) Local

          g) Pain/tenderness

          h) Presence of foreign bodies

          i) Immunization status

          j) Other

             (1) Symptoms suggestive of more extensive facial injuries

             (2) Symptoms suggestive of CNS injury

             (3) Symptoms suggestive of multisystem injuries

      2) Medical history

          a) Blood dyscrasias

          b) Previous dental, ENT, or facial trauma, fractures, or surgeries

   b. Objective data

      1) Physical examination

          a) Facial wounds

          b) Facial asymmetry/swelling

          c) Bleeding

          d) Motor deficits

             (1) Systemic

             (2) Local (e.g., facial muscle movement)

          e) Sensory deficits

             (1) Systemic

             (2) Local: gustatory changes of anterior two thirds of tongue, and other sensory or functional changes (excessive salivation or bleeding at parotid duct opening and excessive lacrimation)

          f) Pain/tenderness

          g) Other

             (1) Signs suggestive of more extensive facial injuries

             (2) Signs suggestive of CNS injury

             (3) Signs suggestive of multisystem injuries

      2) Diagnostic procedures

          a) Radiographs

          b) CT scan

          c) Aerobic and/or anaerobic wound cultures

2. Analysis: differential nursing diagnosis/collaborative problems

   a. Impaired skin integrity related to soft tissue injury

   b. Risk for infection related to soft tissue injury

   c. Pain related to injury

   d. Knowledge deficit related to wound care

3. Planning/interventions

   a. Control bleeding

   b. Copiously irrigate wounds with normal saline

   c. Clean intact skin and wound edges

   d. Replace tissue flaps in proper position

   e. Wrap avulsed part in normal saline, place in plastic bag, and then place in basin with normal saline and ice

  f. *Position patient for comfort and suturing*
  g. *Prepare suture equipment and materials*
    1) Minor surgery or laceration tray
    2) Suture materials
      a) Absorbable
      b) Nonabsorbable
    3) Topical skin adhesive
    4) Anesthetic
      a) Topical
      b) Local
        (1) Lidocaine with epinephrine (for most facial wounds, excluding tip of nose and ears)
        (2) Lidocaine without epinephrine (for tip of nose and ears)
      c) Systemic
        (1) Conscious sedation
        (2) Nitrous oxide
    5) Papoose board or other restraint method for pediatric patients
    6) Proper lighting
    7) Scissors to clip hair as need: never shave or cut eyebrows
    8) Gauze
    9) Dressing materials
  h. *Administer tetanus immunization as indicated*
  i. *Administer narcotics/analgesics as per physician's orders*
  j. *Apply ice to area of trauma but not directly to avulsed part*
  k. *Reassure patient and provide emotional support*
  l. *Assist with definitive treatment of injury*
  m. *Explain all discharge instructions concerning wound care to patient/significant others*
  n. *Give written discharge instructions concerning wound care to patient/significant others*
  o. *Inform patient that final result of laceration (e.g., scarring) cannot be evaluated until approximately 6 months after accident or injury*
  p. *Assist patient in recognizing his or her sensory and perceptual deficits*
4. **Expected outcomes/evaluation** (see Appendix B)

F. Mandibular fractures

Of the multiple causes of mandibular fractures, the most common are vehicular crashes and interpersonal altercations. The types of situations most likely to cause mandibular fractures are sustaining direct blows to the mandible (e.g., with fists or clubs), falling forward on the chin, and catapulting forward, as would the driver in a motor vehicle crash.

The mandible's facial prominence and U shape make it one of the most frequently fractured facial bones. The mandible is also susceptible to multiple fractures, when force at one site is transmitted to another area distant from the impact site. Common fracture sites are the body of the mandible, the angle adjacent to a wisdom tooth, the subcondylar area, and the condyle. TMJ dislocation may accompany mandibular fractures.

1. **Assessment**
  a. *Subjective data*
    1) History of present illness
      a) Injury
      b) Pain/tenderness

      c) Malocclusion

      d) Facial asymmetry

      e) Bleeding around mouth

      f) Paresthesia/numbness of lower lip

      g) Trismus: inability to open mouth

      h) Edema or hematoma formation

      i) Ruptured tympanic membrane

   2) Medical history

      a) Blood dyscrasias

      b) Previous dental, ENT, and/or facial trauma, fractures, or surgeries

      c) TMJ disorder (chronic)

      d) Immunization status

  b. *Objective data*

    1) Physical examination

      a) Facial wounds

      b) Facial swelling and/or facial asymmetry

      c) Malocclusion or lateral crossbite

      d) Point tenderness at fracture site

      e) Bony defects palpable at fracture sites

      f) Mobility of fracture fragments

      g) Ecchymosis in floor of mouth

      h) Sublingual edema

      i) Tearing of gingival tissues/oral bleeding

      j) Trismus: inability to open mouth

      k) Possible ruptured tympanic membrane on side of injury or hemotympanum

      l) Decreased or altered sensation on affected side

    2) Diagnostic procedures

      a) Posteroanterior, lateral, and lateral oblique radiographs of face and skull

      b) Panorex views of mandible

      c) Waters' and Towne's views: can also provide valuable information

      d) CT scan

2. Analysis: differential nursing diagnosis/collaborative problems

  a. *Risk for ineffective airway clearance related to facial injury resulting in edema or hemorrhage*

  b. *Pain related to fracture*

  c. *Risk for infection related to possible soft tissue injury*

  d. *Knowledge deficit related to management of mandibular fractures*

3. Planning/interventions

  a. *Ensure patent airway, assess C-spine, and maintain airway, breathing, circulation*

    1) Position patient for optimal airway clearance and comfort (e.g., high Fowler's position if no concurrent spinal injury)

    2) Prevent aspiration of teeth, bone fragments, blood clots, vomitus, etc.

      a) Ensure proper positioning (e.g., side-lying and high Fowler's positions unless contraindicated)

      b) Have suction equipment readily available to prevent secretions or blood from pooling in oral cavity

      c) Have emergency intubation and tracheostomy equipment readily available

    3) Control bleeding and swelling

  b. *Closely monitor patient*

    1) Airway patency

2) Vital signs

3) Degree of swelling

c. *Ensure ongoing explanations to patient/significant others regarding treatments, prognosis, and so forth*

d. *Administer narcotics or analgesics as per physician's orders*

e. *Position patient for comfort; elevate head (if spinal injury ruled out)*

f. *Apply ice*

g. *Reassure and provide emotional support*

h. *Assist with definitive treatment of fracture*

    1) Displaced symptomatic fractures necessitate reduction and occlusion fixation (intermaxillary or direct wiring of fracture fragments may be indicated)

i. *Provide oral rinses with half-strength hydrogen peroxide and water*

j. *Administer antibiotics as per order*

k. *Monitor for signs and symptoms of infection*

l. *Culture wounds*

m. *Administer tetanus immunization as indicated*

n. *Prepare patient for home discharge if fracture is undisplaced and asymptomatic*

    1) Mechanical soft diet

    2) Immobilization orders

    3) Medication instructions

    4) Follow-up care

o. *Instruct patient to use a straw and drink plenty of liquids*

p. *Prepare patient for admission if fracture is displaced and symptomatic*

4. Expected outcomes/evaluation (see Appendix B)

G. Maxillary fractures

The most common causes of maxillary fractures are motor vehicle crashes, interpersonal altercations, and other trauma. The types of situations most likely to cause maxillary fractures are sustaining direct blows to the maxilla (e.g., with fists or clubs), catapulting forward, as would the passenger in a motor vehicle crash, and being involved in high-speed vehicular decelerating crashes. Maxillary fractures are less common than mandibular fractures; therefore, they are considered to reflect massive facial trauma and are frequently associated with multisystem injuries. Maxillary fractures may involve the maxilla alone; however, they frequently occur in conjunction with fractures of other bones of the midface. These fractures are categorized as the following: (1) LeFort I (transverse fracture): maxillary fracture causing transverse detachment of the entire maxilla above the teeth at the level of the nasal floor; (2) LeFort II (pyramidal fracture): fracture of the midface that involves a triangular segment of the midportion of the face and the nasal bones; (3) LeFort III (craniofacial disjunction): complete separation of the cranial attachments from the facial bones (Fig. 6–1). Maxillary fractures are not always so clearly defined, and frequently, they may occur in combination (completely or partially) with one another (e.g., left LeFort II and right LeFort III).

1. Assessment

a. *Subjective data*

    1) History of present illness

        a) Accident or injury

        b) Pain/tenderness

        c) Bleeding

        d) Swelling/asymmetry of face

        e) Infraorbital mobility and/or paresthesia

        f) Ecchymosis

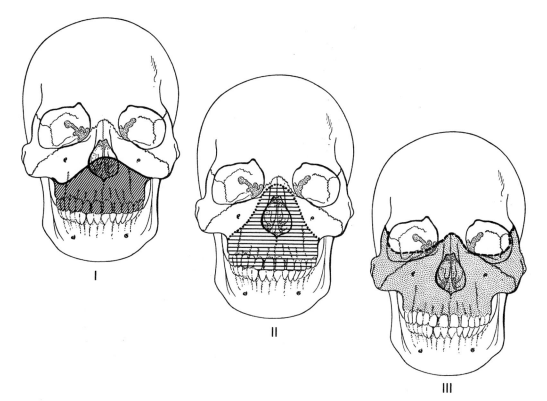

FIGURE 6–1. LeFort classification of maxillary fractures. I, Transverse fracture; II, pyramidal fracture; and III, craniofacial disjunction. Reprinted with permission from Lewis, M. B. (1989). Maxillofacial and soft tissue injuries. In E. W. Wilkins (Ed.), Emergency medicine (p. 791). Baltimore: Williams & Wilkins.

g) Epistaxis

h) Malocclusion

i) Visual disturbances

j) Cerebrospinal rhinorrhea (LeFort II and III)

k) Cervical spine pain

l) Immunization status

2) Medical history

   a) Blood dyscrasias

   b) Previous dental, ENT, and/or facial trauma, fractures, or surgery

b. *Objective data*

1) Physical examination

   a) Facial wounds

   b) Severe pain over injury site

   c) Facial swelling and massive soft tissue injury

   d) Facial asymmetry/distortion (elongation of midface)

   e) Malocclusion or anterior open bite

   f) Intraoral ecchymosis

   g) Periorbital edema/periorbital ecchymosis

   h) Bony defect at orbital rims

   i) Subconjunctival hemorrhage

   j) Epistaxis

   k) Cerebrospinal rhinorrhea (LeFort II and III)

   l) Midface maxillary mobility

   m) Infraorbital paresthesia

          n) Symptoms of intracranial and/or spinal injuries

          o) Symptoms of multisystem injuries

      2) Diagnostic procedures

          a) Waters' view radiographs

          b) Radiographs of individual facial bones (anterior, posterior, and lateral views)

            (1) Mandible

            (2) Zygomatic arches

            (3) Nasal bone

            (4) Orbits

          c) CT scan

2. Analysis: differential nursing diagnosis/collaborative problems

    a. Risk for ineffective airway clearance related to edema or hemorrhage

    b. Pain related to fracture

3. Planning/interventions

    a. Ensure patent airway, assess C-spine, and maintain airway, breathing, circulation

      1) Position patient for optimal airway clearance and comfort (e.g., high Fowler's position if no concurrent spine injury)

      2) Prevent aspiration of teeth, bone fragments, blood clots, vomitus, etc.

          a) Ensure proper positioning (e.g., semi-Fowler's or high Fowler's positions unless contraindicated)

          b) Have suction equipment readily available

          c) Have emergency intubation and tracheostomy equipment readily available, and assist as needed

      3) Control bleeding and swelling

    b. Closely monitor patient

      1) Airway patency

      2) Vital signs

      3) Degree of swelling

      4) Amount of bleeding

      5) ABG values

    c. Administer narcotics/analgesics and antibiotics as per physician's orders

    d. Position patient for comfort and elevate head (if spinal injury ruled out)

    e. Apply cold packs to face

    f. Explain all diagnostic tests, procedures, and treatments to patient/significant others

    g. Reassure patient and provide emotional support

    h. Prepare for definitive treatment of fractures

      1) Open reduction

      2) Internal wiring for stabilization

      3) Prophylactic antibiotic therapy

    i. Encourage patient to express emotion

    j. Offer reassurance (realistic) regarding eventual outcome or healing of facial bones and soft tissue injuries

    k. Prepare patient for hospital admission

    l. Administer tetanus immunization as indicated

4. Expected outcomes/evaluation (see Appendix B)

H. Zygomatic fractures

    Motor vehicle crashes, interpersonal altercations, and other types of trauma are the most common causes of zygomatic fractures. The types of situations most likely to result in zygomatic fractures are direct blows to the prominence of the zygoma or malar eminence (e.g., with fists or clubs) and falling on the side of the face. Some zygomatic fractures are called *tripod fractures* and involve all of the zygomatic suture lines. Fractures of the zygoma are frequently associated with orbital floor fractures. These are called blow-out fractures (see Chapter 14).

1. **Assessment**
   a. *Subjective data*
      1) History of present illness
         a) Accident or injury
         b) Pain/tenderness
         c) Bleeding
         d) Swelling
         e) Pain with jaw movement
         f) Visual disturbances
         g) Immunization status
      2) Medical history
         a) Blood dyscrasias
         b) Previous dental, ENT, and/or facial trauma, fractures, or surgery
   b. *Objective data*
      1) Physical examination
         a) Facial wounds
         b) Bleeding
         c) Local swelling or edema
         d) Asymmetry of face
            (1) Flatness of cheek on affected side or reduction in height of malar eminence
            (2) Depression of infraorbital rim with downward displacement of globe of eye on affected side
            (3) Palpebral fissure slanted on affected side
         e) Epistaxis, probably unilateral
         f) Diplopia
         g) Subconjunctival hemorrhage
         h) Periorbital ecchymosis (most common)
         i) Point tenderness along zygomatic arch and lateral and infraorbital rim
         j) Bony defect over zygomatic arch
         k) Limited movement of lower jaw
         l) Paresthesia of cheek, nose, and upper lip of affected side
         m) Subcutaneous emphysema of face may indicate that fracture extends to paranasal sinuses
      2) Diagnostic procedures
         a) Waters' view radiographs (for evaluation of malar eminence)
         b) Submentovertical view (for evaluation of zygomatic arch)
2. **Analysis: differential nursing diagnosis/collaborative problems**
   a. *Pain related to fracture*
3. **Planning/interventions**
   a. *Administer narcotics/analgesics as per physician's orders*
   b. *Position patient for comfort and elevate head (if spinal injury is ruled out)*
   c. *Apply ice to fracture site*
   d. *Explain all diagnostic tests, procedures, and treatments to patient/significant others*
   e. *Reassure patient and provide emotional support*
   f. *Prepare for definitive treatment of fracture by physician*
      1) Open reduction

      2) Internal wire fixation
    g. Encourage patient to express emotion
    h. Offer reassurance (realistic) regarding eventual outcome (e.g., healing of facial bones and soft tissue injuries)
    i. Prepare patient for probable hospital admission
  4. Expected outcomes/evaluation (see Appendix B)

BIBLIOGRAPHY

Adler, R. J. (1989). Trigeminal glycerol chemoneurolysis: Nursing implications. *Journal of Neuroscience Nursing, 21*(6), 337–341.

Blake, G. J. (1991). Carbamazepine for trigeminal neuralgia and pain. *Nursing 91, 21(3),* 102.

Brenner, P. H. (1986). When sinusitis is not obvious. *Patient Care, 20*(19), 49–64.

Bobb, J. K. (1988). Trauma in the elderly. In V. D. Cardona, P. D. Hurn, P. J. Bastnagel Mason, A. M. Scanlon-Schilpp, & S. W. Veise-Berry (Eds.), *Trauma nursing: From resuscitation through rehabilitation* (pp. 692–706). Philadelphia: W. B. Saunders.

Counselman, F. L. (1989). The dangers of an inflamed sinus. *Emergency Medicine, 21*(21), 87–100.

Crumley, R. L. (1992). Maxillofacial & neck trauma. In C. E. Saunders & M. T. Ho (Eds.), *Current: Emergency diagnosis and treatment* (4th ed.). Norwalk, CT: Appleton & Lange.

Deli, S. L., & Bower, T. C. (1988). Maxillofacial and soft tissue injuries. In V. D. Cardona, P. D. Hurn, P. J. Bastnagel Mason, A. M. Scanlon-Schilpp, & S. W. Veise-Berry (Eds.), *Trauma nursing: From resuscitation through rehabilitation* (pp. 570–597). Philadelphia: W. B. Saunders.

Dickens, J. H., & Jacobs, J. R. (1987). Chronic sinusitis. *Hospital Medicine, 23*(10), 59–86.

Dollins, C. M. (1990). Bell's palsy: Signs, symptoms, outcomes. *Journal of Practical Nursing, 40*(3), 36–40.

Dudley, J. P. (1989). Ear, nose, throat, and sinus infections. *Topics in Emergency Medicine, 10*(4), 43–51.

Dyck, P. J., Hasse, G., & May, M. (1988). Diagnosis and care of Bell's palsy. *Patient Care, 22*(17), 107–121.

Gantz, N. M., Gwaltney, J. M., & Sogg, A. J. (1988). Questions and answers on sinusitis. *Patient Care, 22*(13), 53–75.

Gisness, C. M. (1998). Maxillofacial trauma. In L. Newberry (Ed.), *Sheehy's emergency nursing: Principles and practice.* St. Louis, MO: C. V. Mosby.

Howell, E., Sherer, C., & Leyden, A. (1988). Face and neck trauma. In E. Howell, L. Widra, & M. G. Hill (Eds.), *Comprehensive trauma nursing: Theory and practice* (pp. 470–494). Glenview, IL: Scott, Foresman.

Lewis, M. B. (1989). Maxillofacial and soft tissue injuries. In E. W. Wilkins (Ed.), *Emergency medicine* (p. 791). Baltimore: Williams & Wilkins.

Lewis, T. (1988). Temporomandibular joint disorders. *Radiologic Technology, 59*(4), 351–352.

Lower, J. (1986). Maxillofacial trauma. *Nursing Clinics of North America, 21*(4), 611–628.

Raff, M. J. (1988). The acutely infected sinus. *Emergency Medicine, 20*(6), 24–34.

Selfridge-Thomas, J. (1997). *Emergency nursing: An essential guide for patient care.* Philadelphia: W. B. Saunders.

Simon, R. P. (1992). Headache. In C. E. Saunders & M. T. Ho (Eds.), *Current: Emergency diagnosis and treatment* (4th ed.). Norwalk, CT: Appleton & Lange.

Tami, T. A., Crumley, R. L., & Mills, J. (1992). ENT emergencies: Disorders of the ears, nose, sinuses, oropharynx, and teeth. In C. E. Saunders & M. T. Ho (Eds.), *Current: Emergency diagnosis and treatment* (4th ed.). Norwalk, CT: Appleton & Lange.

Vallerand, A. H., Russin, M. M., & Vallerand, W. P. (1989). Taking the bite out of TMJ syndrome. *American Journal of Nursing, 89*(5), 688–690.

Widner-Kolberg, M., & Moloney-Harmon, P. (1988). Pediatric trauma. In V. D. Cardona, P. D. Hurn, P. J. Bastnagel Mason, A. M. Scanlon-Schilpp, & S. W. Veise-Berry (Eds.), *Trauma nursing: From resuscitation through rehabilitation* (pp. 664–691). Philadelphia: W. B. Saunders.

Woods, C. A. (1995). Treatment of common infections. In G. Bosker, D. A. Talan, H. B. Goldman, & J. M. Albrich (Eds.), *The manual of emergency medicine therapeutics.* St. Louis, MO: C. V. Mosby.

Sharon Pierce Peabody, MS, CEN, FNP

CHAPTER **7**

General Medical Emergencies: Part I

MAJOR TOPICS

I. GENERAL STRATEGY

A. Assessment

    1. **Primary survey/resuscitation** (see Chapter 1)

    2. **Secondary survey** (see Chapter 1)

    3. **Psychological, social, and environmental factors**

        a. Age: illness more severe in very young and very old

        b. Family history

        c. Race and socioeconomic status: may determine increased incidence

        d. Lifestyle

            1) Alcohol and street drug (especially intravenous [IV]) use

      2) Homosexual or bisexual sexually active men

      3) Acquired immunodeficiency syndrome (AIDS) or human immunodeficiency virus (HIV) infection in patient, family member, or sexual partner

      4) Bisexual or IV drug user sexual partner

      5) Sexual practices, multiple sexual partners

      6) Intrauterine exposure of fetus

      7) Prostitution: male or female

      8) High-risk occupation for disease contact

      9) Day care center utilization

      10) Military recruit camp residents

      11) Homelessness, institutional residence

      12) Sedentary lifestyle

      13) Nutritional status: obesity and dietary excess or lack

   e. Chronic illness (e.g., hypertension, renal disease, diabetes, cancer, thyroid disease)

   f. Inadequately treated disease process

   g. Exposure to illness

   h. Splenectomy: changes immune response

   i. Infection: viral, bacterial, or fungal

   j. Contact with blood or contaminated needles

   k. Blood transfusion, hemodialysis

   l. Recent diet (seafood or untreated water)

   m. Recent out-of-country travel

   n. Inadequate immunizations

   o. Vaccine failures in high school and college students

   p. Emigration from country with high incidence of tuberculosis (TB)

   q. Stressors: surgery, trauma, illness, and psychosocial factors

   r. Climate or environment

   s. Medications: interactions and adverse reactions

  4. Focused survey

   a. Subjective data

     1) Chief complaint

     2) History of present illness

       a) Pain: PQRST

         (1) Provocation

         (2) Quality

         (3) Region/radiation

         (4) Severity

         (5) Time

       b) Injury: mechanism and time

       c) Fatigue, malaise

       d) Vomiting

       e) Altered mental status or decreased level of consciousness

       f) Fever

       g) Dyspnea

       h) Rash

       i) Edema: location and type

       j) Weakness

       k) Weight loss

       l) Cough

       m) Sore throat

       n) Other symptoms: anorexia, pruritus, diarrhea

       o) Current medications

        (1) Anticoagulants
        (2) Insulin or oral hypoglycemic agents
        (3) Thyroid hormone
        (4) Diuretics
        (5) Oral contraceptives
        (6) Acetaminophen or aspirin
        (7) Antiretroviral agents and protease inhibitors
        (8) Steroids or cancer drugs
      p) Allergies: medications
   3) Medical history
     a) HIV
     b) Diabetes
     c) Alcoholism
     d) Renal disease
     e) Recent illness or major trauma
     f) Previous similar episodes
     g) TB exposure
     h) Recent animal or tick bites
     i) Blood transfusions
     j) Thyroid disease or surgery
     k) Immunizations
     l) Measles, varicella
 b. *Objective data*
   1) Physical examination
     a) General survey
       (1) Level of consciousness or mental status
       (2) Skin: color, temperature, moisture, turgor, rash
       (3) Vital signs, including orthostatic blood pressure/pulse
       (4) Odors: breath and body
       (5) Gait
       (6) General appearance: grooming and general health
       (7) Weight
     b) Inspection
       (1) Neck veins
       (2) Rash
       (3) Edema
       (4) Eye signs
       (5) Mucous membranes
       (6) Skin lesions
       (7) Kaposi's sarcoma lesions
       (8) Evidence of trauma
       (9) Areas of erythema
     c) Auscultation
       (1) Breath sounds: clear, wheezes, crackles, other sounds
       (2) Bowel sounds: normal, hyperactive, hypoactive, absent
       (3) Heart sounds: S_1 and S_2, other sounds (e.g., murmurs)
     d) Percussion
       (1) Sinus tenderness
       (2) Chest: tone of percussion note
       (3) Abdominal distention
     e) Palpation
       (1) Areas of tenderness
       (2) Areas of edema

        (3) Areas of hyperthermia

        (4) Arteries: equality of peripheral pulses

        (5) Veins: venous filling and varicosities

        (6) Lymph nodes

  2) Diagnostic procedures

    a) Laboratory

        (1) Complete blood count (CBC)

        (2) Serum electrolyte levels

        (3) Creatinine and blood nitrogen urea (BUN) levels

        (4) Arterial blood gas (ABG) values

        (5) Serum glucose level

        (6) Urinalysis

        (7) Ethanol level

        (8) Drug screen: therapeutic level and toxic ingestions

        (9) Clotting studies, partial thromboplastin time (PTT), and prothrombin time (PT)

        (10) Blood type and cross-match

        (11) Liver enzyme levels

        (12) Mono spot

        (13) TB skin test and sputum

        (14) Hepatitis screen

        (15) Serum ketone levels

        (16) Cerebrospinal fluid: cell count, glucose and protein content, culture

        (17) Serum osmolality

        (18) Cultures: blood, sputum, wound, throat, nasopharyngeal, viral

        (19) HIV

        (20) CD4 cell count

        (21) Thyroid function studies

        (22) Cortisol level

    b) Radiology

        (1) Chest radiograph

        (2) Extremity, rib, pelvis radiographs

        (3) Skull and cervical spine radiographs

        (4) Arteriogram

        (5) Venogram

        (6) Computed tomography (CT) scan

        (7) Magnetic resonance imaging (MRI) scan

    c) 12- to 15-lead electrocardiogram (ECG)

    d) Electroencephalogram (EEG)

    e) Preparation of patient and family for diagnostic procedures

        (1) Physical preparation

        (2) Emotional support

        (3) Patient/family teaching

        (4) Written consent

B. Analysis: differential nursing diagnosis/collaborative problems

    1. Anxiety/fear

    2. Decreased cardiac output

    3. Fluid volume deficit

    4. Impaired gas exchange

5. Impaired tissue integrity
6. Impaired tissue perfusion
7. Impaired verbal communication
8. Ineffective airway clearance
9. Ineffective breathing pattern
10. Knowledge deficit
11. Pain
12. Risk for aspiration
13. Risk for injury
14. Risk for infection

C. Planning/interventions

1. **Determine priorities**
   a. *Control and maintain airway, breathing, circulation*
   b. *Prevent complications*
   c. *Control pain*
   d. *Prevent spread of infection or disease*
   e. *Maintain fluid and electrolyte balance*
   f. *Maintain acid-base status*
   g. *Stabilize thermoregulatory system*
   h. *Reverse disease process*
   i. *Relieve anxiety*
   j. *Protect patient*
   k. *Educate patient/significant others*
2. **Develop nursing care plan specific to patient's presenting emergency**
3. **Obtain and set up necessary equipment and supplies**
4. **Institute appropriate interventions based on nursing care plan**
5. **Document and record data as appropriate**

D. Expected outcomes/evaluation

1. **Monitor patient's responses and outcomes, adjusting nursing care plans as indicated**
   a. *Specific interventions*
   b. *Disposition/discharge planning*
2. **If positive outcomes are not demonstrated, re-evaluate assessment and/or plan of care**
3. **Record data as appropriate**

E. Age-related considerations

1. **Pediatric**
   a. *Growth and developmental related*
      1) Neonates, infants, and toddlers are more susceptible to illness and injury but also have more recuperative capacity
      2) Immune systems not completely developed
      3) Brain development not complete until about age 20 years, so more susceptibility to injury exists
      4) More exposure to illness: children are exposed to day care center attendees, siblings, school classmates; understanding of hygiene and infection control is lacking

5) Fluid and electrolyte composition: 75 to 80% of body weight in infants is fluid, making them more susceptible to dehydration

b. *"Pearls"*

1) Pediatric patients are developmentally unable to care for themselves during illness (e.g., maintaining adequate fluid intake)
2) Parents know their children better than anyone: listen to them
3) Most therapeutic choice is often reassurance

2. Geriatric

a. *Aging related*

1) In healthy elderly people, physiological decreases in function are usually apparent only under stress
2) Reserve capacity for responding to stress decreases
3) Immune system is compromised
4) Reduced ability to metabolize and clear medications leads to frequent occurrence of toxicity and adverse reactions
5) Neurological system: loss of nonreplicating cells (neurons) may lead to permanent deficit
   a) Dopaminergic neurons are lost, impairing gait and balance and increasing susceptibility to side effects of medication
   b) Loss of other neurotransmitter systems leads to autonomic dysfunction and alterations in neuroendocrine control and mental function
6) Cardiovascular system
   a) Decreases in heart rate are accompanied by increased end-diastolic and end-systolic volumes: reserve mechanisms to increase cardiac output are used routinely and may be overwhelmed by illness
   b) Baroreceptor reflex sensitivity decreases, altering response of system to changes in intravascular volume
      (1) Greater risk exists during rapid volume expansion
      (2) Orthostatic hypotension is more prevalent
7) Pulmonary system: elasticity of small airways is lost
   a) Increasing tendency for alveoli to collapse
   b) By age 65 years, not all airways are open during regular breathing, increasing susceptibility to atelectasis and pneumonia
8) Endocrine system
   a) Glucose intolerance, insulin resistance, and abnormal regulation of insulin secretion occur
   b) Metabolic clearance of thyroid hormone decreases: in thyroid disease, must decrease dose of exogenous thyroxine (thyroid medication)
   c) Decreased estrogen level alters bone metabolism, leading to osteoporosis
9) Fluid and electrolytes: adaptive mechanisms are impaired, although balance (volume and number of solutes) is unchanged
   a) Nephron loss and decrease in renin and aldosterone levels contribute to increased sodium loss before compensatory mechanisms can be fully activated
   b) Decreased glomerular filtration rate, baroreceptor reflex sensitivity, and insulin and beta-adrenergic responsiveness increase risk of hyperkalemia
   c) Water conservation and urine-concentrating ability, as well as thirst mechanism, are impaired, resulting in increased susceptibility to dehydration
   d) Increased osmoreceptor sensitivity with higher setpoint for vasopres-

sin (antidiuretic hormone) increases risk of syndrome of inappropriate antidiuretic hormone (SIADH) in patients taking certain drugs and in pulmonary and neurological diseases

    10) Renal system: renal blood flow, glomerular filtration rate, and creatinine clearance are decreased

    11) Vision and hearing

       a) Decreased visual acuity, changes in refractive power, loss of accommodation, cataracts, and decreased tear secretion influence ability to see adequately

       b) Hearing loss occurs as a result of changes in peripheral auditory system and cerebral cortex

  b. *"Pearls"*

    1) Decreased activity and less emotional involvement in activity or roles occur

    2) Elderly patients have increased concern with immediate environment, health, and factors affecting them directly

II. COMMUNICABLE AND INFECTIOUS DISEASE EMERGENCIES

A. HIV infection and AIDS

HIV infection and subsequent AIDS result from infection by a retrovirus. The Centers for Disease Control and Prevention has categorized HIV infection into multiple groups and subgroups. HIV-1 is found in the United States; HIV-2 is found primarily in Africa. Acute infection is characterized by a mononucleosis-like or other viral syndrome occurring 2 to 6 weeks after exposure. Antibody seroconversion usually takes place within 45 days, but rarely may not occur for up to 6 months after infection. It is followed by a clinically asymptomatic period lasting months to years, during which time the virus is replicating, mutating, and destroying the immune system. Then development of persistent generalized lymphadenopathy occurs, and finally other diseases develop, including constitutional disorders, neurological disorders, secondary infection, secondary cancer, and other infections such as pneumonitis. Development of these problems signals the beginning of AIDS. At this time, it is believed that all HIV infection will result in AIDS. At this writing, the mean length of time between exposure to HIV and development of AIDS is about 10 years and between development of AIDS and death, 2 to 10 years. The sooner treatment begins after infection, the better is long-term survival.

HIV infection causes a defect in cell-mediated immunity and results in decreased resistance to other opportunistic infections. Specifically, it attacks the CD4 cell, which is the cornerstone of the immune system that identifies everyday infections and starts an immune response. All patients are profoundly immunodeficient at the onset of AIDS. There is aberration in the number and function of T lymphocytes, with a decrease in T helper cells, B lymphocytes, and macrophages. Syphilis and drug-resistant TB frequently occur. Extrapulmonary TB is more common in HIV patients, affecting in particular the meninges, bones, joints, and urinary tract. Opportunistic infections, commonly *Pneumocystis carinii* pneumonia, cytomegalovirus infection, and Kaposi's sarcoma are the usual causes of death.

1. Assessment

  a. *Subjective data*

    1) History of present illness

       a) Generalized lymphadenopathy, persistent

       b) Fever for longer than 1 month

        (1) Episodic spiking

        (2) Persistent low-grade fever

    c) Diarrhea for longer than 1 month

    d) Weight loss

    e) Anorexia

    f) Night sweats

    g) Malaise or fatigue, arthralgias, myalgias

    h) Mild opportunistic infections

        (1) Oral candidiasis

        (2) Herpes zoster

        (3) Tinea

    i) Skin lesions, rashes

    j) Cough

    k) Broad range of neurological complaints, both focal and global, including dementia

    l) Current medications

        (1) Antiretroviral agents: zidovudine (AZT), zalcitabine (ddC), didanosine (ddI), stavudine (d4T), lamivudine (3TC), nevirapine, delavirdine

        (2) Pneumocystis prophylaxis: trimethoprim-sulfamethoxazole, pentamidine, dapsone

        (3) Protease inhibitors: indinavir, saquinavir mesylate, nelfinavir, ritonavir

2) Medical history

    a) Blood transfusions, especially before 1985

    b) Hemophilia

    c) Occupational needle sticks or blood exposure

    d) Sexually transmitted diseases (STDs)

    e) Tissue transplantation

    f) Infant with HIV-positive mother

    g) Sexual contact with IV drug user

    h) Sexual contact with HIV-positive partner

    i) Sexual practices including multiple partners, anal sex, oral-anal sex, or fisting

    j) Recent TB exposure

b. *Objective data*

1) Physical examination

    a) Chronically ill appearance

    b) Kaposi's sarcoma skin lesions

    c) Chest: crackles and wheezes

    d) Dyspnea

    e) Abnormal vital signs

    f) Lymphadenopathy

    g) Dementia

    h) Wasting syndrome; signs of volume depletion

    i) Withdrawn, irritable, apathetic, depressed

    j) Slow, unsteady gait; weakness; poor coordination

2) Diagnostic procedures

    a) Chest radiograph

    b) CBC

        (1) Anemia

        (2) Lymphopenia

        (3) Thrombocytopenia

      c) ABGs

      d) Electrolytes, liver function tests

      e) Determination of HIV antibodies (e.g., via enzyme-linked immuno-sorbent assay [ELISA] and Western blot analysis)

      f) Decreased CD4 cell count

      g) Immunological studies

      h) Blood cultures

      i) Urinalysis

      j) TB skin test (purified protein derivative [PPD]): 5 mm is positive in HIV-infected person

  2. **Analysis: differential nursing diagnosis/collaborative problems**

    a. Impaired gas exchange related to ventilation-perfusion imbalance

    b. Risk for infection related to immune system malfunction

    c. Knowledge deficit related to disease process

    d. Anxiety/fear related to disease entity, treatment, prognosis

3. **Planning/interventions**

    a. Maintain airway, breathing, circulation

    b. Provide humidified oxygen

    c. Monitor respiratory rate, breath sounds, skin color

    d. Elevate head of bed to 30 degrees

    e. Prepare to assist with aggressive ventilatory support as necessary

    f. Monitor vital signs; use pulse oximetry

    g. Health care providers wear masks if patient coughing (TB concern)

    h. Administer antipyretic medication as ordered

    i. Initiate administration of isotonic IV solutions to maintain body hydration

    j. Monitor intake and output

    k. Minimize contact with blood and body secretions: use standard precautions with every patient; health care workers who have percutaneous exposure from known HIV should receive as prophylaxis mono-antiretroviral or combination antiretroviral therapy until testing completed

    l. Disinfect body fluid spills (e.g., with 10% solution of household bleach in water): teach patient and family to do this

    m. Provide discharge instructions

      1) Adhere to safer health and sex practices

        a) Know your sexual partner

        b) Engage in mutually monogamous sexual relationship

        c) Use condoms if sexually active

        d) Do not share drug paraphernalia

        e) Do not share razors, toothbrushes

        f) Avoid pregnancy to prevent fetal transmission

        g) Avoid high-risk sexual practices

      2) Report any fever, cough, or unusual fatigue immediately to health care provider

      3) Avoid contact with persons who are ill

      4) Take medicines correctly

      5) Drink adequate oral fluids and eat well

    n. Allow patient to express feelings

    o. Allow significant others to be present during emergency treatment, if practical

    p. Refer to local support group if possible

    q. Discuss home and work safety

    r. Provide written reminders of tasks, medicines, appointments

4. **Expected outcomes/evaluation** (see Appendix B)

B. Diphtheria

Diphtheria is an acute, highly contagious disease caused by a gram-negative bacillus, *Corynebacterium diphtheriae*, that usually causes membranous nasopharyngitis or obstructive laryngotracheitis. Cutaneous lesions may also occur. It is spread by airborne respiratory droplets or direct contact with respiratory secretions or skin lesion exudate. The exotoxin of this rapidly progressive illness can result in widespread organ damage and complications, including myocarditis, thrombocytopenia, vocal cord paralysis, acute tubular necrosis, and an ascending paralysis similar to Guillain-Barré syndrome. Diphtheria is rare in the United States, seen most often in the South and the Pacific Northwest among the urban and rural poor. It occurs in immunized as well as nonimmunized persons; severity of illness is directly related to immunization status. The only effective control of this disease is universal immunization. Incidence is greatest in fall and winter; transmission occurs by intimate contact, typically in crowded living conditions. The incubation period is 2 to 5 days. Treated illness is communicable for up to 4 days; untreated illness can be spread for up to 2 weeks. Occurrence of active disease does not confer immunity. Pseudomembranous inflammation develops on mucosal surfaces, which may lead to airway obstruction. Death usually results from respiratory (asphyxia) or cardiac (myocarditis) complications. Death is most common in the very young and very old, usually within 3 or 4 days of onset of illness.

1. **Assessment**
   a. *Subjective data*
      1) History of present illness
         a) Onset lasting 1 to 2 days
         b) Sore throat
         c) Difficulty in swallowing or breathing
         d) Fever: low grade or high (rarely > 103°F [39.4°C]), chills
         e) Headache
         f) Nausea
         g) Malaise
         h) Travel to endemic areas in previous week
         i) Crowded living conditions
      2) Medical history
         a) Childhood diseases
         b) Immunization status
         c) Allergies
   b. *Objective data*
      1) Physical examination
         a) Cervical lymphadenopathy
         b) Dirty, gray-white, rubbery membrane covering structures of pharynx and larynx (removal of membrane leaves bleeding surface)
         c) Swelling of structures of pharynx
         d) Respiratory distress
            (1) Cyanosis
            (2) Use of accessory muscles
            (3) Nasal flaring
            (4) Stridor
            (5) Aspiration (from paralysis of soft palate and posterior pharynx)
         e) Vital signs
            (1) Rapid, thready pulse
            (2) Temperature above 101°F (38.3°C)
            (3) Hypercapnia

        f) Alteration in neurological functions
           (1) Lethargy
           (2) Withdrawal
           (3) Confusion
           (4) Cranial nerve neuropathies
        g) Alteration in cardiac functions
           (1) ST- and T-wave changes
           (2) First-degree heart block
           (3) Dyspnea, heart failure, circulatory collapse
        h) Anxiety
     2) Diagnostic procedures
        a) Throat culture: specimen swabbed from beneath membrane or piece of membrane
        b) Notify laboratory that *C. diphtheriae* is suspected: requires special media and handling

2. Analysis: differential nursing diagnosis/collaborative problems
   a. Ineffective airway clearance related to obstruction
   b. Pain related to inflammatory disease process
   c. Anxiety/fear related to disease process and respiratory distress
   d. Risk for aspiration related to paralysis of soft palate and posterior pharynx

3. Planning/interventions
   a. Provide strict respiratory isolation
   b. Maintain airway, breathing, circulation
      1) Monitor vital signs and pulse oximeter
      2) Assemble emergency cricothyrotomy equipment at bedside
      3) Administer oxygen for dyspnea or cyanosis
   c. Establish IV catheter for administration of intravenous fluid
   d. Administer prescribed medication
      1) Diphtheria antitoxin
        a) Equine serum
        b) Test for sensitivity (intradermal or mucous membrane) before administration
        c) Often administered before diagnosis is confirmed because of virulence of disease
      2) Antibiotic: erythromycin or penicillin G
      3) Antitussive
      4) Antipyretic
      5) Topical anesthetic agent
   e. Minimize environmental stimuli
   f. Instruct patient on importance of complete bed rest
   g. Provide immunization
      1) Regular booster every 10 years, combined with tetanus booster, after completion of initial series of three doses
      2) Identify close contacts
        a) Culture and prophylactic antibiotics
        b) Booster of tetanus and diphtheria toxoid if none within 5 years
        c) Active immunization for nonimmunized persons (series of three doses)

4. Expected outcomes/evaluation (see Appendix B)

C. Encephalitis

    Encephalitis is a viral infection of the brain causing an inflammatory response of brain tissue. It often coexists with meningitis and has a broad range of signs and symptoms, ranging from unrecognized mild cases to profound neurological involvement. Most cases in North America are caused by arboviruses, herpes simplex type I, varicella-zoster virus, Epstein-Barr virus, and rabies. Transmission may be by animal bites (rabies) or may occur seasonally from vectors (e.g., mosquitos, ticks, and midges carry arboviruses, Lyme disease, Rocky Mountain spotted fever, and so on). The more common human viruses are airborne and are transmitted via droplet or lesion exudate to the person, in whom replication takes place, and then the virus enters the nervous system through the blood. In the brain, the virus enters the neuron, causing inflammation, neurological dysfunction, and damage. Encephalitis occurs in all age groups, and mortality ranges from 5 to 10% from arbovirus infection to nearly 100% for rabies.

1. **Assessment**
   a. *Subjective data*
      1) History of present illness
         a) Recent viral illness or herpes zoster
         b) Recent animal or tick bite
         c) Travel to endemic area; season of year
         d) Fever
         e) Headache
         f) Photophobia
         g) Nausea, vomiting
         h) Confusion, lethargy, coma, other alterations in sensorium
         i) New psychiatric symptoms
      2) Medical history
         a) Immune disorders
         b) Allergies
         c) Medications
   b. *Objective data*
      1) Physical examination
         a) Altered level of consciousness
         b) Rash specific to cause
         c) Meningism
         d) Altered reflexes
         e) Focal neurological findings
         f) Abnormal movements
         g) Seizures
   c. *Diagnostic procedures*
      1) Lumbar puncture, CT scan, MRI, EEG
      2) CBC: results variable, depends on cause
      3) Blood cultures
      4) Serology
2. **Analysis: differential nursing diagnosis/collaborative problems**
   a. *Risk for injury related to altered level of consciousness*
   b. *Ineffective airway clearance related to altered level of consciousness*
   c. *Impaired verbal communication related to altered level of consciousness*
3. **Planning/interventions**
   a. *Institute standard precautions and isolation until causative agent identified*
   b. *Monitor airway, breathing, circulation*
   c. *Monitor vital signs and pulse oximeter*
   d. *Administer oxygen*
   e. *Prepare to assist with intubation*
   f. *Insert large-bore IV catheter, and administer isotonic solutions as ordered*
   g. *Administer medications as ordered*

    h. Administer antimicrobial/antiviral agents
    i. Administer steroids
    j. Monitor blood sugar and electrolytes
    k. Insert urinary catheter, as needed
    l. Monitor intake and output
    m. Institute seizure precautions
    n. Monitor for cerebral edema and treat as ordered
    o. Elevate head of bed 30 degrees
    p. Restrict IV fluids
    q. Keep body temperature normal
    r. Administer diuretics as ordered
    s. Explain procedures and disease process to patient/family
    t. Allow patient/significant others to verbalize fears
    u. Prepare patient/family for admission to hospital
  4. Expected outcomes/evaluation (see Appendix B)

D. Hepatitis

    Hepatitis is a viral syndrome involving the hepatic triad (bile duct, hepatic venule, and arteriole) and the central vein area. Cellular inflammation leads to disruption of the hepatic architecture. Hepatitis type A virus is transmitted primarily via the fecal-oral route. It is found in serum and stool and is infectious 2 weeks before and 1 week after jaundice. Hepatitis type B virus (HBV) is transmitted most commonly by blood and sexual contact and consists of three antigens. Hepatitis B surface and hepatitis B e antigens appear early in the disease process. Following them is the Dane particle, which is a two-part antigen: an inner core (hepatitis B core antigen) and the surface antigen (hepatitis B surface antigen). Antibodies are produced for each antigen. Persistence of core antibody indicates chronic infection. Persistence of surface antibody indicates immunity to reinfection. Hepatitis B surface antigen in the serum without symptoms is indicative of a carrier state. Hepatitis type C is identified by the presence of antihepatitis C virus antibody. As many as 50% of Hepatitis C infections become chronic, and no immunity is developed. Hepatitis C causes about 90% of hepatitis cases transmitted by blood transfusion. Hepatitis E is an epidemic, enterically transmitted infection from shellfish and contaminated water and is similar to hepatitis A. Hepatitis D is found in patients with acute or chronic HBV infection. All forms have the same clinical features; specific diagnosis is made in the laboratory. Chronic infection results in cirrhosis and liver cancer. At this time there is no specific treatment, although studies using interferon are underway.

  1. Assessment
    a. Subjective data
      1) History of present illness
        a) Prodrome: preicteric phase, occurs 1 week before jaundice
          (1) Low-grade fever
          (2) Malaise: earliest, most common symptom
          (3) Arthralgias
          (4) Headache
          (5) Pharyngitis
          (6) Nausea, vomiting
          (7) Rash, with type B usually
          (8) May or may not progress to icteric phase
          (9) Incubation: type A, 15 to 45 days; type B, 30 to 180 days; and type C, 15 to 150 days

(10) Duration: type A, 4 weeks; type B, 8 weeks; type C, 8 weeks
  b) Icteric phase
    (1) Disappearance of other symptoms
    (2) Anorexia
    (3) Abdominal pain
    (4) Dark urine
    (5) Pruritus
    (6) Jaundice
  2) Medical history
    a) Immunizations
    b) Alcohol consumption
    c) Allergies
    d) Medications: all medications are significant because they pass through liver
    e) Blood transfusions
    f) Chronic medical problems
    g) Travel
    h) Living in institution
    i) IV drug use
    j) Hemophilia or dialysis
    k) Living in area of recent floods or other natural disasters
  b. *Objective data*
  1) Physical examination
    a) Posterior cervical lymph node enlargement
    b) Enlarged, tender liver
    c) Splenomegaly in 20% of cases
    d) Jaundice
    e) Vital signs: usually normal; may have tachycardia, hypotension if volume depleted
    f) Fever
  2) Diagnostic procedures
    a) Liver enzymes: serum glutamic oxaloacetic transaminase (SGOT) and serum glutamate pyruvate transaminase (SGPT) levels: elevated
    b) Direct and indirect bilirubin levels: elevated
    c) Alkaline phosphatase and γ-glutamyl transpeptidase levels: elevated
    d) Differential leukocyte count: leukopenia with lymphocytosis, atypical lymphocytes
    e) CBC
    f) Antigen and/or antibody titers
    g) Abdominal radiograph
    h) Urinalysis: elevated bilirubin level
    i) PT: prolonged

2. **Analysis: differential nursing diagnosis/collaborative problems**
   a. *Fluid volume deficit, risk for related to nausea and anorexia*
   b. *Knowledge deficit related to disease process and therapeutic regimen*
   c. *Anxiety/fear related to disease process and prognosis*

3. **Planning/interventions**
   a. *Provide increased calories*
   b. *Monitor for signs of dehydration*
   c. *Give fluids: may need to initiate IV replacement of isotonic solution for dehydration*
   d. *Record intake and output*
   e. *Assess support systems of patient*

f. Hospitalize if unable to care for self or PT greater than 15 seconds

g. Initiate prophylaxis

  1) Type A

    a) Immune serum globulin 80 to 90% effective if given within 7 to 14 days after exposure (family members and close personal contacts); use if exposed to fecal-oral secretions and contaminated food, water, or shellfish

    b) Vaccine administered in two doses: given to high-risk population: foreign travel, endemic areas (e.g., Alaska), military, immunocompromised or at risk for HIV, chronic liver disease, hepatitis C

  2) Type B: hepatitis B immune globulin plus vaccination, for exposure to serum, saliva, semen, vaginal secretions, breast milk

  3) Type B: vaccination with HBV vaccine inactivated (Recombivax HB)

    a) Vaccinate high-risk persons

      (1) Health care and public safety workers who have exposure to blood in work place

      (2) Clients and staff at institutions for developmentally disabled

      (3) Hemodialysis patients

      (4) Recipients of clotting factor concentrates

      (5) Household contacts and sexual partners of HBV carriers

      (6) Adoptees from countries where HBV infection is endemic: Pacific Islands and Asia

      (7) IV drug users

      (8) Sexually active homosexual and bisexual men

      (9) Sexually active men and women with multiple partners

      (10) Inmates of long-term correctional facilities

    b) Vaccinate all infants (universally) regardless of hepatitis B surface antigen status of mother (administer first dose in newborn period, preferably before leaving hospital)

h. Report to appropriate health department officials

i. Limit exposure of medical personnel to blood, secretions, feces

j. Instruct patient/significant others

  1) Strict hygiene

  2) Private bathroom at home, if possible

  3) Diet of small, frequent feedings low in fat, high in carbohydrates; patient should avoid handling food to be consumed by others

  4) Signs and symptoms that necessitate return to emergency care setting: bleeding, vomiting, increased pain

  5) Take medications as prescribed

  6) Weekly or biweekly follow-up with health care provider

  7) Activity as tolerated

  8) Avoid intake of alcohol during acute illness

  9) Take medications only if absolutely necessary

  10) Avoid steroids: they delay long-term healing

  4. Expected outcomes/evaluation (see Appendix B)

E. Herpes: disseminated

Herpes simplex virus (HSV) infection is a relatively benign disease when confined to cutaneous regions. However, it has the capability of invading all body systems, leading to serious illness and death. Primary viremia occurs from spill-over of the virus at its site of entry, infecting the susceptible organ. During the second stage, HSV disappears from the blood but grows within cells of infected organs. A secondary viremia results from increasing virus production, causing seeding to other organ systems. The organ systems involved and the extent of damage are variable. Dissemination occurs in susceptible persons: newborns, malnourished children, children with measles and other illnesses, and people with skin disorders such as burns and eczema, immunosuppression, and immunodeficiency, especially HIV. HSV seems to have a predilection for the temporal lobe of the brain. Encephalitis is the most common infection, with a 70% mortality rate without treatment. Even with treatment, one half of survivors have residual neurological deficit. Virus may have a latency period within sensory nerve ganglion sites, resulting in mild or life-threatening infection years later.

1. **Assessment**
    a. *Subjective data*
        1) History of present illness
            a) Onset: usually acute
                (1) After other illness
                (2) After outbreak of cutaneous infection
                (3) After any stressor
            b) Symptoms depend on organ system affected
                (1) Neurological system: headache, confusion, seizures, coma, olfactory hallucinations
                (2) Liver: abdominal pain, vomiting
                (3) Lung: cough, fever
                (4) Esophagus: dysphagia, substernal pain, weight loss
        2) Medical history
            a) HSV infection
            b) Chronic illness, cancer, HIV
            c) Medications: immunosuppressants
            d) Allergies
    b. *Objective data*
        1) Physical examination
            a) Fever
            b) Other vital sign abnormalities depend on organ system involved
            c) Focal neurological signs
                (1) Anosmia
                (2) Aphasia
                (3) Temporal lobe seizures
                (4) Confusion, somnolence, coma
            d) Respiratory system: crackles
            e) Other physical examination findings depend on organ system involved
        2) Diagnostic procedures
            a) Viral cultures: blood and skin
            b) Lumbar puncture: cerebrospinal fluid for culture
            c) Biopsy of target organ, especially brain
            d) Clotting studies for disseminated intravascular coagulation (DIC)
            e) Liver function studies
            f) CBC
            g) Other studies as indicated by organ system involved
2. **Analysis: differential nursing diagnosis/collaborative problems**
    a. *Ineffective airway clearance related to inflammatory response, herpetic lesions, and altered level of consciousness*
    b. *Ineffective breathing pattern related to edema or herpetic lesions*
    c. *Risk for injury related to altered level of consciousness*
    d. *Anxiety/fear related to disease process and prognosis*

3. **Planning/interventions**
    a. *Maintain airway, breathing, circulation*
    b. *Supply oxygen as needed*
    c. *Prepare to assist with endotracheal intubation*
    d. *Monitor*
        1) Vital signs and pulse oximetry
        2) Neurological status
        3) Intake and output
    e. *Establish IV infusion of isotonic solution at rate to maintain blood pressure and fluid balance*
    f. *Administer IV antiviral medications as ordered*
    g. *Insert urinary catheter as needed*
    h. *Protect from injury resulting from seizures*
    i. *Restrain confused patient as indicated*
    j. *Explain procedures and illness to patient or significant others*
    k. *Prepare for hospital admission*
    l. *Practice standard precautions*
4. **Expected outcomes/evaluation** (see Appendix B)

F. Measles

Measles (rubeola) is an acute, highly contagious viral illness caused by rubeola virus occurring in late winter and early spring. It is transmitted by airborne droplets or direct contact with respiratory secretions; its incubation period averages 10 to 14 days. The patient is contagious from a few days before to a few days after the onset of rash. Most persons recover completely from the disease, but there is a significant incidence of complications such as otitis media, diarrhea, pneumonia, and encephalitis. Permanent brain damage often results from encephalitis. The disease is more serious in infants and in malnourished children. It is also a serious illness in pregnant women, with an increase in spontaneous abortion and preterm delivery. Most persons born before 1957 had the illness and are permanently immune. The vaccine, usually given as measles, mumps, and rubella (MMR) vaccination at age 12 to 15 months, is effective, with a booster dose given at entrance into elementary school or some time during the grade school years. In addition, all high school or college-age persons should be revaccinated unless they had the active disease or two immunizations in childhood.

1. **Assessment**
    a. *Subjective data*
        1) History of present illness
            a) Exposure to measles
            b) Prodrome
                (1) Fever
                (2) Cough
                (3) Coryza
                (4) Photophobia
                (5) Anorexia
                (6) Headache
                (7) Rarely seizures
        2) Medical history
            a) Immunizations
            b) History of measles
            c) Current age: born before 1957
            d) Allergies

    e) Medications
  b. *Objective data*
    1) Physical examination
      a) Fever
      b) Koplik's spots on buccal mucosa (bluish-gray specks on red base)
      c) Conjunctivitis
      d) Harsh cough
      e) Red, blotchy rash
        (1) Appears on third to seventh day
        (2) Maculopapular, then becomes confluent as progresses
        (3) Starts on face, then becomes generalized, occurring on extremities last
        (4) Mild desquamation
        (5) Lasts 4 to 7 days
      f) Vital signs: normal, except fever
      g) Neurological system: may have altered level of consciousness, encephalitis
      h) Respiratory system: may have otitis media, pneumonia
    2) Diagnostic procedures
      a) Viral cultures (expensive and difficult, so not usually done)
      b) Immunoglobulin M antibodies: measles specific
      c) CBC: leukopenia
      d) Other studies if seriously ill

2. Analysis: differential nursing diagnosis/collaborative problems
  a. *Risk for injury related to altered level of consciousness (encephalitis)*
  b. *Knowledge deficit related to disease process and self-care*

3. Planning/interventions
  a. *Provide respiratory isolation*
  b. *Isolate patient/significant others from other people in waiting room*
  c. *Advise patient to avoid school, day care centers, and people outside immediate family until after contagious period*
  d. *Initiate immunization of high-risk contacts*
    1) Live vaccine if given within 72 hours of exposure (use monovalent vaccine in infants younger than 12 months; need reimmunization at 15 months with MMR vaccine)
    2) Immune globulin up to 6 days after exposure
    3) Immunocompromised persons should receive immune globulin even if previously immunized
  e. *Encourage rest in darkened room*
  f. *Administer acetaminophen for fever and discomfort as ordered*
  g. *Encourage parents to have children immunized at appropriate times*
  h. *Instruct patient/parent about signs/symptoms of serious illness or complications*
    1) Persistent fever or cough
    2) Change in mental status or seizures
    3) Difficulty in hearing

4. Expected outcomes/evaluation (see Appendix B)

G. Meningitis

    Meningitis is a bacterial or viral infection of the pia and arachnoid meninges occurring with or without antecedent illness. It usually occurs in late winter and early spring. Viral infections are usually mild and short lived, whereas bacterial infections are severe and life threatening. *Streptococcus pneumoniae, Haemophilus influenzae* (H. flu), and *Neisseria meningitidis* serogroups A, B, and C are the common bacterial agents. H. flu incidence has decreased dramatically because of vaccination of infants. Bacteria enter via the blood, basilar skull fracture, infected facial structures, and brain abscesses. Bacteria initially colonize in the nasopharynx. In bacterial disease, the subarachnoid space is filled with pus, which may obstruct cerebrospinal fluid circulation, resulting in hydrocephalus and increased intracranial pressure. Infants and the elderly often do not exhibit classic signs of meningeal irritation and fever. Death is most common within a few hours after diagnosis, especially in children. Up to one third of pediatric survivors are left with some type of permanent neurological dysfunction. Any infant younger than 2 months old with fever must be evaluated for meningitis.

1. **Assessment**
   a. *Subjective data*
      1) History of present illness
         a) Antecedent illness or exposure
         b) Onset: sudden
         c) Headache, especially occipital
         d) Fever and chills
         e) Anorexia or poor feeding
         f) Vomiting and diarrhea
         g) Malaise, weakness
         h) Neck and back pain
         i) Restlessness, lethargy, altered mental status
         j) Disinclination to be held: infants
         k) Seizures
         l) Recent basilar skull fracture
      2) Medical history
         a) Medications
         b) Allergies
         c) Immunizations if child
         d) Chronic disease: liver or renal, diabetes mellitus (DM), multiple myeloma, alcoholism, malnutrition
         e) Asplenic
         f) Recurrent sinusitis, pneumonia, otitis media, mastoiditis
   b. *Objective data*
      1) Physical examination
         a) High-pitched cry in infants
         b) Hyperthermia greater than 101°F (38.3°C) or hypothermia less than 96°F (35.6°C)
         c) Petechiae that do not blanch: 1 to 2 mm on trunk and lower portion of body; also mouth, palpebral and ocular conjunctiva
         d) Purpura
         e) Cyanosis, mottled skin, and pallor
         f) Vital signs
            (1) Tachycardia, hypotension, tachypnea
            (2) Bradycardia in neonates
         g) Meningeal irritation: persons older than 12 months, seen in about 50% of people
            (1) Contraction and pain of hamstring muscles occur after flexion and extension of leg: Kernig's sign
            (2) Bending of neck produces flexion of knee and hip; passive flexion

of lower limb on one side produces similar movement on other side: Brudzinski's sign

    (3) Nuchal rigidity

    (4) Opisthotonos

  h) Infants with meningeal irritation cry when held and are more quiet when left in crib

  i) Photophobia

  j) Focal neurological signs, cranial nerve palsies, and generalized hyper-reflexia

  k) Altered mental status

    (1) Confusion, delirium, decreased level of consciousness

    (2) Lethargy and confusion may be only signs in elderly

  l) Papilledema: unusual

  m) Bulging fontanelle

  n) Irritability

2) Diagnostic procedures

  a) Blood glucose level: infants younger than 6 months old are prone to hypoglycemia

  b) Electrolyte levels: hyponatremia

  c) BUN and creatinine levels

  d) Serum osmolality

    (1) Low because of inappropriate vasopressin secretion

    (2) High because of dehydration

  e) CBC

    (1) Bacterial: high white blood cell (WBC) count

    (2) Viral: normal or low WBC

    (3) Meningococcal: WBC tends to be less than 10,000

  f) Blood cultures

  g) ABGs: if severely ill

  h) Clotting studies (e.g., PT, PTT, fibrinogen, fibrin split products)

  i) Lumbar puncture: cerebrospinal fluid

    (1) Bacterial infection: cloudy appearance; elevated pressure; WBC, 2000 to 20,000 with increased polymorphonuclear cells; glucose level decreased; protein level elevated; bacteria present on Gram's stain

    (2) Viral infection: clear appearance; WBC, less than 500; normal pressure; glucose level normal; protein level normal; no bacteria present on Gram's stain

  j) Urinalysis

  k) Chest and skull radiographs

  l) Latex agglutination

2. Analysis: differential nursing diagnosis/collaborative problems

  a. Pain related to meningeal irritation and inflammation

  b. Fluid volume deficit related to decreased intake, vomiting, fever

  c. Impaired cerebral tissue perfusion related to increased intracranial pressure

  d. Injury, risk for related to altered level of consciousness

  e. Anxiety/fear related to disease process and prognosis

3. Planning/interventions

  a. Ensure that health care providers wear masks if infection with meningococcus is suspected

  b. Undress patient completely to check for petechiae

  c. Supply oxygen via nasal cannula

    d. *Monitor vital signs, including respirations, breath sounds, and skin color, and pulse oximetry every 15 minutes to 1 hour, depending on patient's stability*

    e. *Prepare to suction and assist with aggressive ventilatory support as needed*

    f. *Observe for airway obstruction and respiratory distress after seizure*

    g. *Prepare to assist with lumbar puncture, monitor pulse oximetry during procedure*

    h. *Insert nasogastric tube, if necessary, to prevent aspiration*

    i. *Establish IV catheter: intraosseous route in infants if necessary*

    j. *Monitor IV fluids as related to intake and output or excessive secretion of antidiuretic hormone*

    k. *Administer potassium replacement as ordered*

    l. *Administer antiemetics as ordered*

    m. *Infuse prescribed antibiotics (usually ampicillin, aminoglycosides, cephalosporins) IV or intraosseously*

    n. *Administer benzodiazepines IV, as prescribed*

    o. *Administer corticosteroids, as prescribed*

    p. *Control fever with antipyretics and/or tepid baths as ordered*

    q. *Reduce intracranial pressure*

       1) Use hyperventilation with caution to avoid cerebral ischemia

       2) Elevate head of bed 30 degrees

       3) Administer barbiturates and diuretics as prescribed

    r. *Insert urinary catheter, and monitor intake and output*

    s. *Monitor for signs of dehydration or fluid excess*

    t. *Monitor mental status and neurological signs every 15 minutes to 1 hour, depending on patient's stability; be alert for cerebral edema*

       1) May need to restrain confused patient

       2) Protect seizing patient from physical injury (raise side rails)

    u. *Explain disease process*

    v. *Allow significant others to verbalize feelings of fear and helplessness*

    w. *Explain procedures and need for intensive care unit admission or transfer to pediatric care center as needed*

    x. *Administer prescribed chemoprophylaxis (e.g., rifampin, ceftriaxone) within 24 hours of disease identification to household contacts, day care center contacts, and health care providers if bacterial disease (anyone exposed directly to oral secretions, e.g., kissing, mouth-to-mouth resuscitation, endotracheal intubation, suctioning)*

       1) Side effects include gastrointestinal (GI) disturbance, lethargy, ataxia, chills, fever, and red-orange discoloration of urine, feces, sputum, tears, sweat

       2) Soft contact lenses may be permanently stained with rifampin use

       3) Medication may need to be taken with food for GI intolerance, although it is best absorbed on empty stomach

       4) Birth control pills may not work: need secondary birth control method

       5) Do not give to pregnant women

    y. *Educate parents to have infants immunized against H. influenzae B beginning at age 2 months*

  4. Expected outcomes/evaluation (see Appendix B)

H. Mononucleosis

    Infectious mononucleosis is an acute viral illness with a broad range of signs and symptoms lasting 2 to 3 weeks. It is caused most often by Epstein-Barr virus (EBV), a member of the herpesvirus family, which is transmitted in the saliva.

Incubation period is 2 to 5 weeks. Cytomegalovirus (CMV) is the other most frequent causative agent. About 50% of the population seroconverts to EBV before 5 years of age with subclinical infection or mild illness. There is another wave of seroconversion in midadolescence. Peak incidence is in the 15- to 24-year group; illness in older people is uncommon because of prior immunity. It occurs 30 times more often in whites and in higher socioeconomic groups. It is not very contagious and is often transmitted by a nonsymptomatic carrier of EBV. Most people who become ill do not know anyone who recently had mononucleosis. Complications include glomerulonephritis, autoimmune hemolytic anemia, pericarditis, hepatitis, Guillain-Barré syndrome, meningitis, erythema multiforme, and pneumonia. Rarely death may occur from splenic rupture or airway obstruction as a result of tonsillar hypertrophy.

1. **Assessment**
   a. *Subjective data*
      1) History of present illness
         a) Prodrome lasting 3 to 5 days: malaise, anorexia, nausea and vomiting, chills/diaphoresis, distaste for cigarettes, headache, myalgias
         b) Subsequent development of fever 100.4 to 104°F (38–40°C) lasting 10 to 14 days, sore throat, diarrhea, earache
      2) Medical history
         a) Exposure to mononucleosis, usually not known
         b) Allergies
         c) Medications
   b. *Objective data*
      1) Physical examination
         a) May appear acutely ill
         b) Red throat with exudate; tonsils may be hypertrophied
         c) Tender lymphadenopathy, particularly posterior cervical
         d) Petechiae on palate
         e) Fine red macular rash in 5% of adults: if given ampicillin, 90 to 100% of patients will experience rash
         f) Abdominal tenderness with hepatomegaly
         g) Splenomegaly in 50% of patients
      2) Diagnostic procedures
         a) Heterophile antibody titer (Monospot): positive by second week of illness; may remain negative in children younger than 5 years
         b) Throat culture to rule out group A streptococcus
         c) CBC: neutropenia, thrombocytopenia, lymphocytosis with atypical lymphs, leukocytosis
         d) Liver functions: may be abnormal
         e) Chest x-ray film if pneumonia suspected
         f) Other studies as indicated

2. **Analysis: differential nursing diagnosis/collaborative problems**
   a. *Pain related to inflammatory nature of illness*
   b. *Risk for fluid volume deficit related to decreased intake and fever*
   c. *Knowledge deficit related to disease process and self-care*

3. **Planning/interventions**
   a. *Isolation not necessary*
      1) Avoid kissing on mouth
      2) No sharing eating or drinking utensils
   b. *Activity as tolerated*
      1) Extra rest early in illness

2) Avoid heavy lifting and contact sports for at least 4 weeks if splenomegaly present

c. *Administer antipyretics and analgesics as prescribed (avoid aspirin)*

d. *Administer corticosteroid therapy for severe pharyngitis, evolving airway obstruction, chronic or disabling symptoms, or profound splenomegaly*

e. *Warm salt water gargles for sore throat*

f. *Encourage fluids to avoid dehydration*

g. *Diet as tolerated*

   1) Liquids initially

   2) Soft foods

h. *Do not donate blood for 6 months*

i. *Instruct patient about signs/symptoms of serious illness or complications*

   1) Increasing fever

   2) Cough, chest pain

   3) Progression of illness

   4) Difficulty breathing

   5) Signs of dehydration

   6) Increasing abdominal pain

4. **Expected outcomes/evaluation** (see Appendix B)

I. Mumps

Mumps is an acute generalized, usually benign, viral infection caused by a virus from the *Paramyxoviridae* family, causing nonsuppurative swelling and tenderness of salivary glands and one or both parotid glands. It is transmitted via direct contact, droplet nuclei, or fomites, which enter through the nose or mouth. Incubation averages 16 to 18 days (range, 2–4 weeks). Peak incidence is January to May. It is most contagious just before swelling of the parotid gland occurs. Up to one third of cases are subclinical. Mumps occurs primarily in school-age children and adolescents and is uncommon in infants younger than 1 year. It is usually a more severe illness in the postpubertal age group; 20 to 30% of adult men experience epididymo-orchitis. Impotence is not a sequela, and sterility is rare. Complications include viral meningitis, arthritis, arthralgias, and pancreatitis.

1. **Assessment**

a. *Subjective data*

   1) History of present illness

     a) Exposure to mumps

     b) Prodrome: fever ($< 104°F$ [$40°C$]), anorexia, malaise, headache within 24 hours

     c) Earache and tenderness of ipsilateral parotid gland

     d) Citrus fruits or juices increase pain

     e) Fever, chills, headache, vomiting if meningitis

     f) Testicular pain if orchitis

     g) Abdominal pain if pancreatitis

   2) Medical history

   3) Childhood immunizations

   4) Previous mumps

   5) Allergies

   6) Medications

b. *Objective data*

   1) Physical examination

     a) Swelling of gland, maximal over 2 to 3 days, with earlobe lifted up and out and mandible obscured by swelling

        b) Opening of Stensen's duct red and swollen

        c) Trismus with difficulty in pronunciation and chewing

        d) Testicle warm, swollen, tender

        e) Scrotal redness

    2) Diagnostic procedures

        a) CBC: WBC and differential normal or mild leukopenia

        b) Serum amylase elevated for 2 to 3 weeks

        c) Other studies if seriously ill

2. Analysis: differential nursing diagnosis/colloborative problems

  a. Knowledge deficit related to disease process and self-care

  b. Pain related to inflammatory nature of illness

3. Planning/interventions

  a. Provide respiratory isolation

  b. Isolate patient/significant others from other people in waiting room

  c. Advise patient to avoid school/work until swelling is gone

  d. Administer acetaminophen for fever and discomfort as ordered

  e. Administer other analgesics as ordered

  f. Encourage rest until feeling better

  g. Encourage fluids and avoid citrus and other foods that increase discomfort

  h. Warm or cold packs to face

  i. For orchitis

    1) Bed rest

    2) Scrotal elevation

    3) Ice packs

    4) Take pain medicine as prescribed

  j. Interferon for orchitis is being tested; not available at this time

  k. Administer IV fluids as ordered for acutely ill patients, with meningitis or pancreatitis

  l. Recommend considering immunization for male family members who have no history of mumps

  m. Consider immunization of male health care workers who have no mumps antibodies

4. Expected outcomes/evaluation (see Appendix B)

J. Pertussis

    Pertussis (whooping cough) is an acute, widespread, highly contagious bacterial disease of the throat and bronchi caused by the gram-negative coccobacillus *Bordetella pertussis* and spread by airborne droplets from sneezing and coughing. Infants and children up to 4 years of age who have not been immunized against pertussis are most frequently affected, although it may occur at any age. Females have a higher incidence of morbidity and mortality. Partially immunized children have less severe illness. Adults have only minor respiratory symptoms and persistent cough, and probably represent the majority of cases (often unrecognized) in the United States. The duration of vaccine immunity is less than 12 years, so most adults are not protected. The incubation period is approximately 7 to 10 days but can vary from 6 to 21 days. The peak incidence is during late summer and early fall. The pertussis bacteria invade the mucosa of the upper respiratory tract and produce symptoms. Complications include pneumonia (a common cause of death), pneumothorax, seizures, and encephalitis. Children also frequently experience laceration of the lingual frenulum and epistaxis.

1. Assessment

  a. Subjective data

1) History of present illness
   a) Exposure to pertussis
   b) Three stages: catarrhal: lasts up to 2 weeks
      (1) Conjunctivitis and tearing
      (2) Fever/chills
      (3) Rhinorrhea, sneezing
      (4) Irritability
      (5) Fatigue
      (6) Dry nonproductive cough, often worse at night
   c) Paroxysmal: lasts 2 to 4 weeks
      (1) Severe cough with hypoxia, unremitting paroxysms, and clear, tenacious mucus; patient appears well between paroxysms of coughing; cough often triggered by eating and drinking
      (2) Apnea can occur in rare cases
      (3) Vomiting follows cough
      (4) Anorexia
   d) Convalescent: residual cough
2) Medical history
   a) Recent illness or infection
   b) Medications
   c) Allergies
   d) Immunization status
b. *Objective data*
   1) Physical examination
      a) Paroxysmal explosive coughing ending in prolonged high-pitched crowing inspiration
      b) Coryza
      c) Clear, tenacious mucus in large amounts
      d) Temperature greater than 101°F (38.3°C)
      e) Restlessness
      f) Crepitus from subcutaneous emphysema
      g) Periorbital/eyelid edema
   2) Diagnostic procedures
      a) Culture and sensitivity testing of nasopharynx using calcium alginate Dacron-tip swab
      b) Immunofluorescent antibody staining of nasopharyngeal specimens
      c) CBC with differential leukocyte count: lymphocytosis

2. **Analysis: differential nursing diagnosis/collaborative problems**
   a. *Ineffective breathing pattern related to paroxysmal coughing*
   b. *Ineffective airway clearance related to increased mucus production and paroxysmal coughing*
   c. *Pain related to irritation of mucous membranes and increased use of respiratory muscles*
3. **Planning/interventions**
   a. *Maintain respiratory isolation*
   b. *Monitor vital signs and respiratory status*
   c. *Be prepared to assist with endotracheal intubation*
   d. *Administer oxygen as needed*
   e. *Isolate patients with active disease from school or work until they have taken antibiotics for 14 days*
   f. *Monitor for signs of dehydration or nutritional deficiency secondary to vomiting*
   g. *Administer prescribed medication*

      1) Antibiotic: erythromycin

      2) Antitussive

      3) Analgesic

      4) Antipyretic

  h. Position comfortably

  i. Admit patients younger than 1 year to hospital: prepare for nasotracheal suctioning

  j. Initiate immunization

      1) Education of parents about importance of complete immunization

      2) Household and other contacts younger than 1 year: prophylactic erythromycin

      3) Household and close contacts ages 1 to 7 years who had less than four diphtheria, tetanus, and pertussis (DTP) vaccine doses or more than 3 years since last dose

         a) Erythromycin for 14 days

         b) DTP immunization

  k. Review signs and symptoms that necessitate return to emergency care setting

      1) Difficulty in breathing recurs or worsens

      2) Blue color of lips or skin occurs

      3) Restlessness or sleeplessness develops

      4) Medicines are not tolerated

      5) Fluid intake decreases

4. Expected outcomes/evaluation (see Appendix B)

K. Shingles (herpes zoster)

    Shingles is an acute localized infection caused by varicella-zoster virus (VZV). During an episode of chickenpox, VZV travels from skin lesions to sensory nerve ganglia, where it sets up a latent infection. It is postulated that when immunity to VZV wanes, the virus replicates. The virus moves down the sensory nerve, causing dermatomal pain and skin lesions, which may last up to 3 weeks. The exact triggers are unknown, but old age and immunosuppression are risk factors. Up to 20% of the population will experience shingles in a lifetime; about 4% will have a second episode. Fluid from lesions is contagious, but likelihood of transmission is low. Susceptible exposed persons may develop varicella (chickenpox). Complications include postherpetic neuralgia, a debilitating pain syndrome that may last several months, blindness, disseminated disease, and occasionally death.

1. Assessment

  a. Subjective data

      1) History of present illness

         a) Pain, itching, tingling, burning of involved dermatome precede rash by 3 to 5 days

         b) Rarely headache, malaise, fever

      2) Medical history

         a) History of chickenpox, HIV infection, cancer, chronic steroid use

         b) Allergies

         c) Medications

  b. Objective data

      1) Physical examination

      2) Tenderness over involved dermatome

      3) Rash

         a) Unilateral; does not cross midline

         b) Usually thoracic or lumbar dermatome

c) Small fluid-filled vesicle on red base

d) May become hemorrhagic

e) New lesions occur for about 1 week

4) Fever (low grade if present)

5) Visual acuity, if eye involved

  c. *Diagnostic procedures*

1) Viral culture

2) Other studies if seriously ill

2. Analysis: differential nursing diagnosis/collaborative problems

  a. *Pain related to irritation and inflammation*

  b. *Risk for infection related to skin lesions*

  c. *Knowledge deficit related to disease process and self-care*

3. Planning/interventions

  a. *Provide contact isolation*

  b. *Advise patient to avoid school/work until all lesions are crusted over*

  c. *Recommend immunization of high-risk contacts*

  d. *Varicella-zoster immune globulin (VZIG)*

1) Postexposure prophylaxis

2) Immunocompromised persons (HIV, AIDS, cancer, steroid therapy)

3) Effective up to 96 hours after exposure, but the sooner given the better

4) Susceptible health care workers should be vaccinated

  e. *Administer medications as prescribed*

1) Analgesics for fever and discomfort

2) Antihistamines for itching: use with caution in elderly

3) Antivirals (acyclovir, famciclovir) IV or orally (PO) will lessen disease severity and incidence of postherpetic neuralgia if administered within 72 hours of onset of rash

  f. *To prevent infection of lesions, cut fingernails short*

  g. *Topical baking soda paste or baths and calamine lotion may help with itching*

  h. *Ophthalmological consult if facial/eye involvement*

  i. *Instruct patient about signs/symptoms of serious illness or complications*

1) Increased fever

2) Cough

3) Becoming more ill

4) Signs of skin infection

4. Expected outcomes/evaluation (see Appendix B)

L. Skin infestations: lice

Three types of lice infest humans: *Pediculus humanus* var *corporis* (human louse, body lice); *P. humanus* var *capitis* (human head louse); and *Phthirus pubis* (pubic or crab louse). Head and body lice are 2 to 4 mm grayish-white, flattened, wingless, and elongated insects with pointed heads. Pubic lice are wider and shorter and resemble a crab. Eggs (nits) laid by the female are firmly glued to body hairs or clothing fibers and look like white protrusions, which may be mistaken for dandruff. This problem is important because lice can cause significant cutaneous disease, and they may serve as vectors for infectious diseases such as typhus, relapsing fever, and trench fever. The head louse infects all socioeconomic groups and is more common among whites, females, and children. It is transferred by close personal contact and possibly by sharing hats, combs, and brushes. The body louse is seen with overcrowding and poor sanitation. The louse lays its eggs and resides in seams of clothing rather than on skin; it leaves clothing only to feed on a blood meal from its host. Nits are viable in clothing for up to 1 month. The pubic louse is transmitted by sexual or close body contact. It resides primarily in pubic hair, but can also be seen in eyebrows, eyelashes, axillary hair, and coarse hair on the back and chest of men. It may also occasionally infest hair. Up to one third of persons with pubic lice may have another STD.

1. **Assessment**
    a. *Subjective data*
        1) History of present illness
            a) Itching in infected area; may be severe on scalp
            b) Fever, malaise in severe infection
            c) Exposure to lice
            d) Recent sharing of clothing, beds, combs/brushes
            e) Previous treatment for current infestation, including over-the-counter medications
            f) Symptoms of concurrent STDs
        2) Medical history
            a) Previous infestations
            b) Allergies
            c) Medications
            d) Objective data
        3) Physical examination
            a) Excoriation of scalp and skin
            b) Secondary bacterial infection, especially of scalp
            c) Weeping and crusting of skin
            d) Lymphadenopathy
            e) Small, red macules, papules on trunk
            f) Small, gray to bluish macules measuring less than 1 cm on trunk (maculae ceruleae) from anticoagulant injected into skin by biting louse
            g) Nits on hairs
            h) Thick, dry skin; brownish pigmentation on neck, shoulder, back from chronic infection
            i) Signs of concurrent STDs
        4) Diagnostic procedures: studies appropriate for possible STDs
2. **Analysis: differential nursing diagnosis/collaborative problems**
    a. *Risk for impaired skin integrity related to disease process*
    b. *Risk for infection related to impaired skin integrity*
    c. *Knowledge deficit related to disease process and self-care*
3. **Planning/interventions**
    a. *Contact isolation*
    b. *Advise patient/parent to avoid school/work until one treatment completed*
    c. *Administer analgesics, antihistamines, antibiotics as prescribed*
    d. *Use pediculicides as prescribed*
        1) Lindane: avoid in children 2 years of age or younger and pregnant or lactating women
        2) Pyrethrin liquid
        3) Permethrin creme
    e. *Treat sexual contacts*
        1) Administer medications for other STDs as prescribed
        2) Instruct patient/parent that itching may continue after treatment: do not re-treat without physician order
    f. *Instruct patient/parent to*
        1) Remove nits from hair
        2) Soak hair with equal parts warm vinegar and water

3) Mechanically remove nits with fine-toothed comb
4) If nits in eyelashes or eyebrows, apply layer of petroleum jelly; repeat two times a day for 10 days; do not have parents mechanically remove nits from eyelashes
5) Soak combs and brushes in pediculicide for 1 hour
6) Launder clothing/bedding in hot water; dry in hot drier if possible; discard clothing and linen if practical
7) Iron seams of clothing if body lice
8) Put socks over hands of small children at bedtime to decrease scratching
9) Cut fingernails short
10) Put hats, coats, other nonlaunderable items away for at least 72 hours
11) Avoid sharing hats, combs, brushes
12) Instruct patient/parent about signs/symptoms of serious illness or complications: signs of infection

    4. Expected outcomes/evaluation (see Appendix B)

M. Skin infestations: scabies

Scabies is a highly contagious infestation of the skin caused by the itch mite *Sarcoptes scabiei* var *hominis*. Eggs are laid in burrows several millimeters in length at the base of the stratum corneum layer of the epidermis. The mite causes significant cutaneous disease but is not a vector for other infectious diseases. It is transmitted usually by intimate personal or sexual contact; however, it may be spread to health care workers by even causal contact. Scabies should always be considered whenever a patient complains of rash with intense itching.

1. Assessment
    a. Subjective data
        1) History of current illness
            a) Intense itching, worse at night
            b) Rash
            c) Previous treatment for current problem
            d) Exposure to scabies
        2) Medical history
            a) Previous infestations
            b) Allergies
            c) Medications
    b. Objective data
        1) Physical examination
            a) Rash
                (1) Red papules, excoriations, and occasionally vesicles
                (2) More common in interdigit web spaces, wrists, anterior axillary folds, periumbilical skin, pelvic girdle, penis, ankles
                (3) For infants and small children, soles, palms, face, neck, and scalp are often involved
                (4) Patient scratching
                (5) Signs of infection of lesions
    c. Diagnostic procedures: skin scrapings for mite

2. Analysis: differential nursing diagnosis/collaborative problems
    a. Risk for impaired skin integrity related to disease process
    b. Risk for infection related to impaired skin integrity
    c. Knowledge deficit related to disease process and self-care

3. Planning/interventions
    a. Contact isolation

     b. Advise patient/parent to avoid school/work until one treatment completed

     c. Administer analgesics, antihistamines, and antibiotics as prescribed

     d. Use pediculicides as prescribed

       1) Lindane: avoid in children 2 years of age or younger and pregnant or lactating women

       2) Pyrethrin liquid

       3) Permethrin creme

     e. Instruct patient/parent

       1) Itching may continue for up to 1 week after treatment; do not retreat without physician order

       2) Launder clothing/bedding in hot water; dry in hot dryer if possible; discard clothing and linen if practical

       3) Put socks over hands of small children at bedtime to decrease scratching

       4) Cut fingernails short

       5) Put hats, coats, and other nonlaunderable items away for at least 72 hours

     f. Instruct patient about signs/symptoms of serious illness or complications: signs of infection

  4. Expected outcomes/evaluation (see Appendix B)

N. Skin infestations: myiasis

     Myiasis is the invasion of living, necrotic, or dead tissue by fly larvae (maggots). They do not carry infectious agents, but can cause significant disease of the tissues.

  1. Assessment

     a. Subjective data

       1) History of present illness

         a) Skin lesions or wounds

         b) Social history

         c) Living conditions

         d) Ability to care for self

         e) Substance abuse

       2) Medical history

         a) Previous myiasis

         b) Allergies

         c) Medications

     b. Objective data

       1) Physical examination

         a) Skin wound or lesion

         b) Boil-like lesion

         c) "Creeping eruption" of open wounds

         d) Poor hygiene: may see maggots in skinfolds or on intact skin surface

         e) Diagnostic studies: as indicated by underlying problem

  2. Analysis: differential nursing diagnosis/collaborative problems

     a. Risk for impaired skin integrity related to disease process

     b. Risk for infection related to impaired skin integrity

     c. Knowledge deficit related to disease process and self-care

  3. Planning/interventions

     a. Contact isolation

     b. Advise patient/parent to avoid school/work until treatment completed

     c. Administer analgesics and antibiotics as prescribed

     d. Prepare to assist with surgical debridement of wounds

     e. Apply petroleum jelly to cutaneous boils as prescribed

     f. Instruct patient about prevention

1) Eradicate flies
2) Keep open wounds properly dressed
3) Stay indoors, away from fly-infested areas

g. *Instruct patient about signs/symptoms of serious illness or complications: signs of infection*
h. *Refer to social services as indicated*
i. *Refer for substance abuse counseling as indicated*

4. **Expected outcomes/evaluation** (see Appendix B)

O. Tuberculosis

TB has made a resurgence in recent years after being well controlled. It is caused by *Mycobacterium tuberculosis*, which is an acid-fast bacillus (AFB). It is not highly infectious and requires close, frequent exposure for transmission to occur. TB is spread from the respiratory tract through exhaled air and by droplet nuclei that are small enough to be inhaled directly into the alveoli and bronchioles. Droplets may remain suspended on still air for days. Susceptibility of the host usually determines whether infection occurs. TB infection is defined as exposure resulting in a positive PPD, with no symptoms and no evidence of disease, and is noninfectious. TB disease occurs when the patient becomes symptomatic and is infectious. Two to 10 weeks after infection, the body develops an immunological response, which allows healing and results in a positive PPD test result. The risk of acquiring disease in greatest in the first 2 years after infection. TB in adults is often due to reactivation of an old focus after years or decades. The lung is the primary site of disease; however, 15% of cases are extrapulmonary. Most commonly affected are the kidney, lymphatic system, pleura, bones or joints, and blood (disseminated or miliary). Diagnosis is made by one of two groups of criteria: (1) culture of the bacteria from sputum or other body fluid and (2) positive tuberculin test result, signs and symptoms of TB, and unstable chest radiographic findings. Noncompliance with medication regimens is the main difficulty in treating TB, and has resulted in a growing number of drug-resistant cases.

1. **Assessment**
   a. *Subjective data*
      1) History of present illness
         a) Exposure to TB
         b) Productive prolonged cough
            (1) Longer than 2 weeks
            (2) Becoming progressively worse
         c) Fever and chills
         d) Night sweats
         e) Easy fatigability and malaise
         f) Anorexia
         g) Weight loss
         h) Hemoptysis
         i) Recent tuberculin skin test conversion
         j) Foreign born from, or travel to, high-prevalence country: Vietnam, Philippines, Mexico, Haiti, China, Korea
         k) Resident or staff member of nursing home, prison, or homeless shelter
         l) Alcoholic or other substance abuser
         m) Racial/ethnic minority: African-American, Hispanic, Alaska native, American Indian
      2) Medical history
         a) DM

b) Malignancy
c) Silicosis
d) Chronic renal failure
e) Immunosuppression
f) HIV infection or AIDS
g) Medications, especially prolonged steroid therapy
h) Allergies
i) Bacille Calmette-Guérin (BCG) vaccination (person usually from another country)

b. *Objective data*
1) Physical examination
a) Healthy or ill appearance
b) Chest: decreased breath sounds
c) Fever
d) Signs of underlying disease
2) Diagnostic procedures
a) Tuberculin testing
(1) PPD: induration of 5 mm or greater is considered positive if patient has HIV, is in close contact with person with newly diagnosed TB, or has abnormal radiograph with old healed TB scar; induration of 10 mm or greater is considered positive in all other persons (redness not a factor)
(2) Discard opened PPD vial after 1 month
(3) May repeat PPD immediately if first attempt went subcutaneous: place second one at least 2 inches away; if second attempt fails, wait 1 month to repeat
(4) Only contraindication to PPD is previous positive test
(5) Mono-Vacc Test: same criteria as for PPD; when administering, press hard enough to leave impression of points and base of device on forearm; use for mass screening only, never diagnosis; any palpable erythema is positive, even 1–2 mm, and warrants PPD
b) Chest radiograph: infiltrate, especially of upper lobe
c) Sputum for AFB and culture: three successive early-morning specimens
d) Gastric aspiration for obtaining swallowed sputum in young children
e) Aspartate aminotransferase (AST) level: obtain before starting isoniazid (INH) in persons older than 35 years or who have increased hepatotoxicity risk
f) Other cultures and tests as ordered and indicated by history and physical examination findings

2. **Analysis: differential nursing diagnosis/collaborative problems**
a. *Impaired gas exchange related to ventilation-perfusion mismatch and ineffective breathing pattern*
b. *Knowledge deficit related to disease process and self-care*

3. **Planning/interventions**
a. *Decrease transmission of disease*
1) Isolate coughing patient from waiting room, preferably in negative-pressure treatment room
2) Teach patient to cover nose and mouth with tissue when coughing or sneezing: reduces droplet nuclei
3) Educate patient to dispose of tissue properly and wash hands after coughing

      4) Isolate patient at home for first 2 weeks of therapy for active disease; patient is considered infectious until

        a) After 14 days of directly observed therapy

        b) Decrease in cough and afebrile

        c) Three consecutive negative AFB smears

      5) Surgical masks are helpful for patient to wear; not effective for health care staff or family; need special TB mask

      6) Ventilate living quarters (e.g., house and apartment) with fresh air and exhaust old air to outside: need about 20 air changes per day

      7) Unnecessary to dispose of clothes and linen; unnecessary to boil dishes or utensils

      8) Unnecessary for health care provider to wear caps, gowns, gloves

  b. Use correct technique to administer tuberculin testing

  c. Encourage patient/significant others to return for reading of TB test

  d. Encourage compliance with medication regimen through education about disease and its transmission

  e. Report patient and contacts to proper public health authorities

  f. Administer and educate about medications

      1) All patients with active disease should have directly observed therapy (DOT), even if the patient is a health care worker

      2) Preventive therapy given for 6 months and recommended for

        a) Patients with HIV or suspected HIV with PPD induration of 5 mm or greater: treat for 12 months

        b) Household members and close contacts of newly diagnosed patient

        c) Recent tuberculin test converter

        d) Intravenous drug users known to be HIV negative with PPD induration of 10 mm or greater

        e) Persons with past TB not treated

        f) Persons with chronic medical conditions known to pose increased risk of TB who have PPD induration of 10 mm or greater (e.g., diabetes, renal failure, leukemia, underweight, malnourishment)

        g) Persons younger than 35 years with PPD induration of 10 mm or greater and no other risk factors

      3) Medications: both preventive and therapeutic; generally a four-drug regimen

        a) Isoniazid

        b) Pyridoxine: to prevent peripheral neuropathy from isoniazid

        c) Rifampin: discolors body fluid and permanently stains soft contact lenses

        d) Pyrazinamide

        e) Ethambutol

  g. Encourage testing for HIV

  h. Provide social service referral as indicated

4. Expected outcomes/evaluation (see Appendix B)

P. Varicella (Chickenpox)

    Chickenpox is a highly contagious disease caused by VZV. It is transmitted by direct contact, droplet, or aerosol from skin lesion fluid or respiratory tract secretions. Average incubation is 14 to 16 days (range, 10–21 days). The contagious period starts 1 to 2 days before the rash and ends when all the lesions are crusted over, usually 4 to 5 days after onset of rash. More than 90% of cases occur in children younger than 3 years. Adolescents, adults, and immunocompromised persons are at risk for more severe disease and complications. Less than 5% of varicella cases occur in persons older than 20 years, but they account for 55% of deaths from varicella. Complications include bacterial infection of lesions, pneumonia, DIC, renal failure, and encephalitis. Congenital varicella syndrome may occur from infection during the first half of pregnancy, and there is a 31% mortality rate among neonates born to infected mothers.

1. **Assessment**
    a. *Subjective data*
        1) History of present illness
            a) Exposure to chickenpox
            b) Prodrome: 48 hours before rash: fever, malaise, headache, rash often with itching
        2) Medical history
            a) Immunizations
            b) Pregnant or trying to become pregnant
            c) HIV, cancer, or other immunocompromised state
            d) Allergies
            e) Medications
    b. *Objective data*
        1) Physical examination
        2) Rash, typically 250 to 500 lesions
            a) Starts on trunk as faint, red macules
            b) Becomes teardrop vesicles on a red base, which dry and crust over
            c) New crops appear over several days
            d) Palms and soles are spared
            e) Vesicles may occur in mucous membranes, rupture, and become shallow ulcers
        3) Fever, low grade
        4) Skin excoriations from scratching
        5) Signs of lesion infection: red, swollen, tender
        6) If other complications, may appear acutely ill
        7) Altered mental status
        8) High temperature
        9) Dehydration
        10) Cough
    c. *Diagnostic procedures*
        1) Generally none: diagnosis made clinically
        2) If diagnosis in doubt, Tzanck smear of vesicle contents
        3) Other studies of seriously ill
2. **Analysis: differential nursing diagnosis/collaborative problems**
    a. *Pain related to skin lesions/inflammation*
    b. *Risk for fluid volume deficit related to decreased intake and fever*
    c. *Knowledge deficit related to disease process and self-care*
3. **Planning/interventions**
    a. *Provide respiratory and contact isolation*
    b. *Isolate patient/significant others from other people in waiting room*
    c. *Advise patient to avoid school/work until all lesions are crusted over*
    d. *Recommend immunization of high-risk contacts*
        1) VZIG
            a) Postexposure prophylaxis
            b) Immunocompromised persons (HIV, AIDS, cancer, steroid therapy)
            c) Effective up to 96 hours after exposure, but the sooner given, the better
            d) Susceptible health care workers should be vaccinated

2) Administer medications as prescribed
   a) Acetaminophen for fever and discomfort
   b) Never use aspirin (risk of Reye's syndrome)
   c) Antihistamines for itching
   d) Antivirals, IV or PO, to older children and adults will lessen disease severity
3) To prevent infection of lesions
   a) Suggest putting socks over small children's hands at bedtime to decrease scratching and excoriation
   b) Cut fingernails short
   c) Topical baking soda paste or baths and calamine lotion may help with itching
   d) Encourage parents to have children immunized at appropriate times
   e) Instruct patient/parent about signs/symptoms of serious illness or complications
      (1) Increased fever
      (2) Cough
      (3) Becoming more ill
      (4) Signs of skin infection
4) Susceptible health care workers exposed to varicella should not work days 10 to 21 after exposure to prevent inadvertent spread of disease

4. Expected outcomes/evaluation (see Appendix B)

III. ENDOCRINE EMERGENCIES

A. Adrenal crisis

Adrenal insufficiency (Addison's disease) is a chronic disorder in which the adrenal cortex ceases to produce glucocorticoid and mineralocorticoid hormones. Acute adrenal insufficiency or adrenal crisis occurs in response to an acute stressor, such as major or minor infection, hemorrhage, trauma, surgery, burns, pregnancy, or abrupt cessation of therapy for Addison's disease. Crisis is due primarily to cortisol deficiency. It is life threatening because adrenal glucocorticoids and mineralocorticoids are necessary for the maintenance of blood volume, blood pressure, and glucose hemostasis. Adrenal crisis should be suspected in patients who have septicemia with unexplained deterioration; adults with major illness who have abdominal, flank, or chest pain; patients with dehydration, fever, hypotension, or shock; and patients who may experience adrenal hemorrhage. Death often occurs because of circulatory collapse and hyperkalemia-induced dysrhythmia.

1. Assessment
   a. *Subjective data*
      1) History of present illness
         a) Rapid worsening of symptoms of adrenal insufficiency (see Medical history, which follows)
         b) Fever
         c) Nonspecific abdominal pain; may simulate acute abdomen
         d) Nausea and vomiting
      2) Medical history
         a) Primary adrenal insufficiency
         b) Hyperpigmentation of skin
         c) Weakness, fatigue, lethargy
         d) Anorexia and weight loss
         e) Nausea, vomiting, diarrhea

  f) Salt craving

  g) Postural hypotension

  h) Allergies

  i) Medications

 b. *Objective data*

  1) Physical examination

   a) Appears acutely ill

   b) Signs of shock as a result of dehydration

    (1) Hypotension, but may have warm extremities

    (2) Tachycardia

    (3) Tachypnea

    (4) Orthostatic hypotension

   c) Fever

   d) Altered mental status, confusion

   e) Hyperpigmentation of skin

   f) Very soft heart sounds

  2) Diagnostic procedures

   a) CBC: anemia of chronic disease

   b) Electrolyte levels

    (1) Hyponatremia

    (2) Hyperkalemia

   c) Blood glucose level: hypoglycemia

   d) BUN: elevated (azotemia secondary to dehydration)

   e) Urinalysis

   f) Blood cultures

   g) Plasma cortisol level

   h) ECG

    (1) Low voltage

    (2) Flat or inverted T wave

    (3) Prolonged QT, QRS, or PR intervals

   i) Chest radiograph

   j) CT scan of abdomen: if diagnosis not clear

2. Analysis: differential nursing diagnosis/collaborative problems

 a. *Fluid volume deficit related to fluid shifts*

 b. *Tissue perfusion, altered cardiopulmonary and cerebral related to decreased fluid volume/blood flow*

3. Planning/interventions

 a. *Supply oxygen*

 b. *Insert large-bore IV catheter*

 c. *Administer rapid infusion of normal saline or lactated Ringer's solution*

 d. *Monitor vital signs, including orthostatic blood pressure and pulse*

 e. *Monitor intake and output*

 f. *Obtain initial weight if possible, especially if patient will be in emergency care area for prolonged period*

 g. *Monitor other signs of adequate tissue perfusion: capillary refill and skin temperature and moisture*

 h. *Administer medications as ordered: usually given IV because hypotension results in poor intramuscular absorption*

  1) Dexamethasone

  2) Hydrocortisone

  3) Corticotropin

  4) Glucose

  5) Vasopressors

       i. Monitor levels of electrolytes and glucose
       j. Monitor cardiac function
       k. Prepare patient/significant others for admission and other procedures as indicated by underlying cause of crisis (acute stressor)
       l. Instruct patient or significant others about disease process
   4. Expected outcomes/evaluation (see Appendix B)

B. Diabetic ketoacidosis

Diabetic ketoacidosis is a result of insulin deficiency and stress hormone excess. It typically occurs in insulin-dependent diabetes (type I) but may also be seen in non–insulin-dependent diabetes (type II). Insulin lack causes decreased cellular glucose uptake, release of free fatty acids, and increased gluconeogenesis by the liver. Hyperglycemia promotes osmotic diuresis with dehydration, hyperosmolality, and electrolyte depletion. Counter-regulatory (stress) hormones (glucagon, catecholamines, cortisol, and growth hormone) have anti-insulin effects and stimulate the release of free fatty acids. Free fatty acids are converted to ketone bodies, which release hydrogen ions, thereby contributing to metabolic ketoacidosis. Acidosis decreases myocardial contractility and cerebral function. Infection and stressful events are the usual precipitating factors, along with omission of insulin and new-onset diabetes. The goal of therapy is a gradual, even return to normal metabolic balance. Complications of therapy such as cerebral edema, hypoglycemia, and electrolyte imbalance may contribute to death during treatment.

  1. Assessment
    a. Subjective data
      1) History of present illness
        a) Onset: gradual, 24 hours to 2 weeks
        b) Preceding bacterial or viral illness, current infectious process, or significant stress
        c) Nausea and vomiting
        d) Abdominal pain, usually generalized
        e) Fever
        f) Polyuria, polydipsia, polyphagia
        g) Lethargy, weakness, and fatigue
        h) Decreasing level of consciousness and altered mental status
        i) Weight loss
      2) Medical history
        a) Administration of insulin or oral hypoglycemic agents
        b) Discontinuance or decreased dose
        c) Other medications
        d) Allergies
        e) Previous similar episodes
    b. Objective data
      1) Physical examination
        a) Tachycardia
        b) Orthostatic or frank hypotension
        c) Kussmaul's respirations if pH less than 7.2
        d) Dry, hyperthermic, flushed skin
        e) Dry mucous membranes
        f) Poor skin turgor
        g) Acetone breath odor
        h) Confusion, coma, and decreased mental status
      2) Diagnostic procedures

a) Serum glucose level: greater than 300 mg/dL
b) Electrolyte levels
   (1) Sodium, chloride, and bicarbonate: decreased
   (2) Potassium: normal or elevated initially; falls rapidly during treatment
   (3) Serum phosphate: elevated to 6 to 7 mg/dL as a result of insulin deficiency and prerenal azotemia; total body phosphate depletion as a result of osmotic diuresis
c) Serum osmolality: greater than 310 mOsm/kg
d) Serum acetone level: elevated
e) BUN and creatinine levels: normal unless advanced renal disease or severe dehydration is present
f) ABGs
   (1) Normal partial pressure of arterial oxygen (PaO_2)
   (2) Metabolic acidosis and anion gap acidosis: pH < 7.3; bicarbonate (HCO_3) < 15 mEq/L
   (3) Respiratory alkalosis
g) Urinalysis: increased glucose and ketone levels
h) Chest x-ray film
i) ECG
j) CBC: WBC greater than 25,000 if infection present
k) Cultures as indicated

2. **Analysis: differential nursing diagnosis/collaborative problems**
   a. *Tissue perfusion, altered cerebral related to decreased fluid volume/blood flow*
   b. *Fluid volume deficit related to osmotic diuresis*
   c. *Anxiety/fear related to disease process and prognosis*
   d. *Knowledge deficit related to disease process and self-care*

3. **Planning/interventions**
   a. *Establish two IV catheters for infusion of normal saline at rate of 1 L in 1 to 2 hours*
   b. *Administer oxygen, maintain airway, breathing, circulation*
   c. *Administer regular insulin as prescribed*
      1) *Bolus IV push of 10 units; if patient awake, may give half IV and half subcutaneous (SC) (0.1–0.3 U/kg IVP)*
      2) *IV maintenance with infusion pump 6 to 10 units/hr; discard first 50 mL of insulin drip to saturate tubing*
      3) *Children: 0.1 units/kg/hr IV drip*
   d. *Administer HCO_3 as prescribed: if pH less than 7.0*
   e. *Potassium: added to IV fluid when serum level less than 5.5 mEq/dL (hypokalemia develops rapidly with insulin treatment)*
   f. *Add dextrose as prescribed when blood glucose level is less than 250 mg/dL to prevent hypoglycemia*
   g. *Administer phosphate replacement as ordered (usually several hours into treatment before needed)*
   h. *Administer antibiotics or antiemetics as ordered*
   i. *Insert urinary catheter; insert nasogastric tube to help control vomiting if decreased level of consciousness*
   j. *Monitor vital signs every 15 to 60 minutes until patient stable*
   k. *Monitor glucose every hour and potassium every 2 hours*
   l. *Monitor and record intake and output; monitor for signs of dehydration*
   m. *Maintain flow sheet of measurements*
   n. *Institute use of cardiac monitor until patient is stable*

        (5) Areas of erythema

    c) Auscultation

        (1) Breath sounds: clear, wheezes, crackles

        (2) Bowel sounds: normal, hyperactive, hypoactive, absent

        (3) Heart sounds: S_1 and S_2, other sounds (e.g., murmurs), dysrhythmias

    d) Percussion

        (1) Sinus tenderness

        (2) Chest: note tone of percussion

        (3) Abdominal

    e) Palpation

        (1) Areas of tenderness

        (2) Areas of edema

        (3) Areas of hyperthermia

        (4) Arteries: equality of peripheral pulses

        (5) Veins: venous filling and varicosities

        (6) Lymph nodes

2) Diagnostic procedures

    a) Laboratory

        (1) Complete blood count (CBC)

        (2) Serum electrolyte levels

        (3) Creatinine and blood nitrogen urea (BUN) levels

        (4) Urinalysis

        (5) Arterial blood gases (ABGs)

        (6) Serum glucose level

        (7) Drug screen: therapeutic level and toxic ingestion

        (8) Clotting studies: partial thromboplastin time (PTT), prothrombin time (PT)

        (9) Blood type and cross-match

        (10) Serum ammonia level

        (11) Carboxyhemoglobin level

        (12) Serum uric acid level

        (13) Liver enzyme levels

        (14) Sickle cell screen

        (15) Hepatitis screen

        (16) Serum ketone levels

        (17) Cerebrospinal fluid (CSF): cell count, glucose and protein count, culture

    b) Radiology

        (1) Chest radiograph

        (2) Computed tomography (CT) scan

        (3) Magnetic resonance imaging (MRI) scan

    c) Twelve- to 15-lead electrocardiogram (ECG)

    d) Electroencephalogram (EEG)

    e) Preparation of patient and family for diagnostic procedures

        (1) Physical preparation

        (2) Emotional support

        (3) Patient/family teaching

        (4) Written consent

B. Analysis: differential nursing diagnosis/collaborative problems

  1. Anxiety/fear

  2. Decreased cardiac output

    o. Continually assess neurological status; monitor for signs of cerebral edema (occurs from too-rapid resolution of acidosis and hypoglycemia)

    p. Monitor for respiratory distress syndrome; occurs with overzealous fluid administration

    q. May need to restrain confused patient

    r. Discuss sick day rules as related to insulin and diet

    s. Review preventive fluid therapy

        1) Must keep self-hydrated during any illness, no matter how minor

        2) If unable to retain fluids, contact physician immediately

    t. Review disease process and medication regimen

    u. Instruct in signs and symptoms that necessitate return to emergency care setting: inability to drink fluids and persistent vomiting, diarrhea, fever

    v. Teach to identify and manage symptoms of hypoglycemia or hyperglycemia

    w. Allow significant others and patient to express anxiety and verbalize feelings in situations of newly diagnosed disease

    x. If noncompliance is suspected, alert hospital nursing staff to pursue when patient recovers

    y. Refer to social service or local diabetes organization as indicated

    z. Arrange appropriate medical follow-up care

4. Expected outcomes/evaluation (see Appendix B)

    a. Fluid and electrolyte balance achieved: pH that gradually returns to normal range, serum glucose level of 100 to 200 mg/dL, potassium level of 4.0 to 5.0 mEq/dL, serum osmolality of 285 to 300 mOsm/kg

C. Hyperglycemic hyperosmolar nonketotic coma

    This is a syndrome, occurring in type II (non–insulin-dependent) diabetes, of profound dehydration because of hyperglycemia and resultant osmotic diuresis. The patient is unable to drink a sufficient amount of fluid to prevent dehydration. Ketoacidosis does not develop because there is enough endogenous insulin present to inhibit ketogenesis. Often it is precipitated by infection, stroke, or sepsis. It may also be the initial presentation in a patient with new-onset type II DM. Dehydration predisposes the patient to widespread thrombosis and DIC. The mortality rate is high despite aggressive therapy, probably because the patient is usually elderly with impaired renal, cerebral, or cardiac function. This illness rarely occurs in infants and children and is usually due to gastroenteritis.

1. Assessment

    a. Subjective data

        1) History of present illness

            a) Insidious onset from days to weeks

            b) Recent illness or infection

            c) Thirst

            d) Reduced fluid intake

            e) Polyuria or oliguria

        2) Medical history

            a) Non–insulin-dependent diabetes

            b) Elderly patient with undiagnosed diabetes

            c) Medications: oral hypoglycemic agents, diuretics

            d) Allergies

    b. Objective data

        1) Physical examination

            a) Hypotension

            b) Tachycardia

  c) Normal respirations

  d) Confusion and altered mental status are most prominent physical findings; may be comatose

  e) Dry skin and mucous membranes: dehydration

  f) May have fever

  g) Seizures

  h) Hemiparesis/hemisensory deficits

 2) Diagnostic procedures

  a) Serum glucose level: greater than 800 mg/dL, often greater than 1000 mg/dL

  b) Serum osmolality: greater than 350 mOsm/kg

  c) Hypernatremia resulting from dehydration

  d) Potassium level: normal to high initially; hypokalemia develops with insulin therapy

  e) BUN and creatinine levels: elevated as a result of prerenal azotemia

  f) ABGs

   (1) Normal PaO_2

   (2) Mild metabolic acidosis as a result of dehydration

   (3) Serum ketone level: normal or slightly elevated

  g) Urinalysis: elevated glucose level

  h) Chest x-ray film

  i) ECG

  j) Cultures of blood, urine, sputum if infection source not obvious

  k) Creatine kinase (CK) elevated as a result of rhabdomyolysis

2. Analysis: differential nursing diagnosis/collaborative problems

 a. Risk for injury related to altered level of consciousness

 b. Tissue perfusion, altered cerebral related to decreased fluid volume/blood volume

 c. Fluid volume deficit related to osmotic diuresis

3. Planning/interventions

 a. Supply oxygen, maintain airway, breathing, circulation

 b. Assist with endotracheal intubation if PaO_2 less than 70 to 80 mm Hg

 c. Establish large-bore IV catheter for rehydration

  1) Adults: normal saline at 500 to 1000 mL/hr until blood pressure stabilizes

  2) Child: normal saline (20 mL/kg bolus if hypotensive) to prevent cerebral edema from too-rapid correction of hyperosmolality

 d. Prepare for central venous pressure or Swan-Ganz catheter insertion

 e. Elevate head of bed to 30 degrees if possible

 f. Observe for peripheral cyanosis

 g. Monitor vital signs every 15 to 60 minutes until patient stable

 h. Administer regular insulin as indicated

  1) Bolus IV push of 10 units; if patient awake, may give half IV and half SC (0.1–0.3 U/kg)

  2) Intravenous maintenance with infusion pump 6 to 10 units/hr; discard first 50 mL of insulin drip to saturate tubing

  3) Children: 0.1 units/kg/hr IV drip

 i. Administer potassium replacement as indicated

 j. Administer low-dose heparin as ordered

 k. Add dextrose when blood glucose level is less than 300 mg/dL

 l. May need to restrain confused patient

 m. Continually reassess neurological status, and monitor for signs of cerebral edema and seizures

 n. Monitor intake and output

o. *Insert urinary catheter*

p. *Monitor for signs of fluid overload (major problem in elderly) or dehydration; assess breath sounds as indicated for pulmonary edema*

q. *Allow time for significant others to vent feelings*

r. *Discuss disease process with significant others*

s. *Refer to social service agency as necessary*

4. **Expected outcomes/evaluation** (see Appendix B)

a. *Fluid and electrolyte balance achieved: serum glucose level of 100 to 200 mg/dL, potassium level of 4.0 to 5.0 mEq/dL, serum osmolality of 285 to 300 mOsm/kg*

D. Hypoglycemia

Hypoglycemia is a decrease in the serum glucose level to less than 50 mg/dL and is the most common endocrine emergency. A rapid reduction in glucose levels does not allow time for activation of ketogenesis to provide an alternative energy substrate. At levels below 35 mg/dL, the brain is unable to extract oxygen adequately, resulting in hypoxia and eventually coma. The very young and very old are more susceptible to experiencing low blood sugar. Because hypoglycemia occurs for multiple reasons (mainly diabetes and alcohol ingestion) and lack of glucose causes permanent brain dysfunction, any person with an altered level of consciousness should be considered to have hypoglycemia until proven otherwise.

1. **Assessment**
   a. *Subjective data*
      1) History of present illness
         a) Rapid onset
         b) No recent food intake
         c) Alcohol ingestion within 36 hours followed by fasting
         d) Hunger, nausea
         e) Weakness, dizziness
         f) Lethargy
         g) Shakiness
         h) Anxiety
         i) Headache
         j) Altered mental status
      2) Medical history
         a) Diabetes
         b) Insulin: increased dosage (easily reversed)
         c) Oral hypoglycemic agents: long half-life (difficult to reverse)
         d) Adrenal insufficiency
         e) Liver disease
         f) Propranolol, salicylates, sedatives
         g) Increase in physical exercise
   b. *Objective data*
      1) Physical examination
         a) Cool, diaphoretic skin
         b) Pale appearance
         c) Dilated pupils
         d) Confusion
         e) Hypothermia
         f) Shallow respirations but normal rate
         g) Normal blood pressure and pulse
         h) Combative behavior or coma

  i) Seizures
  j) Hemiplegia or other signs of stroke
  2) Diagnostic procedures
  a) Blood glucose level: less than 50 mg/dL
  b) Electrolyte levels: normal
  c) Urinalysis: normal
  d) ABGs: normal pH
  e) Serum alcohol level
 2. **Analysis: differential nursing diagnosis/collaborative problems**
  a. *Altered nutrition: less than body requirements, related to decreased intake or altered metabolism of glucose*
  b. *Knowledge deficit related to disease process and self-care*
 3. **Planning/interventions**
  a. *Supply oxygen*
  b. *Monitor respiratory rate, breath sounds, signs of adequate oxygenation; maintain airway, breathing, circulation*
  c. *Suction as necessary*
  d. *Assist with endotracheal intubation if PaO_2 is less than 70 to 80 mm Hg*
  e. *Determine blood glucose level (e.g., fingertip venous blood glucose level)*
  f. *Administer thiamine IM or IV if patient is malnourished*
  g. *Give oral glucose solution if gag reflex present*
  h. *Initiate IV administration of 5% dextrose in water if patient is unresponsive or unable to take oral solution*
  i. *Give IV 50% dextrose in water; if no response, repeat; dextrose 25% if less than 2 years old*
  j. *Give glucagon IM or SC if unable to establish an IV: 0.5 to 2 mg and may repeat twice; not effective in alcohol-induced hypoglycemia (no glycogen stores left)*
  k. *Monitor mental status continually*
  l. *May need to restrain combative patient*
  m. *Educate patient and significant others*
  1) Review mechanism of disease process with patient and significant others
  2) Reinforce need to eat regularly
  3) Carry quick glucose foods: simple carbohydrates (hard candy, sugar, orange juice, soft drinks made with sugar), not complex carbohydrates (e.g., candy bars) because fat retards ability to use glucose
  4) Decrease insulin dosage if exercising
  5) Avoid alcohol consumption while fasting; alcoholics need to eat when bingeing
  n. *Prepare patient for hospitalization if hypoglycemia is due to oral agents because of prolonged drug half-life*
  o. *Refer to social service or appropriate community agency as necessary*
  p. *Allow time for patient/significant others to verbalize feelings about diet restrictions*
  q. *Instruct patient in signs and symptoms that indicate inadequate nutrition and necessitate return to emergency care setting*
  1) Persistent symptoms of hypoglycemia in spite of adequate food intake
  2) Seizure
  3) Failure to return to normal mental status after hypoglycemic episode
 4. **Expected outcomes/evaluation** (see Appendix B)
  a. *Blood glucose level of 90 to 140 mg/dL*

E. Myxedema coma

Myxedema coma is the most severe form of hypothyroidism, causing marked impairment of central nervous system function and cardiovascular decompensation. Recognition of this illness is hampered by its insidious onset and rarity. It is usually seen in winter in elderly women with a history of hypothyroidism. Precipitating factors include serious infection (pneumonia and urinary tract infection are common), recent sedative or tranquilizer use, stroke, exposure to cold environment, and termination of thyroid hormone replacement. Death is common, but many patients can survive if they receive prompt adequate care.

1. **Assessment**
   a. *Subjective data*
      1) History of present illness
         a) Recent illness
         b) Progressive decline in intellectual status
         c) Apathy, self-neglect
         d) Emotional lability
         e) Anorexia
         f) Recent weight gain
      2) Medical history
         a) Hypothyroidism or thyroid surgery
         b) Allergies
         c) Medications: thyroid replacement hormone, recent use of tranquilizers and sedatives
   b. *Objective data*
      1) Physical examination
         a) Decreased mental status
         b) Depressed mental acuteness
         c) Confusion or psychosis
         d) Pale, waxy, edematous facies with periorbital edema
         e) Macroglossia
         f) Dry, cold, pale skin
         g) Nonpitting extremity edema
         h) Thin eyebrows
         i) Deep, coarse voice
      2) Vital signs
         a) Hypothermia, usually above 95°F (35°C)
         b) Bradycardia with distant heart sounds, stroke volume, and cardiac output decreased
         c) Hypoventilation
         d) Hypotension
         e) Scar from prior thyroidectomy
      3) Diagnostic procedures
         a) Electrolytes: hyponatremia
         b) ABGs: hypoxia and hypercarbia
         c) Thyroid studies: low thyroxine (T_4), elevated thyrotropin (thyroid-stimulating hormone [TSH])
         d) ECG
            (1) Low voltage
            (2) Sinus bradycardia
            (3) Prolonged QT interval
         e) CBC: anemia and decreased WBC
         f) BUN and creatinine: elevated

> g) Blood sugar: variable hypoglycemia
> h) Chest x-ray film
> i) Urinalysis
> j) Obtain pretreatment plasma cortisol level

2. **Analysis: differential nursing diagnosis/collaborative problems**
   a. *Impaired breathing pattern related to slowed metabolism*
   b. *Decreased cardiac output related to decreased myocardial contractility, decreased venous return*
   c. *Thermoregulation, ineffective: hypothermia related to decreased tissue perfusion*

3. **Planning/interventions**
   a. *Monitor airway, breathing, circulation, and other vital signs*
   b. *Administer high-flow oxygen as ordered*
   c. *Prepare to assist with intubation and mechanical ventilation*
   d. *Attach pulse oximeter and cardiac monitor*
   e. *Insert large-bore IV catheter*
   f. *Administer IV fluids as ordered*
      1) Hypertonic saline
      2) Crystalloids
      3) Whole blood
   g. *Administer medications as ordered*
      1) Intravenous thyroid hormone
      2) Glucocorticoids (to prevent adrenal crisis)
      3) Vasoconstrictors
   h. *Rewarm patient*
      1) Use passive rewarming with blankets and increased room temperature
      2) Avoid rapid rewarming
      3) Be prepared for seizures
   i. *Insert urinary catheter*
   j. *Monitor intake and output*
   k. *Prepare patient/significant others for admission and other procedures as indicated*
   l. *Instruct patient/significant others about disease process*

4. **Expected outcomes/evaluation** (see Appendix B)

F. Thyroid storm

Thyroid storm is an extreme and rare form of thyrotoxicosis with a high mortality rate. It may occur in the patient with untreated or inadequately treated hyperthyroidism who experiences a stressor such as surgery, infection, trauma, or emotional upset; thyroid surgery; and radioactive iodine administration. The elderly patient may have apathetic hyperthyroidism in which the symptoms go unrecognized and is at higher risk for thyroid storm. The patient experiences cardiac decompensation with congestive heart failure (often a terminal event), central nervous system dysfunction, and GI disorders. It is a life-threatening emergency, which must be treated early and aggressively if the patient is to survive.

1. **Assessment**
   a. *Subjective data*
      1) History of present illness
         a) Fever
         b) Nausea, vomiting, diarrhea
         c) Abdominal pain

d) Worsening of thyrotoxicosis symptoms (see Medical history and Physical examination, which follow)

e) Anxiety

f) Restlessness, nervousness, irritability

g) Generalized weakness

h) Possible coma

i) Precipitating event or intercurrent illness

2) Medical history

a) Thyrotoxicosis

b) Thyroid disease

c) Easy fatigability

d) Weight loss

e) Sweating

f) Body heat loss and heat intolerance

b. *Objective data*

1) Physical examination

a) Fever: temperature may exceed 104°F (40°C)

b) Tachycardia (120–200 bpm), systolic hypertension, widened pulse pressure

c) Hyperdynamic precordium

d) Chest: crackles secondary to congestive heart failure

e) Warm, moist, velvety skin; becomes dry as dehydration develops

f) Spider angiomas

g) Tremulousness

h) Delirium, agitation, confusion, coma

i) Thin, silky hair

j) Enlarged thyroid gland with thrill or bruit

k) Eye signs

(1) Lid lag

(2) Stare

(3) Exophthalmos

(4) Periorbital edema

l) Hepatic tenderness or jaundice

2) Diagnostic procedures

a) Cardiac monitoring/ECG: sinus tachycardia and atrial fibrillation/flutter

b) Thyroid function studies

(1) T_4: elevated level

(2) Triiodothyronine (T_3): elevated resin uptake

(3) TSH: decreased level

c) Serum cholesterol level: decreased

d) Electrolyte levels

e) Serum glucose increased

f) CBC: increased WBC with left shift

g) BUN or creatinine level

h) Hepatic studies: increased liver enzymes

i) Urinalysis

j) Cultures as indicated

k) Radiographs as indicated

2. **Analysis: differential nursing diagnosis/collaborative problems**

a. *Decreased cardiac output related to hypermetabolic state and imbalance between myocardial oxygen supply and demand*

b. *Impaired gas exchange related to decreased cardiac output c. Tissue perfusion, altered related to hypermetabolic state and decreased cardiac output to meet demands*

    d. Risk for fluid volume deficit related to fluid shifts, hyperthermia, and increased respiratory rate

    e. Hyperthermia related to hypermetabolic state

    f. Knowledge deficit related to disease process

    g. Anxiety/fear related to disease process and prognosis

3. Planning/interventions

    a. Administer oxygen

    b. Maintain airway, breathing, circulation

    c. Establish large-bore IV catheter for administration of 5% dextrose and isotonic solution

    d. Initiate cardiac monitoring

    e. Prepare patient for central venous pressure or Swan-Ganz catheter insertion

    f. Administer medication as ordered

        1) Vasopressors: given if volume replacement is not adequate or cardiac dysfunction limits large volume replacement

        2) Antipyretics: acetaminophen only; avoid aspirin because it displaces thyroid hormone from binding sites

        3) Dextrose 50%

        4) Propylthiouracil every 8 hours by mouth, nasogastric tube, or rectally

        5) Glucocorticoids; hydrocortisone

        6) Iodine: Lugol's solution, potassium iodide

        7) Digitalis

        8) Propranolol: given IV to keep heart rate less than 100 bpm

        9) Antibiotics

        10) Vitamins and thiamine

        11) Sedatives

    g. Use cooling blanket and cold packs to decrease temperature

    h. Monitor vital signs and pulse oximeter

    i. Monitor signs of hydration

    j. Monitor cardiac status, including breath sounds

    k. Monitor electrolyte levels

    l. Prepare patient/significant others for patient's admission to intensive care unit

    m. If noncompliance with medication regimen is suspected, alert hospital staff to pursue after patient recovers

    n. Explain procedures to patient/significant others

    o. Allow patient to rest and prohibit strenuous activity

    p. Maintain calm, efficient atmosphere

    q. Allow significant others to be at bedside when possible

    r. Allow patient/significant others to verbalize fears

4. Expected outcomes/evaluation (see Appendix B)

VI. OTHER MEDICAL EMERGENCIES

A. Fatigue and malaise

    Fatigue and malaise are symptoms of an underlying disorder, either physical or psychological, or the result of chronic overwork without adequate personal or social time. There is a feeling of weariness and loss of a sense of well-being. Depression is the prominent psychiatric cause of fatigue and malaise, and its possible existence should not be overlooked. Some of the physical causes of malaise include infection prodrome, viruses, Lyme disease, progressive cardiopulmonary disease, neoplasm, anemia, endocrine disorders, neurological disorders, and obscure disorders such as tuberculosis and parasitic infections. Chronic fatigue syndrome is frequently diagnosed in patients with malaise and extreme fatigue without other cause. Research is ongoing to determine the causes and treatment of chronic fatigue syndrome; EBV is not a cause of this syndrome. Once life-threatening and acute disorders are ruled out, finding the underlying cause of fatigue and malaise is best done in a nonemergency care setting, where consistent follow-up and continuity of care can be maintained.

1. **Assessment**
    a. *Subjective data*
        1) History of present illness
            a) Onset
                (1) Rapid
                (2) Prolonged over days or weeks
            b) Associated symptoms, including
                (1) Fever
                (2) Vomiting and diarrhea
                (3) Headache
                (4) Polyuria and polydipsia
                (5) Pharyngitis
                (6) Weight loss or gain
                (7) Dyspnea
                (8) Fatigue
            c) Altered sleep patterns
        2) Medical history
            a) Previous similar episodes
            b) Viral illness
            c) Chronic illness or depression
            e) Medications
            f) Allergies
    b. *Objective data*
        1) Physical examination
            a) Vital signs
                (1) Temperature: elevated or depressed
                (2) Pulse: elevated or depressed
                (3) Respirations: elevated or depressed
            b) Behavior
                (1) Subdued
                (2) Depressed, with flat affect
            c) Skin
                (1) Jaundice
                (2) Signs of dehydration
            d) Lymphadenopathy
            e) General appearance
                (1) Debilitated
                (2) Signs of nutritional deficiencies
        2) Diagnostic procedures
            a) CBC
            b) Electrolyte levels
            c) Creatinine and BUN levels
            d) Serum glucose level
            e) Urinalysis
            f) Chest radiograph

      g) ECG

      h) Serum viral cultures

      i) Other studies as indicated by history and physical examination findings

2. Analysis: differential nursing diagnosis/collaborative problems

    a. Activity intolerance related to manifestations of fatigue and malaise

    b. Anxiety/fear related to unknown diagnosis, treatment, or prognosis

    c. Knowledge deficit related to therapeutic regimen

3. Planning/interventions

    a. Provide oxygen if indicated

    b. Monitor vital signs, level of consciousness, and cardiac rhythm and rate

    c. Assist with in-depth assessment of depression or high-level stress after evaluation of physiological causes of malaise

    d. Ensure calm, efficient performance of activities

    e. Explain all procedures

    f. Allow significant others or patient to express concerns or anger

    g. Allow significant others to be present with patient in treatment room

    h. Provide appropriate referral to psychiatrist, crisis intervention nurse, social worker, or community groups that deal with stress

    i. Instruct patient in causes of general malaise

    j. Instruct patient in signs and symptoms that necessitate return to emergency care setting: acute depression with suicidal thoughts

    k. Discuss appropriate follow-up arrangements

4. Expected outcomes/evaluation (see Appendix B)

BIBLIOGRAPHY

Barkin, R. M. (Ed.). (1997). *Pediatric emergency medicine.* St. Louis: Mosby-Year Book.

Bates, B. M. (1990). *A guide to physical examination.* Philadelphia: J. B. Lippincott.

Centers for Disease Control and Prevention. (1997). Control and prevention of meningococcal disease and control and prevention of serogroup C meningococcal disease: Evaluation and management of suspected outbreak. *Morbidity and Mortality Weekly Report, 46*(RR-5).

Centers for Disease Control and Prevention. (1996). Prevention of varicella. *Morbidity and Mortality Weekly Report, 45*(RR-11).

Centers for Disease Control and Prevention. (1997). Varicella-related deaths among adults-United States. *Morbidity and Mortality Weekly Report, 46*(19).

Department of Health and Social Services. (1996). *Tuberculosis control in Alaska.* Anchorage, Alaska.

Hardy, W. D. (1996). The human immunodeficiency virus. *Medical Clinics of North America, 80*(6), 1239–1261.

Henderson, D. K. (1995). Risks for exposures to and infection with HIV among health care providers in the emergency department. *Emergency Medicine Clinics of North America, 13*(1), 199–208.

Jordan, R. M. (1995). Myxedema coma: Pathophysiology, therapy, and factors affecting prognosis. *Medical Clinics of North America, 79*(1), 185–193.

Kim, M. J. (1989). *Pocket guide to nursing diagnosis.* St. Louis, MO: C. V. Mosby.

Kitabchi, A. E., & Wall, B. M. (1995). Diabetic ketoacidosis. *Medical Clinics of North America, 79*(1), 9–34.

Marco, C. A. (1995). Presentations and emergency department evaluation of HIV infection. *Emergency Clinics of North America, 13*(1), 61–71.

Mandell, G. L., Bennett, J. E., & Dolin, R. (Eds.). (1995). *Principles and practice of infectious diseases.* New York: Churchill Livingstone.

McEvoy, G. K. (Ed.). (1997). *AHFS drug information.* Bethesda, MD: American Society of Health-System Pharmacists.

Moran, G. J. (1995). Managing the HIV-related medical emergency. *Emergency Medicine, 27*(4), 18–30.

Newberry, L. N. (Ed.). (1997). *Sheehy's emergency nursing principles and practice* (4th ed.). St. Louis, MO: Mosby-Year Book and Emergency Nurses Association.

Rosen, R., & Barkin, R. M. (Eds.). (1998). *Emergency medicine concepts and clinical practice* (4th ed.). St. Louis, MO: C. V. Mosby.

Schleicher, S. M., & Stewart, P. (1997). Scabies: The mite that roars. *Emergency Medicine, 29*(6), 54–58.

Service, F. J. (1995). Hypoglycemia. *Medical Clinics of North America, 79*(1), 1–4.

Tietgens, S. T., & Leinung, M. C. (1995). Thyroid storm. *Medical Clinics of North America, 79*(1), 169–181.

Tintinalli, J. E., Krome, R. L., & Ruiz, E. (Eds.). (1996). *Emergency medicine, a comprehensive study guide* (4th ed.). New York: McGraw-Hill.

Wyngaarden, J. B., Smith, L. H., & Bennett, J. C. (Eds.). (1992). *Cecil textbook of medicine* (19th ed.) Philadelphia: W. B. Saunders.

Lorene Newberry, RN, MS, CEN

CHAPTER **8**

General Medical Emergencies: Part II

MAJOR TOPICS

General Strategy

Specific Medical Emergencies

  Reye's Syndrome

  Gout

  Fever

Allergic Reaction

Fluid and Electrolyte Emergencies

Coma

Hematological Emergencies

I. GENERAL STRATEGY

A. Assessment

1. **Primary survey/resuscitation** (see Chapter 1)
2. **Secondary survey** (see Chapter 1)
3. **Psychological, social, environmental factors**
    a. *Age: illness more severe in very young and very old*
    b. *Family history*
    c. *Gender: some disorders are gender linked*
    d. *Race: may determine increased incidence*
    e. *Lifestyle*
        1) Sedentary lifestyle
        2) Nutritional status: obesity and dietary excess or deficit
    f. *Inadequately treated disease process*
    g. *Exposure to illness*
    h. *Splenectomy: alters immune response*
    i. *Infection: viral, bacterial, fungal, rickettsial, or parasitic*
    j. *Stressors: surgery, trauma, illness, psychosocial factors*
    k. *Vitamin deficiency*
    l. *Malabsorption syndromes*
    m. *Climate or environment*
    n. *Immobilization*
    o. *Medications: interactions and adverse reactions*

4. Focused survey
  a. *Subjective data*
    1) History of present illness
      a) Pain: PQRST
        (1) *Provocation*
        (2) *Quality*
        (3) *Region/radiation*
        (4) *Severity*
        (5) *Time*
      b) Injury: mechanism and time
      c) Fatigue, malaise
      d) Nausea, vomiting
      e) Altered mental status or decreased level of consciousness
      f) Fever
      g) Dyspnea
      h) Urticaria
      i) Edema: location and type
      j) Weakness
      k) Rash
      l) Cough
      m) Sore throat
      n) Other symptoms: anorexia, pruritus, diarrhea
      o) Current medications
        (1) Anticoagulants
        (2) Insulin or oral hypoglycemics
        (3) Decongestants
        (4) Acetaminophen or aspirin
        (5) Phenothiazines
      p) Allergies: medications, environmental factors, food
    2) Medical history
      a) Vascular disease
      b) Diabetes
      c) Alcoholism
      d) Recent illness or major trauma
      e) Previous similar episodes
      f) Sickle cell anemia
      g) Hemophilia
      h) Immunizations
  b. *Objective data*
    1) Physical examination
      a) General survey
        (1) Level of consciousness/mental status
        (2) Skin: color, temperature, moisture, turgor, rash
        (3) Vital signs, including orthostatic blood pressure and pulse
        (4) Odors: breath and body
        (5) Gait
        (6) General appearance: grooming and general health
        (7) Weight
      b) Inspection
        (1) Neck veins
        (2) Rash or urticaria
        (3) Mucous membranes
        (4) Evidence of trauma

3. Fatigue
4. Fluid volume deficit/excess
5. Impaired gas exchange
6. Impaired skin integrity
7. Ineffective airway clearance
8. Knowledge deficit
9. Pain
10. Risk for infection
11. Risk for injury
12. Tissue perfusion, altered

C. Planning/interventions

1. **Determine priorities**
   a. *Control and maintain airway, breathing, circulation*
   b. *Prevent complications*
   c. *Control pain*
   d. *Prevent spread of infection or disease*
   e. *Maintain fluid and electrolyte balance*
   f. *Maintain acid-base status*
   g. *Stabilize thermoregulatory system*
   h. *Reverse disease process*
   i. *Relieve anxiety*
   j. *Protect patient*
   k. *Educate patient/significant others*
2. **Develop nursing care plan specific to patient's presenting emergency**
3. **Set up necessary equipment and supplies**
4. **Institute appropriate interventions based on the nursing care plan**
5. **Record data as appropriate**

D. Expected outcomes/evaluation

1. **Monitor patient's responses and outcomes, adjusting nursing care plans as indicated**
   a. *Specific interventions*
   b. *Disposition/discharge planning*
2. **Record data as appropriate**
3. **If positive outcomes not demonstrated, re-evaluate patient and/or plan of care**

E. Age-related considerations (see Chapter 7)

II. SPECIFIC MEDICAL EMERGENCIES

A. Reye's syndrome

Reye's syndrome is an acute noninflammatory encephalopathy characterized by hepatic, metabolic, and neurological dysfunction. The condition is seen in children after viral illnesses such as influenza B and varicella. Peak age is 11 years after influenza B and 6 years after varicella. Salicylate ingestion may be a predisposing factor. The greatest incidence occurs in later winter and early spring; more cases are reported in white patients living in rural or suburban areas. The primary defect is mitochondrial injury. Glycogen stores are depleted as a result of starvation from prolonged vomiting and dysfunction of gluconeogenesis enzymes pathways. An alternative energy source is not available because fatty acid breakdown does not occur normally. Consequently, acids build up because the body cannot eliminate waste products effectively. The liver enzyme system that converts ammonia to urea is damaged so ammonia also builds up. Additionally, the liver and renal tubules become edematous and infiltrated with fat droplets. Fatty infiltrates develop in the heart with petechiae throughout the epicardium. Hyperammonemia, hypoglycemia, and acidosis contribute to neurological dysfunction, cerebral edema, and coma.

1. **Assessment**
    a. *Subjective data*
       1) History of present illness
          a) Onset
             (1) Antecedent viral illness
             (2) Recovery from viral illness followed by prolonged vomiting
             (3) Subtle change in mental status/behavior
       2) Medical history
          a) Salicylate, phenothiazine, decongestant use
          b) Exposure to pesticides and insecticides
          c) Medications
          d) Allergies
    b. *Objective data*
       1) Physical examination
          a) Neurological status
             (1) Lethargy, restlessness, delirium, combativeness, slurred speech
             (2) Pupils are dilated and react sluggishly
             (3) Engorged retinal veins with loss of venous pulsation
             (4) Hypertonic to hypotonic muscle tone with abnormal flexion or extension
             (5) Seizures
          b) Gastrointestinal (GI) status
             (1) Persistent vomiting
             (2) Hepatomegaly
             (3) GI bleeding: late finding
             (4) Jaundice not usually present
          c) Staging
             (1) Stage 0: Awake and alert
             (2) Stage I: vomiting and lethargy or sleepiness, ability to obey commands, hepatic dysfunction, and EEG changes
             (3) Stage II: delirium, combativeness, hyperreflexia, appropriate response to noxious stimuli, hepatic dysfunction, and continued EEG abnormalities
             (4) Stage III: hyperventilation, coma, decorticate posturing, normal pupillary and oculovestibular responses, continued hepatic and EEG changes
             (5) Stage IV: deeper coma, decerebrate rigidity, dilated pupils, loss of oculocephalic reflex, abnormal oculovestibular reflex, minimal liver dysfunction, abnormal EEG
             (6) Stage V: seizure; flaccidity; areflexia; dilated, nonreactive pupils; apnea; isoelectric EEG
       2) Diagnostic procedures
          a) Hyperammonemia determination

          (1) Less than 48 mg/dL (normal)

          (2) Greater than 300 mg/dL (poor prognosis)

          (3) Use heparinized blood tub on ice to laboratory

     b) Enzyme levels

          (1) Serum glutamic oxaloacetic transaminase (SGOT) and serum glutamate pyruvate transaminase (SGPT) elevated 2 to 3 times normal

          (2) Skeletal and cardiac isoenzymes elevated

     c) Hypoprothrombinemia: prolonged PT and PTT

     d) Hypoglycemia (i.e., more common in children younger than 5 years because of greater metabolism and lower glycogen stores)

     e) Elevated amino and free fatty acid levels

     f) ABGs

          (1) Metabolic acidosis

          (2) Respiratory alkalosis

     g) Cerebrospinal fluid (CSF): normal, except pressure elevation in late stages

     h) Creatinine and BUN levels: mild to moderate elevation, reflecting dehydration and acidosis

2. **Analysis: differential nursing diagnosis/collaborative problems**

     a. Impaired gas exchange related to pulmonary injury/metabolic changes

     b. Risk for fluid volume deficit related to vomiting

     c. Impaired tissue perfusion, cerebral related to dehydration and cerebral edema

     d. Ineffective family coping: compromised related to sudden unanticipated onset of disease process

3. **Planning/interventions**

     a. Monitor respiratory and circulatory status

     b. Administer oxygen

     c. Endotracheal intubation as indicated

     d. Elevate head of bed 10 to 30 degrees to control cerebral edema

     e. Suction as necessary

     f. Place intravenous (IV) catheter for administration of fluid as needed

     g. Maintain fluid volume (e.g., fluid challenge may be necessary): avoid fluid overload in presence of cerebral edema

     h. May give dextrose to counteract hypoglycemia

     i. Monitor intake and output (insert Foley catheter)

     j. Administer prescribed medication therapy

          1) Osmotic diuresis (mannitol IV with filter)

          2) Steroids

     k. Ensure body temperature is normothermic or slightly hypothermic

          1) Antipyretics (i.e., acetaminophen), as prescribed; do not administer salicylates)

     l. Prepare family for possible insertion of intracranial screw for monitoring

     m. Protect patient from injury (e.g., protective devices may be necessary if patient is combative)

     n. Explain all procedures

     o. Clarify behavior of patient

     p. Encourage family to touch and talk to patient

     q. Refer to National Reye's Syndrome Foundation, if diagnosis is confirmed

4. **Expected outcomes/evaluation** (see Appendix B)

B. Gout

Gout is characterized by increased serum urate concentration, recurrent attacks of acute arthritis with crystals of monosodium urate in synovial fluid; deposits of monosodium urate (called tophi) in and around joints; nephropathy involving interstitial tissue and blood vessels; and uric acid nephrolithiasis. The condition is caused by inadequate excretion or overproduction of uric acid. Three stages of gout occur: asymptomatic hyperuricemia, acute gout, and tophaceous gout. Nephrolithiasis may occur at any time. The first bout of gouty arthritis usually occurs at the first metatarsophalangeal joint.

1. **Assessment**
   a. *Subjective data*
      1) History of present illness
         a) Location of pain
            (1) First episode monoarticular, usually first metatarsophalangeal joint (podagra)
            (2) Recurrent episodes polyarticular, usually lower extremities
            (3) Affects insteps, ankles, heels, knees, wrists, fingers, elbows
            (4) Other joints rarely involved except in established disease
         b) Timing/onset of pain: often at night
         c) Characteristics of pain
            (1) Intolerable pain
            (2) Any clothing, movement, or weight bearing is intolerable
         d) Fever
            (1) Low-grade first episode
            (2) Significant with recurrent episodes (101°F [38.3°C] or greater)
      2) Medical history
         a) Thiazide diuretics
         b) Hypertension
         c) Hypertriglyceridemia
         d) Other medications
         e) Allergies
      3) Objective data
         a) Physical examination
            (1) Erythematous, hyperthermic, edematous joint
            (2) Fever
            (3) Reluctant to use extremity
         b) Diagnostic procedures
            (1) Arthrocentesis: monosodium urate crystals in white blood cells (WBCs) of synovial fluid of inflamed joint (affected joint tapped to remove fluid)
            (2) Hyperuricemia: serum uric acid level greater than 7 mg/dL in males and greater than 6 mg/dL in females
2. **Analysis: differential nursing diagnosis/collaborative problems**
   a. *Pain related to gout inflammation*
   b. *Anxiety/fear related to disease process and pain*
   c. *Knowledge deficit related to therapeutic response and health maintenance*
3. **Planning/interventions**
   a. *Administer anti-inflammatory agents, as prescribed*
      1) Colchicine
         a) IV: dilute well, administer slowly, avoid extravasation
         b) Orally: give with food; stop if nausea, vomiting, or diarrhea occurs

2) Indomethacin: give orally with meals (therapeutic level after 3 to 5 days of therapy)
   b. *Provide prophylaxis and education*
      1) Explain disease process
      2) Discuss weight reduction in obese patients
      3) Avoid precipitating factors: consumption of substantial amounts of alcohol, high-purine diet, use of thiazide diuretics
      4) Take colchicine or indomethacin as directed
      5) Maintain adequate hydration to prevent stone formation/nephropathy
      6) Take antihyperuricemic agents, as prescribed
         a) Underexcretion
            (1) Probenecid
            (2) Sulfinpyrazone
            (3) Avoid acetylsalicylic acid, which interferes with uric acid excretion
         b) Overproduction of uric acid: allopurinol
      7) Place extremity in most comfortable position possible
      8) Explain all procedures
      9) Reassure patient that disease can be controlled
      10) Have supportive significant other present
      11) Allow time for patient to verbalize feelings
      12) Maintain calm, efficient manner
      13) Describe signs and symptoms that indicate need to return to emergency care setting (e.g., repeated attacks with uncontrollable pain, medication side effects)
      14) Arrange appropriate follow-up appointment with health care provider
   4. Expected outcomes/evaluation (see Appendix B)

C. Fever

Fever may accompany bacterial, viral, rickettsial, and parasitic infections, as well as neoplasms, diseases of the immune system, vascular inflammation, acute metabolic disorders, tissue infarction, and trauma. Infection is possible when fever is associated with abrupt onset of respiratory symptoms; nausea, vomiting, and diarrhea; severe malaise; myalgias; arthralgias; acute enlargement of lymph nodes and spleen; meningeal signs; leukocyte count greater than 12,000/mm³ or less than 5,000/mm³; and dysuria or flank pain.

Tissue inflammation in response to bacteria causes release of histamine, bradykinin, and serotonin, which increase local blood flow and permeability of capillaries. Large quantities of leaked fluid, protein, and fibrinogen form a clot around injured tissue and isolate the area. Some bacteria are walled off quickly because of extreme tissue toxicity. Others migrate throughout the body before isolation can occur. Neutrophilia (leukocytosis) occurs within a few hours as a result of release of leukocytosis-inducing factor from inflamed tissue, which stimulates increased bone marrow production of neutrophils.

Fever is present in a child when the rectal temperature is greater than 100°F (37.2°C) and axillary temperature is 99°F (37.2°C) or greater. Febrile seizures generally occur between 5 months and 5 years; peak incidence is between 8 and 20 months. Fever increases the irritability of neurons, making the young more sensitive to seizure because of their immature nervous systems. Seizures occur because of the rapidity with which the temperature rises rather than the actual temperature level.

1. Assessment
   a. *Subjective data*
      1) History of present illness

      a) Onset
        (1) Rapid
        (2) Slow
      b) Prodrome
      c) Previous similar episode
      d) Pain
        (1) Ear and throat
        (2) Chest or pleuritic
        (3) Abdomen
        (4) Headache
        (5) Dysuria
        (6) Myalgias and arthralgias
      e) Fever: degree and persistence
      f) Seizure
      g) Nausea or vomiting and diarrhea
      h) Rash
      i) Illness of other family members or friends
      j) If child, level of activity and fluid intake
      k) Recent travel to another country
      l) Recent immunizations
      m) Recent surgical or other invasive procedure
      n) Ingestion of untreated water
  2) Medical history
      a) Chronic illnesses
      b) Medications
      c) Allergies
 b. *Objective data*
  1) Physical examination
      a) Tachycardia and tachypnea
      b) Chest
        (1) Crackles
        (2) Decreased and/or abnormal breath sounds
        (3) Wheezing
      c) Abdomen: tenderness or guarding
      d) Nuchal rigidity
      e) Flank tenderness (i.e., costovertebral angle tenderness)
      f) Local cellulitis with erythema, edema, tenderness, and hyperthermia; lymphangitis
      g) Rash
      h) Postictal state
      i) Inflammation of ears and pharynx
      j) Pelvic examination: tender cervix and adnexa; vaginal discharge
  2) Diagnostic procedures
      a) CBC
      b) Urinalysis
      c) Chest and abdominal radiographs
      d) Cultures: blood, urine, wound, cervical, sputum, nasopharyngeal, joint fluid
      e) Lumbar puncture
        (1) Always done if first seizure before 12 months of age or temperature 106°F (41°C) or higher
        (2) Indicated for adults with nuchal rigidity, headache, and fever of unknown origin

(3) Child who remains irritable and lethargic after aggressive antipyretic therapy

f) Serum glucose level

2. Analysis: differential nursing diagnosis/collaborative problems

a. *Risk for infection related to exposure to bacteria, viruses, parasites*

b. *Risk for fluid volume deficit related to hyperthermia or vomiting*

c. *Risk for injury related to seizure*

d. *Knowledge deficit related to therapeutic regimen and health maintenance*

3. Planning/interventions

a. *Maintain airway, breathing, circulation; monitor vital signs*

b. *Observe for airway obstruction and respiratory distress*

c. *Control temperature greater than 101°F (38.3°C) with antipyretics (e.g., use acetaminophen or ibuprofen); no aspirin for children younger than 16 years (because of association with Reye's syndrome)*

d. *Administer medications as prescribed*

1) Antibiotics

2) Dextrose IV if seizure activity

e. *Administer prescribed anticonvulsants IV for status seizure: diazepam, lorazepam, phenobarbital, phenytoin, fosphenytoin*

f. *Elevate extremity and use heat for cellulitis*

g. *Replace fluids IV or orally*

h. *Limit activity during acute phase*

i. *Hospitalize infants and elderly if no definitive source of fever or infection is identified*

j. *Monitor for*

1) Signs of dehydration

2) Intake and output

3) Seizure activity

k. *Protect patient from physical injury (e.g., put side rails up)*

l. *Instruct patient or significant other about*

1) Fever control measures

2) Drug therapy (e.g, antipyretics, antibiotics, anticonvulsants)

3) Need for adequate fluid replacement to prevent dehydration

4) Signs and symptoms that necessitate return to emergency care setting

a) Inability to control fever

b) Recurrence of seizures

c) Change in mental status

d) Illness does not improve or increases in severity

m. *Reassure parents/significant other of patient with seizure*

n. *Allow parents/significant other to vent feelings of fear and frustration*

4. Expected outcomes/evaluation (see Appendix B)

D. Allergic reaction

Allergic reactions may be immediate and life threatening or occur over hours or days. Four specific types of allergic reactions occur: anaphylactic, cytotoxic, immune complex–mediated, and delayed hypersensitivity. Anaphylactic reactions are the most common allergic reaction seen in the emergency department. These reactions occur in individuals who are sensitive to specific allergens (e.g., insect, food medication, animal fur). The capacity for individuals to experience hypersensitivity to various allergens appears to be an inherited trait. An estimated 20% of the population has an inherited tendency for sensitivity to environmental allergens; one quarter of the population is allergic to Hymenoptera (wasps, hornets, yellow jackets, and fire ants).

1. **Assessment**
    a. *Subjective data*
        1) History of present condition
            a) Description of precipitating event if known (i.e., sting, ingestion, or contact with allergen)
            b) Location of allergen contact
            c) Elapsed time since contact
            d) Patient/family allergy history
            e) Prehospital care
        2) Medical history
            a) Immunization status
            b) Allergies
            c) Medications
    b. *Objective data*
        1) Physical examination
            a) Appearance of contact site
                (1) Redness
                (2) Warmth
                (3) Wheal formation
            b) Complaints of discomfort
                (1) Pinprick sensation
                (2) Continued irritation
                (3) Pruritus
            c) Signs and symptoms of anaphylaxis
                (1) Pruritus, urticaria, angioedema
                (2) Weakness, dizziness, restlessness, disorientation, altered level of consciousness
                (3) Nausea, vomiting, abdominal cramps, diarrhea, incontinence
                (4) Respiratory difficulties
                (5) Wheezing, stridor
                (6) Hypotension, cardiac dysrhythmias, cyanosis
                (7) Collapse, seizures, unconsciousness
        2) Diagnostic procedures: as indicated by clinical symptoms
2. **Analysis: differential nursing diagnosis/collaborative problems**
    a. *Ineffective airway clearance related to airway edema*
    b. *Pain related to response to allergen*
    c. *Anxiety/fear related to pain, circumstances of contact, possible outcomes*
    d. *Knowledge deficit related to prevention of allergic reactions and therapeutic regimen*
3. **Planning/interventions**
    a. *If allergic reaction or evidence of poisoning*
        1) Maintain airway, breathing, circulation; use advanced life support measures if needed
        2) Administer epinephrine
        3) Administer high-flow oxygen
        4) Monitor vital signs
        5) Insert IV catheter and administer normal saline solution
        6) Administer antihistamine if indicated: diphenhydramine hydrochloride (Benadryl) PO or IV
        7) Administer histamine-2 blockers
        8) Administer corticosteroids

     9) Administer beta agonists for bronchospasm

    10. Keep patient warm

    11) Observe patient for several hours

  b. Distinguish between symptoms of fear and those indicating allergic reaction

  c. Minimize physical and emotional stress on patient

  d. Permit calm significant others to remain with patient in treatment area

  e. Treat site of contact

    1) Keep affected part at rest

    2) Remove stinger, if present, but avoid pinching because this releases more venom

    3) Apply cool packs

    4) Apply paste of papain using meat tenderizer to inactivate venom

    5) Wash site with mild antiseptic soap and water

  f. Administer appropriate immunizations

  g. Maintain calm, efficient manner

  h. Provide verbal/written instructions to patient and significant others, including directions to

    1) Apply cold, as needed

    2) Observe for signs of infection

    3) Avoid

      a) Use of perfumes, sprays, brightly colored clothing, and sweet, sticky substances because these attract insects

      b) Extensive skin exposure, especially around the neck

      c) Lying down or sitting in areas with many flowers, trees, and bushes

      d) Going barefoot

  i. Obtain and familiarize self with emergency insect bite kit

  j. Return or make appointment for follow-up care, if indicated

  4. Expected outcomes/evaluation (see Appendix B)

E. Fluid and electrolyte emergencies

1. Dehydration

    Dehydration refers to a disorder of water loss with or without loss of sodium. Three types of dehydration occur: isotonic, hypotonic, and hypertonic. The type of dehydration is based on serum sodium concentration. Isotonic dehydration is the most common type of dehydration, resulting in a loss of plasma volume.

    The serum sodium in isotonic dehydration is normal. Hypotonic dehydration is characterized by a serum sodium level of less than 130 mEq/L. This dehydration is most commonly caused by abnormal GI losses. Hypernatremic dehydration is characterized by a serum sodium level greater than 150 mEq/L. The most common cause is inadequate fluid intake with loss of hypotonic fluid (e.g., diarrhea).

    Loss of fluid, with or without electrolyte depletion, occurs from the GI tract (vomiting, diarrhea, nasogastric suction, and fistula); the renal system (diuretics, osmotic diuresis, adrenal insufficiency, nephropathies, and diabetes insipidus); the skin (insensible water loss, perspiration, burns, and lesions); and third-space sequestration (intestinal obstruction, peritonitis, crush injury or skeletal fractures, pancreatitis, bleeding, and major venous obstruction). Signs and symptoms depend on rapidity of loss, electrolyte levels, development of acid-base imbalance, patient age and gender, and ability to replace loss. Decreased intake for several days without concomitant loss rarely causes dehydration. Infants and small children have a large intrinsic fluid volume and become dehydrated rapidly, often within 6 to 12 hours.

a. Assessment
   1) Subjective data
      a) History of present illness
         (1) Nausea, vomiting, diarrhea
         (2) Decreased intake
         (3) Bleeding from any source
         (4) Weight loss
         (5) Polyuria, polydipsia, excessive thirst
         (6) Lassitude, fatigability, muscle cramps
         (7) Postural dizziness and syncope
         (8) Seizures, coma, confusion
         (9) Unusual salt craving
         (10) Trauma
         (11) Abdominal or chest pain (i.e., attributable to pancreatitis and decreased organ perfusion)
         (12) Alcohol ingestion
         (13) Fever
      b) Medical history
         (1) Medications
         (2) Allergies
         (3) Diabetes or other chronic illness
         (4) Previous similar episodes
   2) Objective data
      a) Physical examination
         (1) Poor skin turgor (sternum or inner thigh in the elderly)
         (2) Dry skin and mucous membranes
         (3) Orthostatic vital sign changes
         (4) Tachycardia and hypotension
         (5) Diminished peripheral pulses
         (6) Weight loss
         (7) Flattened external jugular veins
         (8) Shock
         (9) Sunken fontanelle and sunken eyes
         (10) Confusion, lethargy, coma
         (11) Fever may be present
         (12) Increased respiratory rate and depth
         (13) Decreased urine output
         (14) Skeletal muscle weakness
      b) Diagnostic procedures
         (1) Serum osmolality
         (2) Hematocrit and BUN: elevated
         (3) Serum sodium level: high, normal, or low
         (4) Creatinine level: normal
         (5) ABG analysis: metabolic alkalosis or metabolic acidosis
         (6) Urinalysis
            (a) Osmolality: increased or decreased
            (b) Sodium level: increased or decreased
         (7) Culture blood, urine, or CSF as appropriate
         (8) Radiographic studies as determined by history to rule out infection and trauma
b. Analysis: differential diagnosis/collaborative problems
   1) Fluid volume deficit related to inability to match intake and/or output
   2) Decreased cardiac output related to diminished circulatory blood volume

        3) Knowledge deficit related to therapeutic regimen
- c. *Planning/interventions*
    1) Initiate IV catheter for administration of isotonic solution until laboratory values available
        a) Wide open (1–2 L) in adults without cardiovascular disease
        b) Fluid challenge in older adults; monitor closely for fluid overload (crackles and respiratory distress)
        c) Administer 20 mL/kg bolus in children in shock (may repeat once)
        d) Replace appropriate electrolytes as indicted
    2) Administer oxygen; maintain airway, breathing, circulation
    3) Control causes of dehydration
        a) Administer antiemetics, as prescribed
        b) Administer antidiarrheal agents, as prescribed
        c) Withhold oral fluids for 2 to 6 hours if severe vomiting
    4) Give clear liquids for 24 hours: advance diet as tolerated
    5) Monitor
        a) Heart rate, peripheral pulses, capillary refill
        b) Orthostatic vital signs
        c) Skin turgor and dryness of skin
        d) ABGs
    6) Ensure strict intake and output documentation
    7) Administer prescribed sodium bicarbonate IV if metabolic acidosis (pH <7.1) present
    8) Instruct patient/significant others about dehydration and rehydration
    9) Instruct patient/significant others in use of prescribed medications
    10) Instruct patient/significant others regarding signs and symptoms that indicated need to return to emergency care setting
        a) Continued vomiting
        b) Continued diarrhea
        c) Elevated temperature
        d) Dry mucous membranes and skin
        e) Decreased urine output
        f) Sunken fontanelle and sunken eyes
        g) Crying without tears (i.e., after 2–3 months old)
        h) Lethargy
        i) Postural dizziness
    11) Arrange appropriate follow-up care
- d. *Expected outcomes/evaluation* (see Appendix B)

2. Electrolyte abnormalities

    An electrolyte is an ion with a positive or negative charge that is found in intracellular and extracellular fluid. A cation is an electrolyte with a positive charge; an anion has a negative charge. Electrolytes are critical for normal cellular metabolism and function. Sodium is the major extracellular cation and is responsible for maintaining plasma osmolarity, propagation and transmission of action potentials, maintaining acid-base balance, and maintaining electroneutrality. Potassium is the major intracellular cation responsible for maintaining electrical membrane excitability, maintaining plasma acid-base balance, and regulating intracellular osmolarity. Calcium has several major roles: it is an essential component in contractile processes (i.e., cardiac skeletal and smooth muscle), provides strength and density of teeth and bones, stabilizes excitable membranes, and is a cofactor in the blood-clotting cascade.

    Direct measurement of intracellular electrolytes is not possible in the clinical setting, so these values are determined indirectly. Electrolyte abnormalities may be due to dietary excesses or deficits, prescribed medications, excess water ingestion or lack of water ingestion, vomiting, and diarrhea.

a. *Sodium abnormalities*

Sodium is responsible for normal water balance and impulse conduction. Sodium is the primary extracellular cation. Active transport via adenosine triphosphate is necessary to keep sodium in the extracellular space. Sodium is regulated by the renin-angiotensin-aldosterone system, sympathetic nervous system (SNS), and a less well-defined system mediated by atrial natriuretic factor (ANF). Baroreceptor stimulation of the SNS leads to vasoconstriction, decreased glomerular filtration rate, and retention of sodium and water. Release of ANF by the atria leads to excessive sodium excretion and diuresis.

1) Hyponatremia

Hyponatremia may be due to either actual sodium deficits or dilutional causes. Sodium deficits resulting from dilutional effects can be caused by excess water intake, freshwater drowning, inappropriate antidiuretic hormone secretion, and psychogenic polydipsia or true sodium loss from diuretics, salt-wasting nephropathies, GI losses, adrenal insufficiency, hyperglycemia, congestive heart failure, or burns. Causes of actual sodium deficits resulting from increased sodium excretion can include diaphoresis, diuretic use, wound drainage, decreased secretion of aldosterone, hyperlipidemia, and renal disease. Causes of actual sodium deficits resulting from inadequate sodium intake can include nothing by mouth (NPO) restrictions and a low-sodium diet. Symptoms related to hyponatremia usually do not occur unless sodium level is less than 120 mEq/dL.

a) Assessment

(1) Subjective data

(a) History of present illness
- Anorexia, nausea, vomiting, diarrhea
- Altered oral intake: immobility or inability to obtain oral fluids
- Altered dietary intake of sodium
- Excessive water consumption
- Trauma, burns, or neurological injury or surgery
- Lethargy and apathy
- Thirst, nausea
- Confusion, personality changes
- Seizures and coma
- Weight change
- Fatigue and muscle cramps
- Dizziness
- Headache
- Poor peripheral pulses
- Skeletal muscle weakness

(b) Medical history
- Diuretics
- Previous similar episodes
- Medications
- Allergies

(2) Objective data

(a) Physical examination
- Altered mental status
- Poor skin turgor
- Sunken fontanelle and eyes
- Dry mucous membranes and skin
- Orthostatic vital sign changes
- Hypotension and tachycardia
- Seizures: sodium level less than 110 mEq/L
- Neck veins: flat

- Fever may be present
- Diminished deep tendon reflexes
- Shallow respirations
- Moist crackles
- Increased urine output

(b) Diagnostic procedures
- CBC
- Electrolyte levels
- Sodium: less than 135 mEq/dL
- Chloride: usually decreased
- Bicarbonate: elevated or decreased to replace chloride
- Potassium: normal range, 3.5 to 5.0 mEq/dL; may be normal, decreased, or elevated
- Magnesium: normal range, 1.5 to 2.0 mEq/dL; may be normal, decreased, or elevated
- BUN: elevated if dehydration present
- Creatinine level: normal
- Serum osmolality: normal, increased, or decreased
- Infants: normal value, 275 to 285 mOsm/kg
- Adults: normal value, 285 to 295 mOsm/kg
- Urinalysis
- Blood glucose level
- Definitive neurological studies (CT scan, EEG, and lumbar puncture) as indicated

b) Analysis: differential nursing diagnosis/collaborative problems

(1) Fluid volume excess related to increased intake or inappropriate antidiuretic hormone secretion

(2) Fluid volume deficit related to diuretic use or inadequate replacement of body fluid loss

(3) Cerebral tissue perfusion, altered related to electrolyte imbalance and decreased circulatory blood volume

(4) Risk for injury related to restlessness, seizures, or confusion

(5) Knowledge deficit related to therapeutic regimen and health maintenance

c) Planning/interventions

(1) Initiate IV catheter for administration of isotonic or hypertonic solution until electrolytes results are available

(2) Determine blood glucose level to rule out hypoglycemia

(3) Monitor
  (a) Maintain airway, breathing, circulation
  (b) Intake and output
  (c) Vital signs
  (d) Signs of dehydration or overhydration
  (e) Mental status and neurological status
  (f) Seizure activity

(4) Insert urinary catheter if patient incontinent

(5) May need to restrain combative patient

(6) If seizure occurs
  (a) Protect patient from injury
  (b) Prepare to suction as needed
  (c) Maintain airway by positioning on side as soon as seizure stops

(7) Replace sodium orally or IV as ordered

(8) Instruct patient/significant others regarding disease process

(9) Reinforce instructions regarding use of medications such as diuretics and side effects

(10) Instruct regarding prevention of hyponatremia by reviewing dietary sodium intake

(11) Instruct regarding replacement of fluids and electrolytes after exercise or illness

d) Expected outcomes/evaluation (see Appendix B)

(1) Serum sodium level 135 to 145 mEq/L

2) Hypernatremia

Hypernatremia is less common than hyponatremia and can be due to actual sodium excess or, indirectly, decreased water intake or increased water loss. Indirect causes of decreased water intake are often caused by NPO status. Increased water loss in excess of sodium can occur as a result of sweating, hyperventilation, infection, diaphoresis, diarrhea, diabetes insipidus, and fever. A true increase in sodium volume can be related to administration of sodium bicarbonate and normal saline, near drowning in salt water, renal failure, use of corticosteroids, increased sodium ingestion, and hyperaldosteronism (Cushing's syndrome).

Symptoms of hypernatremia are due to hyperosmolarity. As sodium level rises, cellular dehydration occurs. Brain cells shrink, resulting in central nervous system symptoms. As the brain shrinks, intracranial hemorrhage may occur from mechanical stress that tears vessels. The similarity of signs and symptoms among sodium disorders makes it impossible to differentiate condition without laboratory data.

a) Assessment

(1) Subjective data

(a) History of present illness
- Anorexia, nausea, vomiting, diarrhea
- Altered oral intake
- Altered dietary intake of sodium
- Lethargy and apathy
- Thirst
- Confusion, seizures, coma (agitation may be present if hypovolemia also present)
- Weight change
- Fatigue and muscle cramps
- Dizziness
- Headache
- Thirst
- Immobility or inability to obtain oral fluids

(b) Medical history
- Diuretics
- Diabetes insipidus
- Previous similar episodes
- Medications
- Allergies

(2) Objective data

(a) Physical examination
- Altered mental status
- Poor skin turgor
- Hyperreflexia, spontaneous muscle twitches
- Dry mucous membranes and skin
- Orthostatic vital sign changes
- Hypotension and tachycardia
- Seizures
- Neck veins: flat or full
- Muscle weakness, diminished deep tendon reflexes with severe hypernatremia
- Tremor
- Decreased urine output

(b) Diagnostic procedures
- CBC
- Electrolyte levels
- Sodium: greater than 158 mEq/L
- Chloride: decreased or increased with sodium
- Bicarbonate: elevated or decreased to replace chloride
- Potassium: normal range, 3.5 to 5.0 mEq/dL; may be normal, decreased, or elevated
- Magnesium: normal range, 1.5 to 2.0 mEq/dL; may be normal, decreased, or elevated
- BUN: elevated if dehydration present
- Creatinine level: normal
- Serum osmolality: increased
- Infants: normal value, 275 to 285 mOsm/kg
- Adults: normal value, 285 to 295 mOsm/kg
- Symptoms develop at 320 mOsm/kg
- Coma occurs at 360 mOsm/kg
- Urinalysis
- Blood glucose level
- Definitive neurological studies (CT scan, EEG, and lumbar puncture) as indicated

b) Analysis: differential nursing diagnosis/collaborative problems
  (1) Fluid volume excess or deficit related to elevated sodium levels
  (2) Impaired tissue perfusion, cerebral related to cellular dehydration
  (3) Risk for injury related to restlessness, seizure, or confusion
  (4) Knowledge deficit related to therapeutic regimen and health maintenance

c) Planning/interventions
  (1) Initiate IV catheter for administration of isotonic solution until electrolyte results are available
  (2) Determine blood glucose level to rule out hypoglycemia
  (3) Monitor
      (a) Maintain airway, breathing, circulation
      (b) Intake and output
      (c) Vital signs
      (d) Signs of dehydration or overhydration
      (e) Mental status and neurological status
  (4) Insert urinary catheter if patient incontinent
  (5) Monitor for seizure activity
      (a) Protect patient from injury
      (b) Prepare to suction as needed
      (c) Maintain airway by positioning on side as soon as seizure stops
  (6) May need to restrain combative patient
  (7) Limit sodium intake as ordered (i.e., one teaspoon of salt equals 2 g of sodium)
  (8) Instruct patient/significant others about
      (a) Disease process
      (b) Medications such as diuretics and their side effects
      (c) Prevention of hypernatremia by reviewing dietary sodium intake
      (d) Replacement of fluids and electrolytes after exercise or illness

d) Expected outcomes/evaluation (see Appendix B)
  (1) Serum sodium level between 135 and 145 mEq/L

b. *Potassium abnormalities*

Potassium is the primary intracellular cation. Potassium regulates cell membrane potential, cellular osmolality, and volume. Renal tubules are the primary control for potassium excretion. However, potassium can also be found in sweat, gastric juices, pancreatic juice, and bile. Acute acidosis moves potassium from the cell in exchange for hydrogen ions, whereas alkalosis drives potassium into the cells in exchange for hydrogen ions. Potassium abnormalities may be the result of vomiting and diarrhea, may be associated with diabetic ketoacidosis, or may be caused by massive crush injuries, which frees intracellular potassium.

1) Hypokalemia

Hypokalemia refers to serum potassium below 3.5 mEq/L. Potassium decreases can be due to inadequate potassium intake (e.g., NPO status) and excessive losses of potassium; gastrointestinal losses (vomiting, diarrhea, suction); excessive renal losses (diuretics, increased mineralocorticoid levels); wound drainage; diaphoresis; and use of various drugs (e.g., digitalis, diuretics, corticosteroids). Potassium decreases can also be related to intracellular shifts in which potassium moves from the ECF to intracellular space: diabetic acidosis treatment, alkalosis, burns, and use of hyperalimentation. Potassium decreases can result from relative deficits caused by overhydration (e.g., water intoxication, IV therapy without potassium replacement). Hypokalemia in patients receiving digitalis preparations can result in digitalis toxicity.

a) Assessment

(1) Subjective data

(a) History of present illness
- Nausea, vomiting, anorexia (major causes of hypokalemia in pediatric population)
- Weakness, fatigue
- Cramps
- Shortness of breath
- Frequency of urination
- Poor dietary intake of potassium: related to poorly fitting dentures in the elderly; access to potassium-rich foods may be limited because these may be expensive
- Constipation

(b) Medical history
- Cardiovascular disease
- Congestive heart failure
- Diuretic use
- Renal disease
- Ulcerative colitis
- Use of steroids
- Diabetes

(2) Objective data

(a) Physical examination
- Shallow respirations; weak, thready pulses; orthostatic hypotension
- Muscle tenderness, hyporeflexia, eventual flaccid paralysis
- Dysrhythmias (heart blocks)
- Abdominal distention
- Paralytic ileus
- Low osmolality and specific gravity of urine
- Confusion, depression, lethargy, anxiety, coma
- Metabolic alkalosis
- Paralytic ileus, hypoactive bowel sounds
- Polyuria

(b) Diagnostic procedures
- Serum electrolytes
- Serum potassium normal range, 3.5 to 5.0 mEq/L
- ABG: alkalosis
- ECG
- Depressed ST segments

- Flattened T waves
- U waves
- Ventricular irritability

b) Analysis: nursing diagnosis/collaborative problems
  (1) Decreased cardiac output related to hypokalemia-induced rhythm disturbances
  (2) Knowledge deficit related to health maintenance and diet
c) Planning/interventions
  (1) Maintain airway, breathing, circulation
  (2) Obtain IV access
  (3) Administer IV potassium chloride as ordered; maximum dose, 10 to 40 mEq/hr; dilute before use
  (4) Correct acid-base imbalance
  (5) Continuously monitor and assess
    (a) Cardiac rhythm
    (b) Vital signs
    (c) Heart, lung sounds
    (d) Level of consciousness
    (e) Peripheral perfusion
    (f) Intake and output
    (g) Serum potassium
  (6) Assess knowledge of patient or significant other regarding signs and symptoms of hypokalemia
  (7) Review signs and symptoms that may warrant medical attention
    (a) Nausea, vomiting, anorexia
    (b) Weakness, fatigue
    (c) Muscle cramps
  (8) If patient is using potassium supplement, review and assess patient's knowledge of
    (a) Indications for use
    (b) Proper dosage
  (9) If patient is using diuretics, assess knowledge regarding
    (a) Indications for medication
    (b) Proper dosage
  (10) Review instructions and precautions
    (a) Indications for medications such as diuretics and potassium supplements
    (b) Proper dosages, side effects
  (11) Review potential for digitalis toxicity in presence of hypokalemia for patient using digitalis preparations
  (12) Answer patient's questions concerning information given
d) Expected outcomes/evaluation (see Appendix B)
  (1) Serum potassium level between 3.5 and 5.5 mEq/L
2) Hyperkalemia

Hyperkalemia is characterized by excess serum potassium, exceeding 5.5 mEq/L. Effects of elevated serum potassium on the cardiovascular system are the most important manifestations of the condition, resulting in cardiac dysrhythmias. Hyperpolarization from excess extracellular potassium causes an inability of action potential. Asystole is the terminal result, after development of dysrhythmias. Etiologies of hyperkalemia include excessive potassium input, both exogenous (IV potassium use, penicillin G therapy, transfusions with long-stored blood) and endogenous (severe tissue injury, acidosis, hyperuricemia, hypercatabolism, insulin deficiency). Hyperkalemia also results from decreased potassium excretion (decreased glomerular filtration rate, acute renal failure) and decreased sodium and potassium exchange (Addison's disease, drugs, isolated aldosterone deficiency). Geriatric patients, in general, have lower estimated dietary potassium; therefore, elevation is poorly tolerated. In the pediatric population, hyperkalemia is usually related to trauma or acute renal failure precipitated by exposure to nephrotoxic substances (or ingestion), near drowning, dehydration, or acute glomerulonephritis.

a) Assessment
  (1) Subjective data
    (a) History of present illness
      • Confusion
      • Hyperexcitability
      • Muscle weakness
      • Numbness
      • Abdominal distention
      • Diarrhea
      • Crush/burn injury
    (b) Medical history
      • Renal disease
      • Addison's disease
      • Potassium-sparing diuretic use
  (2) Objective data
    (a) Physical examination
      • Mental confusion
      • Neuromuscular excitability
      • Weakness
      • Paresthesia
      • Ascending flaccid paralysis
      • Dysrhythmias (Fig. 8–1)
      • Abdominal distention
      • Oliguria
      • Intestinal colic
      • Bradycardia
      • Hypovolemia
      • Hypoactive bowel sounds
    (b) Diagnostic procedures
      • Serum potassium greater than 5.0 mEq/L.
      • ECG
      • Peaked T waves
      • Depressed ST segment
      • Depressed or flat P wave
      • Widening QRS segment
      • Prolonged PR interval
b) Analysis: differential nursing diagnosis/collaborative problems
  (1) Decreased cardiac output related to cardiac dysrhythmias secondary to hyperkalemia
  (2) Anxiety/fear related to altered health status
  (3) Knowledge deficit related to symptomatology of hyperkalemia and health maintenance
c) Planning/interventions
  (1) Maintain airway, breathing, circulation
  (2) Establish IV access
  (3) Administer medications as ordered (i.e., used to drive potassium back into the cells)
    (a) Sodium bicarbonate
    (b) Glucose 50%

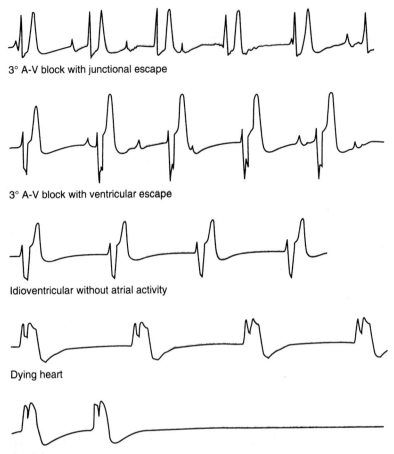

3° A-V block with junctional escape

3° A-V block with ventricular escape

Idioventricular without atrial activity

Dying heart

Asystole

FIGURE 8–1. Electrocardiographic changes associated with hyperkalemia. (A-V, atrioventricular.) (Modified with permission from John M. Clochesy.) (From Ignatavicius, D. D., Workman, M. L., & Mishler, M. A. [1997]. *Medical surgical nursing* [2nd ed., p. 298]. Philadelphia: W. B. Saunders. Used with permission.)

      (c) Insulin
  (4) Administer cation exchange resin sodium polystyrene sulfonate plus sorbitol solution as ordered
  (5) Prepare patient for peritoneal dialysis or hemodialysis if necessary
  (6) Continuously monitor and assess
      (a) Cardiac rhythm
      (b) Vital signs
      (c) Heart, lung sounds
      (d) Level of consciousness
      (e) Peripheral perfusion
      (f) Intake and output
      (g) Serum potassium
  (7) Maintain a calm, efficient manner
  (8) Explain all procedures to patient
  (9) Allow significant other at bedside, if possible
 (10) Assess patient's knowledge regarding
      (a) Potential causes of hyperkalemia
      (b) Signs and symptoms of hyperkalemia
 (11) Review symptoms that may indicate need for medical interventions

(a) Nausea, diarrhea

(b) Abdominal distention

(c) Mental confusion

(d) Weakness

(12) Assess patient's understanding of and compliance with dietary restrictions: identify barriers to compliance; obtain dietary consultation if necessary

(13) Answer patient's questions

d) Expected outcomes/evaluation (see Appendix B)

(1) Serum potassium within 3.5 to 5.5 mEq/L

c. *Calcium abnormalities*

Almost 100% of the body's calcium is combined with phosphorus and stored in the skeletal system. Calcium and phosphorus levels are inversely related: as one increases, the other decreases. Calcium levels are regulated by the endocrine system through parathyroid hormone (PTH) and thyrocalcitonin (Table 8–1). Calcium is factor IV in the body's clotting cascade and is required at various stages of coagulation. Other calcium effects are normal membrane permeability, transmission of normal neuromuscular impulses, and bone formation.

1) Hypocalcemia

Hypocalcemia can occur primarily as a result of deficits of calcium intake, inhibition of calcium absorption from the GI tract, or increased calcium excretion: decreased dietary intake or decreased vitamin D, lactose intolerance, malabsorption syndromes (e.g., celiac sprue, Crohn's disease), renal failure (i.e., polyuria phase), diarrhea/steatorrhea, and wound drainage.

Indirect causes of calcium deficits can be conditions that decrease the ionized fraction of calcium: alkalosis, massive transfusion of citrated blood (e.g., decreases serum calcium because citrate binds with calcium), hyper-

Table 8–1 HORMONAL REGULATION OF CALCIUM

	Action
Parathyroid Hormone (PTH)	
Secreted in response to low or low-normal serum calcium levels	Increases bone resorption of calcium (leaching of stored calcium)
Secretion results in a rise in serum calcium concentration	Increases the absorption of ingested calcium from the gastrointestinal tract into extracellular fluid
	Increases renal reabsorption of calcium at the proximal convoluted tubule
Thyrocalcitonin (TCT)	
Secreted by the thyroid gland in response to high or high-normal serum calcium levels	Increases bone uptake of calcium
	Inhibits the absorption of calcium from the gastrointestinal tract so that ingested calcium is excreted from the body in feces
Secretion results in a reduction of the serum calcium concentration	Inhibits renal reabsorption of calcium at the proximal convoluted tubule so that more calcium is excreted in the urine

From Ignatavicius, D. D., Workman, M. L., & Mishler, M. A. (1997). *Medical-surgical nursing: A nursing process approach* (2nd ed.). Philadelphia: W. B. Saunders.

phosphatemia, immobility, acute pancreatitis, use of calcium chelators/binders (e.g., sodium cellulose phosphate [Calcibind], pamidronate disodium [Aredia], penicillamine, mithramycin). Indirect deficits of calcium can also be due to endocrine disturbances, which reduce PTH levels: removal or destruction of parathyroid glands (e.g., thyroidectomy, radiation therapy of thyroid glands, neck injuries).

Loss of extracellular calcium increases sodium entry into neurons so excitation threshold decreases and spontaneous firing occurs. Alkalosis decreases the percentage of free calcium by encouraging protein binding. Clinical symptoms occur when total serum calcium is 5 mg/dL or less.

a) Assessment
  (1) Subjective data
    (a) History of present illness
      • Paresthesias followed by numbness
      • Muscle cramps
      • Altered dietary intake
      • Acute anxiety and stress
      • Infants: seizure, irritability, and vomiting
    (b) Medical history
      • Recent thyroidectomy or parathyroidectomy
      • Pancreatitis
      • Renal failure
      • Transfusion
      • Tumors
      • Toxic shock syndrome
      • Infant
      • Prematurity or low birth weight
      • Feeding cow's milk: elevates phosphate level, which decreases calcium level
      • Allergies
      • Medications
    (c) Physical examination
      • Hypotension
      • Tachycardia
      • Diminished peripheral pulses
      • Decreased respiratory effort
      • Muscle weakness
      • Hyperreflexia
      • Carpopedal spasm, hyperactive deep tendon reflexes
      • Tetany
      • Hyperventilation: causes alkalosis
      • Seizures
      • Trousseau's sign: carpal spasm after blood pressure cuff compression of arm
      • Chvostek's sign: contraction of facial muscles when face tapped at angle of jaw
      • Laryngeal stridor
      • Infants: twitching, vomiting, abdominal distention
    (d) Diagnostic procedures
      • Electrolyte levels
      • Serum calcium: normal range, 8.5 to 10.5 mg/dL; symptoms if 5.0 mg/dL or less
      • Sodium
      • Potassium
      • Magnesium: decreased
      • Phosphate: elevated
      • BUN and creatinine levels
      • ABGs: look for alkalosis
      • Serum albumin level: normal range, 3.5 to 5.5 g/dL
      • Parathyroid hormone level: elevated

- ECG and cardiac monitor
- Prolonged QT and ST intervals
- T-wave inversion may be present
- Radiographs as appropriate

b) Analysis: differential nursing diagnosis/collaborative problems
  (1) Pain related to metabolic neuron excitement and muscle spasms
  (2) Risk for injury related to increased neuromuscular excitability
  (3) Ineffective airway clearance related to possibility of laryngospasm, or seizures

c) Planning/interventions
  (1) Maintain airway, breathing, circulation and suction as needed
  (2) Initiate IV administration of isotonic saline if seizures occur
  (3) Initiate cardiac monitoring
  (4) Assist patient to slow down breathing if hyperventilating
  (5) Instruct patient regarding relationship of hyperventilation and hypocalcemia secondary to alkalosis
  (6) Administer calcium IV as ordered (i.e., administer carefully because exsanguination causes sloughing)
      (a) Calcium gluconate
      (b) Calcium chloride
      (c) Do not combine calcium with bicarbonate
  (7) Administer oral calcium supplement as needed
  (8) Ensure adequate amounts of vitamin D daily
  (9) Administer analgesics as ordered
  (10) Ensure adequate dietary intake of calcium
  (11) Ensure adequate fluid intake

d) Expected outcomes/evaluation (see Appendix B)
  (1) Serum calcium levels between 9 and 11 mg/dL

2) Hypercalcemia

Serum calcium levels are maintained in a narrow range by the kidney and the parathyroid gland. Any decrease in renal function or use of thiazide diuretics can reduce excretion of calcium; this in combination with an influx of calcium results in hypercalcemia. Elevated PTH levels stimulate bone dismantling, releasing calcium into the serum. The most common causes of hypercalcemia are due to increased bone reabsorption of calcium: primary hyperparathyroidism, malignancy, immobility, hyperthyroidism, and use of glucocorticoids. Hypercalcemia is rarely due to increased absorption of calcium (e.g., increased calcium or increased vitamin D intake). Hypercalcemia can occasionally be due to hemoconcentration effects resulting from adrenal insufficiency, dehydration, and use of lithium.

Fluid depletion secondary to hypercalcemic vomiting, anorexia, and reabsorption of sodium ion (to which calcium is tightly bound) in the process of volume deficit correction contributes to the cycle of hypercalcemia. Deterioration of renal function leads to increased calcium levels, which, in turn, cause coma and eventual death. Hypercalcemia is known to occur as an end-stage event in patients with cancer.

a) Assessment
  (1) Subjective data
      (a) History of present illness
          - Anorexia, nausea, vomiting, constipation
          - Abdominal pain
          - Weakness
          - Depression, lethargy, confusion, psychosis, coma
          - Weight loss

- Polyuria and polydipsia
- Pruritus
- (b) Medical history
  - Malignancy
  - Hyperparathyroid disease
  - Other chronic illness
  - Medications
  - Allergies
- (2) Objective data
  - (a) Physical examination
    - Mental status changes
    - Tachycardia
    - Hypertension
    - Increased urine output
    - Profound muscle weakness
    - Hyporeflexia
    - Hallucinations, lethargy, coma
    - Hypoactive bowel sounds
    - Abdominal distention
  - (b) Diagnostic procedures
    - Electrolytes levels
    - Serum calcium: normal range, 8.5 to 10.5 mg/dL; severe elevation, more than 13 to 14 mg/dL
    - Sodium: decreased
    - Potassium: hypokalemia common
    - Magnesium: normal range, 0.8 to 1.2 mmol/L; hypomagnesemia common
    - Phosphate: normal range for adult, 2.7 to 4.5 mg/dL; normal range for child, 4 to 7.1 mg/dL; (hypophosphatemia increases serum calcium level)
    - BUN and creatinine levels: elevated because of volume depletion and renal dysfunction
    - ABGs
    - Serum albumin level: normal range, 3.5 to 5.5 g/dL; 50% of calcium is bound to albumin; if level is low, there is more free calcium
    - Parathyroid hormone level: elevated
    - ECG: short QT interval
    - Serum calcium level greater than 15 mg/dL: widened PR interval, QRS complex, and T wave
    - Serum calcium level greater than 20 mg/dL: bradycardia, heart block, and bundle branch block
    - Other studies as indicated and ordered
- b) Analysis: differential nursing diagnosis/collaborative problems
  - (1) Risk for fluid volume deficit related to vomiting
  - (2) Risk for fluid volume excess related to decreased renal function
  - (3) Risk for injury related to bone degeneration, weakness, confusion
  - (4) Knowledge deficit related to disease process and health maintenance
- c) Planning/interventions (severe disease)
  - (1) Establish large-bore IV access for administration of isotonic saline
    - (a) Dilutes extracellular calcium
    - (b) Expands extracellular volume to increase calcium excretion by kidney
  - (2) Insert urinary catheter
  - (3) Monitor intake and output, keeping urine output greater than 500 mL/hr in adults
  - (4) Cardiac monitor
  - (5) Prepare patient for central venous pressure or Swan-Ganz catheter insertion

  (6) Administer medications as ordered
    (a) Calcitonin IV: inhibits osteoclastic bone resorption and encourages urinary calcium excretion
    (b) Plicamycin IV: inhibits bone resorption
    (c) Loop diuretics: furosemide and ethacrynic acid; given with large volume of fluid to enhance calcium excretion
    (d) Glucocorticoids
    (e) Digitalis: may be toxic in presence of hypercalcemia; usually not used
  (7) Prepare patient/significant others for hemodialysis or peritoneal dialysis if patient is unable to tolerate fluid loading (because of congestive heart failure or renal failure)
  (8) If patient has mild or moderate disease, educate about need for early and persistent weight-bearing exercise to encourage calcium uptake by skeleton
  (9) Protect patient from injury and falling
  (10) Explain procedures to patient/significant others
  (11) Allow significant others to be at bedside when possible
 d) Expected outcomes/evaluation (see Appendix B)
  (1) Serum calcium level between 8.5 and 10.5 mg/dL

d. Magnesium abnormalities

Magnesium is a coenzyme in carbohydrate and protein metabolism and is also involved in the metabolism of cellular proteins. Neuromuscular excitability is profoundly affected by fluctuations in serum magnesium levels. Mechanisms that control magnesium are not well understood; however, it is known that many factors that affect calcium also affect magnesium. Magnesium excretion is regulated through the kidneys.

1) Hypomagnesemia

The primary causes of hypomagnesemia are related to decreased or insufficient intake of magnesium; chronic alcoholism is the most common. Other causes of insufficient intake include prolonged IV feeding without magnesium supplements and excessive loss of magnesium through the GI tract (e.g., Crohn's disease, celiac disease, diarrhea, steatorrhea), starvation, and malnutrition. Magnesium deficiencies can also result from increased renal excretion of magnesium: drug therapy (e.g., cisplatin, aminoglycoside therapy, cyclosporin, diuretics), use of citrate (e.g., found in blood products), and alcohol use. Indirect causes of magnesium deficits can be caused by intracellular shifts resulting from hyperglycemia, insulin administration, alkalosis, and sepsis.

Magnesium deficiency develops slowly, places the patient at risk for dysrhythmias, and may be associated with hypokalemia. Clinical findings of hypomagnesemia resemble those seen in hypocalcemia.

a) Assessment findings
 (1) Subjective data
  (a) History of present illness
   • Paresthesias
   • Muscle cramps, twitches, fasciculations
   • Inadequate nutritional intake
   • Seizure, irritability, vomiting
  (b) Medical History
   • Chronic alcoholism
   • Malnutrition
   • Crohn's disease
   • Medications (diuretics, amphotericin, cisplatin)

- Diabetes
- Renal insufficiency

(2) Objective data
    (a) Physical examination
- Hypertension
- Hypotension, bradycardia may occur with severe hypomagnesemia
- Shallow respirations
- Ventricular dysrhythmias (premature ventricular contractions [PVCs], ventricular tachycardia, torsades de pointes, ventricular fibrillation)
- ECG changes (tall T waves, depressed ST segment)
- Trousseau's sign
- Chvostek's sign
- Hyperreflexia
- Tetany
- Seizures
- Central nervous system irritability, confusion, psychosis
- Coma occurs with severe hypomagnesemia

    (b) Diagnostic procedures
- Electrolyte levels
- Serum magnesium (normal range, 1.5–2.5 mEq/L)
- Serum potassium (normal range, 3.5–5.5 mEq/L): may be low
- Serum calcium (normal range, 8.5–10.5 mEq/L): may be low
- BUN and creatinine levels
- ECG and cardiac monitor
- Radiographs as appropriate

b) Analysis: differential nursing diagnosis/collaborative problems
    (1) Risk for injury related to increased neuromuscular excitability
    (2) Ineffective airway clearance related to seizures, hypoventilation

c) Planning/interventions
    (1) Maintain airway, breathing, circulation and suction as needed
    (2) Initiate IV administration of isotonic saline
    (3) Initiate cardiac monitoring
    (4) Administer magnesium sulfate
        (a) Mild deficits can be corrected with oral supplements and foods high in magnesium (e.g., green vegetables, nuts, bananas, oranges, peanut butter, chocolate)
        (b) Parenterally (IV or intramuscular [IM]) for severe hypomagnesemia; administer slow IV to prevent potential cardiac or respiratory arrest
    (5) Give magnesium supplements as needed
    (6) Administer analgesics as prescribed
    (7) Ensure adequate dietary intake of calcium and vitamin D

d) Expected outcomes/evaluation (see Appendix B)
    (1) Serum magnesium between 1.5 and 2.5 mEq/L

2) Hypermagnesemia
    Conditions such as adrenal insufficiency and renal failure reduce excretion of magnesium through the kidneys. Other causes of hypermagnesemia include overdose of therapeutic magnesium. Patients with renal failure who ingest products containing magnesium (e.g., Maalox, milk of magnesia) experience hypermagnesemia. Treatment of eclampsia in pregnant women can also lead to hypermagnesemia.

a) Assessment findings
    (1) Subjective data
        (a) History of present illness
- Nausea and vomiting
- Drowsiness, lethargy
        (b) Medical History

- Renal insufficiency or failure
- Adrenocortical insufficiency
- Overdose of therapeutic magnesium
- Eclampsia

(2) Objective data

(a) Physical examination
- Somnolence
- Shallow respirations
- Depressed or absent deep tendon reflexes
- Respiratory and/or cardiac arrest

(b) Diagnostic procedures
- Electrolyte levels
- Serum magnesium (normal range, 1.5–2.5 mEq/L)
- BUN and creatinine levels
- ECG and cardiac monitor
- Radiographs as appropriate

b) Analysis: differential nursing diagnosis/collaborative problems

(1) Ineffective airway clearance related to seizures, hypoventilation

c) Planning/interventions

(1) Maintain airway, breathing, circulation and suction as needed if seizures occur

(2) Initiate IV administration of isotonic saline

(3) Initiate cardiac monitoring

(4) Administer calcium chloride or calcium gluconate; follow with continuous infusion

(5) Saline diuresis and furosemide may be used

(6) Hemodialysis is used in extreme cases

d) Expected outcomes/evaluation (see Appendix B)

(1) Serum magnesium within 1.5 to 2.5 mEq/L

F. Coma

Coma is a state of profound unconsciousness in which the patient has no psychologically understandable responses to internal or external stimuli. Adequate function of the cerebral hemispheres (content) and the reticular activating system (arousal) is necessary for consciousness. Widespread disruption of either area results in coma. Coma is classified according to cause: structural, metabolic (i.e., diffuse depression of brain function), toxic, or enzymatic inhibition or psychiatric.

Structural causes can include supratentorial mass lesions in which a primary lesion enlarges, causing brain-swelling shift and compression of reticular activating system (e.g., tumor, abscess, cerebrovascular accident [CVA] with edema, hematoma, fulminating meningitis) or mass subtentorial lesions resulting in compression or destruction of brain stem structures (e.g., CVA, hemorrhage, basilar aneurysm).

Metabolic causes can include hemispherical dysfunction; hypoxia resulting from interference of oxygen supply to the brain (e.g., pulmonary disease, carbon monoxide poisoning, reduced atmospheric oxygen tension, seizures); global ischemia resulting from generalized and diffuse interference of brain's blood supply (e.g., cardiac arrest, decreased cardiac output, orthostatic hypotension, low blood volume, hypertensive encephalopathy); hypoglycemia; and vitamin deficiencies (e.g., thiamine, niacin, pyridoxine, vitamin B_{12}).

Toxic or enzymatic inhibition causes may include uremic; hepatic; diabetic; porphyric; exogenous poisons (e.g., sedatives, acid poisons, cyanide, salicylates); CNS toxins (e.g., meningitis, encephalitis, subarachnoid hemorrhage); and fluid/electrolyte imbalances.

Psychiatric causes may include hysteria and catatonia.

1. **Assessment**
   a. *Subjective data*
      1) History of present illness
         a) Onset: rapid or gradual
         b) Activity at time of onset
         c) Headache or confusion preceding coma
         d) Observation of witnesses (e.g., seizure activity, trauma)
         e) Progression of seizure: focal to general or head to toe
         f) Altered mental status preceding motor dysfunction
      2) Medical history
         a) Medications
         b) Allergies
         c) Seizure disorder
         d) Trauma
         e) Headache and fever
         f) Bacterial or viral illness preceding onset
         g) Cardiopulmonary disease and renal/hepatic disease
         h) Endocrine disorder (e.g., Addison's disease, thyroid disorder, diabetes, hypoglycemia)
         i) Depression and recent behavior or emotional status change
         j) Alcohol/drug use
         k) Environmental exposure; suspect if more than one patient
   b. *Objective data*
      1) Physical examination
         a) Level of consciousness
            (1) Alert
            (2) Response to verbal stimulus
            (3) Response to painful stimulus
            (4) Unresponsive
            (5) Describe specific stimulus and response rather than using general terms such as lethargy or stupor
         b) Respiratory rate: may determine type and level of lesion
            (1) Hyperventilation: acidosis, salicylate ingestion, hypoxia, sepsis
            (2) Cheyne-Stokes respirations: hypertensive or metabolic disorders causing diffuse bilateral hemispheric disruption and abnormal response to carbon dioxide levels
            (3) Hypoventilation: trauma, pulmonary disease, narcotic-sedative ingestion
            (4) Central neurogenic hyperventilation: sustained, rapid, deep respirations: midbrain compression from tentorial herniation resulting in respiratory alkalosis
            (5) Apneusis: inspiratory cramp (i.e., pause in full inspiration); probable lower pons lesion or compression
            (6) Ataxic or cluster respirations: irregular and nonpatterned; probable medullary lesion or compression
            (7) Apnea: profound medullary disruption
         c) Pupils (Fig. 8–2)
            (1) Equality
            (2) Reactivity
            (3) Normal pupillary response usually indicative of metabolic coma
            (4) Eyedrops, eye trauma, blindness, prosthesis, surgery may distort response
            (5) Ten to 20% of population have anisocoria of 1 to 2 mm

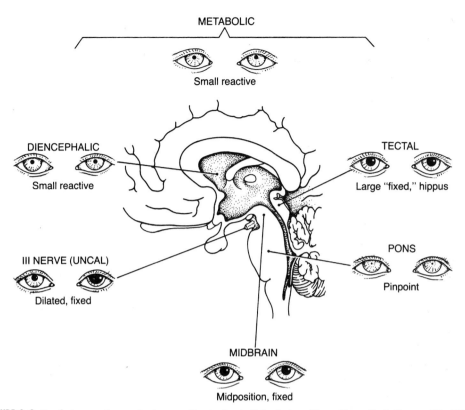

FIGURE 8–2. Pupils in comatose patients according to level of the lesion. (From Plum, F., & Posner, J.B. [1980]. *Diagnosis of stupor and coma* [3rd ed., p. 46]. Philadelphia: F.A. Davis. Used with permission.)

      (6) Hippus: spontaneous rhythmic dilation and contraction, which represents midbrain damage

   d) Eye movements

      (1) Fixed lateral gaze: frontal or pontine injury

      (2) Roving: metabolic coma

      (3) Disconjugate: frontal or pontine injury

      (4) Ocular reflexes

      (5) Oculocephalic reflex: doll's eyes: first rule out cervical spine injury before testing; watch eye movements while turning head horizontally; normal: intact brain stem and conjugate eye deviation opposite direction of head rotation; brain stem injury: eyes remain in their initial position when head rotated; response usually normal in mild to moderate metabolic coma; absence of movement means severe brain stem injury

      (6) Oculovestibular reflex: caloric test: elevate head to 30 degrees; check for intact tympanic membranes and no wax or blood in ear canal; irrigate ear with ice water to inhibit vestibular nerve; observe response: in awake patient, normal response, horizontal nystagmus with rapid movement away from irrigated ear, and possible nausea and vomiting; in comatose patient with intact brain stem, slow, conjugate, ipsilateral eye deviation; in brain stem injury, disconjugate ocular movement; wait 5 minutes and repeat with other ear

      (7) Ciliospinal reflex: sympathetic pathway integrity; painful stimulus to face, neck, and trunk; normal response: asleep or coma with intact

pathway and bilateral pupillary dilation; no response: pathway damage

(8) Corneal reflex: fifth and sixth cranial nerve function; unilateral absence: ipsilateral brain stem or contralateral hemispheric lesion; bilaterally depressed or absent reflexes: posterior fossa or brain stem lesion

(9) Skeletal motor response to application of painful stimulus; purposeful: localization and attempt to remove stimulus; withdrawal: movement away from stimulus; abnormal flexion (decorticate posturing): flexion of any or all extremities, probable lesion of descending motor pathways (pyramidal tracts) above rostral midbrain; abnormal extension (decerebrate posturing): extension of any or all extremities, probable lesion of midbrain or upper pons; flaccidity: no motor response to stimulus; observe and record responses to both sides of the body (Fig. 8–3 illustrates decorticate and decerebrate posturing)

e) Glasgow Coma Scale (see Appendix C)
  (1) Initial evaluation
  (2) Progression of coma
  (3) Prediction of outcome
  (4) Value less than 7 indicative of coma

f) Fever or hypothermia

g) Visible trauma

h) Vital signs

i) Diaphoretic or dry skin

j) Heart and breath sounds

k) Signs of meningeal irritation
  (1) Nuchal rigidity
  (2) Kernig's sign
  (3) Brudzinski's sign

l) Restlessness

m) Sense of impending doom

2) Diagnostic procedures
  a) ABGs
  b) Electrolyte and glucose levels
  c) CBC

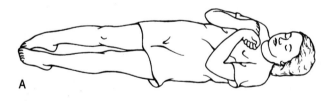

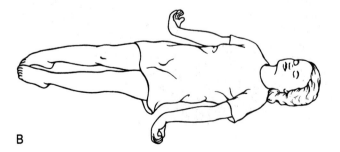

FIGURE 8–3. Posturing. *A*, Decorticate posturing. *B*, Decerebrate posturing. (From Ignatavicius, D. D., Workman, M. L., & Mishler, M. A. [1997]. *Medical-surgical nursing* [2nd ed., p. 1111]. Philadelphia W. B. Saunders. Used with permission.)

    d) Creatinine and BUN levels

    e) Cardiac monitor and ECG

    f) Chest radiograph

    g) Skull and cervical spine radiograph

    h) Head CT scan

    i) Urinalysis

    j) Alcohol and drug screens

    k) Lumbar puncture

    l) Other studies as indicated by history and physical examination

  c. Analysis: differential diagnosis/collaborative problems

    1) Impaired gas exchange related to brain lesion or dysfunction interfering with respiratory center

    2) Impaired tissue perfusion, cerebral related to lesion, hemorrhage, embolus, or thrombus

    3) Risk for fluid volume deficit related to infection, respiratory rate, or inability to take fluids orally

  d. Planning/interventions

    1) Maintain airway, breathing, circulation

    2) Ensure oral or nasal airway: via intubation, cricothyrotomy, or positioning

    3) Provide oxygen

    4) Suction if necessary

    5) Immobilize cervical spine as indicated

    6) Establish IV access for administration of isotonic solution (saline or lactated Ringer's solutions) with large-gauge catheter

    7) Insert nasogastric tube

    8) Use witness, family, and significant others for history

    9) Search for medical alert tags or cards: to avoid injury to medical personnel, do not put hands into pockets

    10) Infuse 50% glucose by IV push after blood studies

    11) Infuse prescribed naloxone by IV push if no response to glucose

    12) Give prescribed thiamine IV or IM in nutritionally depleted or alcoholic patient

    13) Monitor vital signs and neurological status

    14) Monitor intake and output

    15) Set up for potential medical interventions as indicated

    16) Insert urinary catheter

    17) Monitor physical parameters that indicate dehydration

    18) Prepare to administer bolus of fluid (fluid challenge)

  e. Expected outcomes/evaluation (see Appendix B)

G. Hematologic emergencies

    Blood is a suspension of erythrocytes, leukocytes, platelets, and other particulate matter that acts as a medium for exchange between fixed cells in the body and the external environment. Blood provides protection against infection through various leukocytes, transports oxygen and carbon dioxide via erythrocytes, and provides hemostasis through platelets and other clotting factors. The following are the plasma coagulation factors: factor I (fibrinogen), factor II (prothrombin), factor III (tissue thromboplastin), factor IV (calcium), factor V (proaccelerin), factor VII (proconvertin, serum PT conversion accelerator), factor VIII (antihemophilic factor [AHF]), factor IX (plasma thromboplastin component or Christmas factor), factor X (Stuart-Prower factor), factor XI (plasma thromboplastin antecedent), factor XII (Hageman factor), and factor XIII (fibrin-stabilizing factor).

Blood coagulation via the clotting cascade is necessary to prevent loss of volume and essential blood components. However, lysis of a clot that is no longer needed is necessary to restore circulation to the affected area. Hematological function can be affected by diseases such as renal failure or cancer. Various drugs also impair hematological function: drugs that actually cause bone marrow suppression (e.g., amphotericin B, chemotherapeutic agents, interferon, pentamidine, foscarnet [Foscavir], ganciclovir [Cytovene], zidovudine [Retrovir]); drugs that can cause hemolysis (e.g., methyldopa, amoxicillin, penicillin, quinidine polygalacturonate, chlorpropamide [Diabinese], penicillin [Pen-Vee K], procainamide, phytonadione [Aqua-MEPHYTON]); and drugs that disrupt platelet activity (e.g., aspirin, valproic acid, ticlopidine [Ticlid], valproic acid [Depakene], carbenicillin, dipyridamole).

1. **Clotting abnormalities**

   The clotting cascade may be affected by abnormal levels of clotting factors, trauma, or medications. The problem may occur as a primary event, such as hemophilia, or secondary to other problems (e.g., disseminated intravascular coagulation [DIC]). Treatment focuses on identification of the underlying problem and correction of specific deficits within the clotting cascade.

   a. *Disseminated intravascular coagulation*

      DIC, manifested by diffuse microvascular coagulation, depletes clotting factors and impairs hemostasis. DIC is almost never seen as a separate entity, but usually occurs as a complication of, or in association with, other conditions. In DIC, the process of microthrombi formation occurs rapidly and excessively. These clots are deposited in the microvasculature of various organs and cause tissue ischemia. As clots are rapidly lysed, fibrin (split) degradation products (FDP) are released and act as anticoagulants. At the same time, the blood's clotting factors are depleted so abnormal bleeding occurs. DIC also results in a microangiopathic anemia caused by red blood cell fragmentation by fibrin strands.

      1) Assessment
         a) Subjective data
            (1) History of present illness
               (a) Bleeding from any site
               (b) Dizziness
               (c) Weakness
               (d) Rash
               (e) Excessive bruising
               (f) Nausea, vomiting, diarrhea
            (2) Past or current medical history
               (a) Massive blood transfusions
               (b) Abruptio placentae
               (c) Trauma
               (d) Neoplasm
               (e) Malaria
               (f) Snake bite
               (g) Respiratory distress syndrome
               (h) Prolonged extracorporeal circulation
               (i) Hepatic disease
               (j) Medication history: aspirin, anticoagulants, oral contraceptives, estrogen replacement
               (k) Current medications
               (l) Immunization status
               (m) Allergies
               (n) Last menstrual period

b) Objective data
  (1) Physical examination
      (a) Petechiae, purpura
      (b) Ecchymosis
      (c) Bleeding
          • Overt
          • Occult
      (d) Hematuria or anuria
      (e) Altered sensorium
      (f) Acrocyanosis
      (g) Hematemesis
      (h) Adult respiratory distress syndrome (ARDS), interstitial pulmonary bleeders
      (i) Altered sensorium, convulsion, coma
  (2) Diagnostic procedures
      (a) Platelet count: normal 150,000 to 400,000/μL; decreased in DIC
      (b) Thrombin time: control to $\pm$ 3 seconds
      (c) PT: normal 11 to 15 seconds (varies with control); prolonged in DIC
      (d) PTT: activated, 25 to 37 seconds; prolonged in DIC
      (e) Fibrinogen level: 200 to 400 mg/dL; decreased in DIC
      (f) Fibrin degradation products (FDP): normal negative greater than 1:4 dilution; increased in DIC
      (g) Hematocrit: normal, 36 to 45 mL/dL; decreased in DIC
      (h) Hemoglobin level: normal, 12 to 15 m/dL; decreased in DIC
      (i) Urinalysis: blood or hemoglobin in urine
      (j) Type and cross-match for blood and clotting factors
      (k) BUN/creatinine levels: elevated
2) Analysis: differential nursing diagnosis/collaborative problems
  a) Risk for fluid volume deficit related to blood loss
  b) Tissue perfusion, altered related to deposition of fibrin in microcirculation
  c) Risk for injury related to ease of bleeding
  d) Anxiety/fear related to manifestations of disease process and fear of death
3) Planning/interventions
  a) Establish IV access for administration of isotonic solution with large-bore catheter
  b) Maintain adequate fluid volume to prevent renal tubular obstruction from hematuria
  c) Administer supplemental oxygen
  d) Monitor
     (1) Arterial blood pressure
     (2) Peripheral pulses: presence and quality
     (3) Skin and mucous membrane color
     (4) Cardiac rate and rhythm
     (5) Skin temperature
     (6) Mentation
     (7) Urine output
     (8) Clotting time and platelet count
     (9) Serial hematocrit and hemoglobin levels
  e) Guaiac stools and emesis for blood

f) Increase oxygen-carrying capacity of blood by transfusion of blood or red blood cells

g) Replace clotting factors and platelets

h) Insert urinary catheters

i) Administer heparin, as ordered, and monitor response

j) Limit number of venipunctures

k) Handle patient gently

l) Have side rails up on bed

m) Maintain calm, efficient manner

n) Explain all procedures in simple terms

o) Permit calm significant others to accompany stable patient in treatment area

4) Expected outcomes/evaluation (see Appendix B)

b. *Hemophilia*

Hemophilia is an inherited, sex-linked disorder that is almost always seen in males. Females carry the gene and pass it to their children. There are three forms of hemophilia: hemophilia A, hemophilia B, and von Willebrand's disease. Hemophilia A is a coagulation disorder caused by a variant form of factor VIII. Severity of the disease is directly related to activity level of factor VIII. Activity level less than 1% is severe and accompanied by spontaneous bleeding. Activity level of 1 to 5% is moderately severe; there is rare spontaneous bleeding but difficulty during surgery or with trauma. Patients with 5 to 10% or greater activity of factor VIII have mild disease with little risk of spontaneous bleeding, but PTT is prolonged. Bleeding may occur anywhere but characteristically affects joints, deep muscles, urinary tract, and cranial vault. After trauma, bleeding usually is absent at first, because initial coagulation step of platelet plug formation is not affected by hemophilia. Hemophilia B (Christmas disease) results from absent or deficiency of factor IX. The condition is relatively rare, occurring in 1 in 100,000 persons in the United States and is clinically indistinguishable from type A, except for treatment. Von Willebrand's disease occurs in males and females and is less acute than hemophilia A or B. This type of hemophilia is characterized by defective platelet adherence and decreased factor VIII levels.

1) Assessment

a) Subjective data

(1) History of present illness

(a) Unusual, prolonged bleeding after trauma or dental extraction

(b) Spontaneous hemorrhage

(c) Hemarthrosis

(d) Intracranial bleeding

(e) Melena

(2) Medical history: previous hemophilia diagnosis

b) Objective data

(1) Physical examination

(a) Skin
- Ecchymosis
- Hematoma
- Pallor
- Coolness

(b) Joints
- Decreased range of motion
- Tenderness
- Edema
- Abnormal gait

      (c) Pulses in extremity may be abnormal

      (d) Vital signs, including orthostatic blood pressure and pulse

      (e) Assess for occult blood

    (2) Diagnostic procedures

      (a) PTT: prolonged

      (b) PT: normal

      (c) Platelet count: normal

      (d) Factor VIII activity level: decreased in hemophilia A and von Willebrand's disease

      (e) Factor IX activity level: decreased in hemophilia B

      (f) CT scan if neurological symptoms

      (g) Urinalysis

      (h) Hematocrit: normal

2) Analysis: differential nursing diagnosis/collaborative problems

  a) Risk for fluid volume deficit related to bleeding

  b) Knowledge deficit related to therapeutic regimen and health maintenance

3) Planning/interventions

  a) After venipuncture, apply pressure for at least 5 minutes

  b) No intramuscular injections

  c) For hemarthrosis or hematoma

    (1) Apply ice packs

    (2) Immobilize

    (3) Elevate

    (4) Apply mild compressive dressing

  d) Lacerations

    (1) Use local pressure and anesthesia with epinephrine if appropriate

    (2) Observe 4 hours after suturing

  e) Administer topical thrombin for minor wounds and epistaxis as ordered

  f) Mild to moderate disease: administer desmopressin acetate: increases levels of factor VIIIc

  g) Severe disease: factor VIII therapy: cryoprecipitate is preferred over commercial factor VIIIc because of greater risk for infection by hepatitis B virus and human immunodeficiency virus

    (1) Use blood filter

    (2) Platelet concentration infusion set allows IV push administration: should be slow

    (3) After thawing, must be administered within 24 hours, preferably within 3 hours

    (4) Use ABO type–specific blood if available; cross-match not necessary

    (5) Monitor for allergic reaction: urticaria, pruritus, fever

  h) For severe hemorrhage, treat for hypovolemic shock plus cryoprecipitate

  i) Use factor VIII therapy at home to terminate early bleeding episode, decreasing complications

  j) For hemophilia B, use commercial factor IX or fresh frozen plasma

  k) Provide social service referral as needed

  l) Allow time for family to vent feelings

  m) Avoid aspirin and nonsteroidal anti-inflammatory drugs (NSAIDs): inhibits platelet formation; instruct in over-the-counter medications that contain aspirin and NSAIDs

  n) Ensure that tetanus immunization is up to date: IM administration is acceptable

o) Instruct in need for prophylactic dental care

p) Discuss ways to avoid bleeding episodes

    (1) Safety measures

    (2) No contact sports

q) Use medical alert (i.e., MedicAlert) tag

r) Provide referral for appropriate follow-up care

4) Expected outcomes/evaluation (see Appendix B)

c. *Thrombocytopenia purpura*

Congenital disorders or acquired disorders such as decreased bone marrow production, increased splenic sequestration, or accelerated platelet destruction can lead to thrombocytopenia, an abnormal decrease in platelet count. Normal platelet count is 150,000 to 450,000/μL. The most common form of thrombocytopenia is immune thrombocytopenia purpura (ITP). The condition, previously called idiopathic thrombocytopenia purpura, is seen acutely in children several weeks after a viral condition such as rubella or chickenpox. Chronic ITP is seen most often in women 20 to 40 years of age.

1) Assessment findings

  a) Subjective data

    (1) History of present illness

      (a) Bleeding

      (b) Bruising

      (c) Petechiae

      (d) Abdominal pain and tenderness

      (e) Weakness, dizziness, fainting

      (f) Confusion

    (2) Medical history

      (a) Previous episodes unexplained bleeding

      (b) Existing coagulation disease

      (c) Malnutrition

      (d) Infection, sepsis

      (e) Tumors

      (f) Medications (salicylates)

  b) Objective data

    (1) Physical examination

      (a) Ecchymosis

      (b) Petechiae

      (c) Epistaxis, bleeding gums

      (d) Hematuria

      (e) GI bleeding, actual or occult

      (f) Retinal hemorrhage

    (2) Diagnostic procedures

      (a) Platelet count less than 150,000/μL

      (b) Bleeding time prolonged

      (c) PT/PTT normal even with severe thrombocytopenia

      (d) Radiographs and ECG as appropriate

2) Analysis: differential nursing diagnosis/collaborative problems

  a) Risk for altered cardiopulmonary, cerebral, or renal tissue perfusion related to acute or chronic blood loss

3) Planning/interventions

  a) Maintain airway, breathing, circulation and suction as needed

  b) Initiate IV administration of isotonic saline

  c) Initiate cardiac monitoring

  d) Monitor for new or increased bleeding

e) IV immune globulins are used to increase platelet levels rapidly

f) Glucocorticoids may be given if conservative measures fail

g) Splenectomy recommended only for children with severe bleeding

h) Plasmapheresis may be used

i) General nursing care measures

   (1) Handle patient gently

   (2) Use lift sheet when moving and positioning patient in bed

   (3) Avoid intramuscular injections or venipunctures as necessary; use small-gauge needle

   (4) Apply firm pressure to venipuncture site for 5 to 10 minutes or until site does not ooze

   (5) Apply ice to areas of trauma

   (6) Do not take temperatures rectally

   (7) Test all urine and stool for presence of occult blood

4) Expected outcomes/evaluation (see Appendix B)

2. Sickle cell crisis

Sickle cell disease is an inherited genetic disorder affecting primarily blacks. Hemoglobin S makes up 35% of total hemoglobin; normal hemoglobin A accounts for 65%. Fully oxygenated hemoglobin S does not differ from hemoglobin A, so there are few clinical manifestations. Severe hypoxia or dehydration may precipitate a sickling crisis. When deoxygenation occurs, red blood cells containing hemoglobin S change from biconcave disks to crescents, becoming rigid and incapable of traversing the microcirculation and thereby obstructing capillary blood flow. Obstruction leads to tissue hypoxia, which promotes deoxygenation and further sickling. Increasing obstruction results in infarcted tissue and organs. There is occasionally splenic infarction as a result of clumping of abnormally shaped cells. Oxygenation reverses the sickling process in about 80% of cells; the remainder are irreversibly sickled, contributing to severe hemolytic anemia.

a. *Assessment*

1) Subjective data

  a) History of present illness

    (1) Pain

     (a) Location: abdomen, chest, joints, back

     (b) Onset: sudden and explosive

     (c) Frequency: cluster attacks are common; remissions last months to years; recurrence is common

    (2) Impaired growth patterns

     (a) Impaired growth and development

     (b) General failure to thrive

     (c) Retarded puberty, resulting in youthful appearance and long, thin extremities

    (3) Infection

     (a) Increased susceptibility, especially to *Streptococcus pneumoniae*

     (b) Impaired splenic function prevents effective clearance of bacteria

  b) Medical history

    (1) Medications

    (2) Allergies

    (3) Previous diagnosis of sickle cell disease

    (4) Genetic familial history

2) Objective data

  a) Physical examination

    (1) Chronic organ damage

      (2) Congestive heart failure secondary to chronic anemia and hypoxia

      (3) Systolic ejection murmur

      (4) Pulmonary embolus

      (5) Jaundice

      (6) Increased tendency for gallstones

      (7) Isosthenuria: formation of urine at fixed specific gravity of 1.01 leads to dehydration

      (8) Painless hematuria secondary to microinfarction

      (9) Priapism

      (10) Vitreous hemorrhage

      (11) Retinal detachment and infarction

      (12) Skin: chronic ulcers of lower extremities more common in presence of severe anemia

      (13) Neurological function: 25% chance of significant neurological event

      (14) Acute abdomen: frequently overlooked in patient with sickle cell crisis

      (15) Vital signs: tachycardia and tachypnea

      (16) Orthostatic vital signs

      (17) Breath sounds

      (18) Heart sounds

      (19) Assessment of peripheral blood flow

      (20) Capillary blanch test

      (21) Color and temperature of skin

    b) Diagnostic procedures

      (1) CBC

        (a) Hemolytic anemia: hematocrit 20 to 30%

        (b) Elevated reticulocytes

        (c) Peripheral smear: sickled cells

      (2) Hemoglobin electrophoresis: sickle cell hemoglobin (Hb S)

      (3) ABGs: lowered partial pressure of arterial oxygen (PaO_2)

      (4) Bilirubin: elevated secondary to hemolysis

      (5) Chest, abdominal radiograph to rule out infection or acute abdomen

      (6) ECG: to rule out cardiac complications

  b. Analysis: differential nursing diagnosis/collaborative problems

    1) Tissue perfusion, altered cerebral, cardiopulmonary, renal, hepatic, and splenic related to decreased blood flow

    2) Risk for fluid volume deficit related to vomiting or inadequate oral intake

    3) Pain related to decreased oxygen to tissue

    4) Knowledge deficit related to therapeutic regimen and health maintenance

  c. Planning/interventions

    1) Provide low-flow oxygen via nasal cannula to reverse hypoxia and sickling

    2) Monitor for signs of inadequate perfusion

      a) Increased pain

      b) Capillary refill greater than 2 seconds

      c) Skin: cool and pale

      d) Decreased urine output

    3) Initiate IV catheter for administration of isotonic saline

    4) Administer analgesics titrated to pain relief

    5) Transfuse packed red blood cells, as necessary

    6) Administer prescribed IV sodium bicarbonate if metabolic acidosis present

    7) Monitor intake and output

    8) Observe for cardiac overload: person in second decade of life or older

    9) Offer oral fluids if vomiting has subsided

10) Assess and monitor signs of dehydration
11) Help patient assume position of comfort
12) Provide support of extremities with pillows
13) Restrict to bed rest
14) Allow supportive significant others to be present
15) Refer to social service agency or local support group for sickle cell disease
16) Allow time for patient/significant others to vent feelings
17) Assess coping mechanisms of patient/significant others
18) Suggest alternative coping mechanisms of patient/significant others
19) Instruct patient/significant others about disease process
20) Provide preventive suggestions
    a) Ensure adequate fluid intake
    b) Avoid high altitude
    c) Avoid stressful situations
    d) Avoid cold weather
    e) Avoid infection and trauma
    f) Elevate legs
21) Instruct patient in use of prescribed medications
22) Instruct patient regarding signs and symptoms that indicate need to return to emergency care setting, including recurrence of symptoms, severe abdominal pain, and illness with signs of dehydration
23) Arrange appropriate follow-up care

   d. *Expected outcomes/evaluation* (see Appendix B)

3. **Immune compromise**

The immune system may be adversely affected by disease, drugs, or nutritional deficits. Typically, the patient seen in the emergency department with immune compromise is receiving treatment for cancer or is on immunosuppressive therapy after organ transplantation. The patient with immune compromise experiences neutropenia: decrease in total white cell count and neutrophils. Decreased neutrophil counts places the patient at risk for infection from normal body flora as well as opportunistic infection. Classic signs of infection such as redness, heat, and swelling do not occur because the body's phagocytic response is impaired. Pus formation is also absent because white blood cells are the major component of pus. Consequently, the most significant indicator of infection in the patient with neutropenia is fever. The patient is instructed to call the physician any time the temperature is greater than 100°F. Care of the patient with immune compromise in the emergency department focuses on protecting the patient, identifying the source of the infection, and initiating antibiotic therapy immediately.

   a. *Assessment findings*
     1) Subjective data
       a) History of present illness
         (1) Fever
         (2) Cough, sore throat, dysphagia
         (3) Dysuria, urinary frequency
         (4) Pain or tenderness
         (5) Weakness, dizziness, fainting
         (6) Confusion
         (7) Redness or swelling
         (8) Nausea, vomiting, diarrhea, anorexia
         (9) Rectal tenderness
         (10) Vaginal itching or discharge

      b) Medical history

         (1) Cancer, acquired immunodeficiency syndrome (AIDS), or other immune disease

         (2) Chemotherapy, biological therapy

         (3) Radiation therapy

         (4) Infection, sepsis

         (5) Recent surgery

         (6) Medications (phenothiazines, phenytoin [Dilantin], chloramphenicol)

         (7) Recent travel to third-world country

  2) Objective data

      a) Physical examination

         (1) Fever, tachycardia, low to normal blood pressure, increased respiratory effort

         (2) Decreased skin turgor, pallor

         (3) Signs of infection

         (4) Ulcers in mouth (aphthous, herpetic)

      b) Diagnostic procedures

         (1) Total WBC count less than 5000/μL

         (2) Neutrophil count less than 1000 to 1500/μL; absolute neutrophil count less than 50/μL places patient at severe risk

         (3) Peripheral blood smear is done to assess for immature forms of WBCs

         (4) Hematocrit level, reticulocyte count, and platelet count are done to evaluate general bone marrow function

         (5) Chest radiograph

         (6) ECG as appropriate

         (7) Culture blood, urine, stool, wounds, sputum, CSF as appropriate

  b. Analysis: differential nursing diagnosis/collaborative problems

    1) Risk for infection related to decreased neutrophils and altered response to microbial invasion and presence of environmental pathogens

  c. Planning/interventions

    1) Place patient in private room as soon as possible

    2) Establish IV access for administration of antibiotics

    3) Dilute all medications, and administer carefully to minimize vein irritation

    4) Administer antipyretics (acetaminophen)

    5) Prepare for use of cooling blankets and other techniques to lower temperature

    6) Monitor temperature, pulse, and blood pressure carefully; be alert for signs of possible septic shock

    7) Maintain adequate hydration with oral or IV fluids

    8) Observe for new signs of infection

    9) Use good hand-washing techniques, and limit number of personnel in room

   10) Implement nursing care measures for patient with immunosuppression

      a) Do not use supplies from common area for immunosuppressed patient

      b) Obtain specimens of all suspicious areas for culture

      c) Wear mask when entering the room

      d) Avoid use of indwelling urinary catheter

   11) Administer granulocyte colony-stimulating factor (G-CSF; filgrastim [Neupogen]) and granulocyte-macrophage CSF (GM-CSF; sargramostim [Leukine, Prokine]): to stimulate production of neutrophils

  d. Expected outcomes/evaluation (see Appendix B)

BIBLIOGRAPHY

Bowers, A. C., & Thompson, J. M. (1992). *Clinical manual of health assessment* (4th ed.). St. Louis, MO: Mosby–Year Book.

Clochesy, J. M., Breu, C., Cardin, S., Whittaker, A. A., & Rudy, E. B. (1996). *Critical care nursing* (2nd ed.). Philadelphia: W. B. Saunders.

Guyton, A. C., & Hall, J. E. (1996). *Textbook of medical physiology* (9th ed.). Philadelphia: W. B. Saunders.

Ignatavicius, D. D., Workman, M. L., & Mishler, M. A. (1997). *Medical-surgical nursing: A nursing process approach* (2nd ed.). Philadelphia: W. B. Saunders.

Kelley, W. N. (1997). *Textbook of internal medicine* (3rd ed.). Philadelphia: Lippincott-Raven.

Kitt, S., Selfridge-Thomas, J., Proehl, J. A., & Kaiser, J. (1995). *Emergency nursing: A physiologic and clinical perspective* (2nd ed.). Philadelphia: W. B. Saunders.

Lewis, S. M., Collier, I. C., & Heitkemper, M. M. (1996). *Medical surgical nursing* (4th ed.). St Louis, MO: Mosby–Year Book.

Luckmann, J. (1997). *Saunders manual of nursing care*. Philadelphia, PA: W. B. Saunders.

McCorkle, R., Grant, M., Frank-Stromborg, M., & Baird, S. B. (1996). *Cancer nursing: A comprehensive textbook* (2nd ed.). Philadelphia: W. B. Saunders.

Newberry, L. (1998). *Sheehy's emergency nursing principles and practice* (4th ed.). St. Louis, MO: Mosby–Year Book.

Rakel, R. E. (1995). *Textbook of family practice* (5th ed.). Philadelphia: W. B. Saunders.

Rosen, R., & Barkin, R. M. (1998). *Emergency medicine: Concepts and clinical practice* (4th ed.). St. Louis, MO: Mosby–Year Book.

Thompson, J. M., McFarland, G. K., Hirsch, J. E., & Tucker, S. M. (1997). *Mosby's clinical nursing* (4th ed.). St Louis, MO: Mosby–Year Book.

Tierney, L. M., McPhee, S. J., & Papadakis, M. A. (1997). *CURRENT medical diagnosis & treatment 1997* (36th ed.). Stamford, CT: Appleton & Lange.

Tintinalli, J. E., Ruiz, E., & Krome, R. L. (1996). *Emergency medicine: A comprehensive study guide* (4th ed.). New York: McGraw-Hill.

Cynthia S. Baxter, RN, BSN, CCRN, CEN

CHAPTER **9**

Genitourinary Emergencies

MAJOR TOPICS

I. GENERAL STRATEGY

A. Assessment

1. **Primary survey** (see Chapter 1)
2. **Secondary survey** (see Chapter 1)
3. **Psychological, social, and environmental risk factors**
   a. *Personal habits*
      1) Unprotected sexual activity
      2) Multiple sexual partners
      3) New sexual partner in last 2 months
      4) Decreased fluid intake
      5) Immobility
      6) Diet high in oxalates
      7) Poor perineal hygiene
   b. *Other risk factors*
      1) Pregnancy
      2) Diabetes
      3) Gout

        4) Spinal cord injury

        5) Previous infections

        6) Recent genitourinary instrumentation, including Foley catheter insertion

        7) Use of lap restraint over distended abdomen

        8) Presence of pelvic fracture

        9) Extremes of age

4. Focused survey

  a. Subjective data

    1) History of present illness

      a) Pain: PQRST (*p*rovocation, *q*uality, *r*egion/radiation, *s*everity, *t*iming)

      b) Discharge: vaginal, urethral, rectal (onset, color, character, odor, amount)

      c) Change in urine/urinary elimination patterns (frequency, dysuria, urgency, hematuria, odor, oliguria/anuria, dribbling/incontinence, enuresis, nocturia)

      d) Injury (mechanism, treatment before arrival, previous injuries, use of foreign objects)

      e) Fever and chills

      f) Change in eating/feeding patterns (nausea, vomiting, anorexia)

      g) Tissue/skin changes (swelling, rash, turgor, deformity, pallor/cyanosis, open wounds)

      h) Lethargy or irritability

      i) Sexual history (active, orientation, safe sex practices)

    2) Medical history

      a) Trauma

      b) Surgery/urethral instrumentation

      c) Renal disease

      d) Urinary or pelvic infections

      e) Sexually transmitted diseases (STDs)

      f) Other chronic diseases

      g) Current medication history

      h) Medication allergies

      i) Immunization status

  b. Objective data

    1) Physical examination

      a) General survey

        (1) General appearance/activity

        (2) Level of consciousness

          (a) Restless or irritable

          (b) Lethargic

        (3) Vital signs

      b) Inspection

        (1) Guarding with movement

        (2) Wound: open or closed

        (3) Presence of visible foreign objects

        (4) Odor

        (5) Presence of discharge, bleeding, inflammation, rash, lesions

        (6) Asymmetry or deformity of affected part

      c) Auscultation

        (1) Bowel sounds

        (2) Fetal heart tones if pregnant

      d) Percussion
        (1) Bladder distention
        (2) Costovertebral angle tenderness
      e) Palpation
        (1) Areas of tenderness
        (2) Abdomen: soft, nontender; tender, rigid, rebound, mass, guarding
        (3) Testes: should be firm and mobile; presence of swelling or nodules
      f) Focused exam to area of complaint
  2) Diagnostic procedures
      a) Laboratory studies
        (1) Urine dipstick: blood, leukocytes, nitrite
        (2) Urinalysis
        (3) Urine culture and sensitivity
        (4) Urine stone analysis
        (5) Complete blood count with differential and platelets
        (6) Serum electrolytes with BUN/creatinine
        (7) Prothrombin time (PT)/partial thromboplastin time (PTT)
        (8) Type, cross-match blood
        (9) Gram's stain
       (10) Gonococcus (GC) culture
       (11) *Chlamydia* culture
       (12) Wet mount: saline and potassium hydroxide (KOH)
       (13) Cytological smear
       (14) Test for syphilis: rapid plasma reagin (RPR)
      b) Radiographic studies
        (1) Abdomen (kidney, urethra, bladder [KUB]): flat plate, upright
        (2) Retrograde urethrogram
        (3) Cystogram
        (4) Intravenous pyelogram (IVP)
        (5) Ultrasonogram
        (6) Computed tomography scan (CT)/magentic resonance imaging (MRI)
        (7) Renal arteriogram

B. Analysis: differential nursing diagnosis/collaboration problems

1. **Altered urinary elimination**
2. **Anxiety/fear**
3. **Body image disturbance**
4. **Fluid volume deficit**
5. **Fluid volume excess**
6. **Ineffective breathing pattern**
7. **Impaired gas exchange**
8. **Knowledge deficit**
9. **Pain**
10. **Risk for altered tissue perfusion**
11. **Risk for decreased cardiac output**
12. **Risk for infection**

C. Planning/interventions

1. **Determine priorities**
   a. *Control and maintain airway, breathing, circulation (airway, breathing, circulation)*
   b. *Prevent complications*
   c. *Control pain*
   d. *Relieve anxiety or apprehension*
   e. *Educate patient and/or significant others*
2. **Develop nursing care specific to patient's presenting emergency**
3. **Obtain and set up necessary equipment and supplies**
4. **Institute appropriate interventions based on nursing care plan**
5. **Record data as appropriate**

D. Expected outcomes/evaluation

1. **Monitor patient responses and outcomes, adjusting nursing care as indicated**
   a. *Specific interventions*
   b. *Disposition/discharge planning*
      1) Written instructions
      2) Appropriate referrals
2. **Record all pertinent data**
3. **If positive outcomes are not demonstrated, re-evaluate assessment and/or plan of care**

E. Age-related considerations

1. **Pediatric**
   a. *Growth or developmental related*
      1) Increased risk for testicular torsion during the first year of life and during adolescence
      2) Enuresis may be presenting symptom for urinary tract infection (UTI)
      3) Infants may need suprapubic tap
   b. *"Pearls"*
      1) Child may fear punishment for insertion of foreign bodies
      2) Feeling of "immortality" by young adults may explain decreased use of barrier method of contraception (safe sexual practices)
      3) STD in young children may indicate child abuse
2. **Geriatric**
   a. *Age related*
      1) At risk for UTIs/calculi if immobile
      2) Epididymitis associated with bacterial causes
   b. *"Pearls"*
      1) May have decreased fluid intake, increasing risk for UTIs and calculi
      2) Prostatic hypertrophy may be cause of bladder distension
      3) As females age, occurrence of UTIs increases

II. Specific genitourinary emergencies

A. Acute renal failure

Acute renal failure causes an accumulation of waste products in the blood (BUN, creatinine, protein breakdown by-products) in addition to dangerous fluid and electrolyte imbalances. It can occur as a result of prerenal, renal, or postrenal causes (Table 9–1) or as an acute episode in a patient with chronic renal failure. Regardless of the specific cause, prerenal failure develops when the kidney is not adequately perfused with blood and, therefore, the kidney is unable to filter the blood or regulate fluid and electrolytes. The goal is to correct the underlying cause and provide the kidney adequate perfusion. Postrenal failure develops when the outflow of urine output backs up through the urinary system, causing hydronephrosis and pressure on the renal parenchyma and resulting in ischemia. Treatment is aimed at relieving the obstruction. Intrarenal failure can result from untreated prerenal and postrenal causes as well as toxic exposures, trauma, and inflammation. Treatment consists of treating the underlying causes and preventing repeated toxic exposures. Hyperkalemia, hyponatremia, hypocalcemia, hyperphosphatemia, volume overload, and metabolic acidosis are the most common fluid and electrolyte imbalances in acute renal failure. Indications for emergency dialysis are coma or stupor, volume overload and pulmonary edema, life-threatening hyperkalemia, and acidosis. Depending on the underlying cause and treatment course, acute renal failure may be reversed or may result in renal insufficiency or failure.

1. **Assessment**
    a. *Subjective data*
        1) History of present illness
            a) Shortness of breath
            b) Decreased or alteration in urinary output
            c) Chest pain
            d) Nausea, vomiting, diarrhea or constipation, anorexia
            e) Longer bleeding time

Table 9–1   CAUSES OF THE THREE TYPES OF ACUTE RENAL FAILURE

Pathological Change	Causes
Prerenal	
Decreased blood flow to the kidneys leading to ischemia in the nephrons; prolonged hypoperfusion can lead to tubular necrosis and ARF	• Conditions that cause decreased cardiac output: • Shock • CHF • Pulmonary embolism • Anaphylaxis • Pericardial tamponade • Sepsis
Intrarenal (Intrinsic)	
Actual tissue damage to the kidney caused by inflammatory or immunological processes or from prolonged hypoperfusion	• Acute interstitial nephritis • Exposure to nephrotoxins • Acute glomerulonephritis • Vasculitis • Hepatorenal syndrome • ATN • Renal artery or vein stenosis/thrombosis
Postrenal	
Obstruction of the urinary collecting system anywhere from the calices to the urethral meatus Obstruction of the bladder must be bilateral to cause postrenal failure unless only one kidney is functional	• Urethral or bladder cancer • Renal calculi • Atony of bladder • Prostatic hyperplasia or cancer • Cervical cancer • Urethral stricture

ARF, acute renal failure; CHF, congestive heart failure; ATN, acute tubular necrosis. From Ignatavicius, D. D., Workman, M. L., & Mishler, M. A. (1995). *Medical-surgical nursing* (2nd ed., p. 2148). Philadelphia: W. B. Saunders. Used with permission.

f) Lethargy, memory impairment

g) Increase in body weight

h) Edema

2) Medical history

a) History specific to underlying causes

b) Current acute and chronic illnesses

c) Medications

d) Allergies

b. *Objective data*

1) Physical examination

a) General survey

b) Dialysis fistula, graft, or catheter

2) Diagnostic procedures

a) Urinalysis

b) Serum electrolytes, especially serum potassium, BUN, creatinine

c) Electrocardiogram (ECG)

d) Chest x-ray film

e) Renal and/or abdominal ultrasound

f) CT scan of abdomen, kidneys without contrast

g) IVP, retrograde pyelogram

h) Renal arteriogram (may not be performed because of dye load and risk of further renal damage)

i) Hemodynamic monitoring; pulmonary artery catheter

2. **Analysis: differential nursing diagnosis/collaborative problems**

a. *Fluid volume excess related to acute renal failure and hypervolemia*

b. *Ineffective breathing pattern related to fluid volume excess and pulmonary overload*

c. *Altered tissue perfusion related to decreased renal blood flow*

d. *Impaired gas exchange related to pulmonary overload, fluid volume excess*

e. *Altered urinary elimination related to acute renal failure*

f. *Risk for infection related to uremia (causes decreased response of white blood cells)*

g. *Anxiety/fear related to diagnosis, procedures, and prognosis*

h. *Pain related to calculi, obstruction*

3. **Planning/interventions**

a. *Maintain airway, breathing, circulation*

b. *Establish intravenous (IV) catheter for administration of crystalloids at low rates, medication administration*

c. *Continuously monitor*

1) Airway and breathing

2) Hemodynamic status and circulation

3) Neurological status

4) Pain

5) ECG pattern

d. *Prepare for/assist with medical interventions*

1) Radiological examinations

2) Subclavian or femoral dual lumen venous access placement for dialysis

3) Dialysis

4) Surgery

5) Pulmonary artery catheter placement

e. *Administer pharmacological therapy as ordered*

1) Antihypertensives

2) Vasopressors

3) Inotropic agents

4) Potassium binding agents: sodium polystyrene sulfonate (Kayexalate); insulin and glucose, sodium bicarbonate IV (temporary measures, last 4 hours, cause intracellular shift of potassium)

5) Diuretics

6) Analgesics

7) Nitrates

8) Calcium

f. *Allow supportive significant other to remain with patient and participate in care as appropriate*

g. *Encourage verbalization from patient/significant other regarding fear of diagnosis and procedures*

h. *Discuss cause of acute renal failure specific to patient's underlying cause, treatments, complications, outcomes*

4. **Expected outcomes/evaluation** (see Appendix B)

B. Urinary tract infection

A urinary tract infection is defined as symptomatic bacteriuria, which occurs anywhere along the urinary tract, including urethra, bladder, ureters, and kidney. (Lower urinary tract infections are discussed here; upper urinary tract infections are discussed as pyelonephritis). The causative organism for 90% of UTIs is *Escherichia coli*, but adenovirus-related hemorrhagic cystitis and other less common bacteria may be the cause. UTI occurs throughout the life span and, other than in the neonate population, females are affected 10 times more often than males because of a shorter urethra and ascending bacterial invasion. In neonates UTI may be a cause of sepsis. Circumcision reduces the risk of UTI in this population. Childhood UTIs may be related to congenital obstructive lesions and inadequate emptying of the bladder, diabetes, poor hygiene, chemical irritation from soaps and bubble baths, sexual activity, or abuse. UTIs in men younger than 50 years are most frequently associated with STDs. UTIs in men older than 50 years may be related to urethral or prostate infections or prostate obstruction. UTIs in women may be related to sexual activity, and the frequency increases with age. Susceptibility for frequent infections may have a genetic basis that involves the presence of epithelial cells that promote colonization of *E. coli*.

1. **Assessment**

   a. *Subjective data*

      1) History of present illness

         a) Pain: constant or on voiding; spasm may occur at end of urination; burning or suprapubic/lower abdomen cramping

         b) Change in urinary elimination patterns: frequency, urgency, dysuria, oliguria, night enuresis or daytime incontinence in children, hematuria, malodorous urine

         c) Poor weight gain, anorexia or poor feeding in infants and children (may be associated with septic presentation: acidosis, dehydration, pallor, hypothermia)

         d) Irritability or lethargy in infants and children (may be associated with septic presentation)

         e) Nausea, vomiting, diarrhea

         f) Fever, chills

      2) Medical history

         a) Medications

        b) Allergies

        c) Recent surgery or urethral instrumentation

        d) Chronic disease, such as diabetes

        e) Previous UTI

        f) Recent sexual activity

   b. *Objective data*

     1) Physical examination

       a) General survey

         (1) Pulse and blood pressure may be elevated as a result of pain

         (2) Orthostatic vital signs (may have decreased oral intake to avoid urination)

       b) Focused examination

         (1) Suprapubic tenderness on palpation

         (2) May need pelvic exam to rule out gynecological cause of symptoms

     2) Diagnostic procedures

       a) Urine dipstick

       b) Urinalysis (may need catheterization or suprapubic tap if unable to obtain clean catch specimen: menstruation, infants, elderly)

       c) Urine culture and sensitivity

       d) Complete blood count with differential

       e) Blood cultures

2. Analysis: differential nursing diagnosis/collaborative problems

   a. *Altered urinary elimination related to bladder inflammation/infection*

   b. *Pain related to bladder spasms and irritation*

   c. *Knowledge deficit related to cause of disease, treatment, complications, prevention of recurrence*

3. Planning/interventions

   a. *Maintain airway, breathing, circulation*

   b. *Establish IV access for administration of crystalloid solution if dehydrated or for IV antibiotics*

   c. *Continuously monitor*

     1) Urine output

     2) Amount and frequency of voiding

     3) Response to pain medications, urinary analgesics

   d. *Prepare for/assist with medical interventions*

     1) Possible pelvic examination

     2) Suprapubic tap

   e. *Administer pharmacological agents as ordered*

     1) Antibiotics

     2) Analgesics

     3) Antipyretics

   f. *Allow significant other to remain with patient and participate in care as appropriate*

   g. *Discuss cause of UTI, complications, and treatment*

   h. *Provide the following information to prevent recurrence*

     1) Finish all antibiotics

     2) Clean front to back in female perineal area

     3) Void frequently and completely

     4) Avoid bubble baths and perfumed soaps

     5) Void immediately after sexual intercourse

     6) Clean under foreskin in uncircumcised male

     7) Fruit juices and protein increase acidification of urine

     8) Increase fluid intake

9) Return for flank pain, fever, or persistent symptoms, which may indicate pyelonephritis
10) Follow-up urine culture

4. Expected outcomes/evaluation (see Appendix B)

C. Pyelonephritis

Pyelonephritis is an infection in the upper urinary tract that involves the renal parenchyma and pelvis. It is usually caused by ascending *E. coli* from the lower genitourinary tract. It is more prevalent in infants, young women who are sexually active, and older men with obstructive uropathy. Predisposing factors include pregnancy, prolonged symptoms before seeking care, an immunocompromised state, a history of three or more UTIs in the past year, and diabetes. Pyelonephritis is a serious complication of pregnancy. Pyelonephritis may not present with classic signs and symptoms, and it may occasionally be difficult to distinguish between a lower UTI and an upper UTI. Continued and untreated, pyelonephritis may lead to scarring of renal tissue, causing renal insufficiency.

1. Assessment
  a. *Subjective data*
    1) History of present illness
      a) Pain at costovertebral angle/flank, unilateral, dull, increased on palpation/urination; may radiate along subcostal area toward umbilicus, especially in children, or may radiate to lower abdomen
      b) Fever, chills
      c) Recent UTI or STD
      d) Anorexia, feeding difficulties, nausea, and vomiting, especially in young children or infants (may be part of sepsis presentation)
      e) Dysuria, frequency and/or hematuria
      f) Newly developed enuresis in children
      g) Lethargy or irritability, especially in children (may be part of a sepsis presentation)
    2) Medical history
      a) Medications
      b) Allergies
      c) Pregnant or postpartum
      d) Recurrent UTIs
      e) Solitary kidney
      f) History of renal surgery
      g) Any acute or chronic illness
  b. *Objective data*
    1) Physical examination
      a) General survey
        (1) May have elevated temperature and pulse, chills
        (2) Orthostatic vital signs
        (3) Lethargy or restlessness in infants and young children
      b) Focused examination
        (1) Costovertebral angle (CVA) tenderness
    2) Diagnostic procedures
      a) Urinalysis (may need catheterization or suprapubic tap when unable to obtain adequate clean catch such as in menstruation, infant, or elderly)
      b) Urine culture and sensitivity
      c) Complete blood count with differential

    d) BUN and electrolytes

    e) Blood cultures

    f) Abdominal radiograph if obstruction suspected

    g) Renal CT scan

    h) IVP if obstruction or renal disease suspected

2. Analysis: differential nursing diagnosis/collaborative problem

    a. *Fluid volume deficit related to fever, anorexia, nausea and vomiting, diarrhea*

    b. *Pain related to inflammatory process*

    c. *Anxiety/fear related to undiagnosed nature of illness*

    d. *Knowledge deficit related to disease, treatment, complications, prevention of recurrence*

3. Planning/intervention

    a. *Maintain airway, breathing, circulation*

    b. *Establish IV access for administration of crystalloid fluid and medication administration*

    c. *Continuously monitor*

        1) Vital signs and hemodynamic status

        2) Intake and output

        3) Color, clarity, concentration of urine

    d. *Prepare for/assist with medical interventions*

        1) IVP

        2) Suprapubic tap

    e. *Administer pharmacological therapy as ordered*

        1) Antibiotics

        2) Analgesics

        3) Antipyretics

    f. *Allow supportive other to remain with patient and participate in care as appropriate*

    g. *Encourage verbalization from patient and significant other regarding feelings of anxiety related to diagnosis*

    h. *Discuss cause, complications, treatment*

    i. *Provide information regarding prevention of recurrence (see UTIs)*

4. Expected outcomes/evaluation (see Appendix B)

D. Urinary calculi

    Urinary calculi are one of the most common urinary tract diseases. A urinary calculus, or stone, is the abnormal collection of one or many substances, including calcium, struvite, uric acid, or cystine. They vary in size and can occur anywhere along the genitourinary tract but most commonly in the renal pelvis. They may migrate and cause pain all along the genitourinary tract. Ninety percent of stones exit spontaneously. Some calculi may be associated with urinary tract infection. Risk factors for the development of urinary calculi include sedentary lifestyle; history of gout; previous calculi; frequent UTIs; large intake of protein, calcium, or fruit juices; pregnancy; and dehydration.

1. Assessment

    a. *Subjective data*

        1) History of present illness

            a) Pain: severe, colicky flank and CVA pain with a constant, dull underlying pain; may radiate to abdomen, groin, scrotum, or labia as stone migrates; may worsen with voiding; no relieving factors, unable to find a comfortable position; restlessness and irritability

        b) Dysuria

        c) Nausea and vomiting

     2) Medical history

        a) Medications

        b) Allergies

        c) Renal disease or surgery

        d) Previous calculi, history of gout or UTIs

        e) Diet high in proteins, calcium, or fruit juices

        f) Pregnant

        g) Any other acute or chronic illnesses

  b. *Objective data*

     1) Physical examination

        a) General survey

           (1) Fever and chills (if infection present)

           (2) Rapid pulse; elevated blood pressure; cool, clammy skin; pallor

           (3) Restlessness, irritability

        b) Focused examination

           (1) CVA tenderness

           (2) Hematuria (may not be present in complete obstruction)

           (3) May have distended abdomen if obstruction is present

     2) Diagnostic procedures

        a) Urine dipstick (for microscopic hematuria)

        b) Urinalysis

        c) Urine culture and sensitivity

        d) Complete blood count with differential

        e) Serum electrolytes and BUN, creatinine

        f) Serum uric acid

        g) Stone analysis

        h) KUB

        i) Renal CT scan

        j) IVP

2. Analysis: differential nursing diagnosis/collaborative problems

  a. *Pain related to obstruction or stone movement*

  b. *Altered urinary elimination related to obstruction*

  c. *Risk for infection related to urinary stasis caused by obstruction*

  d. *Anxiety/fear related to pain, undiagnosed nature of illness, diagnostic procedures*

  e. *Knowledge deficit related to disease, treatment, complications, and prevention of recurrence*

3. Planning/interventions

  a. *Maintain airway, breathing, circulation*

  b. *Establish IV access for administration of crystalloid fluid for medication administration and volume*

  c. *Continuously monitor*

     1) Pain

     2) Frequency, amount, concentration, color, and clarity of urine: strain all urine and send solids to lab for stone analysis

     3) Hemodynamic status

  d. *Prepare for/assist with medical interventions*

     1) Radiological studies

     2) Admission criteria: pain requiring repeated doses of IV analgesics; infection; inability to take oral fluids; solitary kidney; presence of ileus; high-

grade obstruction; underlying renal insufficiency; stones larger than 6-mm wide

e. *Administer pharmacological therapy as ordered*
  1) Analgesics
  2) Antibiotics
  3) Antipyretics

f. *Allow supportive other to remain with patient and participate in care as appropriate*

g. *Encourage verbalization from patient and significant other regarding anxiety related to diagnosis, pain, treatment*

h. *Discuss cause, complications, treatment*

i. *Provide information regarding recurrence*
  1) Increased risk in majority of patients with previous calculi
  2) Dietary changes depending on stone analysis
    a) Calcium: avoid spinach, rhubarb, parsley, chocolate, cocoa, instant coffee, tea, large amounts of milk
    b) Uric acid: avoid sardines, herring, liver, kidney, goose
  3) Increase fluid intake

j. *Provide information concerning potential complications and need to return for evaluation with recurrence of severe pain, excessive vomiting, fever, chills*

k. *Instruct patients to strain the urine for up to 72 hours after pain relief to retrieve stones for chemical analysis*

4. **Expected outcome/evaluation** (see Appendix B)

E. Testicular torsion

Testicular torsion results from the bilateral maldevelopment of fixation between the testes and the posterior scrotal wall. Unilateral cremaster muscle contraction results in torsion of the unfixated testicle. Testicular circulation is compromised by twisting of the spermatic cord. Two thirds of all cases occur between the ages of 12 and 18 years in conjunction with maximal hormone stimulation at puberty, but it may occur at any age. If detorsion and orchiopexy (surgical fixation of testes to scrotal wall) are performed within 4 hours, the testicular salvage rate is 80%. If more than 12 hours have elapsed, salvage rate drops to 20% and necessitates an orchiectomy (removal of the ischemic testicle). Contralateral orchiopexy is usually performed because of the increased risk of torsion for the contralateral testicle. Less than 50% of patients with testicular torsion will present with the classic clinical manifestations. Diagnosis is made by clinical findings and Doppler ultrasonography to differentiate testicular torsion from epididymitis.

1. **Assessment**
  a. *Subjective date*
    1) History of present illness
      a) Testicular pain: rapid onset; severe; may radiate to lower abdomen and inguinal canal; not relieved by elevation or ice; may occur during exertion or more often during sleep (50%)
      b) Nausea and vomiting possible
    2) Medical history
      a) Medications
      b) Allergies
      c) Previous episode that spontaneously resolved is reported by approximately one third of patients

    b. Objective data
       1) Physical examination
          a) General survey
             (1) May have rapid pulse
             (2) Pallor
             (3) Normal or low-grade fever
          b) Testicular examination
             (1) Variable amount of scrotal swelling, redness, tenderness, firmness on affected side
             (2) Elevated testes on affected side
             (3) Horizontal (vs. vertical) lie of testicle with epididymis displaced anteriorly
             (4) Elevated testis and absence of cremasteric reflex on affected side
       2) Diagnostic procedures
          a) Urinalysis: absence of significant pyuria (inflammatory vs. infectious event)
          b) Complete blood count
          c) Doppler ultrasound flow study

2. Analysis: differential nursing diagnosis/collaborative problems
    a. Tissue perfusion, altered testicular function related to interruption of blood flow
    b. Pain related to ischemia of testicle
    c. Anxiety/fear related to pain, undiagnosed nature of illness

3. Planning/interventions
    a. Maintain airway, breathing, circulation
    b. Establish IV for crystalloid fluid administration, analgesics and/or conscious sedation
    c. Continuously monitor
       1) Pain
       2) Airway and breathing with conscious sedation
    d. Prepare for/assist with medical interventions
       1) Doppler ultrasonography
       2) Manual detorsion
       3) Urologic consultation and surgery
    e. Administer pharmacological therapy as ordered
       1) Analgesics
       2) Sedatives
       3) Preoperative antibiotics
    f. Provide as much privacy as possible
    g. Discuss cause, interventions, and outcomes to alleviate anxiety
    h. Allow parents or significant other to remain with patient and participate in care as appropriate
    i. Encourage verbalization from patient of feelings of anxiety and fear

4. Expected outcomes/evaluation (see Appendix B)

F. Epididymitis

    Epididymitis is an inflammatory process within the epididymis and is generally seen in adult males. In the pediatric population, congenital anomalies of the lower urinary tract may cause a chemical epididymitis from retrograde reflux of sterile urine into the epididymis. In men younger than 40 years, epididymitis is more likely to result from an STD or be a complication of a stricture. For men older than 40 years, common urinary pathogens such as *E. coli* and *Klebsiella* are suspected, and infection may result from the back-up of urine from an enlarged prostate gland. As the inflammation progresses, the patient presents with a large tender mass of the scrotum. Epididymitis may be difficult to differentiate from torsion or carcinoma.

1. **Assessment**
   a. *Subjective data*
      1) History of present illness
         a) Pain: gradual onset; dull ache in the scrotum or lower abdomen; increases with sexual activity; decreases with elevation (Prehn's sign) and application of ice
         b) May have urethral discharge (more common with STDs)
      2) Medical history
         a) Medications
         b) Allergies
         c) Recent urethritis and/or STD
         d) Recent urethral instrumentation
         e) Recent prostatectomy
         f) Unprotected sexual intercourse/multiple partners
   b. *Objective data*
      1) Physical examination
         a) General survey
            (1) May have rapid pulse, elevated blood pressure with pain
            (2) Fever may be present
            (3) "Duck waddle" gait (to avoid touching area while walking and causing pain)
         b) Scrotal examination
            (1) Red, swollen, warm scrotum
            (2) May have urethral discharge
      2) Diagnostic procedures
         a) Urinalysis: may have pyuria (more common with bacterial infection)
         b) Urine culture and sensitivity
         c) Gram's stain and culture of urethral discharge (STD)
         d) Complete blood count
2. **Analysis: differential nursing diagnosis/collaborative problems**
   a. *Pain related to inflammatory/infectious process*
   b. *Anxiety/fear related to concern about loss of sexual function and/or STD*
   c. *Knowledge deficit related to disease, treatment, complications, and prevention of recurrence*
3. **Planning/interventions**
   a. *Maintain airway, breathing, circulation*
   b. *Establish IV for crystalloid fluid and/or medication administration as needed (prn)*
   c. *Continuously monitor pain and response to pain relief measures*
   d. *Prepare for/assist with medical interventions*
      1) Possible ultrasonography
      2) Culture of urethral drainage
   e. *Administer pharmacological therapy as ordered*
      1) Antibiotics
      2) Analgesics
      3) Anti-inflammatories
   f. *Allow supportive significant other to remain with patient and participate in care as appropriate*
   g. *Encourage verbalization of concerns, reassure patient that scrotum will return to normal size and appearance with treatment*

   h. Discuss cause, course, and complications of disease

   i. Provide discharge instructions

     1) Finish medications as prescribed: complete entire course of antibiotics

     2) Follow up with urologist or primary care provider in 5 to 10 days for repeat culture

     3) Bed rest until pain free; begin ambulation with scrotal support

     4) Avoid lifting heavy objects or strain with bowel movements (will increase intra-abdominal pressure and exacerbate inflammatory process)

     5) Return to work will be decided at follow-up visit

   j. Explain how to prevent complications

     1) Complete treatment program

     2) Recognize and return for new or increasing symptoms

       a) Fever

       b) Increasing abdominal pain

       c) Continued dysuria, urethral discharge

     3) Safe sexual practices (condom use with each intercourse, limit sexual partners)

4. Expected outcomes/evaluation (see Appendix B)

G. Urethral injury

    Urethral injury occurs most often as the result of surgery or childbirth and may also occur as an infrequent (6–12%) consequence of blunt or penetrating trauma to the pelvis, perineum, or penis. Urethral rupture should be considered early in the management of pelvic trauma to avoid converting a partial tear to a complete transection of the urethra by insertion of a urinary catheter. The insertion of foreign bodies into the urethra should also raise the suspicion of a urethral injury.

1. Assessment

   a. Subjective data

     1) History of present illness

       a) Suprapubic, perineal, or genital pain related to voiding and/or bladder distention

       b) Feeling unable to void

       c) Hematuria

       d) Mechanism of injury

     2) Medical history

       a) Medications

       b) Allergies

       c) Tetanus status

       d) Genitourinary disease or surgery

       e) Acute or chronic illnesses

   b. Objective data

     1) Physical examination

       a) General survey

        (1) May have increased heart rate, pallor because of pain

       b) Focused examination on the perineum, lower abdomen, urinary meatus

        (1) Blood at urinary meatus

        (2) Swelling of suprapubic area (bladder distention) or genitalia/perineum (trauma or extravasation of urine)

        (3) Hematoma of lower abdomen or perineum (butterfly shaped resulting from straddle injury)

        (4) Local abrasions or lacerations

2) Diagnostic procedures
   a) Complete blood count with differential
   b) Serial hematocrits with suspicion of pelvic fracture
   c) Type and cross-match blood with suspicion of pelvic fracture
   d) PT/PTT
   e) Urinalysis
   f) Abdominal and pelvic radiographs
   g) Retrograde urethrogram
   h) Cystography (to determine minor injury or patency)

2. **Analysis: differential nursing diagnosis/collaborative problems**
   a. *Altered urinary elimination related to edema or injury to urethra*
   b. *Pain related to urethral trauma, inability to void*
   c. *Anxiety/fear related to loss of function, diagnostic tests, surgery*
   d. *Risk for fluid volume deficit related to possible pelvic trauma and blood loss*
   e. *Risk for infection related to altered integrity of the urethra*

3. **Planning/interventions**
   a. *Maintain airway, breathing, circulation*
   b. *Establish IV access for crystalloid fluid, possible blood products (with pelvic fracture), analgesics, diagnostic procedures*
   c. *Continue to monitor intake and output, urinary elimination patterns*
   d. *Prepare for/assist with medical interventions*
      1) Catheterization (defer to physician) or suprapubic tap
      2) Cystography
      3) Prepare for surgery
   e. *Administer pharmacological therapy as ordered*
      1) Analgesics
      2) Antibiotics
   f. *Allow supportive other to remain with patient and participate in care as appropriate*
   g. *Encourage verbalization from patient and significant other regarding anxiety and fear related to diagnostic tests and treatment*
   h. *Discuss cause, treatment, complications (impotence, incontinence, and severe stricture) and self-care: rest, fluids, elevation, and ice packs (for injury without a tear)*

4. **Expected outcomes/evaluation** (see Appendix B)

H. Ruptured bladder

Ruptured bladder is an uncommon injury, occurring only 2% of the time with concomitant abdominal injury and 5 to 10% of the time with pelvic fractures. Children are more susceptible to direct-force bladder injuries because of bladder location. A full bladder increases the risk of injury in all ages. Ruptures may involve extravasation of blood and urine into the abdomen. Seventy to 80% of bladder injuries are associated with pelvic fractures, and hemodynamic instability may be present as a result of large amounts of blood loss from pelvic vessels. The majority of injuries occur secondary to blunt trauma.

1. **Assessment**
   a. *Subjective data*
      1) History of present illness
         a) Pain: suprapubic, dull, constant or sharp; may be related to voiding or inability to void; gradually increases
         b) Possible nausea and vomiting resulting from pain
         c) Inability to void

d) Possible hematuria
2) Medical history
a) Medications
b) Tetanus status
c) Allergies
d) Renal disease
b. *Objective data*
1) Physical examination
a) General survey
(1) May have increased heart rate, low blood pressure as a result of bleeding
(2) Pallor if pain or bleeding is present
b) Focused abdominal, pelvic, and perineum examination
(1) Abdominal tenderness, rebound tenderness, distended or rigid abdomen related to extravasation of urine or intra-abdominal bleeding
(2) Lower abdominal or perineal hematoma
(3) Abrasions or lacerations over suprapubic or perineal area
2) Diagnostic procedures
a) Complete blood count with differential, platelet count
b) Serial hematocrits
c) PT/PTT
d) Type and cross-match blood
e) Urinalysis
f) Abdominal and pelvic radiographs
g) Retrograde urethrogram
h) Cystography
i) Pelvic ultrasonogram, CT scan
j) IVP

2. **Analysis: differential nursing diagnosis/collaborative problems**
a. *Risk for fluid volume deficit related to blood loss from pelvic fracture*
b. *Decreased cardiac output related to potential hemorrhage and diminished circulating blood volume associated with pelvic fracture*
c. *Altered urinary elimination related to bladder injury*
d. *Pain related to bladder injury*
e. *Anxiety/fear related to undiagnosed nature of injury, unknown outcome, and prognosis*
f. *Risk for infection related to loss of bladder integrity related to injury*

3. **Planning/interventions**
a. *Maintain airway, breathing, circulation*
b. *Establish IV access for administration of crystalloid fluid, possible blood administration, diagnostic procedures, and medication administration*
c. *Continuously monitor*
1) Hemodynamic status
2) Urinary output
3) Pain
d. *Prepare for/assist with medical interventions*
1) Radiographical studies
2) Pelvic ultrasonography
3) Surgery
4) Catheterization (defer to physician) or suprapubic tap
e. *Administer pharmacological therapy as indicated*
1) Analgesics
2) Antibiotics

f. *Allow supportive significant other to remain with patient and participate in care as appropriate*

g. *Encourage verbalization from patient and significant other regarding pain and anxiety related to illness/injury and unknown outcome or possible surgery*

h. *Discuss cause and treatment; explain all procedures*

4. Expected outcomes (see Appendix B)

I. Renal trauma

Renal trauma seldom occurs independently, and should be considered in any patient presenting with chest, abdominal, or back trauma. There is a high incidence of occurrence of renal trauma with concomitant vertebral and flank injuries. Blunt trauma accounts for 70 to 80% of renal trauma. Of these injuries, 40 to 68% require surgical repair. The majority of severe renal pedicle injuries occur in children and young adults from an acceleration-deceleration force from motor vehicle crashes. The left renal vein is most often involved. Surgical repair is required within 12 hours to salvage the ischemic kidney. Regardless of the mechanism of injury, extrarenal or intrarenal bleeding can occur as well as urine extravasation, causing hypovolemic shock, pain, and inflammation.

1. Assessment

a. *Subjective data*

1) History of present illness

a) Mechanism of injury

b) Pain: CVA or abdominal, with varying quality depending on severity and mechanism of injury

c) Nausea and vomiting resulting from ileus, pain

2) Medical history

a) Medications

b) Allergies

c) Renal disease

d) Hypertension

e) Solitary kidney

f) History of renal surgery

g) Any other acute or chronic illness

b. *Objective data*

1) Physical examination

a) General survey

(1) May have rapid heart rate, hypotension, pallor, moist and cool skin in presence of hemorrhage

(2) Increased heart rate and blood pressure with pain

b) Focused flank, abdominal examination

(1) May have retroperitoneal hematoma; may be pulsatile

(2) Hematuria: gross, urine dipstick positive (absent in one third of patients)

(3) Oliguria or anuria

(4) Contusions, abrasions, lacerations in area of injury

(5) Decreased or absent bowel sounds as a result of colon injury, ileus

(6) CVA tenderness

2) Diagnostic procedures

a) Complete blood count with differential

b) Serial hematocrits

c) Serum electrolytes

       d) BUN, creatinine
       e) PT/PTT
       f) Urinalysis
       g) Type and cross-match blood
       h) Abdominal radiographs
       i) IVP
       j) CT scan/MRI
       k) Renal arteriogram

2. Analysis: differential nursing diagnosis/collaborative problems

   a. Decreased cardiac output related to hemorrhage and diminished circulating blood volume

   b. Tissue perfusion, altered related to hemorrhage

   c. Pain related to effects of trauma

   d. Risk for infection related to alteration in skin integrity (in penetrating trauma), possible extravasation of urine and blood

   e. Anxiety/fear related to unknown outcome of injury

3. Planning/interventions

   a. Maintain airway, breathing, circulation

   b. Establish large-bore peripheral IV access for administration of crystalloid, medications, possible blood products, and diagnostic procedures

   c. Continuously monitor

      1) Hemodynamic status
      2) Neurological status
      3) Tissue perfusion
      4) Pulse oximetry
      5) Liquid intake and output

   d. Prepare for/assist with medical interventions

      1) Blood products transfusion
      2) Radiographical and diagnostic studies
      3) Surgery

   e. Administer pharmacological therapy as ordered

      1) Tetanus toxoid
      2) Analgesics
      3) Antibiotics
      4) IV pressor support

   f. Allow supportive significant other to remain with patient and participate in care as appropriate

   g. Encourage verbalization of fear and/or anxiety related to injuries, treatment, surgery, and long-term complications (abscess, calculi, chronic pyelonephrosis, renal insufficiency)

   h. Discuss cause of injury, treatment options, complications, and procedures

4. Expected outcomes/evaluation (see Appendix B)

J. Priapism

    Priapism is a persistent, painful erection of the penis that is not associated with sexual desire. Both corpora cavernosa are engorged with stagnant blood, but the corpus spongiosum and glans penis remain soft and uninvolved. Urinary retention occurs in 50% of cases, requiring a Foley catheter. Treatment is aimed at immediate detumescence (subsiding of congestion and swelling to prevent endothelial inflammation and injury). Development of fibrosis and scarring in the cavernous spaces is related to duration of priapism and can cause impotence. Causes of priapism may be categorized as reversible and nonreversible. Reversible causes include sickle cell crisis, medications for impotence (prostaglandin E [PGE], papaverine, phentolamine) or leukemic infiltration. Idiopathic factors, high spinal cord lesions or injury, and some medications (phenothiazines, trazodone [Desyrel]) are considered nonreversible causes. Treatment includes aspiration of corporeal blood, instillation of phenylephrine (Neo-Synephrine), heparin irrigation, and shunt surgery. Shunt surgery includes two techniques: in one, tissue is removed to relieve obstruction; the second technique involves anastomosis of the veins between the glans and cavernosa. Supplemental oxygen, analgesia, IV fluids, and red blood cell transfusion may be included in the treatment of priapism related to sickle cell crisis.

1. **Assessment**
    a. *Subjective data*
        1) History of present illness
            a) Pain: persistent, severe, penile pain related to number of hours of erection; intensity may increase with urinary retention and sexual intercourse
        2) Medical history
            a) Allergies
            b) Medications, including psychotropic drugs
            c) History of leukemia, sickle cell disease
            d) Previous episode that spontaneously resolved
            e) Spinal cord injury
            f) Prolonged sexual stimulation
            g) History of penile or urethral neoplasm
    b. *Objective data*
        1) Physical examination
            a) General survey
                (1) Blood pressure, heart rate, respiratory rate may be elevated because of pain, bladder distention
            b) Focused penile examination
                (1) Penile erection
                (2) Bladder distention
            c) Other findings specific to underlying cause
                (1) Long bone, joint, and spine pain with sickling
                (2) Fatigue, fever, weight loss, bone pain with leukemia
                (3) Paralysis with spinal cord injury
        2) Diagnostic procedures
            a) Complete blood count with reticulocyte count in sickle cell anemia
            b) Radiological studies related to underlying condition
2. **Nursing diagnosis/collaborative problems**
    a. *Pain related to erection, bladder distention*
    b. *Altered urinary elimination related to urethral obstruction*
    c. *Anxiety/fear related to intimate examination, unknown outcome of illness*
    d. *Knowledge deficit related to disease process, treatment, complications, prevention, and recurrence related to primary episode of disease*
3. **Planning/interventions**
    a. *Maintain airway, breathing, circulation*
    b. *Establish IV access for administration of crystalloid solution or analgesics*
    c. *Continuously monitor*
        1) Pain
        2) Urine output
    d. *Prepare for/assist with medical interventions*
        1) Catheterization

2) Aspiration/irrigation of corpora cavernosa

3) Urological consult

4) Surgical intervention

5) Oxygen, hydration, analgesia, transfusion of packed cells for sickle cell cause

e. *Administer pharmacological therapy as ordered*

1) Analgesics

2) Phenylephrine (Neo-Synephrine)

f. *Allow supportive significant other to remain with patient and participate in care as appropriate*

g. *Encourage verbalization from patient and significant other regarding concerns about sexual function; provide information related to impotence and priapism*

h. *Discuss cause, treatment, and prevention with patient and significant other to alleviate fear and knowledge deficit*

i. *Provide as much privacy as possible during exam and treatment*

j. *Provide instructions if discharged from emergency department*

1) Return if recurs

2) Return for signs and symptoms of infection: fever, redness, drainage

3) Follow-up appointment with urologist

4) Physical and sexual activity restrictions per physician

5) Medications as prescribed (antibiotics, anti-inflammatories, analgesics)

4. **Expected outcomes/evaluation** (see Appendix B)

K. Foreign bodies

Foreign bodies may be placed in the urethra by patients of all ages, but more commonly young children. Placement of foreign bodies in or around the urethra may result from innocent exploration, from attempts to heighten sexual experience, or in a patient unable to predetermine the outcome of such an act such as one with psychiatric or learning impairments. Embarrassment or fear of punishment frequently delays the patient's request for help until pain or infection are present.

1. **Assessment**

a. *Subjective data*

1) History of present illness

a) Pain: urethral pain that may be sharp or dull or sensation of pressure without relieving factors; may be constant or occur only on voiding

b) Patient admits to inserting foreign body into urethra

c) Change in urinary patterns: inability to void, dysuria, oliguria

2) Medical history

a) Medications

b) Tetanus status

c) Allergies

d) Previous foreign body placement

e) Psychiatric or learning impairments

b. *Objective data*

1) Physical examination

a) General survey

(1) Increased blood pressure, pulse, or respiratory rate as a result of pain

b) Focused urethral examination

(1) Hematuria, gross or on dipstick

(2) Urethral discharge (color, odor, consistency), blood at meatus

(3) Foreign object may be visible at urethral meatus

2) Diagnostic procedures

a) Urinalysis

b) Urethral culture if object has been present for prolonged time or signs of infection

c) KUB

d) Cystoscope/retrograde urethrography

2. **Analysis: differential nursing diagnosis/collaborative problems**

a. *Pain related to presence of foreign body, trauma, or inflammatory response*

b. *Altered urinary elimination as a result of presence of foreign body*

c. *Risk for infection related to presence of foreign body*

d. *Anxiety/fear related to pain, alteration in elimination patterns, potential loss of sexual function, and procedures*

3. **Planning/interventions**

a. *Maintain airway, breathing, circulation*

b. *Establish IV for administration of crystalloid fluid, analgesics, and/or conscious sedation for removal of foreign body or examination*

c. *Continuously monitor*

1) Urine output

2) Bladder distension

3) Pain

d. *Prepare for/assist with medical interventions*

1) Possible cystoscope/retrograde urethrography

2) Conscious sedation

3) Possible manual removal

4) Surgery

e. *Administer pharmacological therapy as ordered*

1) Conscious sedation

2) Analgesics

3) Antibiotics

4) Tetanus immunization

f. *Allow supportive significant other to remain with patient and provide care as appropriate*

g. *Encourage verbalization from patient and/or significant other regarding concerns about embarrassment or sexual function*

h. *Discuss treatment and outcomes with patient and significant other*

i. *Provide knowledge for self-care on discharge*

1) Medications: antibiotics, analgesics

2) Monitor urine output

3) Hydration, force fluids

4) Return if stream force declines, bloody urine does not resolve/improve, urine output declines

4. **Expected outcomes/evaluation** (see Appendix B)

BIBLIOGRAPHY

Barnett, S. (1997). Urinary tract infection: An overview. *American Journal of the Medical Sciences, 314*(4), 245.

Bellinger, M. (1994). Spermatic cord torsion: A true emergency. *Emergency Medicine, 26*(16), 50.

Drach, G. (1992). *Campbell's urology* (6th ed., vol. 3). Philadelphia: W. B. Saunders.

Miller, K. (1996). Urinary tract infections: Children are not little adults. *Pediatric Nursing, 22*(6), 473.

Newberry, L. (1998). *Sheehy's emergency nursing principles and practice* (4th ed.). St. Louis, MO: Mosby–Year Book.

Propp, D. (1989). Reliability of a urine dipstick in emergency department patient. *Annals of Emergency Medicine, 18*(5), 560.

Ruth-Sand, L. (1995). Renal calculi. *American Journal of Nursing, 95*(11), 50.

Schrier, R. W. (1994). *Manual of nephrology* (4th ed.). Boston: Little, Brown.

Smith, M., & Singer, C. (1992). Sexually transmitted viruses other than HIV and papillomavirus. *Urology Clinics of North America, 19*(1), 47.

Tintinalli, J. E., Ruiz, E., & Kromel, R. L. (1996). *Emergency medicine: A comprehensive review.* New York: McGraw-Hill.

Tonetti, J., & Tonetti, F. (1990). Testicular torsion or acute epididymitis? Diagnosis and treatment. *Journal of Emergency Nursing, 16*(2), 96.

Wirtz, K. M., LaFavor, K. M., & Ang, R. (1996). Managing chronic spinal cord injury: Issues in critical care. *Critical Care Nurse, 16*(4), 24.

Gail E. Polli, RN, MS, CS
Susan Engman Lazear, RN, MN, CEN, CFRN

CHAPTER **10**

Mental Health Emergencies

MAJOR TOPICS

General Strategy

Specific Mental Health Emergencies

Anxiety and Panic Reactions

Ineffective Coping and Situational Crisis

Depression

Grief

Suicide or Suicidal Behavior

Homicidal or Violent Behavior

Psychotic Behavior

Bipolar Disorder

Child Abuse/Neglect

Battered Adult

Elder Abuse/Neglect

I. GENERAL STRATEGY

A. Assessment

1. **Primary survey/resuscitation** (see Chapter 1)
2. **Secondary survey** (see Chapter 1)
3. **Psychological, social, environmental factors**
   a. *Family history of mental health disorders*
   b. *Situational stress*
   c. *Biochemical imbalances*
   d. *Underlying medical or mental health disorder*
   e. *Lack of social support system or network*
      1) Broken family relationships
      2) Gang membership
      3) Disintegration of social relationships
   f. *Lack of knowledge and availability of community support or rehabilitative services*
   g. *Loss of control/violence*
   h. *Fear*
   i. *Guilt or anger*
   j. *Poor self-image or self-esteem*

    k. Unhealthy work life

4. Focused survey

  a. Subjective data

    1) History of present illness: patient's perspective and that of significant others

      a) Behavioral changes

      b) Somatic symptoms

      c) Hallucinations or thought disturbances

      d) Thoughts of harming oneself or others

      e) Precipitating event

      f) Injury: mechanism and time

        (1) Unintentional

        (2) Intentional

    2) Medical history

      a) Previous similar episodes

      b) Mental health history

      c) Hospitalizations: to determine chronicity and frequency of disturbances

      d) Chronic illness (especially affecting neurological function or mental status)

        (1) Diabetes

        (2) Alcoholism/drug dependency

        (3) Central nervous system (CNS) disorders such as Guillain-Barré syndrome, multiple sclerosis, and amyotrophic lateral sclerosis

        (4) Head trauma

      e) Medication history

        (1) Psychotropic drugs

        (2) Anticonvulsants

        (3) Hypoglycemic agents

        (4) Drugs of abuse

  b. Objective data

    1) Physical examination

      a) General survey

        (1) Level of consciousness: alert or lethargic

        (2) Appearance: unkempt/anxious

        (3) Head-to-toe observation for injury

        (4) Psychomotor activity: tics or tremors, which may be evidence of dystonic reaction; altered gait; disequilibrium; agitated or retarded movements

      b) Vital signs

      c) Mental status examination

      d) Pupils: size and reactivity

      e) Musculoskeletal examination to rule out or confirm organic causes of presenting symptoms

        (1) Range of motion

        (2) Deep tendon reflexes

        (3) Coordination and movement

      f) Neurological examination to rule out or confirm organic causes of presenting symptoms (see Chapter 12)

    2) Diagnostic procedures

      a) Electrocardiography (ECG): cardiac monitoring and 12- to 15-lead ECG if tricyclic antidepressant overdose is suspected or somatic symptoms suggest cardiac origin

      b) Laboratory

        (1) Blood glucose level for any change in mental status

(2) Complete blood count (CBC) if trauma or infection suspected

(3) Serum electrolyte levels if imbalance suspected as cause of behavioral symptoms

(4) Toxicology screen: urine levels to determine presence of toxic substances and blood levels to determine toxins identified in urine

(5) Therapeutic drug levels for patients taking prescribed medications

(6) Thyroid function tests to determine whether endocrine abnormalities are producing mental health symptoms

(7) Liver function tests if hepatic insufficiency or failure is suspected

(8) Renal function tests if renal dysfunction is suspected

(9) Arterial blood gas (ABG) values if respiratory difficulties suspected as cause of behavioral change

B. Analysis: differential nursing diagnosis/collaborative problems

1. **Anxiety**
2. **Impaired verbal communication**
3. **Ineffective coping**
4. **Self-esteem disturbance**
5. **Altered family processes**
6. **Sleep pattern disturbance**
7. **Sensory/perceptual alterations**
8. **Altered thought processes**

C. Planning/interventions

1. **Determine priorities of care**
   a. *Control and maintain airway, breathing, circulation*
   b. *Maintain safety of patient, patient's significant others, other patients, staff*
      1) Remove guns, knives, matches, other devices that could harm patient or others
      2) Restrain patient if necessary
      3) For acutely agitated patients, consider chemical restraints
      4) For patient who expectorates, secure surgical mask over patient's face
   c. *Assess for life-threatening emergencies*
   d. *Prevent complications*
   e. *Provide appropriate environmental setting*
   f. *Implement therapeutic modalities*
   g. *Educate patient and family/significant other*
2. **Develop nursing care plan specific to patient's presenting emergency**
3. **Obtain and set up necessary equipment and supplies**
4. **Institute appropriate interventions on basis of nursing care plan**
5. **Record data as appropriate**

D. Expected outcomes/evaluation (see Appendix B)

E. Age-related considerations

1. **Pediatric**
   a. *Growth or development related*
      1) Appropriate behavior varies with age (Table 10–1)
      2) Many disorders have age-specific onset; others cross all age groups or occur at various points along age continuum (Table 10–2)

Table 10–1   DEVELOPMENTAL TASKS OF INFANCY, EARLY CHILDHOOD, CHILDHOOD, AND ADOLESCENCE

Infancy (0–18 months)	Childhood (6–12 years)
• Attempts to develop secure attachments to primary caretaker • Begins to determine own effectiveness in getting others to meet needs • Begins to determine level of trust in relationship to environment	• Developing a sense of competency and achievement • Developing increased responsibility for own behavior • Understanding importance of peer relationships: seeks acceptance from peers, especially same-sexed peers; participates in mutual sharing with peers • Increased initiative and risk taking • Demonstrates concrete problem-solving skills

Early Childhood (10 months–6 years)	Adolescence (12–18 years)
• Begins to develop "sense of self": growing perception of separateness from caretakers • Develops sense of self-discipline (e.g., delayed gratification) • Developing sense of individualism in decision making (e.g., ability to say "no") • Developing cooperative abilities (e.g., play) • Increasing use of language to meet needs • Increasing exploration of own body • Develops increased socializing behaviors with peers	• Testing out family's values and developing own set of standards and values • Increased independent decision making (symbolically moving away from family) • Coming to grips with own sexuality and sexual roles • Increased intimacy in peer relations • Increased ability to utilize abstract problem-solving skills and judgment in life situations

Adapted with permission from McFarland, G. K., & Thomas, M. D. (Eds.). (1990). *Psychiatric mental health nursing: Application of the nursing process*. Philadelphia: J. B. Lippincott.

    b. *"Pearls"*
       1) It is often difficult to determine whether behavior is abnormal or merely part of normal adjustment to life's developmental challenges; if behavior seriously interferes with personal, family, or social adjustment, it is most likely deviant and in need of attention
       2) Many children and adolescents rely on acting-out behaviors to express emotions: signifies a problem when behaviors are socially or culturally unacceptable; these children or adolescents may come to the attention of emergency department (ED) personnel when they are brought in by police, school, or family

2. Geriatric
    a. *Age related*
       1) Declining health may be contributory
       2) Most common problems include depression, suicide potential, suspiciousness and altered perceptions, anxiety, situational crisis, and sleep pattern disturbances
    b. *"Pearls"*
       1) Assessment should include risk determination of drug/alcohol abuse
       2) Thorough assessment of prescribed medication therapy and dosing schedules: certain drugs can cause depression (e.g., propranolol, chloral hydrate, digitalis, corticosteroids, and sulfonamides)
       3) Evaluation must rule out organic cause of mental health manifestations
       4) Personal losses and socioeconomic stressors, frequently seen with the older adult, can precipitate emotional disorders

Table 10–2   RELATIONSHIP BETWEEN AGE AT ONSET AND TYPE OF DISORDER EVIDENT IN CHILDREN AND ADOLESCENTS

Age Group	Disorders with Variable Onset	Disorders with Age-Specific Onset
Infancy (0–1 year)	Depression, Autistic disorder (spanning from Preschool through); Mental retardation, Elective autism, Avoidant disorder, Separation anxiety disorder (from School age); Substance abuse, Obsessive-compulsive disorder (from later School age/Adolescence); Conduct disorders (Adolescence)	Rumination disorder of infancy / Reactive attachment disorder
Toddlerhood (13–36 months)		Pica / Reactive attachment disorder / Developmental coordination disorder / Developmental expressive language disorder
Preschool (3–5 years)		Functional enuresis / Receptive language disorder / Functional encopresis / Gender identity disorder
School age (5–12 years)		Attention deficit disorder / Developmental articulation disorder / Gender identity disorder of childhood / Oppositional disorder / Developmental reading disorder / Expressive writing disorder
Adolescence (12–18 years)		Tourette's syndrome / Anorexia nervosa / Bulimia nervosa / Gender identity disorder of adolescence / Identity disorder

Adapted with permission from McFarland, G. K., & Thomas, M. D. (Eds.). (1990). *Psychiatric mental health nursing: Application of the nursing process.* Philadelphia: J. B. Lippincott.

II. SPECIFIC MENTAL HEALTH EMERGENCIES

A. Anxiety and panic reactions

Anxiety is a subjective individual experience ranging from vague discomfort to a feeling of impending disaster or death. It can be a normal response to certain events or a symptom of some underlying disease. Anxiety occurs as a result of a threat to self, self-esteem, or identity. It can be manifested as apprehension in response to known or unknown threats. Levels of anxiety range from mild to severe, including a state of panic (panic reaction) with corresponding symptoms ranging from mild discomfort to a lack of functional capability. Anxiety may heighten during developmental changes or when extreme effort is needed to cope with a situational crisis. The symptoms range from jumpiness, nervousness, and apprehension to panic states. Objective findings include cool and clammy skin, tachycardia, and tachypnea. A panic reaction is defined as extreme anxiety with personality disorganization and lack of functional abilities.

1. Assessment
  a. *Subjective data*
    1) History of present illness
      a) Previous episodes
      b) Precipitating event
      c) Measures already taken by patient that have or have not helped
      d) Family history of organic disease and anxiety disorders
      e) Occurrence during developmental cycle
        (1) Children: separation from parents
        (2) Adolescents: extreme peer pressure, perceived loss of love, failure to achieve
        (3) Adults: midlife crisis, marriage, divorce, menopause, failure to achieve goals
        (4) Elderly: loss of significant other, loss of home, increased dependence, death of friends
      f) Physical ailments that cause pain or impairment in function
      g) Impaired communication abilities resulting from cerebrovascular accident (CVA), hearing impairment, blindness, lack of language fluency
      h) Insufficiency of previously used coping patterns
      i) Acute changes in health
      j) Lack of knowledge regarding available resources
      k) Inadequate parenting patterns with abuse
      l) Recent life change (e.g., occupation, relationships, responsibilities)
      m) Difficulty with sleep
      n) Events causing anger
      o) Passivity in face of threats
      p) Feeling of impending doom, including sensation of heart attack or choking
      q) Reports of sexual difficulties, including impotence, lack of desire, dyspareunia
    2) Medical history
      a) Phobias
      b) Hyperventilation syndrome
      c) Anxiety disorder
      d) Conversion disorder
      e) Post-traumatic stress disorder
      f) Drug intoxication
      g) Medication history
  b. *Objective data*
    1) Physical examination
      a) Cardiovascular system
        (1) Heart rate increased to 120 bpm, greater than 140 bpm in panic reactions
        (2) Systolic blood pressure elevated
        (3) Temperature normal or slightly elevated
        (4) Skin cool and clammy
        (5) Premature ectopy noted on cardiac monitor
      b) Respiratory system
        (1) Rate may increase to hyperventilation
        (2) Breath sounds are normal unless anxiety has organic cause

c) Neurological system
   (1) Mental status examination results essentially normal with some impairment of judgment; patient may be hyperalert
   (2) Pupillary dilation
   (3) Ptosis (drooping of upper eyelids) may be caused by muscle fatigue, oculomotor nerve dysfunction, chronic lid edema
   (4) Skin hair erect
   (5) Nystagmus: eye movements that result from stimulation of semicircular canals and reflect oculovestibular and cerebral cortex functioning
d) Musculoskeletal system
   (1) Increased reflex responses and clumsy movements
   (2) Tremors: tense musculature
   (3) Startle reaction
   (4) Insomnia
   (5) Pacing
e) Gastrointestinal system
   (1) Dry mouth: sympathetic nervous system stimulation
   (2) Evidence of recent, rapid weight loss
   (3) Nausea and vomiting resulting from sympathetic stimulation
   (4) Cramping and diarrhea resulting from increased motility of gastrointestinal tract
   (5) Abdominal distention: sympathetic nervous system stimulation
f) Assessment for anxiety level
   (1) Level I—mild anxiety state: patient is more aware of multiple environment stimuli; is still able to problem solve; can grasp information, has insight; has slightly elevated vital sign variables
   (2) Level II—moderate anxiety state: patient is aware of environmental stimuli but focuses on immediate problem; voices concern; cooperates with caregiver; is able to follow directions or instructions; exhibits slight increase in physiological responses (facial twitches and trembling lips)
   (3) Level III—severe anxiety state: patient focuses on minute detail and does not grasp entire situation; responds to multiple stimuli, is unable to focus on priority events; demonstrates startle reaction; exhibits regressive behaviors (seen especially with children); exhibits agitation, restlessness, sleeplessness, increased pacing with no purpose; has difficulty following directions and asks for repeated directions; increases tone, pitch, rate of speech; has difficulty sustaining meaningful conversation, exhibits diminished ability to organize; is dependent on staff to problem solve; decreases eye contact; exhibits reactions that may range from total engulfment to dissociation from current problem
   (4) Level IV—panic anxiety state: patient cannot problem solve or think logically; needs safety precautions to be provided by others because of disrupted perceptual fields; appears terrorized, withdrawn, detached or shows intense nervousness and apprehensive with purposeless behavior; is disengaged from environmental situation and is totally absorbed with self; may be noncommunicative; frequently misinterprets stimuli and conversations of others; has shortness of breath, exhibits poor motor coordination, and is accident prone; has pale skin and mucous membrane color and muscle cramping; may experience personality disorganization

2. Analysis: differential nursing diagnosis/collaborative problems

a. *Anxiety/fear related to etiology as determined through assessment*

b. *Impaired gas exchange related to hyperventilation*

c. *Impaired verbal communication related to psychological manifestations of anxiety*

d. *Ineffective individual or family coping related to insufficient resources or inability to manage stressful life situations*

e. *Risk for injury related to inability to make deliberative or thoughtful judgments secondary to anxiety*

f. *Knowledge deficit related to problem solving or coping strategies*

g. *Altered thought processes related to physiological and psychological manifestations of anxiety*

3. Planning/interventions

a. *Rule out organic cause of signs and symptoms*

b. *Build trusting relationship*

   1) Introduce self and explain role to patient

   2) Enhance acceptance and self-esteem by acknowledging patient's anxiety and offering reassurance

   3) Provide for safety and security needs

c. *Communicate in calm manner*

   1) Explain all procedures in simple, understandable terms

d. *Convey attitude of acceptance*

e. *Assist patient in recognizing causes and effects of anxiety*

f. *Direct patient to refocus attention to begin problem-solving process*

   1) Facilitate patient's expression of feelings

   2) Emphasize realistic perceptions

g. *Assist patient with problem-solving activities*

   1) Identify precipitating event

   2) Determine measures already taken to resolve problem

   3) Determine usual coping measures

h. *Determine options available*

   1) Select most desirable option

   2) Offer direct assistance

   3) Verbally acknowledge and comment positively on appropriate problem solving by patient

i. *If patient is hyperventilating, encourage to breathe with paper bag over mouth and nose and/or use behavioral techniques such as breathing control and relaxation exercises, after ruling out organic cause*

j. *Administer antianxiety medications such as diazepam (Valium), long acting; chlordiazepoxide (Librium), medium acting; and lorazepam (Ativan), short acting; clonazepam (Klonopin) is often used as antipanic agent*

k. *Use interpreter when patient's primary language is foreign or when patient is hearing impaired*

l. *Assist patient in determining source of fear and identify means of allaying fear*

m. *If patient has altered health maintenance, identify type of impairment and refer for appropriate follow-up care*

n. *If there is potential for injury related to poisoning or trauma, refer for crisis evaluation and suicide risk assessment*

o. *Place patient in area where he or she can be closely observed*

p. *Ascertain degree of knowledge deficit and provide up-to-date information*

q. *Refer to community resources such as Alcoholics Anonymous, counseling services, social support services, community mental health centers, crisis intervention hotlines as appropriate, depending on patient's underlying problems r.* *If patient expresses distress in parenting, determine severity and make referral to appropriate service: family counseling center, community outreach service, governmental child protective services*

  s. *If sleep disturbance is present, teach sleep hygiene measures; consult with physician regarding prescribed medications*

  t. *Teach patient appropriate use of prescribed medication*

  u. *If thought processes are altered, orient patient to current reality; refer for psychiatric evaluation to determine whether judgment is impaired; help make appropriate and safe discharge disposition*

  v. *Work with health care team to determine whether discharge is appropriate or supportive environment necessary until acute stage of anxiety abates*

 4. Expected outcomes/evaluation (see Appendix B)

B. Ineffective coping and situational crisis

  Failure to fulfill basic physiological and psychosocial needs can lead to increased difficulty in coping with emergency problems and eventually to a crisis. Ineffective individual coping occurs when an individual is unable to solve problems and deal with stressors, whether they are internal or external. Ineffective coping may be precipitated by an increase in the number or frequency of stressors or by diminished resources or coping abilities. Lack of anticipation of an event or the inability to prevent a stressful event can also cause ineffective coping.

  A situational crisis can precipitate the individual's inability to cope and occurs or develops as a response to a specific event in a person's life. The events are frequently unexpected, but they may also be anticipated occurrences that do not meet expectations (e.g., the financial deal that is not as lucrative as planned). There is an initial shock period with an inability to function and an overwhelming emotional response. If there have been concomitant crises during a short time, such as maturational and developmental crises plus other situations, the person may be experiencing fatigue and exhaustion. The situational crisis may precipitate behavior that includes excessive alcohol intake, drug abuse, and suicidal, homicidal, or criminal behavior. The person experiencing the crisis may be so overwhelmed by the situation that he or she is unable to use help effectively.

  Social isolation may be a result of an individual's attempt to cope with anxiety and is often evident in patients with chronic diseases seen in the ED during an exacerbation of the illness.

 1. Assessment

  a. Subjective data

   1) History of present condition

    a) Precipitating event or previous level of functioning

    b) Recent loss or change in body appearance

    c) Persistent stressor or sudden, recent stressors, such as new job, move to new geographical location, frequent illness or accidents

    d) Demands of school or job

    e) Maturational crisis of patient or family member (e.g., birth, marriage, retirement)

    f) Ingestion of substance to alter mood

    g) Reliance on ineffective or inappropriate coping strategies

    h) Natural disaster

   2) Medical history: individuals with chronic diseases or recent changes in health (e.g., chronic obstructive pulmonary disease [COPD], congestive heart disease [CHD], newly diagnosed diabetes), substance abusers (e.g.,

alcoholic), and individuals with stress factors are at risk for ineffective coping

b. *Objective data*
1) Physical examination
   a) Physiological stability
   b) Clothing or appearance may be unkempt
   c) Behavior: altered affect
   d) Poor eye contact
   e) Tense, compulsive, or agitated behavior and tremors
   f) Thought pattern: may be unclear or illogical
   g) Diminished impulse control
   h) Evidence of physical violence or self-destructive behavior (e.g., wrists slashed)
2) Diagnostic procedures
   a) Mental status examination
   b) Neurological diagnostic tests as indicated (see Chapter 12)

2. **Analysis: differential nursing diagnosis/collaborative problems**
   a. *Ineffective individual or family coping related to inadequate resources or inability to manage stressors*
   b. *Self-esteem disturbance related to inability to prevent or control stressful situations*
   c. *Altered thought processes related to physiological and psychological response to stress*
   d. *Dysfunctional grieving related to actual or perceived loss and inadequate or unavailable supports or resources*
   e. *Anxiety/fear related to real or perceived inability to control undesirable event or outcome*
   f. *Altered health maintenance related to ineffective coping with situational crisis*

3. **Planning/interventions**
   a. *Assist patient to identify precipitating event*
   b. *Assist patient to identify measures to resolve problem with usual method of coping*
   c. *Help patient to define and clarify realistic options*
   d. *Develop plan for intervention*
   e. *Structure priorities for problem-solving interventions*
   f. *Provide time and opportunity for communication, and support the patient in coming to ED for assistance*
   g. *If thought processes are disturbed, protect patient from harm*
   h. *Refer to community resources such as Alcoholics Anonymous, counseling service, social support service, and community or mental health center*
   i. *Refer frequently seen patients to social worker, mental health professional, or mental health care team to establish realistic care plan*

4. **Expected outcomes/evaluation** (see Appendix B)

C. Depression

Depression consists of specific alterations in mood, often accompanied by a negative self-concept, and physical changes, along with changes in activity and interest levels. Depression can be suspected when at least five of the following characteristics last for 2 weeks: loss of interest in usual activities, depressed mood, appetite increase or decrease with weight change, insomnia or hypersomnia, fatigue, psychomotor agitation or retardation, decreased ability to think, recurrent thoughts of death, and feelings of worthlessness.

1. **Assessment**
   a. *Subjective data*
      1) History of present illness
         a) Precipitating events
         b) Depressed affect and loss of interest in diversional activities and social relationships
         c) Fatigue and insomnia or hypersomnia
         d) Psychomotor agitation or retardation
         e) Difficulty in concentrating
         f) Recurrent thoughts of death and suicidal ideation
         g) Feelings of worthlessness
         h) Increase in alcohol and prescription and over-the-counter medication use
         i) Situational crisis
            (1) Recent childbirth (postpartum depression)
            (2) Loss of significant other or support system
            (3) Acute health changes
            (4) Chronic illness resulting from perpetual strain of long-term treatment regimens
            (5) Changes in role performance, occupational status, and power base
            (6) Separation from spiritual or cultural background
         j) Occurrence during developmental cycle
            (1) Children may have hyperactivity, enuresis, or regressive behavior
            (2) Adolescents may present as result of delinquency or injuries related to trauma; may be cynical, detached, angry, hostile, disillusioned, lonely; there may also be sexual promiscuity, acting-out behavior, alcohol and drug abuse
            (3) Adults, including elderly, may have symptoms similar to those of adolescent; may be dressed carelessly; and may relay loss of interest in social life, decreased sexual activity, inability to concentrate
            (4) All age groups may have any of just-mentioned symptoms
      2) Toxic ingestion: rule out medical emergency
      3) Medical history
         a) Depression, including family history of depression
         b) Chronic disease that necessitates prolonged and painful treatment regimens or that has no known cure
         c) Medication history and psychotropic therapy
         d) Injury that has caused debilitation/chronic pain
   b. *Objective data*
      1) Physical examination
         a) Affect
            (1) Quiet and withdrawn demeanor
            (2) Restricted affect (limited emotional expression)
            (3) Dysphoric mood
         b) Cardiovascular system
            (1) There may be abnormalities in the context of coexisting disease
         c) Respiratory system: breath sounds normal unless concomitant physical illness
         d) Neurological system
            (1) Mental status examination with possible changes in appearance, behavior, speech, mood, perception, thought process and content, cognitive functioning, and/or judgment
            (2) Generalized psychomotor retardation or agitation

(3) Completion of neurological examination helps to rule out organic cause of depression, such as brain tumor

e) Musculoskeletal system

(1) Poor posture and slow gait

(2) In some patients, psychomotor agitation and increased motor activity with crying, restlessness, increased verbalization

f) Gastrointestinal system

(1) Alteration in elimination patterns: constipation resulting from decreased motility of gastrointestinal tract

(2) Alteration in eating patterns: weight loss or gain

g) Somatizations: must rule out organic causes

(1) Low back pain

(2) Fatigue

(3) Headaches

2) Diagnostic procedures

a) Twelve- to 15-lead ECG if indicated by somatic symptoms

b) Laboratory: normal range unless concomitant illness

(1) Thyroid function tests: normal unless thyroid deficiency

(2) Toxicology screen of urine if drug ingestion is suspected

(3) Blood alcohol level if alcohol ingestion is suspected

c) Other tests depend on somatic symptoms

2. Analysis: differential nursing diagnosis/collaborative problems

a. *Impaired verbal communication related to manifestation of depression*

b. *Ineffective individual coping related to depression in response to stressors*

c. *Risk for injury, poisoning related to depression*

d. *Knowledge deficit related to use of coping strategies and sources of assistance*

e. *Altered thought processes related to depression*

3. Planning/interventions

a. *Rule out organic cause of emergency*

b. *Convey attitude of acceptance*

c. *Encourage patient to identify feelings*

d. *Assist patient in recognizing causes and effects of depression*

e. *Place patient in safe and observable area*

f. *Determine whether poison ingestion has occurred and treat: administration of ipecac, gastric lavage, activated charcoal as indicated*

g. *Refer for crisis evaluation of suicidal risk (see Section II.E.)*

h. *For impaired overall health, help patient identify type of impairment and necessary modifications in lifestyle*

i. *If nutritional sustenance is deficient, determine degree of deficit and initiate therapy as appropriate; provide fluid and electrolyte therapy for dehydration*

j. *If nutritional excess is present, refer to community program for weight control and behavior modification*

k. *Ascertain degree of knowledge deficit and provide up-to-date information*

l. *Refer to community resources such as Alcoholics Anonymous for alcohol dependency, family counseling services or governmental family protective services for difficulty in parenting, social support services for economic difficulties or social isolation, counseling for underlying disturbance in self-concept, and crisis intervention hotlines for use in case of acute distress*

m. *Consult with psychiatrist/physician regarding prescribed medications, and teach patient appropriate use of prescribed medications*

n. *Inquire whether spiritual belief and support systems can be used to affect feelings*

     o. Refer to religious counseling if desired by patient or cultural centers if patient is not in native culture

     p. If thought processes are altered, orient patient to current reality

     q. Work with health care team to determine whether discharge is appropriate or supportive environment is necessary until acute stage of depression abates

  4. Expected outcomes/evaluation (see Appendix B)

D. Grief

     Acute grief is a normal emotional reaction to a loss. Death may be the most significant loss, but other types of losses include changes in health, body function, body parts, mental acuity, self-image, relationships, economic security, material possessions and homes, and independence. The concept of loss involves something that a person once had, or hoped to have, and now has no possibility of possessing. It is usually experienced as a void and evokes feelings of emptiness. As loss occurs, grief work begins and involves the process of letting go, of severing emotional ties, and of gradually reinvesting in new interests and people.

     In the emergency care setting, grief may be experienced by a patient who has survived when others perished or by family members who must cope with the sudden loss of a loved one. Regardless of who is experiencing the grief reaction, acceptance, comprehension of the loss, and the painful process of emotionally detaching oneself should begin in the emergency care setting.

  1. Assessment

     a. Subjective data

       1) History of present condition

         a) Identifies loss as real or threatened

         b) Describes measures or attempts to resolve situation that have been successful or unsuccessful

       2) Medical history

     b. Objective data

       1) Physical examination

         a) Somatic symptoms: overidentification can cause a survivor to experience some symptoms observed in family member, friend, etc. who is now deceased

         b) Syncope, gastrointestinal distress, yawning, hyperventilation, and palpitations

         c) Exacerbation of existing illness to crisis proportions

           (1) Cardiac disease: angina

           (2) Obstructive pulmonary disease: dyspnea

           (3) Hypertension: dizziness and headache

       2) Diagnostic procedures: need to rule out organic basis of signs and symptoms if patient experiences symptoms similar to those experienced by the deceased (e.g., if patient has chest pain, rule out myocardial infarction)

  2. Analysis: differential nursing diagnosis/collaborative problems

     a. Grieving related to actual or anticipated loss

  3. Planning/interventions

     a. Appear confident, establish trusting relationship, and allow for unhurried time

     b. Escort into private room

     c. Facilitate discussion of concerns, worries, feelings

     d. Provide periodic reports to update progress or lack of progress; all information should be honest and delivered in a caring fashion

     e. Use hospital health care team members (e.g., social workers, clergy, psychiatric clinical nurse specialists, and mental health care team members) as needed to assist, support, and stay with individual experiencing grief

f. *Call other persons in the social network (family, friends, and clergy or spiritual advisor) to provide ongoing support and to help survivor work through and prepare for anticipated loss*

g. *Suggest "what if . . . ? " situations to help survivor work through and prepare for anticipated death or loss*

h. *Encourage survivor to talk about impending loss and its meaning*

i. *Actively listen to response*

j. *Accept all behavioral responses (e.g., denial, hope for improved status, and silence); do not insist on talk*

k. *Evaluate survivor's coping ability and express confidence in his or her ability to cope*

l. *When death has occurred*
   1) With physician, inform survivors or significant others of death and refer to deceased by name
   2) Explain course of death in simple and understandable terms
   3) Provide emotional support to bereaved, being aware of religious and cultural needs
   4) Offer opportunity to view body (offer may need to be repeated)
      a) Prepare survivors for alterations in physical appearance (e.g., those caused by trauma) of deceased
      b) Accompany survivors, but remain unobtrusive to provide privacy
   5) Report death to legal authorities
   6) Help survivors to focus attention on decisions requiring immediate action
      a) Organ donation
      b) Postmortem examination, if family has option
      c) Signing for valuables, property, clothing of deceased
      d) Tentative selection of funeral home
   7) Assist survivors to practice how to tell others, especially young children, about death; emphasize use of words "he is dead" or "she is dead"
   8) Help survivors "leave" when the time is right
   9) Plan with survivor for follow-up telephone call in 4 to 6 weeks to assess type of grief reaction
   10) Refer as needed to community agencies

4. **Expected outcomes/evaluation** (see Appendix B)

E. Suicide or suicidal behavior

Suicide is death caused by a self-inflicted act that is willful and a result of planning. Suicidal behavior refers to attempts to cause death by life-threatening acts, thoughts of suicide, and behaviors that indicate there is a risk of suicide. Suicide cannot be predicted, although there are high-risk factors associated with suicidal behavior. Demographical risk factors include adolescence or age older than 45 years and male, white, separated, divorced, widowed, living alone, and unemployed status. Adolescent suicide is becoming a significant problem in the United States; more than 5000 adolescents die each year from self-inflicted means. Antecedent life circumstances that may increase the risk of suicide attempts are previous suicide attempts, family history of suicide or attempts, inadequate or unavailable support systems, and major life changes involving loss or illness. Although females make more suicide attempts, males more often succeed in committing suicide and use violent means, such as self-inflicted gunshots and jumps from buildings. The patient who presents for emergency care may require immediate intervention for life-threatening situations, depending on the methods used for self-harm. The patient who has exhibited suicidal behavior frequently experiences depression.

1. Assessment
   a. *Subjective data*
      1) History of present illness
         a) Precipitating factors
         b) Family history of attempting or succeeding in suicide
         c) Newly diagnosed disease with body changes
         d) Substance abuse
         e) Signs of depression
         f) Suicidal ideation
         g) Previous suicide attempts
      2) Medical history
         a) Debilitating disease, such as multiple sclerosis and amyotrophic lateral sclerosis
         b) Chronic disease, such as cancer, acquired immunodeficiency syndrome, human immunodeficiency virus infection, and Parkinson's disease
         c) Depressive illness
         d) Alcoholism
         e) Schizophrenia
   b. *Objective data*
      1) Physical examination
         a) Respiratory status may be depressed from drug ingestion or hypovolemia
            (1) Rate, depth, symmetry
            (2) Breath sounds
            (3) Pulse oximetry to determine oxygen saturation
         b) Cardiovascular status may be depressed from hypovolemia or drug ingestion that is cardiotoxic or vasotoxic
            (1) Blood pressure: hypotensive
            (2) Pulse: weak and rapid
            (3) Cardiac rhythm: tachycardia with atrial or ventricular dysrhythmias
         c) Neurological system
            (1) Mental status examination results may vary
            (2) Pupillary state depends on substances ingested (see Chapter 20)
            (3) Psychomotor disorders
            (4) Seizure activity
            (5) Deep tendon reflexes may be absent
         d) Other system evaluations reveal abnormalities and are based on method of suicide attempt
      2) Diagnostic procedures
         a) Twelve- to 15-lead ECG when ingestion of medication is known or suspected; with tricyclic antidepressants: QRS and QT interval prolongation, conduction defects, sinus tachycardia, atrial fibrillation, ventricular dysrhythmias
         b) Laboratory tests to rule out organic disease or concomitant illness if suspected by history or symptoms
            (1) Urine toxicology test to screen for substances
            (2) Blood alcohol level if alcohol ingestion is suspected
            (3) Lavage for toxicology test if history reveals oral ingestion

2. Analysis: differential nursing diagnosis/collaborative problems
   a. *Ineffective individual coping related to inadequate resources or inability to manage situational crisis*

  b. *Risk for violence: self-directed, related to inadequate resources or inability to manage situational crisis*
  c. *Altered thought processes related to etiological factors determined by assessment and manifested by suicidal ideation*

3. **Planning/interventions**
  a. *Encourage patient to identify feelings*
  b. *Help patient to determine cause, effect, potential solutions to ineffective coping and fear*
  c. *Orient patient to current reality*
  d. *Provide safe environment to protect patient (situate in observable area and remove guns, knives, sharp objects, matches, or other devices that could harm patient)*
  e. *Restrain patient, per institutional policy, with mechanical restraints for patient safety, if needed*
  f. *Treat poison ingestion*
  g. *Refer for psychiatric consultation*
  h. *Provide information to consultant regarding patient's suicide plan. Is plan specific? Does he or she have available means? How lethal are means? Is patient's behavior impulsive?*
  i. *Administer medication as ordered (e.g., haloperidol [Haldol] intramuscularly or intravenously for chemical restraint if needed)*
  j. *Ascertain degree of knowledge deficit and provide information*
  k. *Provide reality orientation regarding role performance, personal identity, self-esteem, perceived obstacles to health*
  l. *If patient expresses difficulty with home maintenance management, determine severity and make referral to appropriate home health care service: family counseling, community outreach service, governmental agency for family protection*
  m. *Inquire whether spiritual belief and support systems can be used to affect feelings and situation*
  n. *Work with health care team to determine whether discharge is appropriate or inpatient admission is necessary for either medical or psychiatric stabilization*
  o. *Refer to appropriate community resources if discharge is appropriate*

4. **Expected outcomes/evaluation** (see Appendix B)

F. Homicidal or violent behavior

Violence is the acting out of the emotions of fear or anger to achieve desired goals. It may also be the result of psychosis, antisocial behavior, or organic disease. It is an assault on a person or object with an intent to harm or destroy. Homicidal behavior is violence with intent to kill directed at another person. During a violent or homicidal encounter, a high level of panic may be present, with a resultant loss of reasoning ability. Violence may also be used as a defense for self-protection or for the protection of loved ones when a person is feeling attacked either emotionally or physically. The patient may be either the attacker or the victim. Violent behavior in the ED is becoming more prevalent, and the ED staff must take measures to protect themselves and others against injury.

1. **Assessment**
  a. *Subjective data*
    1) History of present illness
      a) Precipitating events

       b) Medication and substance use
       c) Previous homicidal or violent behavior
       d) Suicidal thoughts
       e) Child abuse
       f) Preoccupation with sexual thoughts and fantasies
       g) Childhood history of enuresis, fire setting, cruelty to animals, fighting, school problems
    2) Medical history
       a) Psychosis
       b) Organic disease: temporal lobe epilepsy
       c) Head injury
  b. *Objective data*
    1) Physical examination
       a) Head-to-toe assessment with complete vital signs necessary to identify any injuries sustained during episode
       b) Patient is usually anxious and has signs related to anxiety (see Section II.A.)
       c) Cardiovascular system
          (1) Heart rate increased
          (2) Systolic blood pressure elevated; if decreased or if diastolic pressure elevated, suspect hypovolemia
          (3) Temperature normal unless organic basis for fever or hypothermia
          (4) Premature contractions noted on cardiac monitor
          (5) Skin pale and diaphoretic
       d) Respiratory system
          (1) Respiratory rate increased; patient may be hyperventilating
          (2) Breath sounds normal unless injury affects breathing
       e) Other system evaluations reveal abnormalities according to mechanism of injury
    2) Diagnostic procedures
       a) Twelve- to 15-lead ECG if indicated by somatic symptoms and injury
       b) Laboratory
          (1) CBC: white blood cell count may be slightly elevated secondary to injury
          (2) Electrolyte levels: within normal limits, except potassium level may be elevated with injury
          (3) Urine toxicology screen if substance use is suspected
          (4) Blood alcohol level if alcohol ingestion is suspected
          (5) Other tests if indicated by physical examination results and history
       c) Radiology: to determine injury if suspected from physical examination findings and history

2. **Analysis: differential nursing diagnosis/collaborative problems**
  a. *Ineffective individual coping related to insufficient or inadequate skills to control anger or fear*
  b. *Altered thought processes related to physiological or psychological dysfunction manifested by homicidal ideation*
  c. *Risk for violence related to physiological or psychological dysfunction and inadequate coping abilities*
  d. *Risk for injury related to aggressive or assaultive behaviors*
  e. *Anxiety/fear related to real or perceived threat to life or well-being*
3. **Planning/interventions**
  a. *Ensure safety of self and others before intervening with violent/homicidal patient*

    b. *Encourage patient to identify feelings*
    c. *Help patient to determine cause, effect, possible solutions to ineffective coping*
    d. *Orient patient to current reality (time, place, person)*
    e. *If thought processes are altered to degree that patient or others may be harmed, work with health care team to place patient in supportive environment*
    f. *Administer antipsychotic medications as indicated; haloperidol (Haldol) is usually drug of choice administered intramuscularly, intravenously, or orally*
    g. *Remove guns, knives, matches, or other devices that could harm others; use security or police personnel to assist*
    h. *Restrain patient per institutional policy, as necessary, with mechanical restraints*
    i. *Provide safe environment; patient should be placed away from others whenever possible, yet within observable area for ease in staff monitoring*
    j. *Keep door open to area where patient is being treated to reduce possibility of patient feeling trapped*
    k. *If there has been injury that necessitates treatment, prepare patient*
    l. *If family processes are altered, report to governmental authorities for investigation*
    m. *Facilitate open communication by listening objectively*
    n. *Provide reality orientation regarding role performance, personal identity, self-esteem, body image, obstacles to improved health*
    o. *Help patient decide whether spiritual belief and support systems can be used in current situation*
    p. *Contact spiritual advisor if patient requests*
    q. *Refer to community resources, including psychiatric counselors, mental health centers, and crisis intervention hotlines*
    r. *If patient is in police custody, arrange psychiatric follow-up care*
  4. Expected outcomes/evaluation (see Appendix B)

G. Psychotic behavior

    Psychotic behavior is the result of a pathological process that may be acute or chronic, with resultant distorted perceptions, disorganized thinking, impaired judgment, impaired decision making, and regressive behavior. Manifestations occur in the areas of affect, behavior, perception, and thinking. The mood may range from a flat affect to euphoria. Behavioral effects include acting-out behavior, impulsiveness, and psychomotor retardation or agitation. Illusions, hallucinations, and depersonalization are perceptual effects of psychosis. Impaired thinking is exhibited by delusions, loose associations, and incoherence. Psychoses can be functional or organic. Functional types include schizophrenia, mania, psychotic depression, and brief reactive psychosis. Organic psychoses include dementia, delirium, and toxic drug-induced psychosis.

  1. Assessment
    a. *Subjective data*
      1) History of present illness
        a) Schizophrenia: familial history and onset before age 45 years
          (1) Bizarre behavior, including but not limited to reports of decreased ability to care for self or function in work or social environment
          (2) Delusions
          (3) Auditory hallucinations
          (4) Paranoia
        b) Mania
          (1) Previous episodes

        (2) Decreased need for sleep

        (3) Increased physical activity

        (4) Paranoia may be present

        (5) Impulsive and flamboyant behavior

        (6) Euphoria or elation

        (7) Unrealistic plans or thoughts

    c) Psychotic depression

        (1) Loss of energy and pleasure

        (2) Possible command hallucinations

        (3) Agitation

        (4) Lack of communication with others

        (5) Psychomotor retardation

        (6) Decreased ability or desire to care for self

    d) Delirium (organic disorders must be ruled out)

        (1) Rapid onset of symptoms, fluctuating course

        (2) Restlessness, insomnia, nightmares

        (3) Trouble with thinking clearly and without insight into problems

        (4) Changes in temperament

    e) Dementia

        (1) Gradual onset of symptoms

        (2) Noticeable personality changes

        (3) Memory loss and disorientation

        (4) Possible paranoid delusions

        (5) "Sundowning": lucid in morning with worsening at night

  2) Medical history: may be unremarkable

  b. Objective data

    1) Physical examination

      a) Cardiovascular system

        (1) Heart rate and rhythm normal unless agitated behavior is present, causing increased blood pressure and heart rate

        (2) Skin color, temperature, and moisture normal

      b) Respiratory system

        (1) Rate and rhythm normal unless anxiety is present with tachypnea or hyperventilation

        (2) Breath sounds normal unless concomitant illness is present

      c) Neurological system

        (1) Schizophrenia: auditory or visual hallucinations; bizarre speech content; unimpaired cognition

        (2) Mania: delusions of grandeur, auditory hallucinations; labile and euphoric affect; rapid and fluent speech; sexual content of thought or speech often seen

        (3) Psychotic depression: psychomotor retardation, paucity speech; auditory or olfactory hallucinations; disorganized thinking; preoccupation with death and morbid thoughts; possible impaired cognition

        (4) Delirium: rapid onset/fluctuating course; tactile, visual, olfactory hallucinations; disorientation to time, place, person; memory impairment; blunted affect; confabulation (fictitious stories that fill in memory gaps); must rule out organic basis (e.g., metabolic, infectious, endocrine, or neoplastic cause; substance toxicity; trauma [especially head trauma]; congestive heart failure; COPD; subarachnoid hemorrhage)

        (5) Dementia: repetitive speech; recent memory loss and disorientation; lack of awareness of problem; impaired intellectual cognition

2) Diagnostic data
   a) Twelve- to 15-lead ECG may be abnormal if psychosis has organic basis secondary to acute myocardial infarction or congestive heart failure
   b) Laboratory tests are performed on basis of suspected cause of psychosis
      (1) CBC: elevated white blood cell count if infection
      (2) Urinalysis: white cells present if infection
      (3) Levels of electrolytes, blood glucose, and blood urea nitrogen (BUN) and results of tests for renal and hepatic function may be abnormal with organic psychosis
      (4) Other tests that may be ordered as part of diagnostic work-up include Venereal Disease Research Laboratory (VDRL) (tertiary syphilis can be origin of altered mental status); ABG values to determine whether hypoxemia is causal; thyroid function tests (hypothyroid and hyperthyroid function can produce symptoms that mimic those of psychiatric disorders); stool for occult blood (internal bleeding may contribute to anemia, which, if severe enough, may compromise mental status); cerebrospinal fluid analysis for cells, protein, and white blood cell count to determine infectious origin of altered mental status; toxicology screen of urine and blood drug levels (hallucinogens, amphetamines, cocaine)
   c) Radiology
      (1) Computed tomography scan
      (2) Other films on basis of history and physical examination findings

2. **Analysis: differential nursing diagnosis/collaborative problems**
   a. *Visual or auditory sensory/perceptual alteration related to hallucinations secondary to mental health illness*
   b. *Impaired verbal communication related to psychological barriers*
   c. *Risk for injury related to effects of psychosis*
   d. *Ineffective individual or family coping related to inadequate psychological resources and coping strategies*

3. **Planning/interventions**
   a. *Orient patient to reality (time, place, person)*
   b. *Provide safety per institutional policy by mechanical restraints, as necessary, and by continuous observation; separate patient from heavy traffic areas to avoid escalation that may result from added stimuli*
   c. *Administer prescribed antipsychotic medications; haloperidol (Haldol) is generally drug of choice (intramuscularly, intravenously, or orally)*
   d. *Orient patient with respect to hallucinations or delusions; reinforce absence of visual and auditory phenomena*
   e. *Provide atmosphere for open and objective communication*
   f. *Treat injuries sustained as result of psychotic behavior*
   g. *If possibility of exposure exists, treat patient as outlined in Chapter 5*
   h. *Calm patient by speaking softly and placing away from stimulating environment*
   i. *Remove all implements or objects that may cause harm to patient or others; ask security or police personnel for assistance*
   j. *If patient exhibits delusions of grandeur or other manifestations of distortion in personal identity, orient to and acknowledge reality*
   k. *If coping, family processes, or health maintenance is identified as an issue, refer to appropriate health care provider for individual or family care; refer to counseling or psychiatric services or department of family services*
   l. *Work with health care team to make appropriate disposition to protective*

environment; discharge to home with follow-up services if patient is mentally stable or admit to hospital for continuous supportive environment
4. **Expected outcomes/evaluation** (see Appendix B)

H. Bipolar disorder

Manic-depressive illness, or bipolar affective disorder, is characterized by alternating euphoric moods and depressed periods (see discussion of depression in Section II.C.). Affect can be unpredictable and labile, with mood changes occurring over minutes, hours, days, or there may be lengthy periods of stability between episodes. When in a manic state, the patient can be euphoric, irritable, and social. The mood is infectious, with laughter and smiles elicited from others. The manic patient frequently refers to sexual subjects and may show a familiarity with others that is uncomfortable. Impairment in thinking may be present with flight of ideas and grandiosity. Grandiose auditory hallucinations may also be present. Subtle impairment of thinking may be evidenced by poor social judgment, an inflated self-esteem, and arrogance. Mentation is frequently impaired. The patient may be hostile and paranoid when stressed. Bizarre behavior may be present with flamboyant actions, impulsive behavior, and disorganized activity. There is often a family history of manic-depressive disease and a history of repeated cycles. Antidepressant therapy as well as organic problems may precipitate mania. Patients experiencing bipolar disorder often return to premorbid functioning with medication and therapy.

1. **Assessment**
   a. *Subjective data*
      1) History of present illness
         a) Previous manic and/or depressive episodes
         b) Sleep pattern disturbance, with patient frequently feeling he or she requires very little sleep
         c) Rapid onset of symptoms, usually during 2-week period
         d) Labile emotions; euphoria and depression
         e) Noncompliance with prescribed medication regimen (e.g., lithium, divalproex [Depakote], carbamazepine [Tegretol] may be precipitant)
      2) Medical history
         a) Repeated cycles of mania and depression
         b) Disorders that can cause symptoms that mimic psychiatric illness
            (1) Metabolic disorders
            (2) Infections
            (3) Endocrine disorders
            (4) Neoplastic disorders
            (5) Substance toxicity
   b. *Objective data*
      1) Physical examination
         a) Cardiovascular system: essentially normal unless concomitant illness
         b) Respiratory system: essentially normal unless concomitant illness
         c) Neurological system
            (1) Auditory hallucinations at times
            (2) Rapid and pressured speech
            (3) Grandiose context to speech
            (4) Intact intellect
            (5) Thoughts occur in rapid progression with flight of ideas
         d) Musculoskeletal system
            (1) Altered physical activity patterns; hyperactive or hypoactive
            (2) Other assessments normal

2) Diagnostic procedures
   a) Urine toxicology screen for drugs
   b) Serum alcohol level if alcohol use suspected
   c) Serum drug levels (lithium, divalproex [Depakote], carbamazepine [Tegretol]) if currently receiving medication
   d) Other tests if organic causes of mania are suspected

2. Analysis: differential nursing diagnosis/collaborative problems

   a. *Altered thought processes related to biochemical imbalance and mental disorder*
   b. *Risk for injury related to perceptual-cognitive deficit and lack of awareness of hazards secondary to bipolar disorder*
   c. *Visual or auditory sensory/perceptual alterations related to hallucinations secondary to bipolar disorder*
   d. *Ineffective individual or family coping related to insufficient or exhausted supports, resources, or coping strategies*
   e. *Noncompliance related to poor impulse control secondary to bipolar disorder*

3. Planning/interventions

   a. *If patient is delusional, acknowledge thought disorder and orient to reality*
   b. *If patient is receiving mood stabilizing agents, draw blood to determine level*
   c. *Provide safety by restraints per institutional policy, as necessary, and by continuous observation*
   d. *Treat injuries sustained as result of psychotic behavior*
   e. *Calm patient by speaking softly and placing away from stimulating environment*
   f. *Remove all implements or objects that may cause harm to patient or others*
   g. *Treat medical problems caused by malnutrition if present (e.g., dehydration and electrolyte imbalance)*
   h. *If patient's judgment is affected secondary to mania or depression, protect from external stimuli by removing to area where there is less stimuli; patient must be observable at all times*
   i. *Refer patient to crisis intervention nurse or psychiatrist for evaluation*
   j. *Work with health care team to make appropriate disposition to supportive environment*
   k. *Medicate as prescribed*
   l. *Instruct patient on importance of taking prescribed medication*

4. Expected outcomes/evaluation (see Appendix B)

I. Child abuse/neglect

Child abuse/neglect is a nonaccidental act committed by a caregiver (usually a family member or close and trusted friend) that results in physical, sexual, or emotional injury or deprivation to an individual younger than 18 years, but most likely younger than 6 years. Frequently, the abuser does not have the knowledge to understand the needs of the child, which are based on the child's developmental level. This, combined with the abuser's possible limited ability for delayed satisfaction, can result in unrealistically high expectations of the child. When the child cannot meet the unreasonable standard, he or she may be physically abused. The child may begin to try harder to please the abuser in an effort to prevent a recurrence and may imitate the selected abuser's behaviors in an effort to be like and please the abuser. The child victim may learn to batter and to use violence as a coping method; the battering is likely to be carried on into adulthood, thus repeating the cycle.

Sexual abuse of children is involvement of the child (younger than 18 years) in behaviors that he or she neither understands nor consents to. It is estimated that one in six children will be sexually abused by the time they reach 18 years of age. Many cases go unrecognized and unreported for fear of punishment and retaliation. Recognition of childhood sexual abuse requires knowledge of the physical sexual development of children.

Emotional abuse of the child generally takes the form of verbal abuse. The child's self-worth is impacted, and constant criticism results in lifelong feelings of self-worthlessness. Children who are emotionally abused often become adults with a history of emotional problems.

Recognition of the abused child requires an understanding of the physical and psychological development of children of all ages. Child maltreatment is a reportable crime in all 50 states, and the nurse caring for the child victim can be found liable if the case is *not* reported to the appropriate agency.

1. **Assessment**
    a. *Subjective data*
        1) History of present condition
            a) Parent or caregiver and child interviewed separately about current incident or injury
            b) Describes abuse incident in own words
            c) Child recalls incident, using anatomically correct doll
            d) Parent/caregiver's history of incident may be sketchy, inconsistent over time, or inconsistent with child's version of incident; history may sound rehearsed, with same key words used
            e) Verbatim recording of key quotes from parent/caregiver and child is *critical*
        2) Medical history: separate interviews of child and parent/caregiver to determine
            a) Diminished social network: friends, participation in clubs or church activities, involvement with relatives, and family activities are minimal or nonexistent
            b) Decreased or absent ability to trust
            c) School performance level below child's normal expectation
            d) Regressive behaviors, such as enuresis or encopresis
            e) Family stressors
                (1) Illness or death of family member
                (2) Frequent moves or recent move (in past 6 months)
                (3) Caregiver abused as spouse, teen, or child
                (4) History of substance abuse: drugs/alcohol
                (5) Family inability to cope with multiple stressors
    b. *Objective data*
        1) Physical examination of child
            a) Detachment and lack of expression, especially with painful procedures, interventions
            b) Inappropriate behavior for achieved developmental level and regressive behavior (e.g., thumb sucking)
            c) Malnourishment
            d) Ecchymoses or surface injuries in various planes or stages of healing
            e) Geographical or pattern injuries (e.g., cigarette burns or injuries in wire hanger, belt marks, or curling iron pattern)
            f) Injuries inconsistent with age and development
            g) Parent/caregiver's interactions with child, staff, or family members suspicious or inconsistent
        2) Diagnostic procedures for child

      a) Radiology
        (1) Skull radiograph
        (2) Chest radiograph
        (3) Spinal radiographic series
        (4) Radiographs of long bones
        (5) Radiographs of all other obviously injured sites
      b) Laboratory
        (1) Slide of sperm or acid phosphatase: mouth, nose, vagina, rectum
        (2) Urinalysis: for hematuria and sperm
        (3) Culture and sensitivity testing of all orifices for *Neisseria gonorrhoeae*
        (4) Prothrombin time and partial thromboplastin time for bleeding diathesis
        (5) Complete hematology and chemistry studies, especially if child exhibits malnourishment, significant weight loss, failure to thrive
        (6) Photographs for documentation, preferably color and including identifying features of the child

2. **Analysis: differential nursing diagnosis/collaborative problems**
    a. *Ineffective individual and/or family coping related to emotional conflict and inadequate resources or abilities to meet demands of parenting*
    b. *Anxiety related to perceived threats to health or well-being (manifested by child)*
    c. *Risk for impaired skin integrity related to trauma secondary to physical violence*
    d. *Risk for injury related to altered family processes or dysfunctional family system*

3. **Planning/interventions**
    a. *Remain neutral and keep communication lines open*
    b. *Establish trust by acknowledging stress factors*
    c. *Give positive reinforcement for coming to emergency care facility*
    d. *Inform parents/caregivers about ongoing procedures*
    e. *Allow child to see parent/caregiver and family as needed*
    f. *Use therapeutic touch to provide comfort when appropriate*
    g. *Assure child that emergency care staff will help*
    h. *Establish rapport and reinforce belief of child's story by health care team*
      1) Help child focus on feelings
      2) Offer reassurance
      3) Acknowledge difficulty or reluctance to establish etiology of injuries
    i. *Examine for hidden injuries (e.g., feet, buttocks, back)*
      1) Underneath clothing
      2) Old or internal injuries underlying surface wounds
    j. *Determine whether history is incompatible with injury*
    k. *Clean open wounds (see Chapter 21)*
    l. *Immunize as needed*
    m. *Facilitate emergency team notification of family that child requires admission or hospitalization*
    n. *Hospitalize for therapeutic intervention, diagnostic testing, or protection if safety is compromised*
    o. *Determine whether siblings or spouse is at risk for abuse or neglect*
    p. *Assist family or caregiver to identify stressors and validate need for assistance*
    q. *Notify appropriate authority, as mandated by law*
      1) Child abuse hotline
      2) In-hospital child protection team

3) Local or state protection services

4) Local police department, as indicated

    a) To report incident

    b) To obtain court order to retain custody of child, if needed

r. Refer to resources: parenting skills classes, homemakers, social services, foster grandparents, parent effectiveness training, and Parents Anonymous

4. Expected outcomes/evaluation (see Appendix B)

J. Battered adult

Battering includes the components of physical and psychological assault. Physical assault is any act ranging from a slap to homicide performed by a partner from a previous or present intimate relationship. Psychological assault includes verbal threats and insults aimed at lowering self-worth and implying that the individual is unwanted or unloved. Often, the woman is the victim, and the man is the abuser. In one third of all spouse abuse cases, there is also child abuse. Observing or receiving parental violence may teach another generation to use aggression as a coping behavior.

1. Assessment

  a. Subjective data

    1) History of present condition

      a) Vague: does not adequately explain injury

      b) If of childbearing age, obtain obstetrical history

      c) Acute fatigue: sleep disturbances common, fear of assault while asleep

      d) Record of time and place of injury; use patient's or family's own words

    2) Medical history: domestic violence episodes

  b. Objective data

    1) Physical examination

      a) Physiological instability related to precipitating injury (see chapters relating to specific injury)

      b) Pattern injuries (present and past)

      c) Injuries most often on face, head, trunk, genitalia, abdomen if pregnant

    2) Diagnostic procedures

      a) Tests determined on basis of physiological problem: to ensure physiological stability of patient or fetus

      b) Mental status examination

        (1) Affect or mood: depressed; euphoric; or appropriate

2. Analysis: differential nursing diagnosis/collaborative problems

  a. Pain related to wounds or injuries

  b. Ineffective family coping: compromised, related to emotional conflicts and/or exhaustion of supportive capacity

  c. Potential for violence: directed at others, related to etiological factors determined by assessment and manifested by abuse or battering

3. Planning/interventions

  a. Accept patient and situation; share perceptions and suspicion that patient was assaulted

    1) may be necessary to ask patients whether they have been abused; many do not volunteer information for fear of punishment from abuser

  b. Treat physical source of pain

  c. Use nonpharmacological measures, such as applying ice and positioning, and offer and administer prescribed medication to relieve pain symptoms

  d. Facilitate patient's involvement in and cooperation with interview

  e. Document findings in writing, use patient's own words; obtain photographs when appropriate f. Assist patient to acknowledge situation and mobilize self to secure safe environment, advise patient that abuse invariably worsens (rather than improves) with time; situations rarely improve without some kind of direct intervention

   g. If patient acknowledges assault, initiate crisis intervention plan
     1) Determine or locate safe environment
     2) Mobilize patient to secure safe environment
     3) Arrange for safe transportation
     4) Refer to community resources

   h. Assist patient to determine risk of concurrent violence in family (e.g., child abuse or neglect)

   i. If patient does not acknowledge assault, do not attempt to have patient confront the situation. Instead
     1) Provide telephone number for crisis intervention hotline or local women's shelter
     2) Inform patient of potential for severe physical or psychological injury to self and/or children

   j. Provide situational support to patient and family

   k. Refer to community resources to facilitate healthy family coping (police, legal counsel, vocational training, women's center or groups, assertiveness training, clergy or spiritual advisor, and parent effectiveness training)

   l. Help family or caretaker identify stressors

   m. Provide situational support to patient and family

   n. Refer to appropriate resources, including day care centers, nursing home, counseling, homemaker services, church-affiliated support or clergy, police, legal counsel, assertiveness training

   o. Report to legal authorities when indicated

  4. Expected outcomes/evaluation (see Appendix B)

K. Elder abuse/neglect

Elderly persons, especially women, who are dependent, fragile, and in need of caretaker assistance, are most susceptible to elder maltreatment. The majority of these victims reside with family members and experience neglect or abuse because of increased stressors, multiple demands, and limited resources available to the caretaker, who is often a daughter or daughter-in-law. Elderly abuse can take the form of physical injury, emotional abuse, financial abuse, or neglect. Institutional abuse exists as well, but occurs with significantly less frequency than abuse by family members.

  1. Assessment
   a. Subjective data
     1) History of present condition
       a) Vague: unwilling to place blame
       b) Living situation that can precipitate abuse (dependence on caregiver)
       c) Reports of abuse by family member
       d) Recent household crises or conflicts
     2) Medical history: previous suspected episodes
     3) History of injury as given by caregiver
       a) Knowledge of patient's medical condition and needs
       b) Blaming injury on elderly patient, who is described as "forgetful" and "clumsy"
   b. Objective data
     1) Physical examination
       a) Pattern injuries (recent and previously inflicted)

        b) Mental status: agitated, fearful, overly quiet, passive

        c) Signs of neglect: dehydration, malnutrition, inappropriate or soiled clothing, poor hygiene, lack of care for previous conditions (e.g., decubitus ulcers)

        d) Signs and symptoms of overmedication or undermedication

    2) Diagnostic procedures

        a) Tests determined on basis of physiological problem

           (1) Twelve- to 15-lead ECG

           (2) CBC

           (3) Electrolyte panel

           (4) Radiologic screening for fractures

           (5) Serum drug levels

           (6) Metabolic screening for malnutrition

2. Analysis: differential nursing diagnosis/collaborative problems

    a. Risk for injury related to physical abuse

    b. Anxiety/fear related to potential need for placement in long-term care facility

    c. Risk for impaired skin integrity related to trauma (see Chapter 21) secondary to physical violence

3. Planning/interventions

    a. Provide comforting, safe environment for patient to encourage verbalization (denial is common)

    b. Obtain history when patient is alone; obtain separate history from caregiver

    (1) History taking should not be rushed; save delicate questions for last, after establishing rapport

    c. Document findings in writing; use patient's own words; obtain photographs when appropriate

    d. Provide situational support to patient and family

    e. Refer to community resources to facilitate healthy family coping (elder care centers, adult day care centers, nursing homes, homemaker services, church-affiliated support or clergy)

    f. Determine stressors for family or caretaker

    g. Provide situational support to patient and family

    h. Report to legal authorities: know local rules and regulations regarding elder maltreatment

    i. Recognize that elder patient has right to refuse protective services unless found to be incompetent

4. Expected outcomes/evaluation (see Appendix B)

BIBLIOGRAPHY

Aguilera, D. (1994). *Crisis intervention: Theory and methodology* (7th ed.). St. Louis, MO: C. V. Mosby.

Benter, S. E. (1990). Crisis intervention. In G. W. Stuart & S. J. Sunden (Eds.), *Principles and practice of psychiatric nursing* (4th ed., pp. 270–294). St. Louis, MO: C. V. Mosby.

Buckwalter, K. C. (1992). Psychosocial needs and care of the elderly. In G. K. McFarland & M. D. Thomas (Eds.), *Psychiatric mental health nursing: Application of the nursing process* (pp. 625–642). Philadelphia: J. B. Lippincott.

Campbell, J., & Humphreys, J. (1993). *Nursing care of survivors of family violence.* St. Louis, MO: C. V. Mosby.

Carpenito, L. A. (1997). *Nursing diagnosis: Application to clinical practice* (7th ed.). Philadelphia: J. B. Lippincott.

Hyman, S. (1992). *Manual of psychiatric emergencies* (3rd ed.). Boston: Little, Brown.

Kaiser, J., & Scorza, E. (1990). Psychiatric emergencies. In S. Kitt & J. Kaiser (Eds.), *Emergency nursing: A physiologic and clinical perspective* (pp. 575–609). Philadelphia: W. B. Saunders.

Kunes-Connell, J. (1992). Clients with disorders usually first evident in infancy, childhood, and adolescence. In G. K. McFarland & M. D. Thomas (Eds.), *Psychiatric mental health nursing: Application of the nursing process* (pp. 499–512). Philadelphia: J. B. Lippincott.

Naschinski, C. (1992). Life events of adulthood and related mental health needs and treatment. In G. K. McFarland & M. D. Thomas (Eds.), *Psychiatric mental health nursing: Application of the nursing process* (pp. 615–624). Philadelphia: J. B. Lippincott.

National Center on Elder Abuse. (1996). *Elder Abuse: Questions and answers.* Washington, DC: Author.

Sebree, R., & Popkess-Vawter, S. (1991). Self-injury concept formation in nursing diagnosis development. *Perspectives in Psychiatric Care, 6*(5), 279–280.

Thomas, S. (1991). Psychiatric nursing for the 1990's: New concepts, new therapies. *Issues in Mental Health Nursing, 12*(1), v–vi.

Townsend, M. (1991). *Nursing diagnosis in psychiatric nursing: A pocket guide for care plan construction* (2nd ed.). Philadelphia: F. A. Davis.

Wilson, H., & Kneisl, C. (1993). *Psychiatric nursing* (5th ed.). Menlo Park, CA: Addison-Wesley.

Carol Ann Petersen, RN, BSN, MSA

CHAPTER **11**

Multisystem Trauma and Injury Prevention

MAJOR TOPICS

Bronchoesophageal Fistula

Diabetes Insipidus

Ruptured Innominate Artery

Atelectasis

Empyema

Aspiration

Meningitis

Sensory Deprivation (ICU Psychosis)

Hypovolemia

Sepsis

Neurogenic Shock

Pulmonary Embolism

Adult Respiratory Distress Syndrome (ARDS)

Pneumonia

Wound Dehiscence

Gastrointestinal Fistula

Stress Ulcers

I. OVERVIEW OF THE CRITICALLY INJURED PATIENT

A. Trauma definition

1. **Single-system trauma: an injury to the body from an extrinsic factor involving a single isolated body system**
2. **Multiple-system trauma: an injury to the body from an extrinsic factor that involves two or more body systems**

B. Components of a trauma system

1. **Access**
2. **Prehospital**
3. **Initial resuscitation**
4. **Acute care**
5. **Rehabilitation**

C. Principles that guide a system

1. **Each component is equally important**
2. **Each component affects the next component**
3. **If one component fails, the system fails**

D. Purpose of trauma system

1. **Ensure rapid access to care (e.g., high-risk patient)**
   a. *Methods of scoring*
      1) Trauma Score (refer to Table 11–1)
      2) Pediatric Trauma Score (refer to Table 11–2)
      3) Revised Trauma Score (refer to Table 11–3)
      4) CRAMS (refer to Table 11–4)
2. **Provide for adequate resources (e.g., right hospital)**
   a. *Triage decision schema (refer to Fig. 11–1)*
   b. *Trauma care facilities (refer to Table 11–5)*
   c. *Trauma team (refer to Table 11–6)*
3. **Prevent premature morbidity/mortality (e.g., right time frame)**

Table 11–1   COMPONENTS OF THE TRAUMA SCORE

		Rate	Codes	Score
A.	Respiratory rate	10–24	4	
	Number of respirations in 15 seconds; multiply by 4	25–35	3	
		>35	2	
		<10	1	
		0	0	A. _____
B.	Respiratory effort			
	Retractive: Use of accessory muscles or intercostal retraction	Normal	1	
		Retractive	0	B. _____
C.	Systolic blood pressure	≥90	4	
	Systolic cuff pressure: either arm, auscultate or palpate	70–89	3	
		50–69	2	
		<50	1	
	No carotid pulse	0	0	C. _____
D.	Capillary refill			
	Normal: Forehead or lip mucosa color refill in 2 seconds	Normal	2	
	Delayed: More than 2 seconds capillary refill	Delayed	1	
	None: No capillary refill	None	0	D. _____
E.	Glasgow Coma Scale	Total GCS points	Score	
	1. Eye opening			
	Spontaneous ____ 4	14–15	5	
	To voice ____ 3	11–13	4	
	To pain ____ 2	8–10	3	
	None ____ 1	5–7	2	
		3–4	1	E. _____
	2. Verbal response			
	Oriented ____ 5			
	Confused ____ 4			
	Inappropriate words ____ 3			
	Incomprehensible sounds ____ 2			
	None ____ 1			
	3. Motor response			
	Obeys commands ____ 6			
	Purposeful movements (pain) ____ 5			
	Withdraw (pain) ____ 4			
	Flexion (pain) ____ 3			
	Extension (pain) ____ 2			
	None ____ 1			
Total GCS points (1 + 2 + 3) ____				

Trauma Score _____
(Total points A + B + C + D + E)

From Cardona, V. D., Hurn, P. D., Mason, P. B. M., Scanlon, A. M., and Veise-Berry, S. W. (1994). *Trauma nursing: From resuscitation through rehabilitation* (2nd ed.). Philadelphia: W. B. Saunders.

Table 11–2   PEDIATRIC TRAUMA SCORE

Component	Category		
	+2	**+1**	**−1**
Size	≥20 kg	10–20 kg	<10 kg
Airway	Normal	Maintainable	Unmaintainable
Systolic BP	≤90 mm Hg	90–50 mm Hg	<50 mm Hg
CNS	Awake	Obtunded/LOC	Coma/decerebrate
Open wound	None	Minor	Major/penetrating
Skeletal	None	Closed fracture	Open/multiple fractures
Sum total points			

BP, blood pressure; CNS, central nervous system; LOC, level of consciousness.

Reprinted with permission from Tepas, J. J., Mollitt, D. L., Talbert, J. L., et al. (1987). The Pediatric Trauma Score as a predictor of injury severity in the injured child. *J Pediatr Surg, 22,* 14.

Table 11–3   REVISED TRAUMA SCORE

Assessment	Method	Coding
1. Respiratory rate	Count respiratory rate in 15 seconds and multiply by 4	10–29 = 4 >29 = 3 6–9 = 2 1–5 = 1 0 = 0
2. Systolic blood pressure	Measure systolic cuff pressure in either arm by auscultation or palpation	>89 = 4 76–89 = 3 50–75 = 2 1–49 = 1 0 = 0

3. Glasgow Coma Scale
   score

Eye Opening	**Best Verbal Response**	**Best Motor Response**
Spontaneous = 4	Oriented = 5	Obeys command = 6
To voice = 3	Confused = 4	Localizes pain = 5
To pain = 2	Inappropriate words = 3	Withdraws to pain = 4
None = 1	Incomprehensible sounds = 2	Flexion to pain = 3
	None = 1	Extension to pain = 2
		None = 1

Convert Glasgow Coma Scale score as follows:

13–15 = 4
9–12 = 3
6–8 = 2
4–5 = 1
<4 = 0

To obtain the Trauma Score, add the final scores for respiratory rate, systolic blood pressure, and converted Glasgow Coma Scale score together. Summary of survival probability in a trauma center:

Trauma score	12	11	10	9	8	7	6	5	4	3	2	1	0
Survival	.995	.969	.879	.766	.667	.636	.630	.455	.333	.333	.286	.259	.037

Modified from Cardona, V. D., Hurn, P. D., Mason, P. B. M., Scanlon, A. M., and Veise-Berry, S. W. (1994). *Trauma nursing: From resuscitation through rehabilitation* (2nd ed.). Philadelphia: W. B. Saunders.

Table 11-4   CRAMS SCALE

	Components	Score
C	**Circulation**	
	Normal capillary refill and BP $\geq$ 100	2
	Delayed capillary refill or BP $\geq$ 85 < 100	1
	No capillary refill or BP < 85	0
R	**Respirations**	
	Normal	2
	Abnormal (labored or shallow)	1
	Absent	0
A	**Abdomen**	
	Abdomen and thorax nontender	2
	Abdomen or thorax tender	1
	Abdomen rigid or flail chest°	0
M	**Motor**	
	Normal	2
	Responds only to pain (other than decerebrate)	1
	No response (or decerebrate)	0
S	**Speech**	
	Normal	2
	Confused	1
	No intelligible words	0
	Score $\leq$8: major trauma	
	Score $\geq$9: minor trauma	

°"Penetrating wounds to the abdomen or thorax" was added after the study was published.
BP, blood pressure.
From Gormican, S. P. (1982). CRAMS scale: Field triage of trauma victims. *Annals of Emergency Medicine, 11,* 133. Used with permission.

E. Types of trauma

1. Blunt
2. Penetrating
3. Blast
4. Intentional
5. Nonintentional

F. Types of injury

1. Primary: occur at time of injury
2. Secondary: occur as a result of secondary causes (e.g., hypoxia)

G. Incidence/significance

1. 150,000 deaths/year in United States
2. Leading cause of death for persons aged 1 to 44 years
3. Each year in the United States, 500,000–700,000 persons have permanent disabilities from trauma-related injuries
4. Direct and indirect costs
   a. *Cost of trauma to society is estimated at $150–180 billion annually*
      1) Lives lost and disability costs
      2) Money spent on trauma care (i.e., throughout the continuum from prehospital through rehabilitation)

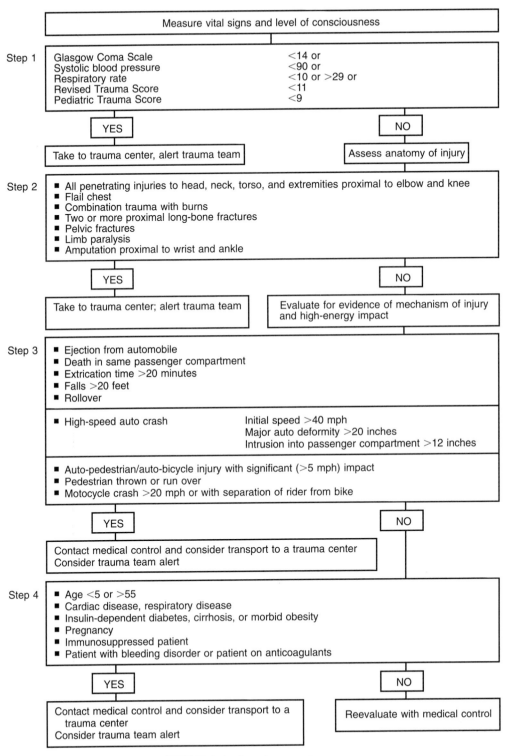

FIGURE 11–1. *See legend on opposite page*

Table 11–5 CHARACTERISTICS OF TRAUMA CARE FACILITIES

Level 1 Trauma Center
Regional resource trauma center
Provides the most sophisticated care as an acute and tertiary center
Provides educational programs for physicians, nurses, paramedics, and other trauma personnel
Conducts major outreach programs, including prevention and public education
Conducts research related to trauma care

Level II Trauma Center
Community trauma center
Provides initial definitive trauma care with the ability to transfer to a level 1 center
Conducts outreach programs, including prevention and public education

Level III Trauma Center
Rural trauma hospital
Commitment to trauma care commensurate with its local resources
Plan of care for the injured includes transfer agreements and protocols

Level IV
Rural clinic or hospital
Commitment to trauma care commensurate with its local resources
Plan of care for the injured includes transfer agreements and protocols

Data from the American College of Surgeons, Committee on Trauma. (1993). *Resources for optimal care of the injured patient.* Chicago: Author. Used with permission.

FIGURE 11–1. Triage decision scheme. (From the American College of Surgeons, Committee on Trauma. [1993]. *Resources for optimal care of the injured patient: 1993.* Chicago: American College of Surgeons. Used with permission.)

NOTES

It is the general intention of these triage guidelines to select severely injured patients for trauma center care. When there is doubt, the patient is best evaluated in a trauma center.

Step 1. Physiologic status thresholds are values of the Glasgow Coma Scale, blood pressure, and respiratory rate from which further deviations from the normal are associated with less than a 90% probability of survival. Used in this manner, prehospital values can be included in the admission trauma score and the quality assessment process.

A variety of physiologic severity scores have been used for prehospital triage and have been found to be accurate. Those scores contained in the triage guidelines are believed to be the simplest to perform and provide an accurate basis for field triage based on physiologic abnormality.

Deterioration of vital signs would necessitate transport to a trauma center.

Step 2. A patient who has normal vital signs at the scene of the accident may still have a serious or lethal injury.

Step 3.° It is essential to look for indications that significant forces were applied to the body.

Evidence of damage to the automobile can be a helpful guide to the change in velocity. Intrusion into the passenger compartment from any direction should prompt consideration of the potential for major injury.

Step 4.° Certain other factors that might lower the threshold at which patients should be treated in trauma centers must be considered in field triage. These include the following:

A. Patients over age 55 have an increasing risk of death from even moderately severe injuries. Those younger than age 5 have certain characteristics that may merit treatment in a trauma center with special resources for children.

B. Comorbid Factors. The presence of significant cardiac, respiratory, or metabolic diseases are additional factors that may merit the triage of patients to trauma centers.

°Each trauma system and its hospitals should use QI programs to determine use of mechanism of injury and cobmorbid factors as activators for bypass and trauma team activation.

Table 11–6 MULTIDISCIPLINARY TRAUMA TEAM

Typical Composition
Trauma surgeon (team leader)
Emergency physician
Anesthesiologist
Trauma nurse team leader—emergency nurse
Trauma resuscitation nurse—critical care nurse
Trauma scribe—emergency nurse
Trauma surgical nurse
Laboratory phlebotomist
Radiological technologist
Respiratory therapist
Social worker/pastoral services
Hospital security officer
Physician specialists as necessary (neurosurgeon, orthopedic surgeon, urologic surgeon)
Inner-Core–Outer-Core Approach
Inner-Core Team
Trauma surgeon (team leader)
Emergency physician
Anesthesiologist
Trauma nurse team leader—emergency nurse
Trauma resuscitation nurse—critical care nurse
Trauma scribe—emergency nurse
Outer-Core Team
Nursing supervisor (team leader)
Laboratory phlebotomist
Radiological technologist
Respiratory therapist
Social worker/pastoral services
Hospital security officer
Registration/emergency clerk
Physician specialist as necessary (neurosurgeon, orthopedic surgeon, urologic surgeon)
(This concept alleviates congestion during initial resuscitation efforts.)

From Clochesy, J. M., Breu, C., Cardin, S., Whittaker, A. A., & Rudy, E. B. (1996). *Critical Care Nursing* (2nd ed., p. 1338). Philadelphia: W. B. Saunders. Used with permission.

H. Factors affecting the outcomes of trauma

1. Persons ≤ 5 years and ≥ 55 years
2. Medical/surgical history
3. Substance abuse
4. Severity of injury
5. Time of injury to definitive care
6. Quality of care

I. Solutions to trauma issues

1. Prevention
2. Education
3. Regionalization of trauma systems

II. INJURY PREVENTION AND EDUCATION

A. Prevention

1. Trauma-related injuries are 50% preventable
2. Methods to improve prevention

    a. Collect data on trauma-related injuries
    b. Analyze the data
    c. Identify specific concerns
    d. Target populations at risk
    e. Identify population characteristics
    f. Develop prevention strategies (i.e., cost effectiveness)
    g. Implement a prevention plan
    h. Evaluate behavioral changes in target population

B. Injury prevention components

1. **Primary: elimination of trauma-related injuries**
2. **Secondary: reduce severity of injury during the incident**
3. **Tertiary: all efforts after trauma to improve the outcome**

C. Intervention strategies

1. **Automatic protection and elimination of environmental hazards**
2. **Legislation**
3. **Education**
4. **Requires multidisciplinary approach**
5. **Age specific**
6. **Reinforced**
7. **Evaluated**

III. GENERAL APPROACH TO CARE OF THE CRITICALLY INJURED PATIENT

A. Assessment

1. **Primary survey/resuscitation (refer to Chapter 1)**
    a. Refer to Table 11–7
2. **Secondary assessment (refer to Chapter 1)**
    a. Refer to Table 11–8
3. **Psychological, social, and environmental factors**

IV. MECHANISM OF INJURY AND KINEMATICS

A. Definitions

1. **Mechanism of injury: refers to detailed cause or type of event**
2. **Kinematics: refers to physics of trauma (how the energy force is dispersed throughout the body during trauma)**

B. Basic laws of physics governing kinematics

1. **Energy cannot be created or destroyed; it simply changes form**
2. **Newton's laws of inertia and momentum**
    a. Inertia: a body at rest will remain at rest until acted upon by an outside force
    b. Momentum: a body in motion will remain in motion traveling in a straight line until acted upon by an outside force

Table 11–7   PRIMARY ASSESSMENT

Assessment		Observations Indicating Impaired Airway, Breathing, Circulation
Airway	Open and patent Maintain cervical spine immobilization	Shallow, noisy breathing Stridor Cyanosis Nasal flaring Accessory muscle use Inability to speak Drooling Anxiety Decreased level of consciousness Trauma to face, mouth, neck Debris of foreign matter in mouth or pharynx
Breathing	Presence and effectiveness	Asymmetrical rise and fall of chest Absent, decreased, or unequal breath sounds Open sucking chest wounds Blunt chest injury Dyspnea Cyanosis Respiratory rate <8–10/min or >40 min Accessory muscle use Anxiety Tracheal shift Distended neck veins Paradoxical chest wall motion

Circulation	Presence of major
	  pulses
	Presence of external
	  hemorrhage
		Weak, thready pulse >120 beats/min
		Pallor
		Blood pressure <90 mm Hg
		Capillary refill >2 seconds
		Obvious external hemorrhage
		Decreased level of consciousness
		Distended neck veins

Disability	Gross neurological
	  status
	Pupil size, equality, and
	  reactivity to light
		Glasgow Coma Scale
		Agitation

Adapted from Clochesy, J. M., Breu, C., Cardin, S., Whittaker, A. A., & Rudy, E. B. (1996). *Critical care nursing* (2nd ed., p. 1343). W. B. Saunders. Used with permission.

C. Detail of mechanism of injury

1. **Data on mechanism of injury collected with primary survey**
   a. *Refer to Table 11–9*
2. **Detail all aspects of mechanism of injury**

V. FUNDAMENTALS OF INITIAL RESUSCITATION

A. Concepts

1. **Assessment and resuscitation occur simultaneously (i.e., a dynamic process)**
2. **Repeat assessment frequently**
3. **Establish priorities and anticipate needs**
4. **Life-threatening injuries take priority over limb-threatening injuries**
5. **Preparedness, organization, and communication are important concepts**

Table 11-8 SECONDARY SURVEY

Area	Inspection	Palpation	Percussion	Auscultation
Head Scalp Skull Face Eyes/ears Nose Mouth	Soft tissue injury Deformities Edema Asymmetry of face Open bite Periorbital edema Otorrhea Rhinorrhea Bloody drainage Extraocular movements Subcutaneous air Visual acuity Eye injuries	Bony deformities of facial bones or skull Scalp wounds Subcutaneous air Crepitus Pain Decreased sensation of face		
Neck	Soft tissue injury Tracheal position Distended neck veins Ask about pain, hoarseness, dysphagia	Crepitus Subcutaneous air Tracheal position Cervical spine tenderness or deformities		
Chest	Soft tissue injury Open sucking wound Subcutaneous air Intercostal retractions Symmetry of chest Respiratory rate, effort Seatbelt marks Impaled objects	Crepitus Subcutaneous air Bony deformities Chest wall excursion	Dullness Hyperresonance	Absent or diminished breath sounds Distant heart or gastric sounds

(Table continued on following page)

Table 11–8 SECONDARY SURVEY *Continued*

Area	Inspection	Palpation	Percussion	Auscultation
Abdomen and flanks°	Soft tissue injury Distension Seatbelt marks Impaled objects Contour Discolorations	Rigidity Distension Pain: diffuse or localized	Dullness Hyperresonance	Bowel sounds in all four quadrants
Pelvis or perineum	Soft tissue injury External genitalia injury Blood at urinary meatus Vaginal bleeding Rectal bleeding Suprapubic masses Priapism	Pelvic instability Femoral pulses Rectal sphincter tone Prostate position Vaginal integrity Open fractures		
Extremities	Soft tissue injury Amputation Crush injury Deformity: open or closed Motor/sensory	Diminished or absent pulses Crepitus Pain or tenderness		
Back	Soft tissue injury to buttocks, posterior thighs, and flanks	Thoracic, lumbar sacral spine pain, tenderness, deformity		

°The sequence of examination of the abdomen is inspection, auscultation, palpation, and percussion.

From Clouchesy, J. M. Breu, C., Cardin, S., Whittaker, A. A., & Rudy, E. B. (1996). *Critical care nursing* (2nd ed., p. 1344). Philadelphia: W. B. Saunders. Used with permission.

Table 11–9 QUESTIONS TO BE ASKED OF PATIENTS WITH VARIOUS TRAUMATIC INJURIES*

Motor Vehicle Crashes
Were you the driver or passenger?
Were you wearing a seatbelt or shoulder harness (or both)?
Did you hit the steering wheel or the dashboard? If so, with what part of your body?
Did you lose consciousness? If so, for how long?
How fast was the vehicle going?
What did the vehicle hit?
Did the vehicle hit a moving object or a nonmoving object? (Paramedics may assist by describing the condition of the car.)
Where is your pain?
How far were you thrown?
What is the condition of the other passengers?
Blunt Trauma From Falls
How far did you fall?
What precipitated the fall?
What did you land on?
Where is your pain?
Did you lose consciousness?
Gunshot Wounds
How long ago did the incident occur?
How many shots did you hear?
What type of gun was it?
From what direction do you think the bullet entered you?
Where is your pain?
Penetrating Wounds or Stab Wounds
How long ago did it happen?
How many times were you stabbed?
How long was the knife?
How far in did it go?
From what direction were you stabbed?
Where is your pain?

*The severity of penetrating trauma will depend on two factors: (1) the anatomical location of the injury and (2) the amount of energy transferred to the body. (This is determined by the force of the penetrating object at the time of impact. Because in general stab wounds are inflicted with less force than gunshot wounds, they have a better prognosis than gunshot wounds inflicted at the same anatomical site.)

From Kitt, S., Selfridge-Thomas, J., Proehl, J. A., & Kaiser, J. (1995). *Emergency nursing: A physiologic & clinical perspective* (2nd ed.). Philadelphia: W. B. Saunders.

6. **Someone must assume control**
7. **Do no further harm**
8. **If condition progressively worsens or remains unstable, definitive care needed (e.g., control bleeding, surgery)**

B. Goal of resuscitation

1. **Primary goal: oxygenation of vital tissues**
   a. *Patent airway and stabilization of cervical spine*
   b. *Adequate ventilation*
   c. *Maximum perfusion/cellular oxygenation*

VI. PRIMARY ASSESSMENT (refer to Chapter 1)

A. Subjective data

1. **Mechanism of injury**
2. **Chief complaint**

B. Airway/cervical spine

1. **Signs and symptoms**
   a. *Decreased level of consciousness*
   b. *Agitation*
   c. *Stridor, airway resistance*
   d. *Cyanosis*
   e. *Use of accessory muscles*
   f. *Abnormal breath sounds*
   g. *Hoarseness*
   h. *No movement of air*
2. **Treatment of nonpatent airway**
   a. *Establish open airway without manipulation of cervical spine; maintain in-line stabilization*
   b. *Simple maneuvers to more complex; manual maneuvers to mechanical*
      1) Manual maneuvers
         a) Modified jaw thrust (chin lift/jaw thrust)
         b) Suction
         c) Clean debris from mouth
         d) Gravity drainage
      2) Mechanical maneuvers
         a) Oral airway
         b) Nasal trumpet
         c) Intubation
         d) Cricothyroidotomy
         e) Tracheostomy

C. Breathing

1. **Signs and symptoms of inadequate ventilation**
   a. *Cyanosis*
   b. *Decreased breath sounds*
   c. *Increased respiratory rate*
   d. *Decreased level of consciousness*
   e. *Noisy respirations*
   f. *Hypoxia*
   g. *Acidosis*
2. **Diagnosis**
   a. *Assessment of clinical presentation*
   b. *Blood gases*
   c. *Oximetry trends*
   d. *Carbon dioxide (CO_2) monitoring*
   e. *Chest x-ray film*
3. **Treatment of inadequate ventilation (refer to Table 11–10)**
   a. *High-flow oxygen*
   b. *Assist ventilation if respiratory rate < 10 or > 30 breaths per minute*
   c. *Treat tension pneumothorax, open pneumothorax, or hemothorax*
   d. *Treat flail chest*
   e. *Pain management*

Table 11–10   INTERVENTIONS FOR INEFFECTIVE BREATHING PATTERNS

Etiology	Interventions
Tension pneumothorax	Prepare for decompression by needle thoracotomy with a 12-gauge to 16-gauge needle in second intercostal space in midclavicular line on affected side Prepare for chest tube insertion
Pneumothorax	Prepare for chest tube insertion on affected side
Open sucking wound	Seal wound with occlusive dressing and monitor chest for signs of tension pneumothorax Remove one corner of dressing if respiratory distress develops; prepare for chest tube insertion
Massive hemothorax	Establish two 14-gauge to 16-gauge IV lines with crystalloids Obtain blood for type and crossmatch Prepare for large chest tube insertion Prepare autotransfusion device Administer blood or blood products as ordered Anticipate and prepare for emergency open thoracotomy
Pulmonary contusion	Prepare for early intubation and mechanical ventilation Administer IV crystalloids at a rate guided by the absence of signs of shock
Flail chest	Stabilize chest wall: may position on affected side with head of bed elevated or apply manual pressure while preparing for definitive internal stabilization Prepare for early intubation and mechanical ventilation Prepare for chest tube insertion Administer IV crystalloids at a rate guided by the absence of signs of shock Administer analgesics as ordered Assist with intercostal nerve block
Tracheobronchial injury	Elevate head of bed to facilitate breathing Prepare for chest tube insertion Anticipate bronchoscopy
Spinal cord injury	Avoid hyperextension or rotation of neck Maintain complete spinal immobilization Prepare for application of cervical traction tongs or halo device Monitor motor and sensory function Monitor for signs of neurogenic shock
Decreased level of consciousness	Position head midline with head of bed elevated Administer osmotic diuretics, steroids, anticonvulsants, or paralytic agents as ordered Anticipate CT scan

IV, intravenous; GA, gauge; CT, computed tomography.
From Clochesy, J. M., Breu, C., Cardin, S., Whittaker, A. A., & Rudy, E. B. (1996). *Critical care nursing* (2nd ed., p. 1347). Philadelphia: W. B. Saunders. Used with permission.

  f. Consider position of comfort to ease respiratory effort, but only after spinal injury is ruled out

  g. Prepare for definitive airway

D. Circulation

 1. **Signs and symptoms of hypovolemic shock**
  a. Altered level of consciousness
  b. Tachycardia
  c. Hypotension
  d. Tachypnea
  e. Cool, diaphoretic skin
  f. Low urine output
  g. Slow capillary refill

 2. **Diagnosis**
  a. CBC, PT, PTT
  b. Radiological examination
  c. Diagnostic peritoneal lavage
  d. Ultrasonogram
  e. Arteriograms

 3. **Treatment of hypovolemic shock**
  a. Apply direct pressure to external bleeding
  b. High flow oxygen
  c. Establish two large-bore intravenous catheters (14- or 16-gauge needles); may consider central catheter
  d. Fluid resuscitation with lactated Ringer's solution or normal saline
   1) Refer to Table 11–11
  e. Prepare to administer crystalloid, colloids, blood, or blood component therapy
  f. Pneumatic antishock garment (PASG) controversial; may be used with pelvic fractures
  g. Rule out tension pneumothorax, cardiac tamponade, myocardial laceration as sources of shock

E. Spinal immobilization

 1. **Immobilization should be based on mechanism, not neurological deficit**
 2. **Fractures of one portion of the spine are often associated with fractures of another area of the spine**
 3. **Spinal cord injuries may occur with or without bony involvement**
 4. **Maintain high index of suspicion based upon**
  a. Pain
  b. Paralysis
  c. Paresthesia
  d. Ptosis
  e. Priapism
  f. Presenting position
  g. Pregnancy (e.g., especially third trimester)
  h. Mechanism of injury
 5. **Spinal immobilization**
  a. Immobilize joint above and below the injury
  b. Immobilization devices alone are only 50% effective

Text continued on page 396

Table 11–11 GUIDE TO PARENTERAL FLUIDS

Type	Description	Composition	Used Indications	Advantages	Disadvantages	Special Considerations
Blood and Blood Products						
Whole blood	500 mL unit of complete blood	Red blood cells Leukocytes Plasma Platelets Clotting factors	To replace blood volume and maintain adequate hemoglobin (Hgb)	Provides intravascular volume Increases the oxygen-carrying capacity of the blood	Possibility of limited supply Potential associated risks of hepatitis and HIV transmission and allergic reactions Delayed administration because of necessary typing and cross-matching Possibility of type and cross-match errors	Whole blood should be stored at 0–10° C, but warmed at least 20–30 minutes before administration (never infuse cold blood) (Use _fresh_ whole blood whenever possible to avoid adverse metabolic changes related to stored blood, i.e., increased ammonia, potassium, and cellular debris)
Red blood cells (packed, concentrate) Fresh	300 mL unit of whole blood minus 80% of plasma (hematocrit 70%)	Red blood cells 20% plasma Some leukocytes and platelets	To increase the hematocrit To correct red blood cell deficiency and improve the oxygen-carrying capacity of the blood	Concentrated form helps prevent excess fluid administration in patients with cardiogenic shock (increases the oxygen-carrying capacity with less volume loading) Associated with fewer risks of metabolic complications when compared with stored whole blood (decreased amount of transfused antibodies, electrolytes, etc.)	Slow infusion rate because of increased viscosity Decreased content of plasma proteins and coagulation factors when compared with whole blood Inadequate (alone) for volume replacement and correction of hypovolemia Altered blood clotting with administration of more than 20 units; clotting factors need to be replenished as necessary	Administer via Y-connector tubing with normal saline to increase infusion flow rate Washed red blood cells (resuspended in saline) can be given in shock to decrease red cell adhesiveness (washing decreases the cell's fibrinogen coating) Administration carries risk of blood-borne disease transmission and allergic reaction

Table continued on following page

Table 11–11 GUIDE TO PARENTERAL FLUIDS *Continued*

Type	Description	Composition	Used Indications	Advantages	Disadvantages	Special Considerations
Blood and Blood Products (continued)						
Frozen (also called leukocyte poor)	200–250 mL unit with 85–90% of red blood cell mass contained in 1 unit of whole blood	Red blood cells No plasma Almost no leukocytes or platelets	Used in anemia and for modest blood loss (when hematocrit is below 25–30%)	Provides economic use of blood as a resource; frees other blood components, such as platelets and clotting factors, to be concentrated and stored	High cost of frozen (thawed) red blood cells	
Human plasma (fresh, frozen, or dried)	200 mL unit of uncoagulated, unconcentrated plasma (separated from 1 unit of whole blood)	Plasma All plasma proteins, including albumin Clotting factors (no red cells, white cells, or platelets)	To restore plasma volume in hypovolemic shock without increasing the hematocrit To restore clotting factors (except platelets)	Effective for rapid volume replacement Contains clotting factors	Expensive Deficient of red blood cells	Human plasma carries the risk of viral hepatitis and HIV transmission and allergic reactions Administer fresh frozen plasma promptly after thawing to prevent deterioration of clotting factors V and VII
Platelets	Platelet sediment from platelet-rich plasma, resuspended in 30–50 mL of plasma	Platelets Lymphocytes Some plasma	To control bleeding due to thrombocytopenia To maintain normal blood coagulability		Deficient of other coagulation factors	

| Plasma protein fraction (e.g., Plasmanate, Plasma-Plex) | 250 mL and 500 mL units of a 5% solution of human plasma proteins in normal saline | Albumin 44g/L, α and β globulins 6 g/L, Sodium 130–160 mEq/L, Potassium 2 mEq/L, Osmolality 290 mOsm/L, pH 6.7–7.3 | To expand plasma volume in hypovolemic shock (while cross-matching is being completed); To increase the serum colloid osmotic pressure | Can be used interchangeably with 5% human serum albumin; Osmotically equivalent to plasma; Associated with low risk of hepatitis or HIV transmission | Expensive; Deficient of clotting factors; Associated with larger number of side effects, such as hypotension and hypersensitivity, than those reported with 5% albumin (due to presence of globulins); Hypotension induced by rapid intravenous administration (greater than 10 mL/min) | Plasma protein fraction is prepared from pooled plasma heated to 60°C for 10 hours; this procedure reduces the risk of transmission of HIV and viral hepatitis; Rapid administration of large doses can alter blood coagulation; This solution should be used cautiously in patients with congestive heart failure (due to added fluid and rapid plasma volume expansion) and in patients with renal failure (due to added proteins) |

Table continued on following page

Table 11–11 GUIDE TO PARENTERAL FLUIDS *Continued*

Type	Description	Composition	Used Indications	Advantages	Disadvantages	Special Considerations
Blood and Blood Products (continued)						
Albumin	Aqueous fraction of pooled plasma prepared from whole blood in buffered normal saline		To increase the plasma colloid osmotic pressure To rapidly expand the plasma volume	Rare allergic reactions (less than 0.011% in all albumin solutions combined) Rare transmission of hepatitis virus due to heating process (transmission only occurs secondary to accidents in its preparation)	Potential leakage from capillaries in shock states associated with increased capillary permeability Possible precipitation of congestive heart failure following rapid infusion in patients with circulatory overload and compromised cardiovascular function	Albumin does not contain preservatives; therefore, each opened bottle should be used at once The rate of administration of 5% albumin should not exceed 2–4 mL/min The rate of administration of 25% albumin should not exceed 1 mL/min 25% albumin is reserved for use in patients with pulmonary or peripheral edema and hypoproteinemia; administer with a diuretic to ensure diuresis
5%	250 and 500 mL units	Albumin 50 g/L Sodium 130–160 mEq/L Potassium 1 mEq/L Osmolality 300 mOsm/L Colloid osmotic pressure 20 mm Hg pH 6.4–7.4				
25% (salt poor)°	25-mL, 50-mL, and 100-mL units	Albumin 240 g/L Globulins 10 g/L Sodium 130–160 mEq/L Osmolality 1500 mOsm/L pH 6.4–7.4				

Pharmaceutical Plasma Expanders

Dextran						
Dextran	Biosynthesized Water soluble, large polysaccharide polymer of glucose		To rapidly expand plasma volume	All dextrans associated with low incidence of anaphylactic reactions (<0.01%) Less expensive than protein solutions	*LMWD* 70% excreted unchanged in the urine, so the urine osmolality and specific gravity are altered	Avoid the use of dextran in patients with active hemorrhage, hemorrhagic shock, coagulation disorders, and thrombocytopenia
Low molecular weight dextran (LMWD; dextran 40; Rheomacrodex; Gentran 40)	500 mL unit of solution that contains 10% dextran in either normal saline or 5% dextrose in water	Glucose polysaccharides with average molecular weight of 40,000		LMWD associated with fewer allergic reactions than HMWD LMWD facilitates blood flow by decreasing red blood cell sludging and platelet aggregation	Potential osmotic-nephrosis and renal tubular shutdown Possible bleeding from raw surfaces due to decreased platelet adhesiveness; side effects include decreased hemoglobin, hematocrit, fibrinogen, and clotting factors V, VIII, and IX	Bleeding times can be prolonged when the correct dose of dextran 70 (1.2 g/kg/day) or dextran 40 (2 g/kg/day) is exceeded
High molecular weight dextran (HMWD; dextran 70; Gentran 70–75; Macrodex)	500 ml unit of solution that contains 6% dextran in either normal saline or 5% dextrose in water	Glucose polysaccharides with average molecular weight of 70,000–75,000		HMWD leaks from the capillaries less readily than LMWD; can effectively increase plasma volume for up to 24 hours	*HMWD* 50% excreted unchanged in the urine, so the urine osmolality and specific gravity are altered Higher incidence of allergic reactions when compared with LMWD Increase blood viscosity and platelet adhesiveness	Administer dextran in dextrose solutions to patients with sodium restriction Dextran administration can interfere with typing and cross-matching of blood when the older (outdated) enzyme method is used

Table continued on following page

Table 11–11 GUIDE TO PARENTERAL FLUIDS *Continued*

Type	Description	Composition	Used Indications	Advantages	Disadvantages	Special Considerations
Pharmaceutical Plasma Expanders (continued)						
Hetastarch (Hespan)	500 mL unit of a 6% solution containing a synthetic polymer of hydroxyethyl starch in normal saline	Globular and branched-chain hydroxyethyl starch prepared from amylopectin Average molecular weight = 69,000–70,000 Sodium 154 mEq/L Chloride 154 mEq/L Osmolality 310 mOsm/L Colloid osmotic pressure 30–35 mm Hg	To expand plasma volume	Same volume expansion characteristics of albumin but with a longer duration of action (up to 36 hours) Associated with low risk of allergic and anaphylactic reactions (0.085%) Cost of hetastarch is about one half that of plasma protein fraction and albumin Nonantigenic No danger of transmission of hepatitis virus	Potential dilution of plasma proteins Potential dilution of clotting factors with resultant coagulation changes Potential circulatory overload in patients with severe congestive heart failure and compromised renal function Increased serum amylase level (>200 mg/100 mL), peaking within 1 hour of intravenous administration of hetastarch and persisting 3 to 4 days (due to action of amylase in hetastarch degradation)	Do not use if the solution is cloudy or deep brown or if it contains crystals Monitor clotting studies and platelet counts, observing for prolonged prothrombin and partial thromboplastin times and thrombocytopenia The safety and compatibility of additives with hetastarch have not been established; the manufacturer recommends infusing hetastarch through a separate line, when possible, or piggybacking the second drug The maximum infusion rate in acute hemorrhagic shock is 20 mL/kg/hr Monitor serum albumin; if it falls below 2 g/100 mL, consider substituting albumin for hetastarch

Solution	Description	Action	Uses	Precautions
Mannitol (Osmitrol)	Solution of mannitol in water or normal saline Mannitol (inert form of sugar mannose)	Reduces intracellular/interstitial swelling Increases urinary output	To raise intravascular volume To reduce interstitial and intracellular edema To promote osmotic diuresis	Potential circulatory overload in patients with congestive heart failure, pulmonary congestion, and renal dysfunction
Crystalloid Solutions ***Isotonic***				
Normal saline	0.9% sodium chloride in water Sodium 154 mEq/L Chloride 154 mEq/L Osmolality 308 mOsm/L	Considered by some to be the single most important salt for maintaining and replacing extracellular fluid Increases plasma volume without altering normal sodium concentration or serum osmolality	To raise plasma volume when red blood cell mass is adequate To replace body fluid	Potential fluid retention and circulatory overload due to sodium content Potential hyperchloremic metabolic acidosis due to high chloride content
Lactated Ringer's solution (Hartman's solution)	0.9% sodium chloride in water with added electrolytes and buffers Sodium 130 mEq/L Potassium 4 mEq/L Calcium 2.7 mEq/L Chloride 109 mEq/L Lactate 27 mEq/L pH 6.5 Osmolality 273 mOsm/L	Lactate is converted to bicarbonate (in the liver), which buffers acidosis Lactate replaces bicarbonate, preventing precipitation of calcium bicarbonate and calcium carbonate Lactate is more stable than bicarbonate and more compatible with ions present in the solution	To replace body fluid To buffer acidosis	Increased lactic acidosis in shock due to lactate Fluid retention and circulatory overload due to sodium content Lactate conversion requires aerobic metabolism; therefore, it should be used cautiously in shock and other hypoperfusion states Use cautiously in patients with liver failure since liver converts lactate

Table continued on following page

Table 11-11 GUIDE TO PARENTERAL FLUIDS *Continued*

Type	Description	Composition	Used Indications	Advantages	Disadvantages	Special Considerations
Crystalloid Solutions (continued)						
Isotonic						
Plasma-Lyte A	0.9% sodium chloride in water with added electrolytes, acetate, and glucagon	Sodium 140 mEq/L Potassium 5 mEq/L Magnesium 3 mEq/L Chloride 98 mEq/L Acetate 27 mEq/L Gluconate 23 mEq/L Osmolality 294 mOsm/L	To replace body fluids	Calcium free, so can be administered with blood Lower chloride content decreases risk of hyperchloremic metabolic acidosis Lacks lactate, so will not exacerbate lactic acidosis Acetate acts to buffer acidosis	Fluid retention and circulatory overload due to sodium content	Give cautiously in patients with renal insufficiency due to potassium and magnesium load
Ringer's solution	0.9% sodium chloride in water with added potassium and calcium	Sodium 147 mEq/L Potassium 4 mEq/L Calcium 5 mEq/L Chloride 156 mEq/L	To replace body fluid To provide additional potassium and calcium	Does not contain lactate, so can be given to patients with hypoperfusion	Potential hyperchloremic metabolic acidosis due to high chloride concentration Potential fluid retention and circulatory overload due to sodium content	
Hypotonic						
1/2 normal saline	0.45% sodium chloride in water	Sodium 77 mEq/L Chloride 77 mEq/L	To raise total fluid volume		Potential interstitial and intracellular edema due to rapid movement of this fluid from the vascular space Dilution of plasma proteins and electrolytes	

| 5% dextrose in water (D₅W) | 5% dextrose | To raise total fluid volume
To provide calories for energy (200 calories/1000 mL) | Distributed evenly in every body compartment (acts like free water)
Reverses dehydration
Prevents hyperosmolar state
Maintains adequate renal tubular flow (facilitates water excretion) | Dilution of plasma proteins and electrolytes due to rapid metabolism of glucose and resultant free water
May cause or exacerbate interstitial and intracellular edema due to rapid movement of this solution from intravascular space |

---

*The term *salt poor* designates the 25% albumin concentration and is a carryover from the days when acetyltryptophan replaced a 1.8% salt solution to increase the thermal stability of the product. The term salt poor is erroneous because both concentrations of albumin contain sodium carbonate or sodium bicarbonate to adjust the pH and sodium caprylate and sodium acetyltryptophan as stabilizers.

Adapted from Rice V. (1984). Shock management. Part I: Fluid volume replacement. *Crit Care Nurse*, 4, 69–73. Used with permission.

    c. If patient has an altered level of consciousness, immobilize

    d. Do not constrict chest or airway

    e. Do not be in a hurry to remove the cervical collar or backboard

  6. Diagnostics

    a. Initial lateral and anteroposterior view to include C-7 and T-1

    b. Consider findings of primary and secondary surveys

    c. Prepare for computed tomography (CT) scan, magnetic resonance imaging (MRI)

F. Neurological assessment (disability)

  1. Subjective data

    a. Altered level of consciousness

    b. Altered motor activity, altered sensation

    c. Anxiety

    d. Altered physiological parameter

  2. Objective data

    a. Level of consciousness (establish baseline)

      1) AVPU: *a*lert, response to *v*erbal stimuli, response to *p*ainful stimuli, *u*nresponsive

    b. Trend Glasgow Coma Scale score

    c. Trend pupillary size, shape, and reactivity

    d. Assess motor function

  3. Diagnostics to

    a. Rule out

      1) Decreased cerebral perfusion and/or direct cerebral injury

      2) Drugs/alcohol

      3) Hypoxia

      4) Hypotension

    b. Clinical presentation

    c. Prepare for radiological studies (e.g., CT scan)

  4. Treatment

    a. Complete primary survey

    b. Continued management of life-threatening injuries

    c. Complete secondary survey

    d. Rapid resuscitation

    e. Prolonged hyperventilation should be avoided unless neurological deterioration occurs

    f. Avoid hypotension (i.e., keep mean arterial pressure [MAP] > 90 mm Hg, cerebral perfusion pressure [CPP] > 70 mm Hg)

    g. Monitor vital signs, Glasgow Coma Scale score; check pupils frequently

    h. Protect patient from further injury

    i. Prepare for possible administration of medications (e.g., naloxone [Narcan], methylprednisolone [Solu-Medrol], mannitol)

    j. Prepare for possible intracerebral pressure monitoring

G. Exposure of the patient during assessment

  1. Must be completely undressed; avoid overexposure, which increases risk of hypothermia, maintain C-spine immobilization

VII. SECONDARY SURVEY

A. Should not be initialized until life-threatening injuries are treated and primary assessment is complete

B. History: pertinent past and present medical history, substance abuse history

1. Allergies
2. Medications
3. Preexisting conditions
4. Last meal
5. Events leading to injury

C. Head-to-toe physical examination

D. Prepare for other diagnostics and laboratory tests

E. Insert Foley catheter and monitor urine outputs hourly

1. Maintain output in adults > 30 mL/hr
2. Contraindications to insertion: blood at meatus, scrotal hematoma, high-riding prostate

F. Decompress the stomach with nasogastric tube

1. Contraindications
   a. *Midface fractures*
   b. *Cerebrospinal fluid leaks*

VIII. SPECIAL POPULATION CONSIDERATIONS

A. Pediatric considerations

1. Assessment and resuscitation considerations
   a. *Immunization status*
   b. *Size/shape of patient (e.g., larger head/body ratio)*
   c. *Greater body surface*
   d. *Age-related functional status*
   e. *Age-related behavioral status*
   f. *Consider abuse and neglect*
   g. *Appropriate size of equipment*
2. Airway concerns
   a. *Potential collapse of posterior pharyngeal area*
   b. *Small oral cavity with large tongue, tonsils*
   c. *Larynx positioned more anteriorly and cephalad*
   d. *Short trachea*
   e. *Insert oral airway directly; more U-shaped epiglottis*
   f. *Use "uncuffed" endotracheal tube in children less than 8 years old*
   g. *Tube sizes appropriate to size of patient*
   h. *Ventilation*
      1) Children: 20 breaths per minute
      2) Infants: 40 breaths per minute
3. Circulation concerns
   a. *Maintain high index of suspicion*
   b. *Increased physiological reserves*

    c. Pediatric patients can have a 25% blood volume loss before they are symptomatic; hypotension is a late and often sudden sign of hypovolemia

    d. Capillary refill, skin color, and temperature are best indicators of tissue perfusion

    e. Tachycardia is a sensitive indicator of tissue perfusion/hypoxia

    f. Treatment of hypotension

        1) Fluid bolus of 20 mL/kg of crystalloid, may repeat; if no improvement, administer blood products (10 mL/kg)

        2) Consider cutdown or interosseous infusion

  4. Thermoregulation

    a. High ratio of body surface area, more susceptible to heat loss

    b. Consider maturity of thermoregulatory mechanisms

B. Geriatric considerations

  1. Assessment and resuscitation concerns

    a. Medical history (e.g., chronic diseases)

    b. Functional status before trauma

        1) Altered perception

        2) Delayed response

  2. Physiological considerations

    a. Airway

        1) Decreased lung mass, elasticity, expansion of rib cage, vital capacity, cough, arterial oxygen tension

        2) Marked tendency to pneumonia

    b. Cardiovascular

        1) Blood pressure unreliable

        2) Frequent monitoring of vital signs imperative

        3) Consider invasive monitoring (i.e., in acute care phase)

        4) Evaluate cause of dysrhythmias

        5) Increased capillary permeability

    c. Cognitive status before trauma

        1) Loss of short-term memory

        2) Dementia

        3) Sensory overload

    d. Musculoskeletal

        1) Limited mobility

        2) Limited joint flexibility

        3) Muscle atrophy

        4) Increased pain threshold

        5) Osteoarthritis of cervical spine

    e. Renal

        1) Decreased renal blood flow

        2) Decreased water absorption

        3) Decreased bladder capacity

        4) Increased incidence of infection

        5) May see increased urinary output with hypotension

        6) Decreased diluting ability

C. Pregnant trauma patient (see Chapter 13)

IX. POTENTIAL COMPLICATIONS

A. Pneumothorax

1. Tension
2. Simple
3. Hemo-pneumothorax

B. Renal failure

C. Bronchoesophageal fistula

D. Diabetes insipidus

E. Ruptured innominate artery

F. Atelectasis

G. Empyema

H. Aspiration

I. Meningitis

J. Sensory deprivation (intensive care unit [ICU] psychosis)

K. Hypovolemia

L. Sepsis

M. Neurogenic shock

N. Pulmonary embolism

O. Adult respiratory distress syndrome (ARDS)

P. Pneumonia

Q. Wound dehiscence

R. Gastrointestinal fistula

S. Stress ulcers

BIBLIOGRAPHY

American College of Surgeons. (1982). *Early care of the injured patient* (3rd ed.). Chicago: Author.

American College of Surgeons, Committee on Trauma. (1993). *Resources for optimal care of the injured patient*. Chicago: Author.

Baker, J. P., O'Neill, B., & Ginsburg, M. (1992). *The injury fact book* (2nd ed.). New York: Oxford University Press.

Cardona, V. D., Hurn, P. D., Mason, P. B. M., Scanlon, A. M., and Veise-Berry, S. W. (1994). *Trauma nursing: From resuscitation through rehabilitation* (2nd ed.). Philadelphia: W. B. Saunders.

Clochesy, J. M., Breu, C., Cardin, S., Whittaker, A. A., & Rudy, E. B. (1996). *Critical care nursing* (2nd ed., pp. 1335–1358). Philadelphia: W. B. Saunders.

Feliciano, D., Moore, D., & Mattox, K. (1996). *Trauma* (3rd ed.). Stanford, CT: Appleton & Lange.

Kitt, S., Selfridge-Thomas, J., Proehl, J. A., & Kaiser, J. (1995). *Emergency nursing: A physiologic & clinical perspective* (2nd ed.). Philadelphia: W. B. Saunders.

Morris J. A., MacKenzie, E. J., Damiano, A. M., et al. (1990). Mortality in trauma patients: The interaction between host factors and severity. *Journal of Trauma, 30*, 1476.

Joan A. Snyder, RN, MS, CEN

CHAPTER **12**

Neurological Emergencies

MAJOR TOPICS

I. GENERAL STRATEGY

A. Assessment

1. **Primary survey/resuscitation (see Chapter 1)**
2. **Secondary survey (see Chapter 1)**
3. **Psychological, social, and environmental risk factors**
   a. *Recent changes in habits (e.g., sleeping, eating, stress levels)*
   b. *Personal habits*
      1) Dependent or independent personality type
      2) Competitive or noncompetitive
      3) Rigid or inflexible behavior
      4) Degree of sensitivity
      5) Sleep habits
      6) Dietary habits

      7) Amount and type of relaxation

      8) Use of oral contraceptives

      9) Substance abuse

    10) Obesity

    11) Excessive use of laxatives in children

    12) Abuse of spouse or child

    13) Failure to use seatbelts

  c. *Cardiovascular factors*

      1) Hypertension

      2) Atherosclerosis

      3) Dysrhythmias

      4) High cholesterol

  d. *Extremes of age*

4. Focused survey

  a. *Subjective data*

    1) History of present illness

      a) Chronological sequence of onset and development of neurological symptoms

      b) Consciousness

        (1) Loss of (time of occurrence, duration, severity)

        (2) Alterations in (fluctuating, steady decline)

      c) Mentation

        (1) Memory (recent and remote)

        (2) Changes in cognitive ability (e.g., problem solving)

        (3) Episodes of getting lost, forgetting everyday information (e.g., names, dates, locations)

      d) Alteration in personality

        (1) Change in affect

        (2) Rages or apathy

        (3) Violent or destructive behavior

      e) Emotional lability or mood swings

      f) Alteration in health or personal habits

      g) Difficulty with activities of daily living

      h) Alteration in communication

        (1) Speech changes

        (2) Hearing difficulties

        (3) Comprehension difficulties

      i) Alteration in motor ability

        (1) Weakness (paresis)

        (2) Paralysis (plegia)

        (3) Loss of coordination

        (4) Tremors

        (5) Twitching or fasciculations

        (6) Difficulty in getting out of a chair or in climbing stairs

      j) Alterations in sensation

        (1) Diminution or loss of

        (2) Hallucinations

      k) Alteration in sexual performance

      l) Alteration in vision

        (1) Loss of or decrease in acuity or visual fields

        (2) Diplopia

      m) Injury or fall

        (1) Mechanism

       (2) Time elapsed since occurrence
       (3) Treatment prior to arrival
       (4) Changes in clinical status
    n) Pain (PQRST)
       (1) *Provocation*
       (2) *Quality*
       (3) *Region*/radiation
       (4) *Severity*
       (5) *Timing*
    o) Headache
    p) Seizures
    q) Vomiting
  2) Medical history
    a) Neurological diseases
    b) Trauma
    c) Fainting, dizziness, "falling-out" spells
    d) Substance abuse (i.e., drugs, alcohol, or nicotine)
    e) Recent stress
       (1) Social
       (2) Occupational
       (3) Personal
    f) Cardiovascular, liver, endocrine, or pulmonary disease
    g) Recent neck or thoracic surgery
    h) Ingestion of or exposure to toxic substances
    i) Fluid or electrolyte imbalances
    j) Current medication history
       (1) Anticonvulsants
       (2) Anti-inflammatory agents, analgesics, aspirin
       (3) Anticoagulants
       (4) Cardiac drugs: antihypertensives, antidysrhythmics, diuretics
       (5) Tranquilizers, sedatives
       (6) Eyedrops
    k) Malignancy
    l) Allergies (food or drug)
b. *Objective data*
  1) Physical examination
    a) General survey
       (1) Inspection
         (a) General appearance (dress and grooming)
         (b) Surface trauma
         (c) Symmetry
       (2) Auscultation
         (a) Heart and lung sounds
         (b) Carotid bruit
       (3) Palpation
         (a) Scalp and skull
         (b) Muscle mass
    b) Level of consciousness using AVPU scale
       (1) Alert, awake; responsive to voice; oriented to person, time, and place
       Verbal; responds to voice but not fully oriented to person, time, or place

Pain; does not respond to voice but responds to painful stimuli

Unresponsive; does not respond to voice or pain

    (2) Awareness (ability to interact with and interpret the environment)

       (a) Orientation (person, place, time)

       (b) Memory (short and long term)

       (c) Judgment and reasoning

       (d) Communication (verbalization and comprehension): content, fluency, rhythm, ability to name objects, articulation, and effort to initiate and to follow one-, two-, and three-step commands with and without cues

       (e) Attention span

       (f) Knowledge of current events

c) Pupillary response

    (1) Size and equality

    (2) Reaction: direct and consensual

    (3) Variance

       (a) Blind eye

       (b) Hippus (failure to hold the constriction with the light on)

       (c) Anisocoria (grossly unequal pupils)

d) Motor response

    (1) Movement

       (a) Normal: follows commands, localizes/purposeful

       (b) Abnormal: withdrawal from stimulus, posturing, rigid flexion (decortication), rigid extension (decerebration), no response

    (2) Tone (increased, decreased)

    (3) Strength

       (a) Symmetry (upper and lower extremity comparison as well as between right and left)

       (b) Grading scale (none = 0, flicker of muscle = 1, joint movement but not against gravity = 2, moves vs. gravity, not resistance = 3, moves vs. resistance, but weak = 4, full strength vs. resistance = 5)

    (4) Gait and posture

       (a) Arm swing (normal or none)

       (b) Balance (ability to turn, ability to stand with feet apart and together)

    (5) Tremors

       (a) Resting

       (b) Intention

    (6) Coordination

       (a) Rapid alternating movement (palm up, palm down)

       (b) Point to point (e.g., finger to nose)

    (7) Reflexes

       (a) Deep tendon

       (b) Abnormal (Babinski's reflex, grasp)

e) Cranial nerves (CN)

    (1) Eye signs/movements (CN II, CN III, CN IV, and CN VI)

       (a) Visual acuity (read or see printed material, count fingers, see dark vs. light, respond to threat)

       (b) Visual fields (central or nasal, peripheral or temporal)

       (c) Extraocular movements: conjugate movement (normal); disconjugate movement (abnormal)

    (2) Speech musculature (CN VII, CN IX, CN X, CN XII)

   (a) Lips (CN VII): "me, me, me"
   (b) Palate (CN IX and X): "ga-ga, ka-ka"
   (c) Tongue (CN XII): "la, la, la"
  (3) Protective reflexes
   (a) Gag/swallow (CN IX and X)
   (b) Corneal (CN V and VII)
  (4) Other
   (a) CN I: sense of smell (rarely tested)
   (b) CN V: response to cotton wisp over forehead, cheek, and chin
   (c) CN VII: facial movement and expression (pucker, raise brow, smile)
   (d) CN VIII: sense of hearing
   (e) CN XI: head turning, shoulder shrugging
 f) Glasgow Coma Scale (see Appendix C)
 g) Brain-stem integrity (Cervical spine and tympanic membrane must be intact before performing these tests)
  (1) Doll's eyes: present when eyes move in the direction opposite that in which the head is moving (found with an intact brain stem but damaged cerebral cortex)
  (2) Caloric testing: present when eyes move toward the ear stimulated with cold water (found with an intact brain stem but damaged cerebral hemispheres; with a brain stem lesion, caloric reflex will be absent or ocular movement will be disconjugate)
  (3) Apnea test: allowing CO_2 to build up to stimulate the respiratory system to determine whether patients will breathe on their own
  (4) Loss of brain-stem reflexes (pupils, gag, cough, corneals)
 h) Vital signs
  (1) Blood pressure (include pulse pressure)
  (2) Pulse (rate and rhythm)
  (3) Respirations (rate, depth, pattern, muscles used)
  (4) Cushing's triad: seen as a *very* late sign with increased intracranial pressure (ICP) and signifies emergency attempt to perfuse the brain
   (a) Increased systolic blood pressure, widened pulse pressure
   (b) Profound bradycardia
   (c) Abnormal respirations
  (5) Temperature (rectal preferred)
 i) Sensory response
  (1) Pain perception (point of a pin)
  (2) Touch and pressure (head of a pin)
  (3) Proprioception (toe up or down?)
 j) Cerebrospinal fluid leaks (otorrhea and/or rhinorrhea)
 k) Meningeal signs
  (1) Stiff neck, photophobia, pain upon neck flexion, positive Brudzinski's sign (knees/hips flex while neck is flexed), positive Kernig's sign (leg is flexed at hip and patient cannot completely extend leg)
  (2) Diagnostic procedures
   (a) 12-lead electrocardiogram (ECG)
   (b) Laboratory studies
    Serum electrolytes and glucose
    Complete blood count (CBC): differential and sedimentation rate
    Toxicology screen

                    Coagulation studies
                    Arterial blood gases (ABGs)
                    Urinalysis
                    Cerebrospinal fluid analysis
            (c) Radiography
                    Radiograph: chest, skull, spine (all seven vertebrae of the
                        cervical spine)
                    Angiogram/arteriogram
                    Computed tomography (CT) scan
                    Magnetic resonance imaging (MRI)
                    Myelogram
                    Brain scan
            (d) Other
                    Lumbar puncture (contraindicated with increased ICP)
                    Electroencephalogram (EEG)
                    Written consent for diagnostic procedures (validate intact
                        short-term memory)

B. Analysis: differential nursing diagnosis/collaborative problems

1. **Ineffective airway clearance**
2. **Tissue perfusion, altered cerebral**
3. **Pain**
4. **Anxiety/fear**
5. **Impaired verbal communication**
6. **Risk for injury**
7. **Impaired gas exchange**
8. **Decreased cardiac output**
9. **Knowledge deficit**
10. **Noncompliance**

C. Planning/interventions

1. **Determine priorities**
   a. *Control and maintain airway, breathing, circulation*
   b. *Prevent further damage or injury*
   c. *Prevent or minimize complications*
   d. *Control pain*
   e. *Relieve anxiety*
   f. *Educate patient and significant others*
2. **Develop nursing care plan specific to patient's presenting emergency**
3. **Obtain and set up necessary equipment and supplies**
4. **Institute appropriate interventions based on the nursing plan of care**
5. **Record data as appropriate**

D. Expected outcomes/evaluation

1. **Monitor patient responses and outcomes, adjusting nursing care plans as indicated**
   a. *Specific interventions*
   b. *Disposition and discharge planning*
2. **Record all pertinent data**

3. **If positive outcomes are not demonstrated, assessment and/or plan of care needs re-evaluation**

E. Age-related considerations

1. Pediatric

   a. *Growth or development related*

   1) Perinatal problems may affect neurological status

   2) Babinski reflex is normal up to age 2 years

   3) Fontanelle closure—anterior fontanel closes between 9 and 18 months of age; posterior fontanel closes by 2 months of age

   b. *"Pearls"*

   1) Assess tone by noting resting position of the infant

   2) Meningeal irritation may show as sharp, shrill cry, irritability, and loss of appetite in infants

   3) Adaptation of the Glasgow Coma Scale for children aged 2 to 5 years (see Appendix C)

   4) History that indicates possible abnormalities: delay or regression in developmental milestones, unusual behavior for age, clumsiness or progressive weakness, learning or school difficulties

2. Geriatric

   a. *Age related*

   1) Gradual slowing of the conscious and reflex reaction time

   2) Impairment of fine discrimination abilities

   3) Decreased corneal sensitivity, slower visual reflexes, decreased visual acuity and depth perception, decreased upward gaze, and smaller pupils

   4) Altered drug response and tolerance

   b. *"Pearls"*

   1) Use stronger stimuli and allow more time to respond

   2) Use sharper contrasts with sensory stimuli

   3) Ensure a protected environment

II. SPECIFIC MEDICAL NEUROLOGICAL EMERGENCIES

A. Headaches

Headache occurs when there is traction, pressure, displacement, inflammation, or dilation of pain receptors (nociceptors) in the brain or surrounding tissues. A primary headache is one for which no organic cause can be consistently identified (e.g., migraines, tension type, cluster). A secondary headache is associated with an organic etiology such as a tumor or aneurysm. Headache is a common problem, affecting up to 75% of the population each year, but of those only 5% of these will seek medical attention. Approximately 50% of all persons with a headache suffer from migraines. Although the exact mechanism is unknown, it is believed that blood vessels supplying the brain and surrounding tissue narrow, which results in reduced blood flow followed by reflex vasodilation, swelling, and inflammation of cerebral blood vessels.

1. Assessment

   a. *Subjective data*

   1) History of present illness

   a) Time frame

   (1) Onset (migraines frequently occur in early morning hours)

    (2) Occurrence (cluster headaches occur in groups followed by a period of remission)

    (3) Aura and awareness (migraines are identified as those with and those without an aura)

    (4) Duration (tension-type headache may last up to 7 days; migraines usually last 4–72 hours)

  b) Pain

    (1) Character and quality (migraine headaches throb, cluster headaches cause burning sensation behind or around the eye, tension-type headaches have constant, nonpulsating pain)

    (2) Intensity (cluster headaches are excruciating)

    (3) Therapeutic measures implemented

    (4) Success of therapeutic measures

  c) Location

    (1) Unilateral or bilateral (migraine headaches are usually unilateral at onset but may switch sides; tension-type headaches are bilateral)

    (2) Occipital, frontal, temporal, neck, or hatband area (typical of tension-type headache)

  d) Symptoms associated with migraine headaches

    (1) Aura (visual or somatosensory)

    (2) Nausea and vomiting

    (3) Photophobia or phonophobia

    (4) Difficulty concentrating

    (5) Visual changes

  e) Precipitating event

    (1) Emotional (stress or depression)

    (2) Metabolic (fever or menses)

    (3) Flickering lights or television

    (4) Alcohol abuse or withdrawal

    (5) Food

    (6) Fatigue or altered sleep-wake cycle

2) Medical history

  a) Family history of headaches

  b) Use of oral contraceptives

  c) Hypertension

  d) Overseas travel

  e) Allergies or sinus problems

  f) Seizure disorder

  g) Medications

  h) Motion sickness as a child

b. *Objective data*

1) Physical examination

  a) Complete neurological examination

  b) Edema over the sinuses

  c) Distended, twitching scalp vessels

  d) Flushed, pale, or shiny skin

2) Diagnostic procedures (if organic disease is suspected)

  a) Skull radiograph

  b) CT scan or MRI

  c) EEG

2. Analysis: differential nursing diagnosis/collaborative problems

  a. *Pain related to vasodilation of cerebral blood vessels, muscle tightness, or ineffective pain relief measures*

    b. *Knowledge deficit related to therapeutic regimen or pain management techniques*

3. **Planning/interventions**
   a. *Physical measures*
      1) Heat (muscular) or cold (vascular)
      2) Darkened room (if photophobic)
      3) Massage
   b. *Psychological measures*
      1) Stress management
      2) Relaxation techniques
      3) Biofeedback therapy
      4) Behavior modification techniques
   c. *Pharmacological measures*
      1) Preventive drugs
         a) Vasoconstrictor agents
         b) Beta blockers
         c) Anticonvulsants
      2) Analgesics
      3) Oxygen
   d. *Instructions regarding medications*
      1) Purpose
      2) Timing
      3) Side effects
   e. *Instructions on triggering factors and measures to decrease or eliminate them*
   f. *Investigation of health profile to determine compliance potential*
4. **Expected outcomes/evaluation** (see Appendix B)

B. Cerebrovascular accidents (CVAs)

    A CVA is a neurological syndrome characterized by a rapid or gradual nonconvulsive neurological deficit that affects a known vascular territory. It occurs when plugging by atherosclerosis or clot creates a narrow lumen, which prevents adequate cerebral blood flow (ischemic stroke) or when a weakened blood vessel ruptures and causes leakage of blood into the brain or subarachnoid space (hemorrhagic stroke). The clinical picture depends on the vessel involved, the extent of the damage, and the collateral flow. There are approximately 500,000 new cases of stroke each year in the United States, and it is most common in those age 65 years and older. Forty percent of persons who experience CVAs are women. Those at greatest risk for CVA include persons with hyperlipidemia, congestive heart failure (CHF), mitral valve disorders, atrial fibrillation, diabetes, and hypertension and those with a history of obesity, smoking, or drug use (e.g., cocaine).

1. **Assessment**
   a. *Subjective data*
      1) History of present illness
         a) Time pattern
            (1) Brief, lasting seconds or hours but less than 24 hours (transient ischemic attack)
            (2) Lasting 48 hours or less, with complete resolution of deficit; reversible ischemic neurodeficit (RIND)
            (3) Progressive development of a deficit over time (stroke in evolution/progressive stroke)
            (4) Immediate maximization of deficit (completed stroke)

    2) Medical history (all conditions related to the high risk of thrombotic or embolic stroke)
      a) Diabetes
      b) Rheumatic heart disease
      c) Recent myocardial infarction (MI)
      d) Migraines
      e) Congestive heart failure
      f) Hypertension
      g) Atrial fibrillation

  b. *Objective data*
    1) Physical examination
      a) Anterior circulation (carotids)
        (1) Alteration in level of consciousness
        (2) Motor deficit: contralateral hemiparesis or hemiplegia
        (3) Sensory deficit: contralateral
        (4) Speech deficit: dysphasia, expressive or receptive (if dominant hemisphere involved)
        (5) Visual deficit: homonymous hemianopia (loss of vision in half of the visual field on the same side)
      b) Posterior circulation (vertebral basilar system)
        (1) Alteration in level of consciousness
        (2) Motor deficit: more than one limb
        (3) Cranial nerve deficit: dysphonia (difficulty in producing voice sounds; dysarthria (difficulty with articulation); dysphagia (difficulty in swallowing)
        (4) Visual deficits: field defects; cortical blindness; diplopia
        (5) Loss of coordination, ataxia
    2) Diagnostic procedures
      a) Doppler flow studies
      b) CT scan
      c) MRI

2. Analysis: Differential nursing diagnosis/collaborative problems
  a. *Tissue perfusion, altered cerebral related to interruption in blood supply (ischemia, edema, or intracranial pressure)*
  b. *Anxiety/fear related to onset of symptoms, unknown prognosis*
  c. *Airway clearance, ineffective related to inability to protect airway or unconsciousness*
  d. *Impaired verbal communication related to cerebral ischemia*
  e. *Knowledge deficit: risk factors and prevention*

3. Planning/interventions
  a. *Maintain airway, breathing, circulation*
  b. *Monitor neurological status for change*
  c. *Maintain venous outflow (head of bed elevated, head in neutral position)*
  d. *Frequently monitor*
    1) Cerebral function
    2) Level of consciousness
    3) Blood pressure
  e. *Supplemental oxygen, pulse oximetry*
  f. *Initiate measures to normalize blood pressure (depending on the etiology of the stroke, pharmacological support for lowering of the blood pressure)*
  g. *Administer anticoagulation therapy (ischemic stroke in evolution only)*
  h. *Administer intravenous (IV) thrombolytics (ischemic stroke only: patient must*

present within 3 hours of onset of symptoms and CT scan must exclude intracranial hemorrhage)
  i. *Prepare for possible surgical intervention*
      1) Carotid endarterectomy (TIAs)
      2) Intra-arterial fibrinolytic therapy
      3) Angioplasty/stent placement
  j. *Allow significant others to be present when feasible*
  k. *Review with patient his or her current lifestyle and health habits*
  l. *Identify need for follow-up care*
  m. *Identify resources for assistance*
  4. Expected outcomes/evaluation (see Appendix B)

C. Dementia

Dementia is global deterioration of acquired cognitive function with a clear sensorium. Memory is the most common cognitive ability that is lost. It results from disorders of cerebral neuronal circuits and is a result of the total quantity of neuronal loss combined with specific location of the loss. It is chronic condition that may be associated with a primary underlying disorder (e.g., drug toxicity, dementia of Alzheimer's disease type, metabolic disorder, neurological condition, hypoxia, brain tumor, infection). Dementia affects more than 4 million persons in the United States each year. Increasing age is the strongest risk factor for dementia; up to 40% of all individuals older than 85 years have clinically identifiable memory loss.

1. Assessment
  a. *Subjective data*
      1) History of present illness
          a) Memory loss
              (1) Onset (acute confusion may represent delirium)
              (2) Duration
          b) Difficulty performing activities of daily living (ADLs) (e.g., managing money, driving, shopping, following instructions)
          c) Agitation or withdrawal
      2) Medical history
          a) Dementia of Alzheimer's disease type
          b) Vascular disease
          c) Head trauma
          d) Chronic alcohol abuse
          e) Parkinson's disease
          f) Chronic drug or medication use
          g) Psychiatric disorder
  b. *Objective data*
      1) Physical examination
          a) Orientation
          b) Recent and remote memory
          c) Calculation
          d) Gait (indicates other disorders)
      2) Diagnostic testing (to rule out other disorders)
          a) Thyroid function
          b) Complete blood count (CBC), electrolytes
          c) CT scan or MRI
2. Analysis: differential nursing diagnosis/collaborative problems
  a. *Injury, high risk for related to altered thought processes*
3. Planning/interventions

> a. *Provide information, explain all procedures, reassure patient, introduce all new personnel*
> b. *Protect patient from injury (provide safe environment, control stressors, do not ask patient to perform beyond skill level)*
> c. *Treat underlying cause (if identified)*
> d. *Consult to appropriate referral services*

4. Expected outcomes (see Appendix B)

D. Shunt problems

Shunts are placed to relieve increased ICP from hydrocephalus by diverting cerebrospinal fluid from the lateral ventricle to the blood or body cavities. This diversion relieves the obstruction by creating alternative pathways for free circulation and/or absorption of cerebrospinal fluid. The two most common complications of shunt insertion are infections and shunt malfunction. Infections may be due to the shunt itself, meningitis, or ventriculitis. Malfunctions are due to obstruction (plugging by the choroid plexus, blood clots, or debris) or to mechanical failure (detachment or malpositioning of the two ends).

1. Assessment
   a. *Subjective data*
      1) History of present illness
         a) Type of shunt
         b) Length of implantation
         c) Neurological status trends
      2) Medical history
         a) Reason for shunt
         b) Previous problems with shunt
      3) Risk factor: child's normal growth ("outgrow" the shunt)
   b. *Objective data*
      1) Physical examination
         a) Shunt malfunction
            (1) Mental status: decreased alertness; decreased intellectual function; behavioral changes
            (2) Eye changes: inability to look up; alteration in visual acuity or fields
            (3) Associated findings: incontinence; gait changes (ataxia); increased motor tone
            (4) Infant: tense fontanelles; shrill cry; placid behavior; loss of appetite
         b) Infection
            (1) Fever
            (2) Meningeal signs
            (3) Altered mental status
      2) Diagnostic procedures
         a) CT scan
         b) Lumbar puncture for cerebrospinal fluid analysis

2. Analysis: differential nursing diagnosis/collaborative problems
   a. *Tissue perfusion, altered cerebral related to increased ICP secondary to shunt malfunction*
   b. *Risk for infection related to the presence of a shunt*

3. Planning/interventions
   a. *Increased ICP may be present (see section on ICP in this chapter)*
   b. *Prepare for, and assist with, intraventricular catheter insertion, if needed*
   c. *Monitor vital signs*
   d. *Prepare patient for, and assist with, diagnostic lumbar puncture*

e. Send cerebrospinal fluid for analysis and culture

f. Initiate antipyretic therapy or antibiotics as ordered

4. **Expected outcomes/evaluation** (see Appendix B)

E. Seizures

A seizure is a sudden, paroxysmal discharge of a group of neurons resulting in transient impairment of consciousness, movement, sensation, or memory. A trigger causes an abnormal burst of electrical stimulus, which disrupts the brain's normal nerve conduction. Seizures may be caused by ionic changes (e.g., pH, electrolyte imbalances, hyperventilation), by metabolic changes (e.g., hyperglycemia, fever, stress, fatigue, menses), and by nerve cell structural changes (e.g., hypoxia, tumors, trauma, vascular insufficiency). Some seizures are idiopathic. Seizures are classified according to EEG and clinical criteria as generalized (synchronous involvement of all regions of brain in both hemispheres) or partial (clinical signs or EEG evidence of a focal onset involving one particular part of the brain).

Status epilepticus is a medical emergency characterized by a series of seizures without recovery of baseline neurological status between seizures that can lead to mortality and morbidity from acidemia, hypoglycemia, autonomic dysfunction, and hypercalcemia. Approximately 120 per 100,000 persons in the United States will have a new seizure each year. The greatest number occur in those younger than 2 years or older than 65 years. Forty percent of all new seizures occur in those younger than 18 years; the majority will have fever-related convulsive seizures. Patients at risk for seizures include those with previous head trauma, CVA, central nervous system (CNS) infections, and degenerative CNS disorders (multiple sclerosis, Alzheimer's disease, Huntington's chorea).

1. **Assessment**
   a. *Subjective data*
      1) History of present illness
         a) Precipitating event (fever, illness)
         b) Site of origin and spread of the seizure
         c) Motor activity
         d) Duration and frequency of seizure
         e) Loss of consciousness (arousability)
         f) Postictal behavior
      2) Medical history
         a) Seizure history
         b) Congenital anomalies
         c) Metabolic abnormalities
         d) Neurological disease (e.g., cerebrovascular, tumor, infectious process)
         e) Recent trauma
         f) Pharmacological history (e.g., excessive laxative use in children)
   b. *Objective data*
      1) Physical examination (during and after seizure)
         a) Level of consciousness
            (1) Responsiveness to stimuli
            (2) Ability to follow commands
            (3) Automatism
         b) Motor activity: type and origin of spread
            (1) Tonic phase: contraction of voluntary muscles, body stiffens
            (2) Clonic phase: violent, rhythmic contractions
         c) Eye deviation
         d) Incontinence

e) Temperature
f) Postictal state
   (1) Level of consciousness
   (2) Weakness of one limb (Todd's paralysis, usually seen after generalized seizures; is time limited)
   (3) Headache, amnesia
   (4) Duration
g) Physical injury sustained
h) Recurrence of the seizure
2) Diagnostic procedures
   a) Therapeutic monitoring of anticonvulsant drug levels (known seizure patient)
   b) If no history of seizure
      (1) CT scan, MRI
      (2) EEG follow-up appointment
      (3) Lumbar puncture
      (4) CBC
      (5) Serum electrolytes, glucose, blood urea nitrogen (BUN), creatinine
      (6) Toxicology screen

2. **Analysis: differential nursing diagnosis/collaborative problems**
   a. *Ineffective airway clearance related to airway obstruction secondary to seizure activity*
   b. *Risk for injury related to seizure activity*
   c. *Noncompliance related to medication therapy*

3. **Planning/interventions**
   a. *Maintain airway, breathing, circulation*
   b. *Turn patient onto his or her side; protect head from injury*
   c. *Loosen tight or restrictive clothing*
   d. *Suction, if necessary*
   e. *Provide supplemental oxygen*
   f. *Establish IV access*
   g. *Pharmacological support to stop the seizures*
      1) Diazepam, IV
      2) Lorazepam, IV
   h. *Pharmacological support to prevent recurrence of seizures*
      1) Phenytoin, IV bolus given no faster than 50 mg/min
      2) Phenobarbital, IV dosage is to effect, given no faster than 50 mg/min
      3) Low-dose barbiturates
      4) Fosphenytoin, IV or IM
   i. *Monitor*
      1) Neurological status
      2) Temperature (no oral temperatures), vital signs
   j. *Pharmacological support to prevent or correct complications*
      1) 50% percent glucose IV
      2) Thiamine, intramuscular (IM) or IV
   k. *Hold for observation until patient has recovered from postictal state*
      1) Monitor neurological recovery
      2) Maintain seizure precautions (bed at low position, side rails up and padded, suction and airway setup at bedside)
   l. *Put side rails up (pad if seizures are generalized and multiple)*
   m. *Perform initial monitoring of therapeutic drug levels*
   n. *Assess patient's perceived compliance*

    o. *Explore social, personal, and health profile to predict potential for compliance*
    p. *Perform discharge teaching*
        1) Knowledge, route, dose, side effects of medications
        2) Discussion of consequences of noncompliance in taking medications as prescribed
        3) Follow-up appointment arranged
            a) Refer patient to social worker/community resource as indicated
    4. **Expected outcomes/evaluation** (see Appendix B)

F. Guillain-Barré syndrome (GBS)

An acute inflammatory polyneuropathy that primarily affects the motor component of peripheral nerves. Although the etiology is uncertain, the source is thought to be an immune-mediated response that triggers destruction of the myelin sheath surrounding axons. This response makes saltatory conduction impossible and nerve transmission is either slowed or blocked completely. The annual incidence of GBS is 1.5 to 2.0 cases per 100,000 population. It occurs with equal frequency in both sexes and in all races. A slight peak in incidence seems to occur in those 16 to 25 years of age. Approximately 50% of all patients with GBS experience a mild febrile illness (usually upper respiratory or gastrointestinal) 2 to 3 weeks prior to the onset of symptoms.

1. **Assessment**
    a. *Subjective data*
        1) History of present illness
            a) Sequence of onset and development of neurological symptoms
                (1) Neuropathy usually begins in lower extremities and ascends in symmetrical pattern
                (2) Symptoms usually peak in 1 week but may progress for several weeks
                (3) Motor function returns in descending fashion
            b) Pain worse at night
            c) No change in level of consciousness or cognitive function
        2) Medical history
            a) Upper respiratory or gastrointestinal disorder 1 to 4 weeks prior to onset of symptoms
            b) Neurological diseases
            c) Trauma
            d) Substance abuse
    b. *Objective data*
        1) Physical examination
            a) Motor weakness or paralysis (usually begins in legs and then progresses upward to trunk and arms)
            b) Paresthesia (hands or feet)
            c) Diminished or absent reflexes (superficial and deep tendon)
            d) Respiratory insufficiency
            e) Autonomic dysfunction (urinary retention, postural hypotension)
        2) Diagnostic procedures
            a) Nerve conduction studies
            b) Pulmonary function testing
2. **Analysis: differential nursing diagnosis/collaborative problems**
    a. *Breathing pattern ineffective, related to neuromuscular weakness of respiratory muscles*
    b. *Impaired physical mobility related to neurological dysfunction*

  c. Anxiety/fear related to change in health status

 3. Planning/interventions

  a. Frequently monitor sensory-motor function

  b. Continuously monitor respiratory status (respiratory rate, vital capacity, tidal volume, pulse oximetry, signs of fatigue)

  c. Elevate head of bed

  d. Supplemental oxygen

  e. Inspect patient's skin for signs of pressure, reposition frequently, and use protective padding as indicated

  f. Pain management (comfort measures, analgesics)

  g. Emotional support

 4. Expected outcomes (see Appendix B)

III. SPECIFIC SURGICAL NEUROLOGICAL EMERGENCIES

A. Increased intracranial pressure

  Intracranial pressure (ICP) is a reflection of three relatively fixed volumes: (1) brain, (2) cerebrospinal fluid, and (3) blood. As the level of any one of these increases, the level of the other two components will decrease in an attempt to compensate and thus keep the ICP within normal limits, despite increasing pathology. Because of this, the brain will demonstrate only slight increases in pressure over a wide range of expansion in volume. However, as the pathology progresses, the compensatory mechanisms are depleted, which results in a rapid increase in ICP with only a small increase in volume. This produces a shift of the brain contents, with herniation of the brain through the tentorial opening, resultant pressure on the brain stem, and a clinical picture of altered level of consciousness as well as pupillary, motor, and vital sign changes. As ICP rises, cerebral perfusion pressure decreases, leading to cerebral ischemia and potential for hypoxia, with secondary insult. Cerebral ischemia can lead to increased concentrations of carbon dioxide and decreased concentrations of oxygen in cerebral vessels. Carbon dioxide vasodilates blood vessels, which further contributes to the problem. Underlying causes for increased ICP include conditions that (1) increase brain volume (e.g., space-occupying lesions, cerebral edema), (2) increase cerebral blood volume (e.g., obstruction of venous outflow, hyperemia, hypercapnia), and (3) increase cerebrospinal fluid (e.g., communication hydrocephalus, subarachnoid hemorrhage, choroid plexus papilloma).

 1. Assessment

  a. Subjective data

   1) History of present illness

    a) Chronological sequence of onset and development of neurological symptoms

    b) Consciousness

     (1) Alterations in

     (2) Loss of

    c) Mentation

     (1) Memory

     (2) Changes in cognitive ability (e.g., problem solving)

    d) Alterations in personality

    e) Alterations in communication

     (1) Speech changes

     (2) Hearing difficulties

     (3) Comprehension difficulties

    f) Alterations in motor ability

         (1) Weakness (paresis)

         (2) Paralysis (plegia)

         (3) Loss of coordination

         (4) Tremors

         (5) Twitching or fasciculations

         (6) Difficulty in getting out of a chair or in climbing stairs

      g) Alterations in sensation

      h) Alterations in vision

         (1) Loss of or decrease in acuity or visual fields

         (2) Diplopia

      i) Injury or fall

         (1) Mechanism

         (2) Time elapsed since occurrence

         (3) Treatment prior to arrival

         (4) Changes in clinical status

      j) Pain (PQRST)

      k) Headache

      l) Seizures

      m) Vomiting (especially in children)

    2) Medical history

      a) Neurological diseases

      b) Trauma

      c) Fainting, dizziness, "falling-out" spells

      d) Substance abuse (drugs, alcohol, or nicotine)

      e) Current medication history

      f) Allergies

  b. *Objective data*

    1) Physical examination

      a) Early picture of increased ICP

         (1) Level of consciousness: more stimulation required to get the same response; loss of finer detail in orientation response; speech less distinct; memory alterations; restlessness; sudden quietness in a very restless patient

         (2) Pupils: sluggish response to light; usually unilateral and ipsilateral to the lesion

         (3) Motor function: usually contralateral to the lesion; pronator drift; loss of one or more grades on the strength scale; increased tone

         (4) Vital signs: occasionally tachycardic; occasionally hypertensive swings

      b) Late picture of increased ICP (herniation)

         (1) Level of consciousness: arousable only with deep pain or unarousable

         (2) Pupils: fixed or dilated

         (3) Motor response to stimuli: dense hemiparesis; posturing; no response

         (4) Vital signs (Cushing's response): elevated systolic blood pressure; profound bradycardia; abnormal respirations; widening pulse pressure

    2) Diagnostic procedures

      a) CT scan or MRI

      b) Insertion of ICP monitoring device

      c) Arterial blood gases (ABGs), specifically $Paco_2$

2. Analysis: differential nursing diagnosis/collaborative problems

a. *Impaired gas exchange related to abnormal breathing patterns secondary to altered brain-stem function*
b. *Tissue perfusion, altered cerebral related to increased ICP*
c. *Sensory/perceptual alterations related to effects of increased ICP*
3. **Planning/interventions**
   a. *Monitor airway, breathing, circulation*
   b. *Administer supplemental oxygen*
   c. *Mechanical airway insertion*
   d. *Mechanical ventilation*
   e. *Assist with medical decompression of cranial vault (goal is to decrease the ICP)*
      1) Diuretics to decrease the water content in the brain
      2) Increase venous outflow through elevation of head of bed, proper head and neck positioning
      3) Hyperventilation (controversial) to decrease cerebral blood flow: in the absence of measured intracranial hypertension, hyperventilation should be reserved for patients demonstrating specific signs of intracranial hypertension such as evidence of herniation or progressive neurological deterioration.
   f. *Ensure adequate cerebral perfusion pressure (goal is to increase the mean arterial pressure to compensate for increased ICP)*
      1) Monitor blood pressure
      2) Blood pressure support by
         a) Cautious administration of IV fluid (depending on cause of decreased blood pressure)
         b) Vasopressor agents
   g. *Decrease metabolic demand of the brain by*
      1) Maintaining normothermia
      2) Preventing seizures
      3) Institution of barbiturate coma (controversial)
      4) Utilization of lidocaine to decrease response to suctioning
   h. *Frequently monitor patient's neurological status*
   i. *Prepare for surgical decompression in the operating room*
   j. *Assist with prevention of complications (if indicated)*
      1) Initiation of anticonvulsants
      2) Initiation of anti-inflammatory agents (steroids)
   k. *Speak to responsive or unresponsive patient while providing care*
      1) Describe procedures
      2) Orient to person, place, and time
      3) Use therapeutic touch while providing care
      4) Continue to assess patient's ability to respond to stimuli
4. **Expected outcomes/evaluation** (see Appendix B)

B. Concussion

A traumatic reversible neurological deficit that results when there is temporary loss of consciousness as well as some degree of retrograde amnesia. Concussion is usually caused by a strong rapid acceleration-deceleration stimulus or sudden blow to the skull. Immediately following blunt trauma, there is a temporary cessation of the functioning of the reticular activating system, the arousal or wakefulness center in the brain stem, as a result of the shock waves from the blow. This results in immediate and transient loss of consciousness, which is reversible in minutes to hours.

1. **Assessment**

      a. *Subjective data*

        1) History of present illness

          a) Mechanism of injury

          b) Level of consciousness immediately following the injury

          c) Duration of loss of consciousness

          d) Changes in neurological status since the event

            (1) Dizziness

            (2) Headache

            (3) Nausea or vomiting

            (4) Memory or recall

        2) Medical history

          a) Neurological disease or injury

          b) Recent fall or trauma

      b. *Objective data*

        1) Physical examination

          a) Complete neurological examination (see Assessment I.A. of this chapter)

          b) Memory

            (1) Retrograde or antegrade amnesia

            (2) Ability to learn new information is present despite amnesia of the event

        2) Diagnostic procedures

          a) Clinical presentation and history are usually diagnostic

          b) Skull films or CT scan to rule out more serious injuries

2. Analysis: differential nursing diagnosis/collaborative problems

      a. *Risk for injury related to change in mental status*

      b. *Knowledge deficit related to complications of head injury and safety precautions*

3. Planning/interventions

      a. *Maintain bed rest*

      b. *Raise side rails*

      c. *Allow significant other to remain with patient*

      d. *Instruct patient/significant others in signs and symptoms requiring an immediate return to medical facilities*

        1) Altered level of consciousness

        2) Change in pupils

        3) Projectile vomiting

        4) Seizure

        5) Inability to arouse

      e. *Instruct patient in postconcussion syndrome*

        1) Clinical presentation

          a) Headache

          b) Dizziness (usually positional)

          c) Tinnitus

          d) Diplopia (usually transient)

          e) Inability to concentrate

          f) Memory disturbance

          g) Personality changes

          h) Decreased energy level

        2) Duration: days to years

        3) Social/occupational consequences

          a) Difficulty with performance in school/work

          b) Negative impact on relationships

4) Any community resources available for help (e.g., support groups)

5) Avoid medications that may worsen signs and symptoms

4. Expected outcomes/evaluation (see Appendix B)

C. Skull fractures

The most common skull fracture, the linear fracture, accounts for about 70% of all fractures. It is usually benign unless it crosses a major vascular channel (sagittal sinus or middle meningeal artery). A depressed skull fracture damages the underlying cerebral tissue by compression or laceration and by retained bony fragments, which may set up a focus for seizures. Basilar skull fractures may occur in any of the three fossae (anterior, middle, or posterior). The clinical picture greatly depends on the fossa affected. The overall complications of skull fractures include infections, hematoma, cerebrospinal fluid leaks, loss of smell (anosmia), loss of hearing, seizures, and pneumocephalus.

1. Assessment

   a. *Subjective data*

      1) History of present illness

         a) Recent trauma

         b) Time elapsed from event to present

         c) Complaint of tasting something sweet or salty in the back of their throat (because of cerebrospinal fluid)

         d) Complaint of "postnasal drip"

      2) Medical history

         a) History of trauma

         b) Malignancy

   b. *Objective data*

      1) Physical examination

         a) Surface trauma (scalp lacerations may lead to significant blood loss, especially in children)

         b) Alteration in level of consciousness

         c) Alteration in pupillary or motor responses

         d) Cerebrospinal fluid leak (otorrhea or rhinorrhea)

         e) Raccoon sign (periorbital ecchymosis)

         f) Battle's sign (mastoid bruising) usually seen after 24 hours

      2) Diagnostic procedures

         a) Skull films

         b) CT scan (if underlying injury suspected)

         c) Test for glucose in the watery nasal discharge

         d) "Cerebrospinal fluid halo" test with otorrhea

2. Analysis: differential nursing diagnosis/collaborative problems

   a. *Risk for infection related to fracture*

   b. *Risk for tissue perfusion, altered cerebral related to increased ICP or other complications of skull fracture*

3. Planning/interventions

   a. *Monitor patient's neurological status for change*

   b. *Monitor patient for seizures*

   c. *Provide drip pads for cerebrospinal fluid rhinorrhea*

   d. *Cleanse the outer ear if otorrhea present (never put anything in the ear)*

   e. *Avoid nasal intubation, nasogastric tube insertion, nose blowing, sneezing, nasal cannula, and so forth*

   f. *Administer anticonvulsant medications as ordered*

   g. *Administer antibiotics as ordered*

        h. Prepare for surgical intervention (depressed skull fracture, especially with a dural tear)

   4. Expected outcomes/evaluation (see Appendix B)

D. Diffuse axonal injury (DAI)

        DAI is the widespread disruption of neurological function without any focal lesions noted, characterized by microscopic damage to axons, diffuse white matter degeneration, global neurological dysfunction, and diffuse cerebral swelling. It is usually caused by an acceleration-deceleration movement to the brain, which results in a shearing injury to axons. Disruption of axons in the cerebrum leads to disconnection of the cortex and the brain-stem reticular formation.

   1. Assessment

      a. Subjective data

         1) History of present illness

           a) Mechanism of injury

           b) Onset of loss of consciousness

           c) Duration of loss of consciousness

         2) Medical history

           a) Neurological disease or injury

           b) Substance abuse

      b. Objective data

         1) Physical examination

           a) Immediate loss of consciousness: lasts days to months

           b) Increased ICP

           c) Brain-stem dysfunction

              (1) Rigid flexion (decorticate posturing) or rigid extension (decerebrate posturing)

              (2) Loss of brain stem reflexes (e.g., cough, gag)

              (3) Hypertension

              (4) Hyperthermia

              (5) Excessive sweating

         2) Diagnostic procedures

           a) CT scan or MRI

   2. Analysis: differential nursing diagnosis/collaborative problems

      a. Tissue perfusion, altered cerebral related to edema, cell destruction, and increased ICP

      b. Risk for injury related to sensory-perceptual alterations

   3. Planning/interventions

      a. Monitor airway, breathing, circulation

      b. Administer oxygen

      c. Mechanical airway insertion

      d. Mechanical ventilation (possible hyperventilation)

      e. Prepare for insertion of ICP monitoring device

      f. Assist with medical decompression of cranial vault (goal to decrease ICP): see Section I.A.

      g. Administer antipyretic medication or use hyperthermia blanket

      h. Psychosocial support for family

   4. Expected outcomes/evaluations (see Appendix B)

E. Cerebral contusion

        A cerebral contusion is an actual bruising of the brain tissue without puncture of pial covering. It is characterized by petechial hemorrhages and extravasation of fluid from the vessels. This results in focal ischemia and edema with the potential for infarction, necrosis, and/or increased ICP. Cerebral contusions are caused by trauma, acceleration or deceleration, high-velocity blows, or the rotation of the brain following such a blow. Frequently the brain has a rebound of its contents following such a blow, resulting in an injury opposite the point of impact (contrecoup injury). The clinical presentation depends on the area involved and the extent of the damage.

1. **Assessment**
   a. *Subjective data*
      1) History of present illness
         a) Mechanism of injury
         b) Changes in neurological status since the event
      2) Medical history
         a) Neurological diseases or injury
         b) Substance abuse
   b. *Objective data*
      1) Physical examination
         a) Alteration in level of consciousness for more than several hours
         b) Presence of surface trauma (occasional)
         c) Brain stem contusion
            (1) Loss of brain stem reflexes
            (2) Unconsciousness
            (3) Posturing
      2) Diagnostic procedures
         a) CT scan
         b) MRI
2. **Analysis: differential nursing diagnosis/collaborative problems**
   a. *Tissue perfusion, altered cerebral related to contusion*
3. **Planning/interventions**
   a. *Assist with medical decompression of cranial vault (goal is to decrease the ICP)*
      1) Hyperventilation to decrease cerebral blood flow
      2) Diuretics to decrease the water content in the brain
      3) Increase venous outflow through evaluation of head of bed and proper head and neck positioning
   b. *Instruct family in potential for swelling and the need for further observation*
   c. *Discuss any bizarre behavior in terms of area injured (e.g., frontal lobe) rather than as an indication of patient's "true" personality*
   d. *Assist family in understanding that a patient with a brain-stem contusion is not merely "sleeping" but has damaged the "awake" center in the brain*
4. **Expected outcomes/evaluation** (see Appendix B)

F. Epidural hematoma

An epidural hematoma is a collection of blood between the skull and dura. It is usually due to a laceration of the middle meningeal artery associated with a temporal skull fracture; the fracture crosses the middle meningeal arterial groove in the temporal bone, lacerates the artery, and allows bleeding into the epidural space. Because the arterial bleed is under high pressure, it does not tamponade but instead rapidly progresses to become a mass lesion causing increased ICP, brain shift, and uncal herniation (a forcing of the medial portion of the temporal lobe, the uncus, to herniate down through the tentorial opening). The mortality for epidural hematomas is approximately 50%.

1. **Assessment**

      a. Subjective data
-    1) History of present illness
  -    a) Mechanism of injury
  -    b) Pattern of unconsciousness following injury (occurs about 30% of the time)
    -    (1) Initial unconsciousness
    -    (2) Lucid interval (5 minutes to 6 hours)
    -    (3) Rapid unconsciousness
  -    c) Course: short (less than 8 hours)
-    2) Medical history
  -    a) Previous trauma
  -    b) Previous head injury

      b. Objective data
-    1) Physical examination (see Assessment I.A.)
  -    a) Alteration in level of consciousness
  -    b) Pupils: unilateral, fixed, and/or dilated
  -    c) Motor: contralateral paresis or paralysis progressing to posturing
  -    d) Cushing's response (late)
-    2) Diagnostic procedure: CT scan

2. Analysis: differential nursing diagnosis/collaborative problems

      a. Impaired gas exchange related to abnormal breathing pattern secondary to increased ICP

      b. Tissue perfusion, altered cerebral related to increased ICP

3. Planning/interventions

      a. Maintain airway, breathing, circulation

      b. Continuously monitor patient's ventilatory ability and ABGs

      c. Intubation and mechanical ventilation with supplemental oxygen

      d. Assist with medical decompression of cranial vault (goal is to decrease the ICP)
-    1) Hyperventilation to decrease cerebral blood flow
-    2) Diuretics to decrease the water content in the brain
-    3) Increase venous outflow through elevation of head of bed and proper head and neck positioning

      e. Frequently monitor patient's neurological status

      f. Prepare for emergency surgery for clot evacuation

4. Expected outcomes/evaluation (see Appendix B)

G. Subdural hematoma

    A collection of blood between the dura mater and the subarachnoid layer of the meninges, usually caused by trauma or occurs as the extension of an intracerebral hematoma into the subdural space. Veins that bridge the subdural space are torn, which allows venous blood to collect beneath the dura. Subdural hematomas are classified based on the onset of clinical signs and symptoms: (1) acute (within 48 hours), (2) subacute (2–14 days), and (3) chronic (more than 14 days).

1. Assessment

      a. Subjective data
-    1) History of present illness
  -    a) Mechanism of injury
  -    b) Time interval
  -    c) Trends in neurological status
-    2) Medical history

      b. Objective data
-    1) Physical examination

    a) Acute subdural

      (1) Headache, drowsiness, confusion

      (2) Steady decline in patient's level of consciousness

      (3) Ipsilateral, unilateral pupillary dilation with lack of response to light

      (4) Contralateral motor changes (hemiparesis)

    b) Chronic and subacute subdural

      (1) Gradual and nonspecific changes

      (2) Alteration in mentation

      (3) Alteration in motor ability (ipsilateral or contralateral hemiparesis)

      (4) Papilledema

      (5) Dilated, ipsilateral pupil sluggish to light

  2) Diagnostic procedures

    a) CT scan

    b) MRI

    c) Angiography

2. Analysis: differential nursing diagnosis/collaborative problems

  a. Impaired gas exchange related to inadequate respiratory effort secondary to increased ICP

  b. Tissue perfusion, altered cerebral related to increased ICP

3. Planning/interventions

  a. Acute

    1) Assist with medical decompression of cranial vault (goal is to decrease the ICP)

      a) Hyperventilation to decrease cerebral blood flow

      b) Diuretics to decrease the water content in the brain

      c) Increase venous outflow through elevation of head of bed and proper head and neck positioning

  b. Nonacute

    1) Elevate head of bed

    2) Monitor neurological status

    3) Maintain adequate oxygenation and ventilation

    4) Maintain adequate blood pressure

    5) Administer anticonvulsants if ordered

4. Expected outcomes/evaluation (see Appendix B)

H. Subarachnoid hemorrhage/aneurysm rupture

Subarachnoid hemorrhage is a diffuse collection of blood between the arachnoid mater and the pia mater. Most aneurysms are the result of a thinning of the medial layer of the arterial wall; the remainder are associated with advanced atherosclerosis or infected emboli. The rupture is usually precipitated by a hypertensive event caused by straining at stool, sexual intercourse, heavy lifting, or excitement. Following a rupture with bleeding into the subarachnoid space, the vessel immediately clamps down to prevent further bleeding (this may also lead to ischemia and infarction, depending on the vessel and size). At the same time, a clot begins to form around the aneurysm. The clinical presentation depends on the vessel involved, severity of bleeding, location of the collection of blood, and amount of collateral circulation. Blood in the subarachnoid space acts like a chemical irritant, producing meningeal signs. Potential complications include increased ICP, vasospasm, rebleeding, ischemia and infarction, and hydrocephalus.

1. Assessment

  a. Subjective data

    1) History of present illness

   a) Sudden alteration in consciousness
   b) Headache
      (1) Patient describes it as "the worst headache of my life"
      (2) Unrelieved by conventional therapy
      (3) Accompanied by nausea and photophobia
   c) Sudden seizure
2) Medical history
   a) Hypertension (may precipitate a rupture in a berry aneurysm)
   b) Atherosclerosis (fusiform aneurysms: large tortuous dilation caused by advanced atherosclerosis)
   c) Infection (mycotic aneurysms resulting from infected emboli; rare)
 b. *Objective data*
1) Physical examination
   a) Grade (based on presentation)
      (1) Grade 1 (minimal bleed): patient alert and awake; mild headache; slight stiff neck; no neurological deficit
      (2) Grade 2 (mild bleed): patient awake and alert; mild to severe headache; nuchal rigidity; mild cranial nerve deficits
      (3) Grade 3 (moderate bleed): patient confused and drowsy; mild focal deficit (motor, speech, vision, depending on vessel)
      (4) Grade 4 (moderate to severe bleed): patient stuporous; mild to moderate hemiparesis
      (5) Grade 5 (severe bleed): patient stuporous with decerebrate posturing *or* comatose
   b) Meningeal signs (e.g., fever, nuchal rigidity)
   c) ECG changes
      (1) T-wave changes: elevation, depression, or inversion
      (2) U waves present
2) Diagnostic procedures
   a) CT scan
   b) Lumbar puncture (*caution*: not performed in patients with Grades 3 to 5 until after CT scan)
   c) Angiography

2. Analysis: differential nursing diagnosis/collaborative problems

 a. *Tissue perfusion, altered cerebral related to interrupted blood supply*
 b. *Pain related to irritation of the meninges secondary to by-products of blood breakdown*

3. Planning/interventions

 a. *Maintain airway, breathing, circulation*
 b. *Provide supplemental oxygen*
 c. *Monitor neurological status*
 d. *Ensure adequate cerebral perfusion pressure*
   1) Cautious volume expansion (0.9 normal saline is preferred because of predisposition of patients with subarachnoid hemorrhage to experience a drop in serum sodium)
   2) Pharmacological manipulation of blood pressure (goal is normotension for the patient until the aneurysm is clipped)
   3) Elevation of head of bed (with caution and if blood pressure is adequate)
 e. *Assist in preventing rebleeding*
   1) Normalize blood pressure
   2) Quiet, nonstressful environment
   3) Sedation
   4) Prevention of Valsalva maneuvers

5) Antifibrinolytic therapy (controversial)

   f. Provide comfort measures to relieve headache

     1) Quiet environment

     2) Cool washcloth over eyes

     3) Analgesic administration, if ordered (non-narcotic agents are preferred to prevent masking a neurological change)

   g. Administer calcium channel blockers, if ordered, to prevent vasospasm

4. Expected outcomes/evaluation (see Appendix B)

I. Spinal cord injuries

Spinal cord injuries (SCIs) involve bruising or tearing of spinal cord substance from penetrating trauma or a fracture/dislocation of the spinal column. Common in the 15- to 35-year age group, SCIs almost always are due to trauma (vehicular, falls, personal violence) and are caused by a variety of mechanisms, including axial loading, hyperflexion, and hyperextension. The resultant injury may involve only the vertebral column, only the spinal cord, or, more commonly, both. Damage to the cord occurs from extrinsic (bony and soft tissue injury) or intrinsic (hemorrhage, edema, hypoxia, or biochemical changes) sources. Injuries are classified as complete (transection of the cord with no preservation of sensorimotor function below the level of the injury) or incomplete (some cord sparing). Incomplete injuries include Brown-Séquard, anterior cord, posterior cord, or central cord syndromes. Respiratory complications occur when the diaphragm, innervated by the phrenic nerve, which exits from the cervical cord at the level of C-3, C-4, and C-5, is damaged. This results in a compromised ability to breathe. Even with the phrenic nerve intact, a low cervical injury causes loss of innervation of the intercostal muscles (T-1 to T-12), which allows one to take a deep breath, cough, and sigh, all of which are important measures in preventing atelectasis.

Neurogenic shock results when a high thoracic or low cervical injury causes loss of the sympathetic nervous system, which exits from the thoracic and lumbar cord. This eliminates the "fight or flight" protective response and permits the parasympathetic system to function unopposed. The result is vasodilation below the level of the injury, pooling of blood, decreased venous return to the heart, and decreased cardiac output.

1. Assessment

   a. Subjective data

     1) History of present illness

       a) Mechanism of injury

       b) Neurological ability at the scene

       c) Trend of neurological status

       d) Stabilization provided at the scene

     2) Medical history

       a) Borderline pre-existing cardiac or respiratory disorders that may be exacerbated by this injury

       b) Chronic disease

   b. Objective data

     1) Physical examination

       a) Surface trauma

       b) Guarding, pain, or tenderness over the spine; there may be no initial signs and symptoms

       c) Respiratory ability

         (1) Muscles used (diaphragm, intercostals, accessory)

         (2) Depth of respiration (shallow, deep)

  (3) Symmetry of chest wall movement
 d) Neurogenic shock (see Chapter 19)
  (1) Hypotension (usually < 90 mm Hg systolic)
  (2) Profound bradycardia
  (3) Warm, dry skin (resulting from loss of sympathetic response)
  (4) Areflexia
  (5) Partial or full loss of motor ability and sensation below the level of the lesion
  (6) Poikilothermy (inability to regulate body temperature by normal mechanisms, so the body temperature becomes variable, based on the external temperature)
 e) Motor ability
  (1) Body position assumed
  (2) Paraparesis/paraplegia or quadriparesis/quadriplegia
  (3) Rectal tone
  (4) No initial deficits
 f) Sensory perception
  (1) Examine distal to proximal
  (2) Response to pain (pinprick)
  (3) Response to pressure (head of pin)
  (4) Proprioception (toe up or down)
 g) Ileus
 h) Atonic bladder
 2) Diagnostic procedures
 a) Spinal films (lateral and oblique)
 b) Odontoid view films
 c) Tomograms
 d) CT scan or MRI
 e) Myelogram (as needed)
 2. **Analysis: differential nursing diagnosis/collaborative problems**
 a. *Ineffective airway clearance related to impaired innervation of diaphragm and intercostal muscles secondary to cervical cord injury*
 b. *Impaired gas exchange related to inadequate respiratory effort secondary to cervical cord injury*
 c. *Decreased cardiac output related to massive vasodilation caused by loss of sympathetic innervation*
 d. *Risk for injury related to sensory-perceptual alterations (tactile, kinesthetic)*
 e. *Ineffective individual or family coping related to implications of SCI*
 3. **Planning/interventions**
 a. *Maintain airway, breathing, circulation*
 b. *Prevent head and neck manipulation during the establishment of an airway*
 1) Jaw lift, mandible thrust
 2) No hyperextension or rotation of the neck
 3) Consider nasopharyngeal intubation
 c. *Cervical spine stabilization*
 1) Manual support/stabilization
 2) Firm cervical collar
 3) Lateral head immobilization
 4) Backboard to entire spine
 d. *Stabilize cervical spine, regardless of examination findings, until cervical films are taken and read as negative (C-1 through C-7)*
 1) Firm collar (prevents hyperextension, flexion, rotation)
 2) Other measures, per individual department or emergency medical service

protocol; some protocols have converted from using sandbags to tape and blanket rolls

    e. Provide supplemental oxygen

    f. Monitor vital capacity, respiratory rate, and PaCO$_2$ by ABG, end-tidal CO$_2$ monitor, pulse oximetry

    g. Provide mechanical ventilation if needed

    h. Monitor level of consciousness and urinary output to determine consequences of hypotension and bradycardia (do not treat the numbers)

    i. Enhance venous return to the heart

        1) Ace wraps, antiembolic hose

        2) Elevate lower extremities

        3) Pneumatic antishock garment (PASG; controversial)

    j. Support blood pressure, if needed

        1) Monitor volume infusion

        2) Pharmacological support (vasoconstrictors)

    k. Give atropine as indicated to elevate heart rate if symptomatic bradycardia occurs

    l. Normalize room temperature to reduce severity of poikilothermy

    m. Prepare for and assist with realignment of the spine (tong insertion)

    n. Administer drugs to preserve, protect, and possibly restore remaining cord: high-dose steroids over a 24-hour period begun within 8 hours after the event

    o. Monitor patient's neurological status for further decline

    p. Insert nasogastric tube to prevent gastric distention and possible resultant aspiration, avoid if suspected

    q. Insert urinary catheter to decompress the bladder

    r. Remove patient from backboard as soon as possible to prevent skin breakdown

    s. Prepare patient for transport to SCI center, if applicable

    t. Do not "take away" patient's denial, but do not reinforce or support it

    u. Attempt to meet identified needs consistently to foster trust

    v. Attempt to have someone with the patient most of the time

  4. Expected outcomes/evaluation (see Appendix B)

J. Autonomic dysreflexia

Autonomic dysreflexia or hyperreflexia is a syndrome that sometimes occurs after the acute phase of SCI in patients with lesions at or above T-6. It is only seen after recovery from spinal shock when reflex activity has returned. Noxious stimuli (bladder or intestinal distention, pressure on glans penis, renal calculi, cystitis, acute abdomen, pressure sores) produce a sympathetic discharge that causes reflex vasoconstriction of blood vessels in the skin and splanchnic bed below the level of the injury. Vasoconstriction of splanchnic bed distends baroreceptors in the carotid sinus and aortic arch, and the body attempts to lower hypertension by superficial dilation of vessels above the level of the injury.

  1. Assessment

    a. Subjective data

        1) History of present illness

            a) Onset

            b) Current bowel/bladder program

        2) Medical history

            a) SCI at or above T-6

    b. Objective data

        1) Physical examination

            a) Severe hypertension

        b) Vasomotor changes: flushed head and neck, pallor, and cool lower extremities

        c) Headache

        d) Visual changes (blurred vision)

        e) Bradycardia

        f) Nasal congestion

        g) Pupil dilation

2. Analysis: differential nursing diagnosis/collaborative problems

    a. Tissue perfusion, altered related to reflex vasoconstriction

    b. Knowledge deficit related to injury and implications

3. Planning/interventions

    a. Elevate head of bed

    b. Relieve trigger mechanism

        1) Check patency of urinary drainage system or insert urinary catheter (if patient did not have one when signs and symptoms began)

        2) Check for fecal impaction, lubricate rectum, or use local anesthetic

        3) Eliminate pressure from skin

    c. Treat hypertension (as needed)

        1) Administer ganglionic blocking agents as directed

    d. Monitor vital signs frequently

    e. Provide resources for patient/family related to self-care

4. Expected outcomes (see Appendix B)

BIBLIOGRAPHY

Allen, T. (1997). Seizure disorders: A primary care guide. *Advanced Nursing Practice, 5,* 32–40.

Bates, B. (1995). *A guide to physical examination and history taking* (6th ed.). Philadelphia: Lippincott-Raven.

Bethel, S. (1997). Intravenous thrombolytic therapy for stroke emergencies. *Journal of Emergency Nursing, 23,* 345–346.

Bullock, R., Chestnut, R., & Clifton, G. (1996). *Guidelines for management of severe head injury.* New York: Brain Trauma Foundation.

Geraci, E., & Geraci, T. (1996). Hyperventilation and head injury: Controversies and concerns. *Journal of Neuroscience Nursing, 28,* 381–385.

Hickey, J. (1997). *Clinical practice of neurological and neuroscience nursing* (4th ed.). Philadelphia: Lippincott-Raven.

Hilton, G. (1995). Diffuse axonal injury. *Journal of Trauma Nursing, 2,* 7–12.

Nussbaum, E. (1996). Clinical snapshot: Migraines. *American Journal of Nursing, 96,* 36–37.

Ozuna, J. (1997). Pharmocologic management of epilepsy: An update. *Journal of Neuroscience Nursing, 29,* 330–335.

Veltman, R., & Jones, S. (1995). Nursing care of patients with mild brain injury. *International Journal of Trauma Nursing, 1,* 82–84.

Kathleen Sanders Jordan, RN, MS, FNP, CCRN, CEN

CHAPTER **13**

Obstetrical and Gynecological Emergencies

MAJOR TOPICS

I. GENERAL STRATEGY

A. Assessment

1. **Primary survey/resuscitation (see Chapter 1)**
2. **Secondary survey (see Chapter 1)**
3. **Psychological, social, environmental factors**
   a. *Age: consider possibility of pregnancy in women 12 to 55 years old*
   b. *Nationality/ethnicity*
   c. *Occupation*
   d. *Economic capabilities and resources*
   e. *Social support system*
   f. *Reproductive history (gravidity, parity, sexually transmitted diseases [STDs], gynecological surgery)*
   g. *Nutritional status*
   h. *Genetic history*
4. **Focused survey**

a. *Subjective data*
   1) History of present illness
      a) Last normal menstrual period (LNMP)
      b) Positive pregnancy test: date and method (serum or urine)
      c) Expected date of confinement (EDC)
      d) Vaginal bleeding: amount, color, presence of clots/tissue
      e) Vaginal discharge: amount, color, quality, odor, itching, burning
      f) Abdominal/pelvic pain: provocation, quality, radiation, severity, timing
      g) Nausea and vomiting
      h) Fever/chills
      i) Visual disturbances, headache, sudden weight gain, dependent/generalized edema
      j) Change in fetal movement
      k) Rupture of membranes: time, color, odor
      l) Uterine contractions: onset, frequency, severity
      m) Urinary frequency, dysuria, urgency, hematuria
      n) Trauma
   2) Medical history
      a) Reproductive history: all pregnancies with dates (include premature deliveries, spontaneous/therapeutic abortions, full-term deliveries, living children)
      b) Prenatal care if appropriate
      c) Date and type of delivery, if postpartum
      d) Abdominal/pelvic surgery
      e) Sexual activity/preference: new sexual partner within last 2 months or multiple sexual partners within last 6 months, high-risk behavior(s)
      f) Contraceptive use
      g) Sexually transmitted diseases (STDs)
      h) Cardiac disease
      i) Pulmonary disease
      j) Hypertension
      k) Diabetes
      l) Thyroid disease
      m) Renal disease
      n) Substance abuse: tobacco, alcohol, recreation drugs
      o) Medications: current and those used in recent past
      p) Allergies
b. *Objective data*
   1) Physical examination
      a) General survey
         (1) Vital signs: orthostatic; left lateral position if patient is greater than 20 weeks gestation
         (2) Skin: color, temperature, moisture
         (3) Respiratory status
         (4) Cardiovascular status
      b) Inspection
         (1) Edema: facial, peripheral or generalized
         (2) Abdominal or perineal wound site
         (3) Vaginal bleeding: color and amount, passage of clots or tissue
         (4) Amniotic fluid: color and pH (amniotic fluid is clear and pH neutral)
      c) Auscultation
         (1) Bowel sounds

          (2) Fetal heart tones if gestational age more than 13 weeks

      d) Palpation

          (1) Abdominal tenderness, rebound tenderness

          (2) Uterine size, fundal height, irritability, contractility

      e) Pelvic exam

          (1) Inspect the external genitalia, noting excoriations, erythema, vesicular lesions

          (2) Inspect vaginal mucosa for color, edema, discharge, lesions; inspect urethra, Bartholin's and Skene's glands for erythema, tenderness, discharge

          (3) Gently insert warm, moist speculum, and assess vagina and cervix for lesions, erosions, ulcerations, bleeding, discharge; obtain specimens and gently remove speculum

          (4) Perform bimanual exam, and palpate for uterine size, shape, consistency, cervical motion tenderness, adnexal tenderness, fullness, masses

  2) Diagnostic procedures

      a) Laboratory

          (1) Complete blood count (CBC)

          (2) Coagulation profile: prothrombin time (PT), partial thromboplastin time (PTT), fibrinogen, fibrin split products

          (3) Serum electrolyte levels

          (4) Urinalysis

          (5) Pregnancy test: urine or serum

          (6) Blood type, Rh factor, cross-match

          (7) Arterial/venous blood gas

          (8) Kleihauer-Betke test (to assess and measure presence of fetomaternal hemorrhage)

          (9) C-reactive protein: nonspecific method for evaluating severity and course of inflammatory diseases; positive reactive protein indicates presence of active inflammation

          (10) STD screening (chlamydia, gonorrhea, hepatitis B, rapid plasma reagin, human immunodeficiency virus [HIV])

          (11) Wet mount (normal saline and potassium hydroxide [KOH])

      b) Radiology

          (1) Chest x-ray film

          (2) Ultrasonography: pelvic and/or transvaginal

          (3) Abdominal x-ray film

          (4) Computed tomography (CT) scan

      c) Other

          (1) Cardiac monitor

          (2) Culdocentesis

          (3) Twelve- to 15-lead electrocardiogram (ECG)

          (4) Cardiotopographic monitoring: uterine contractions and fetal heart rate

          (5) pH reading for amniotic fluid

B. Analysis: differential nursing diagnosis/collaborative problems

  1. Anticipatory grieving

  2. Altered tissue perfusion

  3. Body image disturbance

  4. Anxiety/fear

     5. **Fluid volume deficit**

     6. **Infection**

     7. **Knowledge deficit**

     8. **Pain**

     9. **Rape-trauma syndrome**

C. Planning/interventions

     1. **Determine priorities of care**

       a. Control and maintain airway, breathing, circulation

       b. Provide supplemental oxygen as indicated

       c. Establish intravenous (IV) access for administration of crystalloid fluid and blood products

       d. Continuously monitor and treat as indicated

         1) Hemodynamic status

         2) Vaginal bleeding, passage of clots, tissue, products of conception

         3) Level of pain

       e. Relieve anxiety/apprehension

       f. Educate patient/significant other

       g. Allow significant other to remain with patient if supportive

       h. Develop individualized nursing care plan to meet the physiological and psychosocial needs of patient

       i. Obtain and set up equipment and supplies

       j. Institute appropriate interventions

D. Expected outcomes/evaluation

     1. **Monitor patient response/outcomes, and modify nursing care plan as appropriate**

     2. **If positive patient outcomes are not demonstrated, re-evaluate assessment and/or plan of care**

     3. **Record interventions and patient response**

E. Age-related considerations

     1. **Pediatric**

       a. Growth/development related

       b. "Pearls"

         1) Sexual abuse must always be considered in presence of gynecological complaints; however, many cases of sexual abuse are occult and hard to identify, therefore, a high index of suspicion must be maintained

         2) Vulvovaginitis is not uncommon in prepubertal female; incidence of STDs in prepubertal children is increasing and mandates investigation for possibility of sexual abuse; other causes include chemical irritation, perineal contamination, infections, foreign body, congenital anomaly

         3) Highest rate of STDs is in sexually active adolescents; additionally, this group also at high risk for pelvic inflammatory disease (PID) and least likely to experience or report symptoms; developmental and psychosocial characteristics of adolescent females also increase risk of contracting PID

         4) Pelvic pain in postmenarcheal adolescents is usually due to same causes of pelvic pain as in adults; common cause of pelvic pain in prepubertal females is appendicitis

      5) There is high risk of complications during pregnancy, labor, and delivery in teenage pregnancies
2. **Geriatric**
    a. *Aging related*
      1) Postmenopausal hormonal changes may be responsible for dysfunctional uterine bleeding
    b. *"Pearls"*
      1) Patients in this age group with vaginal bleeding are at increased risk for uterine cancer

II. SPECIFIC OBSTETRICAL EMERGENCIES

A. Vaginal bleeding in early pregnancy: abortion

Abortion is the termination of pregnancy before viability of the fetus (20–24 weeks). Spontaneous abortion should be considered in any woman of childbearing age who presents to the emergency department (ED) with vaginal bleeding. The incidence of spontaneous abortion in the United States is estimated to be 10 to 15% of all recognized pregnancies; the majority occur before 12 weeks gestation. The true incidence of spontaneous abortion is much higher because many pregnancies terminate before diagnosis. The cause of spontaneous abortion is unknown in the majority of cases. Etiological factors that have been implicated include endocrine dysfunction, chromosomal anomalies, maldevelopment of the embryo, and trauma. Additional factors that increase an individual's risk of spontaneous abortion include maternal infections, malnutrition, substance abuse, immunological incompatibility, surgery in pregnancy, and structural anomalies of the reproductive organs. Spontaneous abortions are commonly categorized as threatened, inevitable, incomplete, complete, missed, or septic (Table 13–1).

1. **Assessment**
    a. *Subjective data*
      1) History of present illness
        a) Abdominal pain: crampy in nature, severity
        b) Back pain, pelvic pressure
        c) Vaginal bleeding: color, amount
        d) Passage of clots or tissue
        e) Positive pregnancy test: date and method
        f) Fatigue, dizziness, lightheadedness, syncope
      2) Medical history

Table 13–1   CLASSIFICATION OF SPONTANEOUS ABORTION

Abortion Type	Description
Threatened	Slight vaginal bleeding and mild uterine cramping with a closed cervical os
Inevitable	Moderate vaginal bleeding and moderate uterine cramping with an open cervical os, gross rupture of membranes
Incomplete	Heavy vaginal bleeding and severe uterine cramping with an open cervical os and tissue in the cervix, incomplete expulsion of the products of conception
Complete	Slight vaginal bleeding with mild uterine cramping with a closed cervical os, complete expulsion of the products of conception
Missed	Slight vaginal bleeding and absent uterine contractions with a closed cervical os, prolonged retention of dead products of conception
Septic	Malodorous vaginal bleeding/discharge and absent uterine contractions with a closed cervical os, fever, intrauterine infection

a) Gestational age: LNMP, EDC
b) Reproductive history
c) Contraceptive history
d) Prenatal care
e) Current acute or chronic illness
f) Substance abuse
g) Medications
h) Allergies

b. *Objective data*
1) Physical examination
   a) General survey
   b) Orthostatic vital signs
   c) Auscultation of fetal heart tone (FHT) if gestation age more than 13 weeks
   d) Pelvic exam
2) Diagnostic procedures
   a) Pregnancy test: urine or serum
   b) CBC
   c) Blood type and Rh determination
   d) STD screening
   e) Pelvic ultrasonogram to assess viability of fetus, gestational age

2. **Analysis: differential nursing diagnosis/collaborative problems**
   a. *Fluid volume deficit related to blood loss/hemorrhage*
   b. *Pain related to uterine contractions*
   c. *Anticipatory grieving related to pregnancy loss*
   d. *Knowledge deficit related to self-care*

3. **Planning/interventions**
   a. *Maintain airway, breathing, circulation*
   b. *Establish IV access for administration of crystalloid fluid*
   c. *Continuously monitor*
      1) Hemodynamic status
      2) Vaginal bleeding, passage of clots, tissue, products of conception
      3) Pain
   d. *Prepare for/assist with medical interventions*
      1) Pelvic exam
      2) Pelvic ultrasonogram
      3) Dilation and evacuation
   e. *Administer pharmacological therapy as ordered*
      1) Rh immune globulin (RhoGAM) to all Rh-negative mothers
      2) Oxytocin
      3) Methylergonovine (Methergine)
      4) Analgesics
      5) Antibiotics
      6) Conscious sedation
   f. *Allow supportive significant other to remain with patient and participate in care as appropriate*
   g. *Encourage verbalization from patient and significant other regarding spontaneous termination of pregnancy; facilitate expression of feelings of denial, anger, sadness, guilt, or other emotions*
   h. *Discuss what is known regarding cause of spontaneous abortion to alleviate feelings of guilt in patient and significant other*

    i. Provide patient with appropriate referral for community resources for pregnancy loss

    j. For threatened abortion, provide the following discharge instructions:

       1) Maintain bed rest for 24 to 48 hours or until bleeding subsides

       2) Pelvic rest (no sexual intercourse) until bleeding and cramping stop

       3) Use sanitary pads only: avoid tampons

       4) Return to ED if bleeding or pain increases

       5) Save any clots or tissue that is passed and bring to ED or physician

       6) Ensure appropriate follow-up care with obstetrician

    k. For complete abortion, provide the following discharge instructions:

       1) Mild abdominal pain/cramping is commonly experienced for several days

       2) Use sanitary pads only: avoid tampons

       3) Take temperature four times per day

       4) Take medications as prescribed

         a) Methylergonovine (Methergine)

         b) Analgesics/nonsteroidal anti-inflammatory drugs (NSAIDs)

         c) Antibiotics

       5) Pelvic rest

       6) Ensure appropriate follow-up care with obstetrician

       7) Activity as tolerated

       8) Return to ED if temperature is higher than 100.6°F (38.1°C) or bleeding, pain, or foul-smelling discharge occurs or increases

  4. Expected outcomes/evaluation (see Appendix B)

B. Vaginal bleeding in late pregnancy: placenta previa and abruptio placenta

    Placenta previa and abruptio placenta are the most serious causes of vaginal bleeding in the second and third trimesters of pregnancy. The end result of each of these conditions may be catastrophic for both mother and fetus. Placenta previa is a condition in which the placenta is abnormally implanted in the lower uterine segment and partially or completely obstructs the internal cervical os. It is estimated that approximately 45% of gravid women have a placenta previa during the second trimester of pregnancy; however, the incidence at term is less than 1%. This is because, during the third trimester of pregnancy, the lower uterine segment grows and stretches, which causes the placental site to rise up the uterine wall away from the internal os. Softening of the lower uterine segment and effacement of the cervix in preparation for labor tear the implanted placenta previa, resulting in painless vaginal bleeding. Hemorrhage can result as the cervix continues to efface and dilate. The cause of placenta previa remains unknown. Associated etiological factors include multiparity, multiple gestation, advanced maternal age, previous uterine scarring resulting from prior cesarean section birth or myomectomy, smoking, and placental abnormalities.

    Abruptio placenta occurs when the placenta separates from its normal site of implantation before delivery of the fetus. The incidence is less than 3% of all pregnancies, although it is related to 15% of all perinatal deaths. Partial or complete separation of the placenta may occur, resulting in minimal to copious bleeding that may be seen vaginally or concealed behind the placenta. The vascular placental bed can cause a significant amount of blood loss, resulting in maternal hypotension and hypovolemic shock. The loss of placental circulation can cause fetal distress or demise. Consumptive coagulopathy and progression to disseminated intravascular coagulopathy (DIC) may occur. The primary cause of placental abruption is unknown, but the following conditions have been suggested as etiological factors: maternal hypertension, trauma, illegal drug use (e.g., cocaine, crack, marijuana), premature rupture of the membranes, short umbilical cord, uterine anomaly or tumor, pressure by the enlarged uterus on the inferior vena cava, low socioeconomic status, and dietary deficiency.

1. **Assessment**
    a. *Subjective data*
        1) History of the present illness
            a) Bleeding: onset, duration, quantity, character
                (1) Placenta previa: sudden onset of bright red vaginal bleeding; may be profuse
                (2) Abruptio placenta: dark red vaginal bleeding; amount is variable because bleeding may be concealed
            b) Pain: abdominal, pelvic, and/or back
                (1) Placenta previa: usually absent
                (2) Abruptio placenta: variable intensity
            c) Gestational age (LNMP, EDC)
            d) Recent trauma
            e) Recent sexual intercourse
            f) Decrease/loss of fetal movement
        2) Medical history
            a) Advanced maternal age
            b) Hypertension
            c) Multiparity
            d) Premature rupture of membranes
            e) History of placenta previa, abruptio placenta, previous cesarean section
            f) Illegal drug use
            g) Smoking
            h) Low socioeconomic status
            i) Trauma
    b. *Objective data*
        1) Physical examination
            a) General survey
            b) Orthostatic vital signs
            c) Abdominal exam: tenderness, uterine tone, contractions
            d) Perineal exam: evidence of bleeding (speculum or manual pelvic exam is contraindicated in second- and third-trimester vaginal bleeding until location of placenta is confirmed and previa is ruled out)
            e) Auscultation of fetal heart sounds
        2) Diagnostic procedures
            a) CBC
            b) Coagulation profile: PT, PTT, fibrinogen level, fibrin split products
            c) Type and cross-match (at least four units packed red blood cells in hemorrhaging patient)
            d) Kleihauer-Betke test
            e) Serum electrolytes
            f) Pelvic ultrasonogram
            g) Cardiotopographic monitoring
2. **Analysis: differential nursing diagnosis/collaborative problems**
    a. *Fluid volume deficit related to blood loss/hemorrhage*
    b. *Altered tissue perfusion: maternal and fetal related to hemorrhage and blood loss*
    c. *Anxiety/fear related to possible death of fetus, pain, and surgery/premature delivery*
    d. *Anticipatory grieving related to potential pregnancy loss*

3. Planning/interventions

 a. *Maintain airway, breathing, circulation*
 b. *Provide supplemental oxygen*
 c. *Establish IV access (two large-bore catheters) for administration of crystalloid fluid/blood products*
 d. *Continuously monitor*
   1) Hemodynamic status
   2) Vaginal bleeding: color and amount, passage of clots and tissue
   3) Abdominal pain/uterine contractions
   4) Fundal height (may rise with concealed intrauterine bleeding)
   5) Fetal heart rate
 e. *Maintain patient in left lateral decubitus position*
 f. *Prepare for/assist with medical interventions*
 g. *Pelvic ultrasonogram*
 h. *Administer Rh immune globulin in Rh-negative women*
 i. *Prepare for emergency cesarean section/vaginal delivery if indicated*
 j. *Allow supportive significant other to remain with patient and participate in care as appropriate*
 k. *Provide emotional support to patient and significant others*
 l. *Facilitate appropriate referrals, such as spiritual advisor, social worker*
 m. *Transport to labor and delivery unit when hemodynamically stable*

4. Expected outcomes/evaluation (see Appendix B)

C. Ectopic pregnancy

An ectopic pregnancy (EP) is defined as the implantation of the fertilized ovum outside of the normal uterine cavity. Approximately 95% of EPs are implanted in the fallopian tube, frequently on the maternal right side. If the EP invades the tubal wall too deeply or grows too large, it can rupture the tube. This rupture leads to severe pain, intraperitoneal hemorrhage, and hemorrhagic shock. The remaining EPs implant in the peritoneal cavity, uterine cornu, ovary, or cervix. The incidence of EP has been increasing worldwide. During the last few decades, the rate has nearly quadrupled in the industrialized nations. In the United States, the incidence of EP is approximately 2%; however, complications from EP account for approximately 12% of the maternal mortality. Causes of EPs are classified as mechanical, functional, and assisted reproduction. Mechanical obstruction is due to a narrowing of the fallopian tube, which prevents the normal passage of the ovum. Factors that can lead to mechanical obstruction include PID, salpingitis, fallopian tube surgery, tubal ligation, previous EP, intrauterine device (IUD) use, tumor, or developmental abnormalities of the tube. Functional causes of EP include altered tubal motility from infection or hormonal changes. Reproductive assistance such as the use of ovulation induction agents and in vitro techniques increase the risk of EP. However, it has been estimated that up to 42% of women presenting with EP have none of these risk factors.

1. Assessment

 a. *Subjective data*
   1) History of the present illness
     a) Abdominal pain: character may be nonspecific; may be diffuse, unilateral, or bilateral; may begin as vague discomfort and progress to sharp and colicky; rupture of tube may result in sudden, sharp, severe pain
     b) Referred shoulder pain: phrenic nerve irritation
     c) Vaginal bleeding: irregular, mild

       d) Fatigue, dizziness, lightheadedness, syncope

       e) Symptoms of pregnancy

    2) Medical history

       a) LNMP

       b) Reproductive history (gravidity, parity, previous EPs)

       c) PID or STDs

       d) IUD use

       e) Tubal surgery

       f) Infertility treatment

       g) Current acute or chronic illness

       h) Medications

       i) Allergies

  b. *Objective data*

    1) Physical examination

       a) General survey

       b) Orthostatic vital signs

       c) Abdominal exam

       d) Pelvic exam: cervical motion tenderness; adnexal fullness, masses, or tenderness

    2) Diagnostic procedures

       a) Pregnancy test: quantitative BHcG

       b) CBC

       c) Blood type and cross-match

       d) PT/PTT

       e) Serum electrolytes

       f) Pelvic/transvaginal ultrasonogram

       g) Culdocentesis

2. Analysis: differential nursing diagnosis/collaborative problems

  a. *Fluid volume deficit related to blood loss/hemorrhage*

  b. *Pain related to ectopic pregnancy*

  c. *Grieving related to pregnancy loss*

3. Planning/interventions

  a. *Maintain airway, breathing, circulation*

  b. *Establish IV access (two large-bore catheters) for administration of crystalloid fluid, blood products*

  c. *Continuously monitor*

    1) Hemodynamic status

    2) Level of pain

  d. *Prepare for/assist with medical interventions*

    1) Pelvic exam

    2) Pelvic/transvaginal ultrasonogram

    3) Operative intervention

  e. *Administer pharmacological therapy as ordered*

    1) Methotrexate

  f. *Allow supportive significant other to remain with patient and participate in care as appropriate*

  g. *Encourage verbalization from patient and significant other regarding pregnancy loss; facilitate their expression of feelings of denial, anger, sadness, guilt, other emotions*

  h. *Provide patient with appropriate referral for community resources for pregnancy loss*

4. Expected outcomes/evaluation (see Appendix B)

D. Pregnancy-induced hypertension: preeclampsia and eclampsia

The term *pregnancy-induced hypertension* (PIH) is used to describe hypertension unique to pregnancy. PIH is synonymous with preeclampsia-eclampsia. Preeclampsia is characterized by hypertension, proteinuria, and nondependent edema, which occur after the 20th week of pregnancy. Eclampsia is an extension of preeclampsia characterized by convulsions, coma, or both. The HELLP syndrome is a severe form of preeclampsia characterized by *h*emolysis, *e*levated *l*iver enzymes, and *l*ow *p*latelets. The exact cause of preeclampsia remains unclear; however, the basic underlying pathology is due to vasospasm resulting in an overall increase in peripheral vascular resistance. Vasospasm contracts the intravascular space; therefore, the preeclamptic patient is volume contracted and at risk for complications resulting from any change in intravascular volume. The generalized vasospasm also decreases perfusion in the uteroplacental circulation, thus reducing the delivery of oxygen and nutrients to the fetus. Preeclampsia is the most common medical problem of pregnancy and complicates 5 to 8% pregnancies in the United States. It is primarily a disease of first pregnancies and is the leading obstetric cause of maternal death. Risk factors include extremes of reproductive age, chronic hypertension, history of eclampsia, mother or sister with history of preeclampsia, multiple gestation, diabetes, systemic lupus erythematosus, vascular disease, and molar pregnancy.

1. **Assessment**
   a. *Subjective data*
      1) History of present illness
         a) Headache
         b) Epigastric or right upper quadrant (RUQ) tenderness
         c) Swelling of extremities, face, or generalized edema
         d) Visual disturbances
         e) Anxiety and apprehension
      2) Medical history
         a) Gestational age: EDC, LNMP
         b) Age: young adolescent or older than 35 years, primigravida
         c) Chronic hypertension
         d) Personal or family history of preeclampsia-eclampsia
         e) Multiple gestation
         f) Diabetes
         g) Systemic lupus erythematosus, vascular disease
         h) Medications
         i) Allergies
   b. *Objective data*
      1) Physical examination
         a) General survey
         b) Blood pressure: hypertension is defined as a blood pressure reading of greater than 140/90 mm Hg or a reading that represents an increase of 30 mm Hg systolic or 15 mm Hg diastolic over patient's baseline measurement; to determine this, two blood pressure readings must be taken at least 6 hours apart with patient lying on her left side
         c) Nondependent edema and weight gain
         d) Epigastric and RUQ tenderness
         e) Neurological exam
         f) Auscultation of FHTs
         g) Uterine size, tone
      2) Diagnostic procedures

      a) Urinalysis: proteinuria greater than 1+

      b) CBC

      c) Serum electrolytes, creatinine, liver enzymes

      d) PT/PTT

2. **Analysis: differential nursing diagnosis/collaborative problems**

    a. Altered tissue perfusion related to hypertension and decreased intravascular volume

    b. Altered tissue perfusion, fetal related to decreased ureteroplacental blood flow

    c. Risk for injury related to seizure activity

    d. Anxiety/fear related to diagnosis and prognosis

3. **Planning/interventions**

    a. Maintain airway, breathing, circulation

    b. Provide supplemental oxygen

    c. Establish IV access for administration of crystalloid fluid and pharmacological therapy

    d. Insert Foley catheter to monitor urine output

    e. Administer pharmacological therapy as indicated

      1) Magnesium sulfate IV or intramuscularly (IM) for seizure prophylaxis

      2) Benzodiazepine for seizures resistant to magnesium sulfate

      3) Antihypertensive therapy

    f. Place patient in left lateral decubitus position

    g. Continuously monitor

      1) Airway, breathing, circulation

      2) Blood pressure

      3) Neurological status

      4) FHTs

      5) Signs of magnesium toxicity: loss of patellar reflex, respiratory depression, cardiac arrest (calcium gluconate is the antidote)

    h. Institute seizure precautions

    i. Provide quiet, darkened room to minimize external stimuli

    j. Allow supportive significant other to remain with patient and participate in care as appropriate

    k. Provide the following instructions if patient is discharged:

      1) Maintain reduced activity/bed rest as directed

      2) Take medications as directed

      3) Return to ED for headaches, visual disturbances, increased swelling of face, fingers, or generalized, epigastric or RUQ abdominal pain, tremors, uterine contractions, vaginal bleeding

      4) Follow-up with obstetrician as directed

4. **Expected outcomes/evaluation** (see Appendix B)

E. Hyperemesis gravidarum

    Hyperemesis gravidarum is defined as severe vomiting occurring before the 20th week of pregnancy. Hyperemesis gravidarum occurs in up to 2% of all pregnancies, although the diagnosis is not well defined because the diagnostic criteria used varies from one geographical area to another. This condition usually necessitates hospitalization because both maternal and fetal well-being are threatened. The exact cause of hyperemesis gravidarum remains unclear; however, the following causative factors have been suggested: vitamin B_6 deficiency resulting from a change in protein metabolism, impaired function of the adrenal cortex, hyperthyroidism and excess human chorionic gonadotropin secretion, psychological factors, alterations in gastrointestinal physiology, a hypersensitivity reaction, and poor nutrition. The primary clinical manifestation of hyperemesis gravidarum is frequent, sustained vomiting, often lasting 4 to 8 weeks. This results in significant weight loss and dehydration. Signs of starvation that gradually develop include metabolic acidosis, ketonuria, hypokalemic alkalosis, oliguria, hemoconcentration, and constipation. Complications of hyperemesis gravidarum include gastrointestinal bleeding, Mallory-Weiss tears, and Boerhaave's esophageal disruptions. A few cases of Wernicke's encephalopathy resulting from thiamine deficiency caused by prolonged hyperemesis have been documented. The population at risk includes primiparous, young, nonsmoking women; women with multiple-gestation pregnancies; women with a history of hydatidiform mole pregnancy; and women weighing more than 25% of their ideal body weight.

1. **Assessment**
   a. *Subjective data*
      1) History of present illness
         a) Vomiting: severity and duration
         b) Weight loss
      2) Medical history
         a) Reproductive history
         b) Gestational age: EDC, LNMP
         c) Medications
         d) Allergies
   b. *Objective data*
      1) Physical examination
         a) General survey
         b) Orthostatic vital signs
         c) Weight
         d) FHTs
      2) Diagnostic procedures
         a) CBC
         b) Serum electrolytes
         c) Serum acetone
         d) Urinalysis
2. **Analysis: differential nursing diagnosis/collaborative problems**
   a. *Fluid volume deficit related to nausea and vomiting*
   b. *Nutrition, alteration in: less than body requirements related to nausea and vomiting*
   c. *Knowledge deficit related to disease process and self-care*
3. **Planning/interventions**
   a. *Maintain airway, breathing, circulation*
   b. *Establish IV access for administration of crystalloid fluid and pharmacological therapy*
   c. *Infuse 1 to 2 L of normal saline rapidly followed by dextrose-containing solutions at slower rate of infusion*
   d. *Administer antiemetics as indicated*
   e. *Monitor presence and degree of ketonuria*
   f. *Gradual oral rehydration as tolerated*
   g. *Admit to hospital for continued vomiting*
   h. *Provide the following instructions if patient is discharged:*
      1) Oral fluids as tolerated; advance to small, frequent meals consisting of easily digested high-energy foods
      2) Take medications as directed
      3) Return to ED for persistent vomiting
      4) Moderate activity

5) Follow-up with obstetrician as directed
4. **Expected outcomes/evaluation** (see Appendix B)

F. Postpartum hemorrhage

Postpartum hemorrhage (PPH) is defined as a blood loss exceeding 500 mL or more after the expulsion or extraction of the placenta and membranes. Postpartum hemorrhage is classified as early if it occurs during the first 24 hours after delivery, and late if it occurs after that time. Late PPH usually occurs 6 to 10 days after delivery. The most common cause of early PPH is uterine atony, which accounts for approximately 90% of all cases. Other causes include retained placental fragments, lower genital tract lacerations, uterine inversion, uterine rupture, and maternal coagulopathy. The most common reasons for late PPH are retained products of conception, infection, subinvolution of the placental site, episiotomy breakdown, hematoma, and coital trauma. The following factors place a woman at higher risk of for PPH: overdistention of the uterus as a result of hydramnios, multiple gestation or a macrosomatic fetus; high parity; prolonged difficult labor, especially after oxytocin induction; history of PPH, preeclampsia, placenta previa, or precipitous labor.

1. **Assessment**
   a. *Subjective data*
      1) History of present illness
         a) Recent delivery
         b) Vaginal bleeding: amount and character
         c) Easy bruising/bleeding
      2) Medical history
         a) Reproductive history
         b) Prolonged/complicated labor and delivery
         c) Previous postpartum hemorrhage
         d) Preeclampsia
         e) Placenta previa
         f) Coagulopathy
         g) Medications
         h) Allergies
   b. *Objective data*
      1) Physical examination
         a) General survey
         b) Orthostatic vital signs
         c) Uterine size/tone
         d) Vaginal bleeding: amount, color
         e) Pelvic exam: manual exploration for retained placental fragments
      2) Diagnostic procedures
         a) Complete blood count
         b) Coagulation profile, fibrinogen, fibrin split products
         c) Type and cross-match
         d) Pelvic/vaginal ultrasonogram
2. **Analysis: differential nursing diagnosis/collaborative problems**
   a. *Fluid volume deficit uterine/vaginal bleeding*
   b. *Tissue perfusion, decreased related to blood loss*
3. **Planning/interventions**
   a. *Maintain airway, breathing, circulation*
   b. *Establish IV access (two large-bore catheters) for administration of crystalloid fluid, blood products, and pharmacological therapy*

     c. Uterine atony
1) Perform firm bimanual massage of uterus
2) Administer oxytocin IV to initiate and maintain uterine contractility
3) For persistent bleeding, administer methylergonovine (Methergine) or use prostaglandin IM or vaginal suppository
4) Surgical intervention may be required for persistent bleeding not responsive to medical management (ligation of the uterine, ovarian, or hypogastric arteries; total or subtotal hysterectomy)

     d. Manual removal/curettage to expel retained placental fragments

     e. Surgical repair of genital tract lacerations

     f. Continuously monitor
1) Hemodynamic status
2) Vaginal bleeding, passage of clots, tissue, placental fragments

     g. Allow supportive significant other to remain with patient and participate in care as appropriate

     h. Encourage verbalization from patient and significant other regarding anxiety, fear, and other emotions they may be experiencing

     i. Initiate social service or crisis intervention support for care of newborn and other dependents

     j. Transfer to the labor and delivery unit when hemodynamically stable

4. Expected outcomes/evaluation (see Appendix B)

G. Emergency delivery

When a gravid patient arrives in the ED and delivery appears imminent, it is essential to obtain a rapid obstetric history and physical assessment of the labor status. Contractions alone are not an indication of advanced labor. Uterine contractions must be present with sufficient duration (> 30 seconds), frequency (every 10 minutes), and intensity to produce progressive effacement and dilation of the cervix. The first stage of labor is the time from the onset of regular contractions until complete cervical dilation. The second stage of labor is the time from complete dilation until delivery of the infant. During this stage, the mother will have the urge to push. The third stage of labor is from the delivery of the infant until the delivery of the placenta.

1. Assessment
     a. Subjective data
1) History of present condition
    a) Contractions: frequency, intensity, duration
    b) Rupture of amniotic membranes: time, color, odor
    c) Increase in bloody show
    d) Rectal pressure or passage of feces
2) Medical history
    a) Reproductive history: gravidity and parity, EDC
    b) Obstetrical care received during this pregnancy
    c) Previous labor and delivery history, including complications
    d) Medical problems/medications
    e) Allergies

     b. Objective data
1) Physical examination
    a) General survey
    b) FHTs
    c) Uterine size/tone, irritability, contractility
    d) Vaginal bleeding: amount, color

e) Pelvic exam
  (1) Effacement (thinning) of cervix
  (2) Dilation of cervix
  (3) Consistency (softness or firmness) of the cervix
  (4) Location of cervix
  (5) Station of fetal head
  (6) Status of membranes and color of amniotic fluid if ruptured
2) Diagnostic procedures
  a) pH test of amniotic fluid (amniotic fluid has a neutral pH)

2. **Analysis: differential nursing diagnosis/collaborative problems**
   a. *Pain related to contractions of labor and delivery*
   b. *Anxiety/fear related to emergency delivery*

3. **Planning/interventions**
   a. *Maintain airway, breathing, circulation*
   b. *Assist with delivery process*
      1) Position patient comfortably: side lying or modified Fowler with legs supported
      2) Assist mother with proper breathing: as the head emerges, encourage the mother to "pant like a puppy" to prevent uncontrolled delivery, predisposing to maternal and fetal trauma
      3) Extend fingers of dominant hand on infant's head to allow head to emerge slowly
      4) Once head is delivered, a finger should be passed to neck of infant to ascertain whether it is encircled by umbilical cord; if cord is felt, it should be slipped over infant's head; if cord is tight, it should be clamped in two places and cut
      5) Quickly wipe infant's face, and suction nares and mouth to minimize likelihood of aspiration of amniotic fluid and blood
      6) While supporting infant's head, deliver shoulders: anterior followed by posterior; remainder of infant's body should follow rapidly
      7) While holding infant in a head-dependent position at the level of the introitus, suction mouth and nose
      8) Clamp umbilical cord between two clamps placed 4 to 5 cm from infant's abdomen when the cord stops pulsating
      9) Dry and wrap infant to minimize heat loss
      10) Perform an Apgar score (Table 13–2) at the time of birth and 5 minutes afterward
      11) Do not apply uterine massage or manipulate umbilical cord until placenta is expelled (up to 30 minutes after delivery of infant)
   c. *Allow for early breast-feeding or bonding between mother and infant*

Table 13–2 APGAR SCORING

Objective Sign	Score		
	0	**1**	**2**
Heart rate	Absent	< 100 bpm	> 100 bpm
Respiratory effort	Absent	Irregular, slow	Crying, good
Muscle tone	Flaccid	Some flexion	Active motion
Reflex irritability	No response	Grimace, weak cry	Sneeze, cough, cry
Color	Blue	Pink body, blue extremities	Completely pink

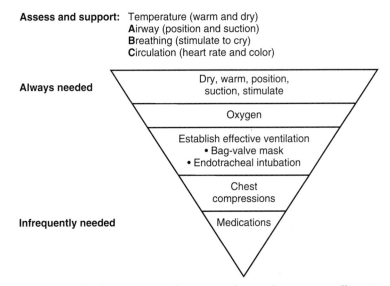

Assess and support: Temperature (warm and dry)
Airway (position and suction)
Breathing (stimulate to cry)
Circulation (heart rate and color)

Always needed

Dry, warm, position,
suction, stimulate

Oxygen

Establish effective ventilation
• Bag-valve mask
• Endotracheal intubation

Chest
compressions

Infrequently needed

Medications

FIGURE 13–1. Inverted pyramid reflecting relatively frequencies of neonatal resuscitation efforts. Reproduced with permission. © *Textbook of Pediatric Advanced Life Support*, 1994. Copyright American Heart Association.

  d. Transport to labor and delivery unit
 4. Expected outcomes/evaluation (see Appendix B)

H. Neonatal resuscitation

  Newborn resuscitation will be required for infants born with any signs of cardiovascular or respiratory compromise. Infants at high risk include those born prematurely (before 37 weeks gestation), breech presentation, multiple gestation, meconium identified before or after delivery, Apgar scores at 1 and 5 minutes lower than 6, or any signs of infant compromise before or after delivery. Neonatal asphyxia is the direct result of conditions that interfere with the placenta's ability to function as the fetal organ of respiration or with the infant's ability to establish extrauterine respiration despite adequate placental functioning. The end result in this setting is an infant who is hypoxic, hypercapnic, and acidotic. However, most infants are not born asphyxiated and only will require maintenance of temperature, suctioning of the airway, and mild stimulation. Six percent of all newborns require further resuscitation. An inverted pyramid illustrates the relative frequencies and priorities of neonatal resuscitation (Fig. 13–1). All neonatal resuscitation efforts should proceed in an orderly and systematic manner, and reassessment should follow each intervention to prevent any further and often unnecessary actions.

 1. Assessment
  a. Subjective data
   1) History of present condition
    a) Gestational age (LNMP, EDC)
    b) Prolonged and/or complicated labor
    c) Prolonged rupture of the membranes
    d) Prolapsed cord
    e) Breech or other abnormal presentation
    f) Meconium-stained amniotic fluid
    g) Multiple gestation
    h) Precipitous delivery
    i) Operative delivery

        j) Medications received during labor and delivery

        k) Signs of distress

    2) Maternal medical history

        a) Reproductive history: gravidity and parity

        b) Obstetrical care received during this pregnancy

        c) Maternal age younger than 16 years or older than 35 years

        d) PIH

        e) Medical problems/medications (e.g., diabetes, cardiovascular, thyroid, substance abuse)

        f) Allergies

  b. *Objective data*

    1) Physical examination

        a) General survey

        b) Apgar scores at 1 and 5 minutes

        c) Meconium-stained amniotic fluid

        d) Birth weight

    2) Diagnostic procedures

        a) Serum glucose

        b) CBC

        c) Venous blood pH/arterial blood gas

        d) Cardiac monitor: 12-lead ECG

        e) Chest and abdominal x-ray film

2. Analysis: differential nursing diagnosis/collaborative problems

  a. *Ineffective airway clearance related to immature airway, secretions, and ineffective thermoregulation*

  b. *Impaired gas exchange related to pulmonary immaturity*

  c. *Tissue perfusion, impaired related to decreased cardiac output*

3. Planning/interventions

  a. *Quickly dry amniotic fluid covering infant, and place infant under a heat source to maintain infant's temperature*

  b. *Maintain infant on his or her back or side with neck in a neutral position; do not hyperextend neck, or airway obstruction may result; if meconium stain is observed, trachea should be gently suctioned before any other resuscitative measures are taken*

  c. *Provide tactile stimulation if necessary by flicking soles of feet and rubbing infant's back*

  d. *Provide blow-by oxygen therapy if respirations are shallow or slow to stimulate infant*

  e. *Institute positive-pressure ventilation at a rate or 40 to 60 breaths per minute with 100% oxygen if respirations are inadequate or gasping is present*

  f. *Monitor heart rate because this is most critical indicator of oxygenation in neonate; if heart rate is less than 60 to 80 bpm and not increasing rapidly despite positive-pressure ventilation within a time period of 30 to 60 seconds, chest compressions should begin*

  g. *Assist with endotracheal intubation if necessary*

  h. *Initiate vascular access via the umbilical vein or intraosseous route*

  i. *Administer pharmacological therapy as indicated*

    1) Epinephrine

    2) Naloxone (Narcan)

    3) Glucose

    4) Sodium bicarbonate (for prolonged resuscitation)

  j. *Administer volume expanders for a hypovolemic infant: normal saline or*

Ringer's lactate; albumin/saline; or whole blood cross-matched with mother's blood
   k. *Continuously monitor infant's response to each intervention*
      1) Cardiovascular status, especially heart rate
      2) Respiratory effort
      3) Color of mucous membranes (compared with general color) and warmth of skin
   l. *Maintain communication with family members regarding infant's status*
   m. *Initiate consultation with social service, chaplain, or other crisis intervention worker*
   n. *Allow family to see infant as soon as possible*
   o. *Transfer to neonatal unit when stable for transfer*
4. **Expected outcomes/evaluation** (see Appendix B)

I. Trauma in pregnancy

Trauma is the primary cause of mortality during pregnancy, accounting for up to 22% of all maternal deaths. It is estimated to occur in 7% of all pregnancies; the majority occur during the third trimester. The most common cause of injury in the pregnant population is blunt trauma as a result of motor vehicle crashes. Other mechanisms include falls, burns and inhalation injury, firearm and stab wound injuries, and domestic violence. Head injury and shock are the most frequent causes of maternal death. The most common cause of fetal death in trauma in pregnancy is maternal death. The second leading cause of fetal death is due to maternal shock. Therefore, the most critical principle in patient management is to direct attention toward maternal well-being. The best chance for fetal survival is to ensure maternal survival. The outcome of trauma in pregnancy is a function of the same factors as with any injured patient: magnitude of the injury, organ systems involved directly and indirectly, success and rapidity of resuscitation, and the ability of the patient's physiological reactions to respond and reach the preinjury state. Assessment of the pregnant trauma patient may be more difficult because of the many anatomical and physiological changes that occur during pregnancy that alter the gravid patient's response to injury (Table 13–3). It is essential to have an understanding of these changes in the approach to the pregnant trauma patient.

1. **Assessment**
   a. *Subjective data*
      1) History of present illness
         a) Mechanism of injury
         b) Loss of consciousness
         c) Vaginal bleeding
         d) Uterine contractions/abdominal pain
         e) Fetal movement
      2) Medical history
         a) Date of LNMP, EDC
         b) Reproductive history
         c) Domestic violence
         d) Current acute or chronic illness
         e) Substance abuse
         f) Medications
         g) Allergies
         h) Tetanus status
   b. *Objective data*
      1) Physical examination

Table 13–3 ANATOMICAL AND PHYSIOLOGICAL CHANGES IN PREGNANCY

System	Alteration	Effect
Cardiovascular	Increased total blood volume	Improved tolerance to hemorrhage
	Increased cardiac output	Increased heart rate 15 to 20 bpm
	Decreased peripheral vascular resistance	Decreased systolic (0–15 mm Hg) and diastolic (10–20 mm Hg) blood pressure
		Increased skin color and temperature
	Aortocaval compression	Supine hypotensive syndrome
	Selective uterine vasoconstriction in response to hemorrhage	Fetal hypoxia
Hematological	Increased plasma volume	Dilutional anemia (hematocrit 32–34%)
	Leukocytosis	WBC up to 20,000/mm^3
	Hypercoagulability	Increase risk of disseminated intravascular coagulation with thromboplastin release
Respiratory	Increased minute ventilation	Decreased P_{CO_2} (30–34 mm Hg)
	Increased tidal volume	Decreased serum bicarbonate (18–22 mEq/L)
		Partially compensated respiratory alkalosis
	Elevation of diaphragm	Decreased functional residual capacity
		Decreased tolerance to hypoxia
	Increased oxygen consumption	Increased risk of maternal and fetal hypoxia
Gastrointestinal	Decreased motility and emptying	Increased risk of vomiting and aspiration
	Compartmentalization of the small intestine into the upper abdomen	Increased risk of injury
	Stretched and laxed abdominal wall	Masked intra-abdominal injury
Urinary	Elevation and compression of bladder	Increased risk of injury

WBC, white blood cell; P_{CO_2}, partial pressure of carbon dioxide

a) General survey: include primary and secondary survey with a thorough understanding of the normal anatomical and physiological changes associated with pregnancy
b) Abdominal exam: tenderness, uterine size and irritability, fundal height, palpable fetal parts
c) Auscultation of FHT if gestation age greater than 13 weeks
d) Pelvic speculum exam: vaginal bleeding or leakage of amniotic fluid
2) Diagnostic procedures
a) CBC
b) Serum electrolytes
c) Blood type and Rh determination
d) Coagulation profile: PT, PTT, fibrinogen, split fibrin products
e) Kleihauer-Betke test: detection of fetomaternal hemorrhage
f) Urinalysis
g) Toxicology screen, blood alcohol level
h) Arterial blood gas
i) ECG
j) Maternal radiographic procedures as indicated (e.g., chest x-ray film, abdominal/pelvic CT scan)
k) Diagnostic peritoneal lavage
l) Pelvic/transvaginal ultrasonogram: fetal assessment, gestational age
m) Cardiotopographic monitoring: fetal heart rate and uterine contractions

2. **Analysis: differential nursing diagnosis/collaborative problems**
   a. *Fluid volume deficit related to blood loss/hemorrhage*
   b. *Cardiac output, decreased related to hemorrhage*
   c. *Impaired gas exchange, high risk for related to pregnancy and trauma*
   d. *Pain related to trauma*
   e. *Risk for injury, fetal compromise related to maternal/fetal trauma*
   f. *Anxiety/fear related to trauma and potential for pregnancy loss*
   g. *Knowledge deficit related to diagnosis and treatment*
3. **Planning/interventions**
   a. *Maintain airway, breathing, circulation*
   b. *Provide supplemental high flow oxygen: fetus is very vulnerable to effects of hypoxia*
   c. *Establish IV access (two large-bore catheters) for administration of crystalloid fluid/blood products*
   d. *Maintain patient in left lateral decubitus position to prevent supine hypotensive syndrome*
   e. *Insert nasogastric (NG) tube and Foley catheter if indicated*
   f. *Continuously monitor*
      1) Hemodynamic status
      2) Vaginal bleeding/amniotic fluid leakage: color and amount
      3) Abdominal pain/uterine contractions
      4) Fundal height: may rise with intrauterine bleeding
      5) Fetal heart rate
   g. *Administer pharmacological therapy as indicated*
      1) Rh immune globulin in Rh-negative women
      2) Tetanus toxoid and tetanus immune globulin as indicated
      3) Antibiotics as indicated
      4) Magnesium sulfate to decrease uterine irritability
   h. *Prepare for/assist with medical interventions*
      1) Diagnostic peritoneal lavage or other diagnostic studies
      2) Emergent cesarean section
   i. *Allow supportive significant other to remain with patient and participate in care as appropriate*
   j. *Encourage verbalization from patient and significant other*
   k. *Transfer to labor and delivery unit when patient is hemodynamically stable*
   l. *Provide the following discharge instructions (all pregnant trauma patients should be monitored for a minimum of 4 hours):*
      1) Activity as ordered
      2) Return to ED or labor and delivery unit for specified symptoms
         a) Abdominal cramping or contractions
         b) Decrease or lack of fetal movement
         c) Vaginal bleeding
         d) Leakage of amniotic fluid
         e) Dizziness and syncope
4. **Expected outcomes/evaluation** (see Appendix B)

III. SPECIFIC GYNECOLOGICAL EMERGENCIES

A. Vaginal bleeding/dysfunctional uterine bleeding

Vaginal bleeding in the nonpregnant patient can be due to a variety of causes, including uterine fibroids, menstrual cycle irregularities, trauma, infection, malignancy, or a coagulopathy. Dysfunctional uterine bleeding (DUB) is a common form of abnormal vaginal bleeding and results from hormonal imbalance. This most frequently occurs secondary to anovulation, which is common at both the beginning and the end of the reproductive years. Causes of DUB may include dysfunction of the hypothalamic-pituitary-ovarian axis, thyroid or adrenal disorders, hormone replacement therapy, or use of steroids, androgens, digitalis, and anticoagulants. Typically, DUB is characterized by steady, painless bleeding and the absence of clots or tissue.

1. **Assessment**
   a. *Subjective data*
      1) History of present illness
         a) Bleeding
            (1) Quantity: spotting versus steady flow; number of pads used per hour; amount compared with normal menses
            (2) Duration: onset; number of hours or days, compared with normal menses
            (3) Quality: color—bright red versus brown; presence of clots/tissue
            (4) Associated with sexual intercourse
         b) Abdominal pain/cramping
         c) Fever/chills
         d) Fatigue, dizziness, lightheadedness, syncope
      2) Medical history
         a) LNMP
         b) Reproductive history
         c) Sexual history
         d) Age-related factors: menarche, precocious puberty, menopause
         e) Contraceptive history (e.g., IUD use, oral contraceptives)
         f) Current acute or chronic illness
         g) Recent trauma or surgery
         h) Medications
         i) Allergies
   b. *Objective data*
      1) Physical examination
         a) General survey
         b) Orthostatic vital signs
         c) Pelvic exam
      2) Diagnostic procedures
         a) Pregnancy test
         b) CBC
         c) Coagulation profile: PT, PTT, fibrin split products
         d) Thyroid function tests, liver function tests, follicle-stimulating hormone (FSH) and luteinizing hormone (LH) levels
         e) Blood type and screen/cross-match
         f) Urinalysis
         g) STD screening
         h) Pelvic/transvaginal ultrasonogram
2. **Analysis: differential nursing diagnosis/collaborative problems**
   a. *Fluid volume deficit related to blood loss/hemorrhage*
   b. *Knowledge deficit related to diagnosis, management, and self-care*
3. **Planning/interventions**
   a. *Maintain airway, breathing, circulation*
   b. *Establish IV access for administration of crystalloid fluid/blood products*
   c. *Continuously monitor*
      1) Hemodynamic status

    2) Vaginal bleeding, passage of clots, tissue

    3) Pain

  d. *Prepare for/assist with medical interventions*

    1) Pelvic exam

    2) Pelvic ultrasonogram

    3) Diagnostic/therapeutic dilation and curettage (D&C)

  e. *Administer pharmacological therapy as ordered (e.g., low-dose combination oral contraceptive therapy, progesterone, estrogen; conscious sedation for D&C)*

  f. *Allow supportive significant other to remain with patient and participate in care as appropriate*

  g. *Prepare for hospital admission as indicated*

  h. *Provide the following discharge instructions as indicated*

    1) Ensure appropriate follow-up care

    2) Activity as tolerated

    3) Return to ED if temperature is elevated above 100.6°F (38.1°C), bleeding, or pain increase

 4. Expected outcomes/evaluation (see Appendix B)

B. Pelvic pain

    Pain in the lower abdomen or pelvis may have a variety of causes. The pain may originate from within the organs anatomically located within the lower abdomen/pelvis, or may be referred from other adjacent body regions, including the urinary and gastrointestinal systems. Poorly localized visceral pain originates in organs and viscera innervated by autonomic nerves. This may be caused by distention of a hollow viscus (e.g., fallopian tube or distended bowel), distention of the capsule of a solid organ, or stretching of pelvic ligaments or adhesions. In contrast, pain that is well localized originates from somatic nerve irritation, such as irritation of the parietal peritoneum caused by an inflamed organ or the presence of blood or purulent fluid (e.g., ruptured EP or acute appendicitis). The causes of pelvic pain can be classified as acute, chronic, and recurrent. Recurrent temporal pelvic pain is related to the menstrual cycle. An accurate history is essential to determine the acuity because the condition causing the pain may be life threatening (Table 13–4).

 1. Assessment

  a. *Subjective data*

    1) History of present illness

      a) Nature of the pain: provocation, quality, region, severity, timing

      b) Fever and/or chills

      c) Nausea and/or vomiting

      d) Relationship to menses

      e) Vaginal discharge

      f) Changes in bowel or bladder function

    2) Medical history

      a) LNMP, menstrual history

      b) History of abdominal pain

      c) Reproductive history

      d) Previous abdominal/pelvic surgery

      e) Trauma

      f) Allergies

      g) Medications

  b. *Objective data*

    1) Physical examination

Table 13–4 CAUSES OF PELVIC PAIN

Cause	Nature of Pain	Fever (+/−)	Nausea and/or Vomiting	Origin (Onset)	Medical History (Contributing Factors)	Pregnancy Test	Region (Location of Pain)	Surgical History	Timing	Undulation (Aggravating)	Vaginal Discharge
Gynecological Degenerating tumor	Fullness to sudden sharp	−	No	Slow	Chronic pelvic vascular congestion, fibroids	−	Midline or generalized	Nonspecific	Constant	Menses, stress, anxiety	None
Ectopic pregnancy (ruptured)	Sharp	−	Nausea possible	Acute	PID, pelvic surgery, previous ectopic pregnancy, infertility surgery, IUD, older first maternal age	+	Pelvis	Tubal, infertility, etc.	Constant	Movement	No, may have light bleeding
Incomplete, threatened, or septic abortion	Sharp or crampy	±	No	Acute	PID, previous abortion	±	Generalized pelvic area	IUD, abortion	Constant	Movement	±
Endometriosis	Sharp	+	No	2–7 days premenses	Familial inherited, delay in childbearing, Asian, congenital anomalies	−	Posterior pelvis, bilateral	Infertility or sterility	Constant during menses	Intercourse, defecation, adhesions	Vaginal bleeding
Mittelschmerz	Sharp	−	No	Acute	Ruptured graafian follicle	−	Generalized midline	Nonspecific	Midcycle	None	None
Ovarian cyst (ruptured)	Sharp	−	No	Acute	Usually occurs during intercourse	−	Pelvis	Nonspecific	Constant	Movement	None
PID*	Sharp	+	Nausea	Acute	Previous PID, STD, frequent sex, multiple partners	−	Bilateral pelvis, (+) CMT	Abortion, IUD	Constant	Intercourse, menses, movement	Yes
PMS	Crampy	−	Nausea possible	Acute	Previous history of PMS	−	Generalized midline	Nonspecific	1–6 days premenses	No	None
Primary dysmenorrhea	Crampy	−	No	Acute	History of primary dysmenorrhea	−	Generalized	Nonspecific	Onset of menses	Movement	None
Septic pelvic thrombosis	Sharp	+	No	Acute	Pregnant or postpartum	±	Pelvis	Nonspecific	Throbbing	Position	None
Torsion of ovary, pedicle, cyst, or tumor	Intense, sharp	±	Nausea and vomiting	Acute	Cyst, fibroid	−	Unilateral or bilateral pelvis	Nonspecific	Constant	Movement, position	None
Tubo-ovarian abscess (TOA)	Sharp	+	Nausea possible	Acute	History of PID, especially if GC	−	Unilateral or bilateral	Nonspecific	Constant	Movement	Purulent

Nongynecological

	Pain quality	Fever	Nausea/Vomiting	Onset	History	±	Location		Timing	Aggravating	Relieving
Appendicitis	Dull, then sharp	Low° grade ±	Nausea	Slow then acute	Noncontributory	–	Periumbilical then RLQ	Nonspecific	Constant	Movement	None
Diverticulitis	Crampy	±°	No	Slow	Peanuts, etc., may obstruct a diverticulum	–	LLQ	±	Intermittent	Dietary	None
DKA	Severe, sharp	±°	Nausea, vomiting	Acute	Diabetes mellitus	–	Diffuse	Nonspecific	Constant	Acidosis, hyperglycemia	None
Gastroenteritis	Crampy	±	Nausea, vomiting	Acute	Viral infection, dietary; diarrhea necessary	–	Diffuse	Nonspecific	Constant	Food, peristalsis	None
Hernia (strangulated)	Dull or sharp	+	Nausea and/or vomiting	Slow	A defect in fascia, muscle, or peritoneum to trap the bowel	–	Generalized peritonitis	Possible	Intermittent	Peristalsis	None
Intussusception	Crampy	±	Vomiting	Slow	Familial history	–	Lower abdomen	No	Intermittent	Eating	None
Leaking AAA	Severe	–	No	Acute	Hypertension, familial history of AAA	–	Site of aneurysm, or may be referred	Nonspecific	Constant	Hypertension hypoxia, bleeding	None
Peritonitis (from ruptured viscus)	Vague then sharp	+	Nausea	Slow or acute	Nonspecific	±	Variable	Nonspecific	Constant	Movement	None
Sickle cell crisis	Severe	+	Nausea, vomiting	Acute	Hypoxia, acidosis, dehydration, infection	–	Diffuse	Nonspecific	Constant	Position	None
Small bowel obstruction	Crampy bloated, severe	–	Nausea, vomiting later stage	Slow	Cancer, adhesions, hernia, fecal impaction, foreign body, volvulus, intussusception	–	Diffuse, may localize	History of surgery	Intermittent, then constant	Movement if perforation, peristalsis, eating	None
Ureteral stone	Sharp	–	Possible	Acute	History of ureteral stones, family history	–	Unilateral flank to groin	Nonspecific	Intermittent	Peristaltic movement of ureter	None
Urinary tract infection	Burning	±	No	Acute	Poor hygiene, frequent coitus, esp. multiple partners	–	Pelvis	Nonspecific	Intermittent	Voiding	None
Volvulus	Sharp	–	Nausea, vomiting	Acute	Previous surgery	–	Diffuse or localized	History of surgery	Intermittent, then constant	Peristalsis	None

*PID includes salpingitis, endometritis, and pelvic peritonitis.

†DKA is often seen as a result of an infection; therefore, a fever may be present.

PID, pelvic inflammatory disease; PMS, premenstrual syndrome; IUD, intrauterine device; STD, sexually transmitted disease; GC, gonococcal; CMT, cervical motion tenderness; DKA, diabetic ketoacidosis; AAA, abdominal aortic aneurysm; RLQ, right lower quadrant; LLQ, left lower quadrant.

Adapted from Howel, J., Altieri, M., Jagoda, A., Prescott, J., Scott, J., & Stair, T. (1998). *Emergency medicine.* Philadelphia: W. B. Saunders. Used with permission.

       a) General survey

       b) Orthostatic vital signs

       c) Abdomen

          (1) Inspection

          (2) Auscultation

          (3) Percussion

          (4) Palpation: light, deep, and rebound

       d) Pelvic exam: abnormal vaginal discharge, cervical motion tenderness, adnexal tenderness

    2) Diagnostic procedures

       a) CBC

       b) Erythrocyte sedimentation rate (ESR)

       c) C-reactive protein

       d) Serum electrolytes

       e) Blood cultures

       f) Pregnancy test

       g) Urinalysis

       h) STD screening

       i) Wet mount (saline, KOH)

       j) Pelvic/transvaginal ultrasonogram

       k) Abdominal CT scan

       l) Diagnostic laparoscopy

2. Analysis: differential nursing diagnosis/collaborative problems

  a. Pain related to inflammation and/or infection

  b. Knowledge deficit related to disease process, treatment, and complications

3. Planning/interventions (see specific diagnosis if known)

  a. Maintain airway, breathing, circulation

  b. Establish IV access for administration of crystalloid fluid and pharmacological therapy

  c. Facilitate diagnostic interventions

  d. Provide pharmacological therapy as indicated

    1) Analgesics

    2) Antibiotics

  e. Prepare for admission as indicated

4. Expected outcomes/evaluation (see Appendix B)

C. Vaginal discharge

    Vaginal discharge may be a normal physiological phenomenon for women of all ages. However, abnormal vaginal discharge is a common reason women seek emergency care. The most common cause of an abnormal vaginal discharge is infection with bacteria, yeast, or parasites. Vaginitis is extremely prevalent and usually results in considerable discomfort for the woman. The most common infections are caused by bacterial vaginosis (40–50%), *Candida albicans* (20–25%), and *Trichomonas vaginalis* (15–20%). Multiple infectious agents may occur simultaneously and may be sexually transmitted (Table 13–5). Vaginitis may also be caused by noninfectious processes, including retained foreign bodies, chemicals, hormonal changes, and alteration in vaginal flora. Predisposing factors leading to an alteration in vaginal flora include pregnancy, recent antibiotic use, diabetes, HIV infection, high-carbohydrate intake, poor hygiene practices, and vaginal hypersensitivity/allergen response.

1. Assessment

  a. Subjective data

Table 13–5 DIFFERENTIAL DIAGNOSIS OF VAGINAL INFECTIONS

Diagnostic Criteria	Condition			
	Normal	Bacterial Vaginosis	Trichomonas Vaginitis	Candida Vulvovaginitis
Vaginal pH	3.8	>4.5	>4.5	<4.5 (usually)
Discharge	White, clear	Thin, homogeneous, white; adheres to vaginal walls	Watery, yellow, gray or green, frothy, or bubbly	White, curdy, "cottage cheese like"; adheres to vaginal walls
Amine odor (KOH whiff test)	Absent	Present (fishy)	May be present (fishy)	Absent
Main patient complaint	None	Discharge, bad odor (possibly worse after intercourse), possible itching	Frothy discharge, bad odor, vulvar pruritus, dysuria	Itching/burning, discharge

KOH, sodium potassium.

    1) History of present illness
       a) Vaginal discharge: color, odor, quality, quantity
       b) Vaginal itching/irritation
       c) Vaginal erythema, edema
       d) Dysuria, urinary frequency
       e) Dyspareunia, bleeding with intercourse
    2) Medical history
       a) LNMP
       b) Reproductive history
       c) Sexual activity
       d) Current acute or chronic illness: diabetes, HIV infection
       e) Recent antibiotic use
       f) Medications
       g) Allergies
  b. *Objective data*
    1) Physical examination
       a) General survey
       b) Pelvic exam
    2) Diagnostic procedures
       a) Vaginal pH: normal, 3.8 to 4.2
       b) Wet mount (saline and KOH)
       c) Amine odor (KOH whiff test)
       d) Endocervical culture and Gram's stain
       e) Pregnancy test: urine or serum
       f) Urinalysis and urine culture

2. Analysis: differential nursing diagnosis/collaborative problems
  a. *Pain related to vaginal irritation/inflammation*
  b. *Knowledge deficit related to disease, treatment, complications, and prevention of recurrence*

3. Planning/interventions
  a. *Prepare for/assist with medical interventions*
    1) Pelvic exam
  b. *Instruct regarding antibiotic therapy as ordered*
    1) Dosage, schedule, and compliance with complete regimen
    2) Side effects
  c. *Instruct in personal hygiene as needed (e.g., cleanse perineum from front to back with mild soap and water; avoid use of sprays, scented soaps, and douches; wear cotton underwear; avoid tight-fitting clothes and pantyhose)*
  d. *Discuss methods to prevent recurrence*
    1) Abstain from sexual activity until treatment is complete and patient is asymptomatic
    2) Facilitate partner's assessment and treatment (e.g., *T. vaginalis*)
    3) Use of prophylactic risk-reducing behavior and methods
    4) Periodic STD examinations if patient is sexually active with multiple partners
    5) HIV counseling and testing if patient is at high risk

4. Expected outcomes/evaluation (see Appendix B)

D. Sexually transmitted diseases

    This group of infectious diseases are classified on the basis of their mode of transmission: sexual activity. The primary STDs include *Neisseria gonorrhoeae, Chlamydia trachomatis, Treponema pallidum* (syphilis), bacterial vaginosis, condyloma acuminatum (venereal wart), herpes simplex virus, and HIV. The major sequelae associated with STDs include vaginitis, cervicitis, PID, urethritis, epididymitis, pharyngitis, proctitis, skin and mucous membrane lesions, and acquired immunodeficiency syndrome (AIDS) associated with the HIV virus (Table 13–6).

E. Pelvic Inflammatory Disease

Pelvic inflammatory disease (PID) is a nonspecific term used to describe infection of the endometrium, fallopian tubes, ovaries, pelvic peritoneum, or pelvic connective tissue. The infection may be acute, subacute or chronic. *N. gonorrhoeae* and *C. trachomatis* are the two most common organisms that cause PID and frequently coexist. Other aerobes and anaerobes may also cause PID. The majority of PID cases result from upward migration of genital infections; the remaining cases are caused by introduction of microorganisms through recent instrumentation. Several factors facilitate the spread of organisms to the upper genital tract, including menses related loss of the cervical barrier; hormonal changes reducing the bacteriostatic properties of cervical mucus; gynecological procedures; and IUD use. *N. gonorrhoeae* infection is frequently menstruation dependent; spread of the disease from the cervix to the endometrium usually occurs within 5 to 7 days of the onset of menses with classic clinical manifestations. In contrast, *C. trachomatis* infection is usually unrelated to menses and may present atypically or insidiously. Severe tubal damage resulting in infertility can result from *C. trachomatis* despite the absence of impressive clinical manifestations. PID can cause significant long-term sequelae, including chronic pelvic pain, dyspareunia, infertility, and ectopic pregnancy. Because the clinical presentation of PID may be insidious, it is essential that the factors associated with an increased risk of PID be identified. Adolescents are at particularly high risk for PID. Predisposing factors for this age group include immature immune systems, larger zones of cervical ectopy, thinner cervical mucus, and greater exposure to multiple sexual partners. The other most common risk factors include individuals with multiple sexual partners, high frequency of intercourse, recent exposure to STDs, nonbarrier contraception, presence of an IUD, recent gynecological procedures, douching, smoking, and proximity to menses.

1. **Assessment**
   a. *Subjective data*
      1) History of present illness
         a) Abdominal pain
            (1) Provocation: exacerbated by movement, intercourse, and the Valsalva maneuver; onset or increase in severity during menstruation
            (2) Quality: may be dull and aching to sharp and persistent
            (3) Region: bilateral lower abdomen; may have RUQ pain in PID-related perihepatitis (Fitz-Hugh–Curtis syndrome)
            (4) Severity: ranges from intermittent and mild to severe and continuous
            (5) Timing: increases in severity over hours or days
         b) Vaginal discharge: mucopurulent, malodorous
         c) Vaginal bleeding: increased menstrual flow, breakthrough bleeding
         d) Dysuria
         e) Fever and chills
         f) Vomiting
      2) Medical history
         a) LNMP
         b) Previous pelvic infection

Table 13–6 STD ASSESSMENT AND INTERVENTION

STD	Incubation Period (Timing)	Discharge	Lesions	Pain	Associated Symptoms	ED Treatment	Home Treatment	Discharge Teaching	Special Instructions
Neisseria gonorrhoeae	3–5 days	Yellow, mucopurulent	None	Males: dysuria Females: may be asymptomatic or have symptoms of PID	Urinary frequency Abnormal vaginal bleeding	Ceftriaxone Cefixime Ciprofloxacin Ofloxacin	None	Abstinence from sexual activity until treatment completed Partner(s) need treatment Use of barrier method to prevent transmission of STD Need to return in 7–10 days for follow-up Consider risk of HIV infection, hepatitis B, syphilis	
Chlamydia trachomatis	5–10 days or longer	Mucopurulent	None	Males: burning on urination, urethral itching, symptoms of epididymitis Females: usually asymptomatic	None	Azithromycin, 1 g	Doxycycline or Erythromycin or Ofloxacin		
Treponema pallidum (syphilis)	3 weeks	None	Indurated ulcer (chancre) found on genitalia, rectum, mouth, or lips	None	May have fever, lymphadenopathy	Benzathine PCN	Doxycycline Erythromycin (will be covered by doxycycline given for *Chlamydia*)		
Trichomonas vaginalis	1 week Worse immediately after menses Most acute during pregnancy	Greenish-gray; thin, frothy; profuse; malodorous	None	Severe pruritus	Genital edema Erythema of vaginal vault	None	Metronidazole		Avoid contact with lesion

Condyloma acuminatum (venereal wart)	3–6 months May flourish during pregnancy	None	Pink-gray soft lesions, taller than they are wide, occur singly or in clusters, may bleed	None	None	Apply to lesions: 10–25% podophyllin in tincture of benzoin (not in pregnancy) or 50% trichloroacetic acid	None	Lesions heal within weeks but are infectious during that time; avoid contact
Chancroid	3–14 days	None	Nonindurated ulcer with undetermined edges May also be found intrameatally	Very painful Increased pain on voiding	Enlarged, tender inguinal glands	Liquid nitrogen Ceftriaxone Azithromycin Erythromycin	Ciprofloxacin, amoxicillin-clavulanate (Augmentin)	
Herpes simplex virus type 2	2–12 days	May have purulent vaginal discharge	Multiple shallow vesicles on genital area, buttocks, or thighs Females: most common sites are cervix, vulva Males: most common sites are glans, prepuce	Very painful dysuria	May have inguinal lymphadenopathy May have urinary retention related to pain May have fever, headache, malaise, myalgias Waddling gait	Famcyclovir Vancyclovir	Acyclovir Warm baths Topical anesthetic ointment Mild analgesics Loose-fitting clothing Antimicrobials for bacterial superinfection may be necessary	About half the patients have recurrence every 2 months Local hyperesthesia usually occurs 24 hours before eruption of vesicular lesions No sexual activity during infectious outbreaks, including 24-hour prodromal period, until lesions dry up

STD, sexually transmitted disease; PID, pelvic inflammatory disease; ED, emergency department; HIV, human immunodeficiency virus;

      c) Sexual activity, new (< 2 months) or multiple sexual partners, nonbarrier contraception

      d) Recent gynecological procedures/instrumentation

      e) Allergies

      f) Medications

  b. Objective data

    1) Physical examination

      a) Fever

      b) Tachycardia

      c) Lower abdominal tenderness, rebound tenderness

      d) Pelvic exam: abnormal vaginal discharge, cervical motion tenderness (chandelier sign), adnexal tenderness

    2) Diagnostic procedures

      a) CBC: leukocytosis with "shift to the left"

      b) ESR: elevated

      c) C-reactive protein: elevated

      d) Serum electrolytes

      e) Blood cultures

      f) Pregnancy test

      g) Urinalysis

      h) Endocervical culture, Gram's stain

      i) Wet mount (saline, KOH)

      j) Pelvic ultrasonogram

      k) Abdominal CT scan

      l) Diagnostic laparoscopy

2. Analysis: differential nursing diagnosis/collaborative problems

  a. Infection related to bacterial invasion of the female reproductive organs

  b. Pain related to inflammation and infection

  c. Knowledge deficit related to PID risk factors, disease process, treatment, and complications

3. Planning/interventions

  a. Maintain airway, breathing, circulation

  b. Establish IV access for administration of crystalloid fluid and pharmacological therapy

  c. Provide pharmacological therapy as indicated

    1) Analgesics

    2) Antibiotics

  d. Prepare for admission as indicated

    1) Temperature greater than 38.5°C

    2) Suspected pelvic or tubo-ovarian abscess

    3) Nausea and vomiting impeding oral antibiotic therapy

    4) Pregnancy

    5) Peritonitis, perihepatitis

    6) Adolescents, children, nulligravidae

    7) IUD use

    8) Immunocompromised patients

    9) Failure to respond to outpatient therapy of 48 to 72 hours

  e. Discuss discharge instructions as indicated

    1) Medication for infection: purpose, dose, schedule, importance of completing course of antibiotics, side effects

    2) Use of analgesics

    3) Follow-up within 72 hours

4) Need to return for persistent or worsening symptoms: fever, chills, abdominal pain, nausea and vomiting
   f. *Discuss methods to prevent recurrence*
      1) Abstain from sexual activity until after post-treatment examination/cultures
      2) Facilitate partner's assessment and treatment
      3) Use of prophylactic risk-reducing behavior and methods
      4) Periodic STD examinations if patient is sexually active with multiple partners
      5) HIV counseling and testing if patient is at high risk
   4. Expected outcomes/evaluation (see Appendix B)

F. Sexual assault

Sexual assault is a common violent crime against a child, woman, or man. Although legal definitions of sexual assault vary in different geographical areas, the common foundation for all definitions is sexual relations imposed against the victim's will. The definition encompasses a broad continuum of violent acts involving nonconsensual sexual activity (e.g., molestation, rape, sodomy). It is estimated that up to 80 to 90% of all cases go unreported. Therefore, accurate statistics are difficult to obtain. Emergency treatment of a victim of sexual assault involves both a medical and forensic examination.

1. Assessment
   a. *Subjective data*
      1) History of present illness
         a) Date, time, and place of assault
         b) Description of assault: document all acts as reported, include the number of assailants, whether force was used, type of assault (i.e., actual or attempted oral, vaginal, or rectal penetration; ejaculation by assailant; use of condom; other assaultive behavior)
         c) Associated injuries
         d) Postassault activity (e.g., change of clothing, bathing, douching, brushing teeth, urination, defecation)
      2) Medical history
         a) LNMP
         b) Reproductive history
         c) Current method of contraception
         d) Consenting intercourse within the last 72 hours
         e) History of STDs or PID
         f) Current or chronic medical/surgical history
         g) Recent trauma or surgery
         h) Medications
         i) Allergies
   b. *Objective data*
      1) Physical examination: perform forensic physical examination for evidence collection if assault occurred less than 72 hours before examination; obtain a sexual assault evidence collection kit and follow step-by-step instructions; maintain chain of evidence
         a) Emotional state and behavior
         b) General survey
            (1) Victim should remove clothing over a large piece of paper
            (2) Clothing should be placed into a paper bag
            (3) Note condition of clothing and skin (e.g., stains, tears, debris); all

foreign material should be carefully removed and placed in a labeled envelope identifying where material was found

(4) Evidence of trauma (e.g., bruises, bite marks): all injuries should be carefully described and diagrammed; photographs may be helpful

c) Oral cavity: swab buccal area and gum line with cotton-tipped swabs; insert small piece of filter paper into patient's mouth and have him/her saturate it with saliva; allow paper to air dry

d) Dried or moist blood/body fluid: scan entire body with Wood lamp in a darkened room to assess for presence of dried or moist blood/body fluid; areas identified to contain dried secretions should be swabbed with moist saline cotton-tipped swab

e) Fingernail scrapings: scrape under each nail with fingernail scraper, allowing any debris to fall onto piece of paper

f) Hair: pull a minimum of 5 full-length head hairs from the scalp; pull a minimum of 15 to 20 pubic hairs; place piece of paper under patient's buttocks and comb pubic hair in downward strokes to allow any debris or loose hair to fall on paper

g) Pelvic exam: observe external genitalia and buttocks for any signs of trauma; perform speculum exam, observing for signs of vaginal/cervical trauma; swab vaginal vault and allow swabs to air dry; swab vaginal folds and allow swabs to air dry; obtain rectal swabs as indicated

2) Diagnostic procedures

a) Pregnancy test

b) HIV, hepatitis B screen, rapid plasma reagin test, ABO group

c) STD screen

d) Wet mount (saline, KOH), wet preparation for sperm mobility

e) Other laboratory/radiographic studies as indicated

2. **Analysis: differential nursing diagnosis/collaborative problems**

a. *Anxiety/fear related to sexual assault, potential for pregnancy and infectious disease*

b. *Rape trauma syndrome related to sexual assault*

c. *Pain related to trauma of assault*

3. **Planning/interventions**

a. *Treat life-threatening conditions as per protocol*

b. *Provide psychosocial support to patient; facilitate consult with rape crisis intervention worker*

c. *Offer prophylactic STD treatment*

d. *Offer pregnancy prevention therapy within 72 hours of assault*

1) Ovral (ethinyl estradiol, 0.1 mg; norgestrel, 1.0 mg) two tablets initially and two tablets in 12 hours or

2) Ethinyl estradiol, 5 mg/day for 5 consecutive days

e. *Discuss discharge instructions as indicated*

1) Medication for STD prophylaxis: purpose, dose, schedule, importance of completing course of antibiotics, side effects

2) Use of analgesics

3) Follow-up in 10 days for repeat STD testing

4) Follow-up for psychosocial counseling

5) Periodic STD examinations if patient is sexually active with multiple partners

6) HIV counseling and testing if patient is at high risk

4. **Expected outcomes/evaluation** (see Appendix B)

REFERENCES

Abbott, J., Emmans, L., & Lowenstein, S. (1993) Ectopic pregnancy: Ten common pitfalls in diagnosis. *American Journal of Emergency Medicine, 11*, 480–482.

Brennen, D. (1995). Ectopic pregnancy—Part 1: Clinical and laboratory diagnosis. *Academic Emergency Medicine, 2*, 1081–1089.

Centers for Disease Control and Prevention. (1993). Sexually transmitted disease treatment guidelines. *MMWR Morbidity and Mortality Weekly Reports, 42*(RR-14), 1–102.

Davis, T., & Anderson G. (1998). Noninfectious pelvic disorders. In J. Howell, M. Altieri, A. Jagoda, J. Prescott, J. Scott, & T. Stair (Eds.), *Emergency medicine* (pp. 1350–1356). Philadelphia: W. B. Saunders.

Druelinger, L. (1994). Postpartum emergencies. *Emergency Medical Clinics of North America, 12*, 219–237.

Dugan, E. (1998). Uncomplicated pregnancy, labor and delivery. In J. Howell, M. Altieri, A. Jagoda, J. Prescott, J. Scott, & T. Stair (Eds.), *Emergency medicine* (pp. 1287–1294). Philadelphia: W. B. Saunders.

Esposito, T. (1994). Trauma during pregnancy. *Emergency Medical Clinics of North America, 12*, 167–199.

Gianopoulos, J. (1994) Emergency complications of labor and delivery. *Emergency Medical Clinics of North America, 12*, 201–217.

Ivey, J. (1997). The adolescent with pelvic inflammatory disease: Assessment and management. *The Nurse Practitioner, 22*(2), 78–93.

Kottman, L. (1995). Pelvic inflammatory disease: Clinical overview. *Journal of Obstetric, Gynecologic, and Neonatal Nursing, 24*(8), 759–767.

Ledray, L. (1992). The sexual assault examination: Overview and lessons learned in one program. *Journal of Emergency Nursing, 18*, 223–230.

Nadel, E., & Talbot-Stern, J. (1997). Obstetric and gynecologic emergencies. *Emergency Medicine Clinics of North America, 15*(2), 389–397.

Neufield, J. (1993). Trauma in pregnancy: What if....

Emergency Medical Clinics of North America, 11, 207–227.

Parker, J. (1994). Obstetrical emergencies. In A. Klein, G. Lee, A. Manton, & J. Parker (Eds.), *Emergency nursing core curriculum* (4th ed., pp. 351–369). Philadelphia: W. B. Saunders.

Pepe, S., & Anderson, G. (1998) Approach to pelvic pain. In J. Howell, M. Altieri, A. Jagoda, J. Prescott, J. Scott, & T. Stair (Eds.), *Emergency medicine* (pp. 1341–1349). Philadelphia: W. B. Saunders.

Quan, M. (1992). Diagnosis of acute pelvic pain. *Journal of Family Practice, 35*(4), 422–432.

Reedy, N., & Brucker, M. (1995). Emergencies in gynecology and obstetrics. In S. Kitt, J. Selfridge-Thomas, J. Proehl, & J. Kaiser (Eds.), *Emergency nursing: A physiologic and clinical perspective* (2nd ed., pp. 265–286). Philadelphia: W. B. Saunders.

Santen, S., & Dugan, E. (1998). Complications of early pregnancy. In J. Howell, M. Altieri, A. Jagoda, J. Prescott, J. Scott, & T. Stair (Eds.), *Emergency medicine* (pp. 1295–1306). Philadelphia: W. B. Saunders.

Sheehy, S., McCall, P., & Varvel, P. (1992). Obstetric and gynecologic emergencies. In S. B. Sheehy (Ed.), *Emergency nursing principles and practice* (3rd ed., pp. 631–647). St. Louis, MO: Mosby–Year Book.

Soper, D. (1994). Pelvic inflammatory disease. *Infectious Disease Clinics of North America, 8*(4), 821–840.

Stovall, T., & Ling, F. (1993). Single-dose methotrexate: An expanded clinical trial. *American Journal Obstetrics Gynecology, 6*(1), 1759–1765.

Sinclair, B., Conner, J., & Heath, J. (1995). Pregnancy. In S. Moskosky (Ed.), *Women's health care nurse practitioner certification review guide* (pp. 338–460). Healthcare Leadership Associates.

Turner, L. (1994). Vaginal bleeding during pregnancy. *Emergency Medical Clinics of North America, 12*(1), 45–54.

Willis, D. (1994). Bleeding in pregnancy. In B. Benrubi (Ed.), *Obstetric and gynecologic emergencies* (pp. 127–133). Philadelphia: J. B. Lippincott.

Patricia C. Epifanio, RN, MS, CEN

CHAPTER **14**

Ocular Emergencies

MAJOR TOPICS

I. GENERAL STRATEGY

A. Assessment

1. **Primary survey (see Chapter 1)**

2. **Secondary survey (see Chapter 1)**

3. **Psychological, social, environmental factors and risk factors**
   a. *Behavior appropriate for age and developmental stage*
      1) Young males at higher risk for serious injury
      2) School-age children susceptible to conjunctivitis because of close contact and contagious nature of disease
      3) Contact lens wearers at greater risk for corneal abrasions and infections
   b. *Occupation or profession*
      1) Exposure to "arc welding" symptoms develop 4 to 8 hours after exposure
      2) Jobs in which metal is struck on metal have potential for embedded foreign bodies

3) Automobile mechanics and service station attendants have potential for acid burns to eye
  c. *Hobbies, avocation, recreational activities*
    1) Injuries occurring in the garden have increased potential for infection
    2) Swimming may increase potential for ocular infections
    3) Home woodworking shop activities increase potential for ocular injuries if safety precautions not taken
    4) Ball sports increase potential for eye injuries, as do contact sports in which no protective eye gear is worn
    5) BB guns and fireworks are frequent causes of eye trauma in children
    6) Cases of child abuse often present with findings of intraocular and/or retinal hemorrhage related to direct trauma and shaking of child
4. **Focused survey**
  a. *Subjective data*
    1) History of present illness/chief complaint
      a) Injury
        (1) Mechanism of injury
        (2) Time elapsed since occurrence
        (3) Treatment before arrival
        (4) Changes in clinical status
      b) Pain (PQRST)
        (1) Provocation
        (2) Quality
        (3) Radiation/region of pain
        (4) Severity
        (5) Time
      c) Abnormal appearance of eye
        (1) Edema
        (2) Erythema
        (3) Change in luster
        (4) Change in configuration
      d) Changes in visual acuity: normal to blindness
        (1) Decreased visual acuity
        (2) Decreased visual field
        (3) Blurring of vision
        (4) Diplopia
        (5) Cloudy or smoky vision
      e) Tearing
      f) Itching
      g) Discharge
    2) Medical history
      a) Ocular
        (1) Corrective lenses
          (a) Contact lenses
          (b) Worn at time of injury
        (2) Glaucoma
        (3) Chronic eye disease
        (4) Past eye disease or injury
        (5) Family history of eye disease
      b) Systemic
        (1) Diabetes
        (2) Cardiovascular disease
        (3) Hypertension

           (4) Allergies

           (5) Immunological diseases

           (6) Last tetanus immunization

    3) Current medication history: medications may cause ocular side effects

        a) Eye medication: prescription or over-the-counter product

        b) Steroids

        c) Parasympatholytic drugs

        d) Opiates

        e) Anticoagulants

  b. Objective data

    1) Physical examination

        a) General survey

            (1) Level of consciousness

            (2) Obvious eye trauma

            (3) Measurement of vital signs

        b) Inspection: always use contralateral eye for comparison

            (1) Spasm of eyelids

            (2) Eye surface, to include upper and lower lids for lesions, foreign bodies, and penetrating wounds

            (3) Tearing

            (4) Discharge: exudate

            (5) Pupils: should be equal, round, reactive to light and accommodation (PERRLA)

            (6) Extraocular movement (EOM)

            (7) Position and alignment of eyes

            (8) Conjunctiva and sclera for color and inflammation

            (9) Edema of lids, conjunctiva, and/or cornea

            (10) Blood in anterior chamber

            (11) Opaque, gray-white area of cornea

            (12) Hazy cornea

            (13) Penetration of globe

            (14) Bleeding or leakage of intraocular fluid to exterior surface of eye

            (15) Nerve, blood vessel, or bony structure involvement

        c) Palpation

            (1) Intraocular pressure: palpation should not be performed if there is concern regarding integrity of globe; may result in extrusion of ocular contents, causing permanent visual loss; procedure should be reserved for ophthalmologist in suspected cases of acute glaucoma

            (2) Deformity of bony structure

        d) Visual acuity: an essential of physical examination process to establish baseline before treatment as well as for medicolegal reasons; exception to this rule involves patient with chemical injury, in which case irrigation first is mandatory; when possible, patients with glasses or contact lenses should have visual acuity tested with correction

            (1) Gross assessment by finger count

            (2) Exact assessment by Snellen's chart (a picture chart or an "E" chart may be necessary for small children and those who cannot read)

               (a) Ambulatory: tested at distance of 20 feet

               (b) Nonambulatory: tested with hand-held card at about 14 inches

            (3) Visual fields

    2) Diagnostic procedures

        a) Direct ophthalmoscopic examination

        b) Tonometry

      c) Fluorescein staining
      d) Slit-lamp examination
      e) Laboratory studies
         (1) Eye culture
         (2) Complete blood count (CBC)
         (3) Urinalysis: if surgery imminent
         (4) Coagulation studies
      f) Radiology
         (1) Computed tomography (CT) scan
         (2) Soft tissue (orbit films) for foreign body
         (3) Facial bones for fracture
         (4) Skull films with Waters' view
      g) Preparation of patient and significant others for diagnostic procedures
         (1) Physical preparation
         (2) Emotional support
         (3) Patient teaching
         (4) Informed signed consent

B. Analysis: differential nursing diagnosis/collaborative problems

1. **Anxiety/fear**
2. **Knowledge deficit**
3. **Noncompliance**
4. **Pain**
5. **Risk for individual ineffective coping**
6. **Risk for infection**
7. **Risk for injury**
8. **Self-care deficit**
9. **Sensory-perceptual alterations: visual**
10. **Tissue perfusion, altered**

C. Planning/interventions

1. **Determine priorities**
    a. Control and maintain airway, breathing, circulation
    b. Prevent further damage and injuries
    c. Prevent or minimize complications
    d. Control pain
    e. Relieve anxiety or apprehension
    f. Educate patient and significant others
2. **Develop nursing care plan specific to patient's presenting emergency**
3. **Obtain and set up necessary equipment and supplies**
4. **Institute appropriate interventions based on nursing care plan**
    a. Removal of contact lenses
    b. Administer medications as ordered
    c. Maintain asepsis
    d. Provide darkened, quiet environment
    e. Provide supportive environment
    f. Explain all procedures in understandable terms
    g. Explain disease process in appropriate terms
    h. Provide discharge instructions
    i. Provide prevention information
    j. Facilitate ophthalmological consultation as appropriate (Box 14–1)

Box 14–1   CONSULTATION CRITERIA

The patients with the following problems should be referred for ophthalmological consultation:

Penetrating ocular truma, including impaled objects, embedded foreign bodies, and ruptured globe

Chemical burns of the eye

Severe lid lacerations

Glaucoma

Central retinal artery occlusion

Retinal detachment

Orbital fracture

Hyphema

Periorbital cellulitis

5. **Document data as appropriate**
   a. *Assessment data to include description of symptoms and any functional deficit*
   b. *Interventions*
      1) Medications
   c. *Reassessment findings and response to interventions*
   d. *Disposition and patient instructions*

D. Expected outcomes/evaluation

1. **Monitor patient responses and outcomes, adjusting nursing care plan as indicated**
   a. *Specific interventions*
      1) Disposition or discharge planning
2. **Record all pertinent data**
3. **If positive outcomes are not demonstrated, re-evaluate assessment and/ or plan of care**

E. Age-related considerations

1. **Pediatric**
   a. *Growth/development related*
      1) May need to use a picture chart or the "E" chart (patient indicates direction to which "E" points)
      2) Delayed presentation may be problematic because children may not notice gradual visual loss
   b. *"Pearls"*
      1) Have great patience
      2) Infants and small children may need to be restrained in a blanket to reduce number of moving parts and facilitate examination
2. **Geriatric**
   a. *Aging related*

1) Vision diminishes gradually until approximately 70 years and then more rapidly thereafter
2) Decreased ability to use the standard charts for visual acuity as a result of physical impairment
3) Decreased accuracy of results from visual acuity testing
4) Decreased near vision is problematic for many older patients
5) Ability of eye to accommodate, or adjust, to distances decreases with age
6) Older patients frequently complain of eye dryness resulting from decrease in lacrimal secretions
7) Cataracts become more common with advancing age, to the point at which approximately one in three people in their 80s are affected
8) Geriatric population more likely to experience glaucoma, detached retina, and retinal bleeds

   b. "Pearls"

1) Older seniors may need home health referrals to help with administration of medications and environmental safety issues
2) Ensure a protected environment

II. SPECIFIC MEDICAL OCULAR EMERGENCIES

A. Conjunctivitis

Conjunctivitis is the inflammation of the conjunctiva. Common causes include bacterial inflammation, viral inflammation, *Chlamydia,* allergies, chemical burns, foreign bodies, ultraviolet or flash burns, exposure to irritants, and some systemic diseases (e.g., it is frequently associated with upper respiratory tract infections). If the conjunctiva is injured or disrupted, the inflammatory process becomes evident with the infection of the cells. Common bacterial organisms that cause conjunctivitis include streptococci, staphylococci, pneumococci, and gonococci. The inflammation causes marked hyperemia and mucopurulent discharge. Young children are at risk because of close proximity with other children and frequent hand-face contact with infrequent and ineffective hand washing.

1. **Assessment**
   a. *Subjective data*
      1) History of present illness/chief complaint
         a) Hyperemia/redness of affected eye(s)
         b) Unilateral or bilateral involvement
         c) Pain, minimal
         d) Foreign body sensation, "gritty" sensation
         e) Discharge
            (1) Purulent or mucopurulent
            (2) Matting of eyelids and lashes after sleeping
         f) Itching
         g) Edema of eyelid(s)
         h) Fever, pharyngitis (associated with viral illness), otitis media
      2) Medical history
         a) Medications
            (1) Steroids may exacerbate local ocular infections; especially danger-ous with herpes infections
            (2) Previous antibiotic use may influence treatment choice
         b) Allergies/hay fever
         c) Recent upper respiratory tract infection
   b. *Objective data*

      1) Physical examination
        a) Visual acuity: normal
        b) Cornea: clear
        c) Pupil: normal
        d) Conjunctiva: red or pink eye from congestion of conjunctival vessels
        e) Discharge: purulent or mucopurulent
        f) Eyelid edema
        g) Enlarged preauricular node(s)
      2) Diagnostic procedures
        a) Culture of discharge if indicated
        b) Fluorescein stain: abnormal; will demonstrate amount of damaged corneal epithelial cells
        c) Gram's stain for identification of bacterial organisms if indicated

2. Analysis: differential nursing diagnosis/collaborative problems
  a. Pain related to inflammatory process
  b. Anxiety/fear related to symptomatology and lack of education regarding disease process
  c. Knowledge deficit related to disease process and self-care

3. Planning/interventions
  a. Administer antibiotic ointment/drops as prescribed
  b. Permit calm significant other to accompany patient in treatment area
  c. Explain disease process in appropriate terms
    1) Contagious nature of disease
  d. Provide discharge instructions
    1) Instillation of medication
    2) Proper asepsis
    3) Eye-cleansing procedure (cleanse lid line with baby shampoo)
    4) Avoid eye makeup
    5) Follow-up care plans
    6) Prevention information
  e. Obtain culture if indicated
  f. Cleanse eyelids gently to remove debris
    1) Wipe from nose to outer corner of eye

4. Expected outcomes/evaluation (see Appendix B)

B. Iritis

    This inflammatory process usually includes the iris or uveal layer of the anterior segment of the eye and sometimes the ciliary body, causing pain, redness, edema, lacrimation, and photophobia. Among the common predisposing conditions are a variety of systemic illnesses, including rheumatic diseases, ankylosing spondylitis, and syphilis. Although iritis may be seen as a sequela of trauma, the condition is usually idiopathic. Pain in the affected eye is experienced when light is directed into the opposite eye because of consensual constriction of the irritated iris.

1. Assessment
  a. Subjective data
    1) History of present illness/chief complaint
      a) Blurring of vision
      b) Unilateral pain: moderate to severe
      c) Edema of upper lid
      d) Red eye
      e) Intense photophobia

        f) Lacrimation
     2) Medical history
        a) Familial history of rheumatic disease
        b) Systemic disease, such as rheumatoid arthritis, ankylosing spondylitis, syphilis
        c) Medications such as steroids and atropine drugs because these types of medications will be used in treatment plan
        d) Allergies
  b. *Objective data*
     1) Physical examination
        a) Visual acuity: decreased
        b) Ciliary flush: redness at eyelashes
        c) Cornea: clear to hazy
        d) Pupils: small, irregular, sluggish reaction
        e) Intraocular pressure: normal to low
        f) Pain on eye pressure
     2) Diagnostic procedures
        a) Fluorescein stain
        b) Slit-lamp examination

2. Analysis: differential nursing diagnosis/collaborative problems
  a. *Pain related to inflammatory ocular disease*
  b. *Sensory-perceptual alteration: visual, related to inflammatory process*
  c. *Anxiety/fear related to lack of education regarding ocular disease and fear of loss of vision*
  d. *Knowledge deficit related to therapeutic regimen*

3. Planning/interventions
  a. *Administer analgesics as prescribed*
  b. *Administer nonsteroidal anti-inflammatory agents as prescribed*
  c. *Administer cycloplegics as prescribed for paralyzing ciliary muscle, thereby paralyzing accommodation and reducing ciliary spasms*
  d. *Provide darkened environment*
  e. *Apply warm compresses*
  f. *Explain need to rest eyes to patient*
  g. *Explain disease process in appropriate terms*
  h. *Provide discharge instruction*
     1) Shielding methods or use of dark glasses
     2) Instillation of medication
     3) Follow-up plan of care

4. Expected outcomes/evaluation (see Appendix B)

C. Periorbital cellulitis

    Periorbital cellulitis is an infection of the cells around the eye. It may occur after trauma such as a laceration or an insect bite. It is usually caused by pneumococcal, staphylococcal, or streptococcal bacteria. In young children, the infection may be secondary to paranasal sinusitis caused by *Haemophilus influenzae.* This represents a major ophthalmological emergency and is potentially life threatening because the infection may extend into the cavernous sinus or the brain.

1. Assessment
  a. *Subjective data*
     1) History of present illness/chief complaint
        a) Marked periorbital erythema

        b) Marked periorbital edema

        c) Aching pain: severe, deep, aggravated by movement of eye

        d) Conjunctival injection

        e) Fever

      2) Medical history

        a) Medications

        b) Allergies

        c) Recent upper respiratory tract infection

    b. Objective data

      1) Physical examination

        a) Visual acuity—decreased

        b) Decreased pupil reflexes

        c) Erythema and swelling of the eyelids and surrounding structures

        d) Paralysis of extraocular muscles

      2) Diagnostic procedures

        a) CT scan of orbit to determine extent of infection

        b) Culture of discharge

        c) Gram's stain for identification of bacterial organisms

        d) Blood cultures

2. Analysis: differential nursing diagnosis/collaborative problems

    a. Pain related to inflammatory process

    b. Anxiety/fear related to symptomatology and disease process

    c. Knowledge deficit related to disease process

3. Planning/interventions

    a. Referral to ophthalmology consultant

    b. Administration of parenteral antibiotics

    c. Instillation of antibiotic ointment

    d. Prepare for hospitalization for bed rest and intravenous (IV) therapy

    e. Application of warm compresses

    f. Provide disposition instructions

4. Expected outcomes/evaluation (see Appendix B)

D. Glaucoma

    Acute angle-closure glaucoma occurs when the distance between the iris and the cornea becomes inadequate or is blocked completely, so that the amount of aqueous fluid produced by the ciliary body is greater than the amount leaving through the canal of Schlemm. The precipitating factors of outflow obstruction are a gradual increase in pressure and sudden dilation of the pupil. Attacks usually occur in a darkened environment. If glaucoma is not recognized and treated early, blindness results when the increase in pressure causes damage to the optic nerve and decreased circulation to the retina. The patient with this condition needs immediate attention because there is only a limited amount of time before permanent damage is incurred. Glaucoma is more common in the geriatric population but may occur in younger people especially those with a history of eye trauma or surgery. This is an emergency situation!

1. Assessment

    a. Subjective data

      1) History of present illness/chief complaint

        a) Red eye: entire conjunctiva is infected

        b) Pain: usually severe, sudden-onset, deep, unilateral eye pain

        c) Intense headache

d) Decreased vision
e) Halos around lights
f) Photophobia
g) Nausea and vomiting
h) Abdominal pain
   2) Medical history
     a) Previous iritis
     b) Trauma to eye
     c) Medications
     d) Allergies to medications
  b. *Objective data*
    1) Physical examination
      a) Visual acuity: decreased
      b) Cornea: hazy, steamy, lusterless
      c) Pupil on affected side: mid-position, poorly reactive, fixed
      d) Increased intraocular pressure (> 20 mm Hg)
      e) Unnatural appearance, rocklike hardness
    2) Diagnostic procedures
      a) Tonometry
      b) Slit-lamp examination

2. Analysis: differential nursing diagnosis/collaborative problems
  a. *Pain related to increased intraocular pressure*
  b. *Sensory-perceptual alteration: visual, related to increased intraocular pressure and decreased visual acuity*
  c. *Anxiety/fear related to potential visual loss and pain*
  d. *Knowledge deficit related to ocular disease*

3. Planning/interventions
  a. *Referral to ophthalmological consultant*
  b. *Administer analgesics as prescribed*
  c. *Administer antiemetics as prescribed*
  d. *Administer pilocarpine eyedrops as prescribed*
  e. *Administer osmotic diuretic agents as prescribed*
  f. *Provide supportive environment*
  g. *Explain all procedures and disease process in understandable terms*
  h. *Provide disposition information regarding medication, activity level, follow-up care*

4. Expected outcomes/evaluation (see Appendix B)

E. Central retinal artery occlusion

Central retinal artery occlusion is a sudden, painless, unilateral loss of vision caused by a blockage of the artery by thrombus or embolus. The embolus usually originates from a carotid artery atherosclerotic plaque or from the cardiac valves. Prompt recognition and intervention within 1 to 2 hours of onset of symptoms are essential for preservation of useful vision. Although such disease generally occurs in the older population, a history of thrombus or embolus may predispose a patient to this condition. This condition is a true ocular emergency!

1. Assessment
  a. *Subjective data*
    1) History of present illness/chief complaint
      a) Sudden unilateral loss of vision
      b) Painless

2) Medical history
   a) History of thrombus or embolus
   b) Diabetes
   c) Hypertension
   d) Arteriosclerotic disease most common underlying cause
   e) Arteritis
   f) Sickle cell disease
   g) Trauma to eye
   h) Medications, especially antihypertensives
   i) Allergies to medications
   b. *Objective data*
      1) Physical examination
         a) Visual acuity limited to light perception in affected eye
         b) Pupil reaction: dilated, nonreactive in affected eye
   c. *Diagnostic procedures*
      1) Funduscopic examination
      2) Digital intraocular pressure measurement
      3) Paracentesis of anterior chamber

2. **Analysis: differential nursing diagnosis/collaborative problems**
   a. *Tissue perfusion, altered to optic nerve related to vascular blockage*
   b. *Anxiety/fear related to sudden loss of vision and prognosis*
   c. *Knowledge deficit related to therapeutic regimen*
   d. *Risk for injury resulting from decreased visual capacity*

3. **Planning/interventions**
   a. *Referral to ophthalmological consultant*
   b. *Digital massage of globe: this therapy should be reserved for physician*
   c. *Provide supportive environment*
   d. *Explain all procedures and disease process in understandable terms*
   e. *Provide carbogen gas (95% oxygen plus 5% carbon dioxide) if available for vasodilation in 3- to 10-minute treatments at 2-hour intervals (potentially harmful to the patient with chronic obstructive pulmonary disease)*
   f. *Interventions may include administration of anticoagulants, tissue plasminogen activator (tPA), and low-molecular-weight dextran*
   g. *Provide disposition instructions*
   h. *Preparation for admission and possible surgery or transfer*

4. **Expected outcomes/evaluation** (see Appendix B)

III. SPECIFIC SURGICAL OCULAR EMERGENCIES

A. Corneal abrasion

Corneal abrasion occurs when there is a partial or complete removal of an area of epithelium of the cornea. The common causes include foreign bodies, contact lenses, and exposure to ultraviolet light. Foreign bodies can scratch the cornea to various depths. Contact lenses can scratch the cornea during insertion or removal when a foreign body becomes trapped between the cornea and the lens; wearing the lenses for a prolonged period can also lead to corneal abrasion. When contact lenses are worn too long and the lens is removed, a part of the cornea adheres to the lens. This is due to the avascular nature of the cornea. Ultraviolet light exposure can occur from the sun, welding arcs, sun lamps, or snow reflecting sunlight, causing a punctate stippling type of abrasion. Corneal abrasion is one of the most common eye injuries seen in the emergency department.

1. **Assessment**

      a. Subjective data

        1) History of present illness/chief complaint

          a) Ocular trauma

          b) Ultraviolet light exposure

          c) Contact lens wearer

          d) Pain ranging from mild to severe

          e) Tearing

          f) Foreign body sensation

          g) Photophobia

        2) Medical history

          a) Previous foreign body in eye

          b) Previous ultraviolet light burn

          c) Medications

          d) Glaucoma

          e) Immunization status

      b. Objective data

        1) Physical examination

          a) Visual acuity: normal to slightly decreased

          b) Fluorescein stain: abnormal; enhances abrasion pattern

          c) Injected conjunctiva

          d) Tearing

          e) Ciliary muscle spasm

        2) Diagnostic procedures

          a) Fluorescein stain

          b) Slit-lamp examination

2. Analysis: differential nursing diagnosis/collaborative problems

      a. Pain related to corneal injury

      b. Anxiety/fear related to therapeutic regimen and self-care

      c. Knowledge deficit related to lack of education or experience regarding eye injury

      d. Risk for infection related to nature of injury

3. Planning/interventions

      a. Administer analgesics as prescribed

        1) Topical

      b. Administer topical ophthalmic antibiotics

      c. Patch affected eye to provide rest for 12 to 24 hours

        1) Small lesions with minimal discomfort may not necessitate patching

        2) Tight patching to prevent upper lid movement

      d. Provide supportive environment

      e. Explain all procedures and disease process in understandable terms

      f. Provide discharge instructions

        1) Importance of follow-up care

        2) Proper patching techniques

        3) Instillation of medications as prescribed

        4) Signs and symptoms of infection

        5) Use of extra precautions for activities requiring accurate depth perception (e.g., use of handrails on stairs)

      g. Provide prevention information

4. Expected outcomes/evaluation (see Appendix B)

B. Extraocular foreign bodies

Foreign bodies can enter the eye as a result of hammering, grinding, working under cars, or working above the head. Patients usually describe the sensation of "something going into the eye," and foreign bodies can range from metal to sawdust to dust particles. Foreign bodies with a metallic component are of specific concern because these objects may form a rust ring in the cornea. If the rust ring is not removed, it may continue to invade the cornea and may interfere with vision. Ocular penetration with single or multiple foreign bodies must be considered with corneal injuries. This type of injury is usually related to occupation or avocation.

1. **Assessment**
   a. *Subjective data*
      1) History of present illness/chief complaint
         a) Pain
         b) Foreign body sensation
         c) Tearing
         d) Redness
      2) Medical history
         a) Glaucoma
         b) Medications
         c) Allergies to medications
         d) Immunization status
   b. *Objective data*
      1) Physical examination
         a) Visual acuity: normal to slightly abnormal
         b) Fluorescein stain: abnormal; enhances scratch pattern if one is present
         c) Foreign body visualized: evert lid to inspect adequately; frequently lodged on dorsal surface of upper lid
      2) Diagnostic procedures
         a) Examination using magnifying glasses
         b) Fluorescein stain
         c) Slit-lamp examination
2. **Analysis: differential nursing diagnosis/collaborative problems**
   a. *Pain related to injury*
   b. *Anxiety related to injury and treatment*
   c. *Knowledge deficit related to therapeutic regimen and self-care*
   d. *Self-care deficit related to bilateral eye patches*
3. **Planning/interventions**
   a. *Administer topical anesthetic*
   b. *Gentle irrigation with normal saline*
   c. *Prepare for foreign body removal with a moist cotton swab, needle, or eye spud if irrigation is unsuccessful*
   d. *Administer analgesics as prescribed*
      1) Topical
         a) Use caution in having patient discharged home with topical analgesics
            (1) Topical anesthetics inhibit wound healing and are toxic to corneal epithelium
            (2) Topical medication may mask symptoms of complications
            (3) Patient may save medication and self-medicate inappropriately in future
      2) Systemic
   e. *Patch both eyes to reduce consensual movement*
   f. *Explain all procedures and disease process in understandable terms*
   g. *Explain disease process in appropriate terms*
   h. *Instillation of medications*
   i. *Provide discharge/disposition instructions*

1) Patching techniques if necessary
2) Plan for follow-up care
3) Preparation for admission/surgery if necessary
4) Provide prevention information
   j. *Assist patient in identifying help that will be needed for self-care and necessary resources*
4. **Expected outcomes/evaluation** (see Appendix B)

C. Retinal detachment

Retinal detachment involves separation of the two primitive retinal layers, with accumulation of serous fluid or blood between the sensory retina and the retinal pigment epithelium, which decrease blood and oxygen supply to the retina. The most common cause of detached retina is degenerative changes in either the retina or the vitreous body in the elderly; however, direct head trauma and injuries associated with sports activities may also result in detachment of the retina.

1. **Assessment**
   a. *Subjective data*
      1) History of present illness/chief complaint
         a) Head or facial trauma
         b) Gradual or sudden deterioration of vision unilaterally
            (1) Cloudy, smoky vision
            (2) Flashing lights
            (3) Curtain or veil over visual field
            (4) No pain
      2) Medical history
         a) Head or facial trauma
         b) Diabetes
         c) Medications, especially antihypertensives
         d) Allergies to medications
         e) Past eye surgery
   b. *Objective data*
      1) Physical examination
         a) Visual field deficit
         b) Visual acuity deficit
         c) Patient may be asymptomatic
      2) Diagnostic procedures
         a) Funduscopy
         b) Visual acuity
         c) Slit-lamp examination
2. **Analysis: differential nursing diagnosis/collaborative problems**
   a. *Sensory-perceptual alteration: visual, related to disease process*
   b. *Anxiety/fear related to disease process, treatment, and prognosis*
   c. *Knowledge deficit related to therapeutic regimen*
   d. *Self-care deficit related to bilateral eye patches and bed rest*
3. **Planning/interventions**
   a. *Referral to ophthalmological consultant*
   b. *Patch both eyes or shielding to reduce eye movement*
   c. *Maintain patient on bed rest, lying quietly*
   d. *Permit calm significant other to accompany patient in treatment area*
   e. *Provide supportive environment*
   f. *Explain all procedures and disease process in understandable terms*

    g. Ensure appropriate level of assistance with self-care by helping patient identify resources and/or by community health agency referral

    h. Provide discharge/disposition instructions

        1) Instillation of medication

        2) Follow-up plan of care

        3) Preparation for admission or transfer as indicated

  4. Expected outcomes/evaluation (see Appendix B)

D. Orbital fracture

    This is a fracture of the orbit without a fracture of the orbital rim produced by a blow on the orbit. A common cause of orbit fracture is blunt trauma to the orbit from a fist, ball, or other nonpenetrating contact. This results in an increase in the intraorbital, hydrostatic pressure with dissipation of the force through the area of least resistance, usually the ethmoid bone on the orbital floor and the medial or lateral wall of the orbit. Contents of the inferior orbit may herniate through the fracture site. These fractures are associated with entrapment and ischemia of nerves or penetration into a sinus.

  1. Assessment

    a. Subjective data

        1) History of present illness/chief complaint

           a) Blunt trauma

           b) Diplopia: functional

           c) Facial anesthesia

           d) Pain

           e) Enophthalmos: sunken appearance of eye

           f) Limited vertical eye movement

        2) Medical history

           a) Previous facial nerve injury

           b) Medications

           c) Allergies

           d) Immunization status

    b. Objective data

        1) Physical examination

           a) EOM abnormal: inability to look upward or downward with affected eye

           b) Paresthesia of infraorbital nerve

           c) Crepitus in area of fracture site

           d) Periorbital edema, hematoma, ecchymosis

           e) Subconjunctival hemorrhage

           f) Assess for associated injuries

        2) Diagnostic procedures

           a) Visual acuity

           b) Funduscopy

           c) CT scan

           d) Radiographs: orbit, facial views; Waters' view, tomography

  2. Analysis: differential nursing diagnosis/collaborative problems

    a. Pain related to injury

    b. Anxiety related to injury, visual changes, and prognosis

    c. Knowledge deficit related to therapeutic regimen

    d. Risk for infection related to break in bony integrity

  3. Planning/interventions

      a. *Ophthalmology consultation*
      b. *Administer analgesics and antibiotics as prescribed*
      c. *Apply ice to injured orbit*
      d. *Explain all procedures and disease process in understandable terms*
      e. *Provide discharge/disposition instructions*
        1) Instillation of medication
        2) Refrain from blowing nose
        3) Follow-up plan of care
        4) Preparation for admission/surgery
   4. Expected outcomes/evaluation (see Appendix B)

E. Chemical burns

     Chemical burns constitute a true ocular emergency. All chemical injuries to the eye should be evaluated by an ophthalmologist. A distinction between acid and alkali exposure to the eye needs to be made to facilitate prognosis; however, such a determination need not be made before treatment is initiated. Acids, except hydrofluoric acids and those with heavy metals, cause immediate denaturation of tissue proteins, which act as a barrier against further penetration and damage. Alkaline agents combine with cellular lipids and produce coagulation necrosis, with total cellular disruption. Immediate irrigation is imperative because of the seriousness of this injury; assessment must be secondary. Risk factors include certain occupations (i.e., chemical workers, auto mechanic, service station workers), environments, and some types of domestic violence.

   1. Assessment
      a. *Subjective data*
        1) History of present illness/chief complaint
          a) Pain
          b) Variable degrees of visual loss
          c) Chemical exposure
        2) Medical history
          a) Medications
          b) Allergies
          c) Occupational hazards
          d) Immunization status
      b. *Objective data*
        1) Physical examination
          a) Visual acuity impaired
          b) Burns of varying degrees
          c) Corneal whitening: inability to define specific eye structures
        2) Diagnostic procedures
          a) Funduscopy
          b) Fluorescein stain
          c) Slit-lamp examination
   2. Analysis: differential nursing diagnosis/collaborative problems
      a. *Sensory-perceptual alteration: visual, related to injury and patching*
      b. *Pain related to injury*
      c. *Fear/anxiety related to permanence of visual loss*
      d. *Knowledge deficit related to therapeutic regimen and self-care*
      e. *Risk for infection related to tissue destruction*
   3. Planning/interventions
      a. *Referral to ophthalmological consultant*

b. *Irrigate thoroughly with copious amounts normal saline (including eversion of upper lid) for 20 to 30 minutes and continue until the pH is 7.0 (normal range, 6.9–7.2)*

c. *Administer cycloplegic agent for paralyzing the ciliary muscle, thereby paralyzing accommodation and reducing ciliary spasm as prescribed*

d. *Administer analgesics as prescribed*
   1) Topical
   2) Oral

e. *Administer antibiotics as prescribed*

f. *Apply eye patch*

g. *Provide supportive environment*

h. *Explain all procedures and disease process in understandable terms*

i. *Administer tetanus prophylaxis*

j. *Provide discharge/disposition instructions*
   1) Preparation for admission or transfer

4. **Expected outcomes/evaluation** (see Appendix B)

F. Hyphema

Hyphema, or blood in the anterior chamber, is usually the result of blunt trauma such as a direct blow of a ball or a fist. This increase in the pressure in the aqueous humor will cause the iris to bleed into the anterior chamber. The patient presenting with this condition needs hospitalization to ensure compliance with the therapeutic regimen. The threat of a secondary bleed occurring in 3 to 5 days is a significant risk, and if it occurs, the outcomes are significantly poorer. In the incidence of microscopic hyphemas, some physicians may choose to treat the patient on an outpatient basis.

1. **Assessment**
   a. *Subjective data*
      1) History of present illness/chief complaint
         a) Blunt trauma
         b) Blurred vision
         c) Blood tinged vision
         d) Pain
      2) Medical history
         a) Glaucoma
         b) Medications
            (1) Antihypertensives: aspirin
            (2) Anticoagulants
            (3) Nonsteroidal anti-inflammatory medications
         c) Allergies to medications
   b. *Objective data*
      1) Physical examination
         a) Impairment of visual acuity
         b) Blood in anterior chamber usually can be visualized at bottom of iris because of settling of blood by gravity
         c) Assess for associated injuries
      2) Diagnostic procedures
         a) Soft tissue radiographs of eye for foreign body or fracture
         b) Tonometry
         c) Slit-lamp examination

2. **Analysis: differential nursing diagnosis/collaborative problems**

     a. Sensory-perceptual alteration: visual, related to eye injury
     b. Anxiety/fear related to injury, treatment, or prognosis
     c. Knowledge deficit related to therapeutic regimen
     d. Self-care deficit related to prescribed inactivity and eye patches

3. Planning/interventions
     a. Have patient sit upright or on bed rest with head elevated 30 degrees
     b. Patch or shield both eyes to provide rest and decrease movement
     c. Administer diuretics to reduce ocular pressure as prescribed
     d. Provide supportive environment
     e. Explain all procedures and disease process in understandable terms
     f. Permit calm significant other to accompany patient in treatment area
     g. Have patient refrain from taking aspirin or aspirin-containing compounds
     h. Refer to ophthalmologist
     i. Provide disposition instructions
       1) Prepare for admission

4. Expected outcomes/evaluation (see Appendix B)

G. Eyelid laceration

    Lacerations of the eyelid may result from multiple types of trauma and may range from a simple laceration of the lid to a complex laceration involving the lacrimal canaliculi, central tendons, or lid margins. Although it is important to maintain function and cosmetic outcomes, more serious ocular injury must be ruled out (see Chapter 21).

1. Assessment
    a. Subjective data
      1) History of present illness/chief complaint
        a) Mechanism of injury
        b) Any visual disturbances
      2) Medical history
        a) Medications
        b) Allergies to medications
        c) Immunization status
    b. Objective data
      1) Physical examination
        a) Laceration of lid
        b) Protrusion of fat
        c) Levator muscle deficit (upper lid does not raise)
        d) Assess for associated ocular injuries (e.g., foreign bodies, corneal abrasions, lacerations)
        e) Bleeding
      2) Diagnostic procedures
        a) Facial and eye muscle function testing
        b) Funduscopy
        c) Fluorescein stain
        d) Slit-lamp examination

2. Analysis: differential nursing diagnosis/collaborative problems
    a. Impaired skin integrity related to laceration
    b. Pain related to injury
    c. Anxiety related to treatment and prognosis
    d. Knowledge deficit related to therapeutic regimen and self-care
    e. Sensory-perceptual alteration: visual, related to swelling

f. Risk for infection related to break in skin integrity and mechanism of injury

3. Planning/interventions

   a. Stop bleeding: avoid direct pressure on the eye

   b. Prepare for surgical repair: wound approximation and closure

   c. Administer analgesics as prescribed

     1) Topical

     2) Oral

   d. Provide supportive environment

   e. Explain all procedures and disease process in understandable terms

   f. Refer to ophthalmologist or plastic surgeon for injury with missing tissue or laceration involving lacrimal duct

   g. Administer tetanus prophylaxis

   h. Provide discharge instructions

     1) Wound care instructions

     2) Signs of infection

     3) Plan for follow-up care

4. Expected outcomes/evaluation (see Appendix B)

H. Globe rupture

This condition is an ocular emergency. All penetrating or perforating injuries may threaten vision and require ophthalmology consultation and hospitalization. Globe rupture may be caused by blunt or penetrating trauma. In blunt trauma, the most common site of perforation is beneath the rectus muscles, where the sclera is thinnest. The anterior chamber deepens, and the iris diaphragm falls backward. There is usually a coexistent hemorrhage caused by perforation of the choroid. Penetrating injuries are usually the result of pounding steel, steel-grinding wheels, or an impaled object. Patient history is very important in the diagnosis.

1. Assessment

   a. Subjective data

     1) History of present illness/chief complaint

       a) Mechanism of injury

         (1) Penetrating

         (2) Blunt

       b) Diminished vision

     2) Sudden visual impairment or loss

     3) Pain: minimal to severe

     4) Medical history

       a) Immunization status

       b) Allergies to medications

   b. Objective data

     1) Physical examination

       a) Decreased visual acuity

       b) Shallow anterior chamber and decreased intraocular pressure below 10 mm Hg

       c) Asymmetry of globe

       d) Extrusion of aqueous or vitreous humor

       e) Direct observation of foreign body if located in anterior chamber

       f) Irregularities in pupillary borders

     2) Diagnostic procedures

       a) Soft tissue radiographs for foreign body or fracture

       b) CT scan

   c) Slit-lamp examination

   d) Ultrasonography

   e) Possibly magnetic resonance imaging (MRI)

 2. Analysis: differential nursing diagnosis/collaborative problems

  a. Sensory-perceptual alteration: visual, related to injury and patching

  b. Pain related to ocular injury

  c. Anxiety related to anticipated treatment and prognosis

  d. Knowledge deficit related to therapeutic regimen

  e. Risk for infection related to disrupted integrity of tissue and coexisting injuries

 3. Planning/interventions

  a. Ophthalmological referral

  b. If suspicion of globe rupture, do not open eye

  c. Keep patient in semi-Fowler's position

  d. Patch or shield injured eye lightly, and patch other eye as well to minimize consensual movement

  e. Administer parenteral analgesics as prescribed

  f. Administer antibiotics parenterally

  g. Administer tetanus prophylaxis

  h. Provide a support environment

  i. Explain all procedures and disease process in understandable terms

  j. Permit calm significant other to accompany patient in treatment area

  k. Prepare patient for admission, surgery, or transfer as indicated

  l. If there is an impaled object, secure it. Do not remove it!

 4. Expected outcomes/evaluation (see Appendix B)

REFERENCES

Bates, B., & Hoeckelman, R. A. (1991). *A guide to physical examination and history taking* (pp. 32–33, 146–152, 160–176). Philadelphia: J. B. Lippincott.

Clark, R. B. (1997). Common ophthalmologic problems. In P. Rosen, R. M. Baker, D. Danzl, R. Hockberger, L. Ling, V. Markovchick, J. Marx, E. Newton, R. Walls (Eds.), *Emergency medicine concepts and clinical practice*. St. Louis, MO: C. V. Mosby.

Jarvis, C. (1996). *Physical examination and health assessment* (pp. 300–350). Philadelphia: W. B. Saunders.

Ortiz, J. M., Antoszyk, J. H., & Daniels, M. B. (1991). Orbital and ocular injuries. *Topics in Emergency Medicine, 5,* 202–207.

Parshall, M. (1996). Eye conditions. In P. S. Kidd & P. Sturt (Eds.), *Mosby's emergency nursing reference*. St. Louis, MO: C. V. Mosby.

Ragge, N. K., & Easty, D. L. (1991). *Immediate eye care*. St. Louis, MO: Mosby–Year Book.

Smith, D. (1995). Eye, ear, nose, throat, and dental emergencies. In S. B. Sheehy & J. E. Lombardi (Eds.), *Manual of emergency care*. St. Louis, MO: C. V. Mosby.

ιourtney Cosby, MN, MS

CHAPTER **15**

Organ and Tissue Donation and Post-Transplantation Emergencies

MAJOR TOPICS

Organ and Tissue Donation Process

    Identification of Potential Donor

    Donor Referral

    Brain Death Determination

    Donor Family Consent

    Management of Potential Organ Donors

    Role of the Emergency Department

Nursing Process Considerations

Post-Transplantation Emergencies

    Pathophysiology of Transplant Rejection

I. ORGAN AND TISSUE DONATION PROCESS

Progress has been made in the art and science of organ transplantation since the first kidney transplant in 1954. The advances made in surgical techniques, tissue typing and matching, understanding the immune system, preventing and treating rejection, and organ procurement and preservation techniques have dramatically increased the demand for organs for transplantation. On October 31, 1996, 49,223 people in the United States were on the United Network of Organ Sharing (UNOS) national waiting list for cadaver organ transplants. This number includes 33,980 for kidneys; 1452 for kidney-pancreas; 319 for pancreas; 7191 for liver; 3718 for heart; 223 for heart-lung; 2260 for lung; and 80 for intestine. Bone, ligament, skin, and other tissues are also in high demand for surgical implantation and research.

Organ transplantation has become a viable and accepted treatment modality for many patients suffering from end-stage organ failure. There are two primary sources of transplantable organs: living donors and cadaveric donors. Of the living donors, the living related donor is a family member who, after extensive testing, proves to be compatible with the recipient. This type of donor usually involves kidney patients, but there have been several living related donor liver transplants performed with success. Living unrelated donors are those who are not family members but, through testing, are found to be compatible with others. This type of donation is done mostly for bone marrow recipients. The vast majority of organs for transplant are obtained from cadaveric donors. These are patients who have suffered an irreversible brain injury that leads to brain death.

The Uniform Anatomical Gift Act of 1968 has been passed in all 50 states and provides that an individual 18 years of age or older can give prior consent for removal of any or all organs after death and can carry a signed witness card to that effect. Most states support this and indicate permission on the individual's driver's license. Even with the signed donor consent, family permission must be obtained; only the most available ranking next of kin need sign a consent for removal of organs from a dead relative.

A decade ago, of the major organs transplanted, the 1-year survival rate among heart recipients was 80%, kidney recipients, 91%, and liver recipients, 65 to 70%; today, the success rates are significantly higher. Because of a shortage of donor organs, recipients may wait up to a year or longer. The limiting fact in the provision of this successful mode of therapy remains donor availability.

Organ procurement has developed into a unique medical specialty in response to the critical need for transplantable organs, and programs have been developed across the United States to promote the procurement, preservation, and distribution of organs and tissues to meet that need. Currently, there are two types of procurement programs: hospital-based organ procurement agencies (OPAs) serving their own transplantation center, and independent organ procurement agencies (IOPAs), which are freestanding, nonprofit organizations serving one transplantation center or several centers within a specific geographical area. Any organ procurement agency in the country can belong to UNOS and use their computerized placement system.

The meticulous matching of a donated organ or tissue to a recipient is done at specific tissue-typing laboratories. Testing optimizes the compatibility of organs or tissues to the recipients to influence survival rates positively and reduces the possibility of graft-versus-host disease and rejection. All potential recipients are registered with the tissue-typing laboratory and a transplant center. To do this, the laboratory must have blood samples to determine human leukocyte antigen (HLA) and current serum available to cross-match against potential donors for compatibility. Antibodies of potential recipients can change over the course of their disease process as a result of increased need for dialysis, blood transfusions, pregnancy, or illness.

As potential recipients are identified at the transplant center, they are placed on a waiting list both with the local organ procurement agency and nationally with UNOS. Recipients are listed by blood type, weight range, date of listing, and acuity. Acuity determines where they are placed on that list. As a donor is identified, the donor's blood type and weight are recorded, and potential recipients are matched at that time. In 1989, 31% of heart transplant candidates died while waiting for an appropriately matched organ. Similarly, 23% of liver transplant candidates died while waiting, most of whom were younger than 45 years. As previously stated, currently, more than 49,000 people nationwide are awaiting organ transplant. Unfortunately, the thought of organ donation is not second nature to either health care professionals or the general public at this time in the United States.

To address this imbalance, OPAs are engaged in educating both the public and health care professionals regarding the need for organ donation. Emergency nurses are an important component in identifying potential donors. The Emergency Nurses Association (ENA) position paper, "Role of the Emergency Nurse in Tissue and Organ Procurement," (ENA, 1992) demonstrates the specialty's commitment to organ and tissue procurement.

A. Identification of potential donor

1. Two types of donors

   a. *Nonheartbeating: suffered primary cardiac arrest and death; can donate only tissue (eyes, skin, bones, connective tissues, heart valves)*

   b. *Heartbeating: brain has sustained an insult that causes complete and irreversible cessation of function and results in patient's death*

2. **Medical history**
   a. *Significant hypertension*
   b. *Insulin-dependent diabetes (serum creatinine level greater than 1.5 mg; given the possibility that these patients may have renal failure, this is closely monitored for evaluation as potential donor)*
3. **History of present injury or condition**
   a. *Cause of death:*
      1) Head trauma, 48.8%
      2) Cerebrovascular accident/stroke, 38.3%
      3) Anoxia, 9.7%
      4) Other, 2.1%
      5) Central nervous system tumor, 1%
   b. *Circumstances of death*
      1) Other, 47.9% (death may be from natural causes without specific circumstances)
      2) Motor vehicle collision, 26.3%
      3) Suicide, 10.1%
      4) Accident (non-motor vehicle accident), 7.5%
      5) Homicide, 7.3%
      6) Child abuse, 0.9%
   c. *Mechanism of death*
      1) Intracranial hemorrhage/stroke, 40.4%
      2) Blunt injury, 29.1%
      3) Gunshot/stab wound, 15.7%
      4) Other, 8.4%
      5) Cardiovascular 3.5%
4. **Criteria for acceptable organ donor candidates**
   a. *Nonheartbeating donors*
      1) Eye donors
         a) Any age
         b) Eye condition acceptable
         c) No systemic infection
         d) No intravenous (IV) drug use
         e) No acquired immunodeficiency syndrome (AIDS) or hepatitis
         f) No viral meningitis
      2) Heart valve donors
         a) Age: 38 weeks gestation (1800 g; 4 lb) to 55 years
         b) No malignancy
         c) No transmissible disease
         d) No IV drug use
         e) No systemic infection
      3) Skin and bone donors
         a) Age: 16 to 75 years
         b) No malignancy
         c) No transmissible disease
         d) No IV drug use
         e) No systemic infection
   b. *Heartbeating donors*
      1) Age: newborn to 70 years
      2) Brain death or impending brain death
      3) On ventilator support
      4) No evidence or history of IV drug abuse within past year
      5) No evidence of sepsis (confirmed by blood cultures)

6) No evidence of metastatic disease (except primary brain tumor)
7) No evidence of transmissible disease (e.g., AIDS, hepatitis)
c. *Current physiological condition*
1) Brain death imminent
2) Blood pressure
   a) Hypotensive
   b) Hypertensive
3) Cardiac and/or respiratory arrest (when occurred and duration)
4) Medications
   a) Vasopressors
      (1) Dopamine
      (2) Norepinephrine (Levophed)
   b) Vasopressin (Pitressin)
5) Urine output
   a) Oliguria
   b) Diabetes insipidus
6) Signs of possible infection
   a) Hyperthermia
   b) Current cultures results
      (1) Blood
      (2) Urine
      (3) Sputum
   c) Chest radiograph results
   d) General diagnostic procedures to determine compatibility with potential recipient
      (1) ABO blood typing
      (2) Accurate body weight: to determine size of organ in relation to body size of potential recipient
      (3) Serology testing for AIDS, hepatitis, syphilis, cytomegalovirus, because these can be potentially life threatening in immunocompromised recipient
      (4) Complete blood count (CBC) and differential: hematocrit should be maintained at more than 30

B. Donor referral

1. **All patients who are critically ill or severely traumatized should be considered potential organ donors; in contrast, all lifesaving interventions on behalf of patient are also in interest of successful organ donation**
2. **Role of organ procurement personnel before actual pronouncement of brain death: laws have been enacted to prevent transplant surgeons from participating in certain aspects of patient care; goals of laws are to avoid any conflict of interest and protect both patient and transplant surgeon**
3. **Contact local OPA early**
4. **Role of OPA**
   a. *First establishes whether patient has been declared brain dead; if not, may advise on interventions that are consistent with maintaining patient's life, such as use of vasopressors, correction of acid-base problems, treatment of hypokalemia*
   b. *Assesses potential donors*
   c. *Counsels donor families and obtains informed consent*
   d. *Manages details related to recovery, preservation, transportation of organs*
   e. *Reviews, and arranges for, reimbursement of all hospital charges associated*

with intensive care unit (ICU) management and recovery of all organs and tissues incurred during donation

5. **Donor family not approached until brain death declared**

C. Brain death determination

1. **Guidelines for Determination of Death—Presidential Commission**
   a. *Irreversible cessation of circulatory and respiratory functions*
   b. *Irreversible cessation of all functions of entire brain, including brain stem*
   c. *Confirmatory testing*
      1) Nuclear medicine flow scan: determine whether there is blood flow to brain; if blood flow is absent, brain death is demonstrated
      2) Apnea test: preoxygenate patient for at least 10 minutes with 100% oxygen; adjust ventilator so that partial pressure of carbon dioxide (PCO_2) is normal (35 to 45 mm Hg), then disconnect ventilator and give passive oxygen via tracheal cannula at 8 to 12 L/min for 10 minutes, and observe patient continuously for spontaneous respirations; if there is no respiratory effort, and PCO_2 is greater than 60 mm Hg, the patient is apneic, and the test is conclusive for brain death
      3) Clinical examination: neurological examination that includes testing for unresponsiveness, cranial or brain-stem reflexes, and deep tendon reflexes; these include corneal reflex, oculocephalic (doll's eyes) reflex, oculovestibular (ice calorics) reflex, oropharyngeal (gag) reflex, and pupillary response to light; deep tendon reflexes are absent, but spinal reflexes may remain intact

2. **Complicating conditions (may mimic brain death; must be corrected before brain death can be determined)**
   a. *Drug and metabolic intoxication*
      1) Barbiturates
      2) Alcohol
      3) Neuromuscular blocking agents
   b. *Hypothermia*
   c. *Children younger than 5 years: because there is limited experience in this area, an experienced pediatric neurologist and extended observation period may be required*

3. **Legislation**
   a. *Uniform Anatomical Gift Act of 1968: allows all individuals 18 years of age and older to sign a card donating their body, or any part of it, for purposes of transplantation, medical research, medical education*
   b. *Omnibus Reconciliation Act of 1986 (Required Request): requires all hospitals receiving reimbursement from Medicare and Medicaid to establish protocols to ensure that potential donor families are aware of option of organ and tissue donation, along with notification of OPA; it also prohibits sale of organs*

4. **Notification of local procurement agency or the United Network for Organ Sharing (UNOS) at 1-800-24-DONOR to locate the transplant/ donation coordinator in specified area**

D. Donor family consent

1. **Data suggest that there must be a clear time separation between notification of brain death and request process**
2. **Designated as "decoupling"**
3. **Key issues to be covered with family**

      a. No financial obligations for donor family
      b. Does not delay funeral
      c. No disfigurement with donation
      d. Donation is confidential information

  4. Support family's decision whether or not they accept donation

  5. Consent
      a. Legal next of kin
        1) Spouse
        2) Adult son or daughter
        3) Either parent
        4) Guardian of deceased at time of death
        5) Any person who is authorized to dispose of body
      b. Uniform organ donor card
      c. Driver's license

E. Management of potential organ donors

  1. Shift of emphasis once brain death declared and permission obtained to supporting viability of organs being donated
      a. Adequate hydration of donor
      b. Maintenance of normal blood pressure (BP)
      c. Establishment of diuresis
      d. Maintenance of adequate oxygenation

  2. Once brain death declared, OPA becomes directly involved
      a. Tissue typing to determine histocompatibility
      b. Cross-matching between donor and recipient

  3. Role of emergency department (ED)
      a. Many times first to identify potential donor
      b. Immediate notification of OPA
      c. Make requests and obtain consent

II. NURSING PROCESS CONSIDERATIONS

A. Assessment

  1. Donor: refer to preceding information

  2. Donor's family
      a. Family's definition of death
      b. Family's belief system
      c. Role(s) of prospective donor in family
      d. Meaning of death of loved one to family
      e. Family's understanding of and feelings about organ or tissue donation
      f. Meaning of donation to family
      g. Wishes of prospective donor, if known

B. Analysis: differential nursing diagnosis/collaborative problems

  1. Donor: nursing diagnosis/collaborative problems related to underlying illness or injury
      a. Decreased cardiac output
      b. Risk for fluid volume deficit
      c. Altered tissue perfusion
      d. Impaired gas exchange

2. **Donor's family**
   a. *Altered family processes related to loss of family member*
   b. *Anticipatory grieving related to actual or perceived loss*
   c. *Knowledge deficit related to brain death*
   d. *Family coping: potential for growth related to surviving loss of family member*
   e. *Spiritual distress (distress of human spirit related to loss of loved one)*

C. Planning/interventions

1. **Donor: for organ donation**
   a. *Maintain systolic BP greater than 100 mm Hg*
   b. *Maintain urine output greater than 100 mL/hour*
   c. *Prevent and treat infections*
   d. *Maintain electrolyte balance*
   e. *Maintain normal body temperature*
   f. *Maintain dignity of donor*
2. **Donor's family**
   a. *Information provided to family to make informed decision*
      1) Explanation of brain death
      2) Potential use of and need for organs and tissues
      3) Criteria for determining organ or tissue donation
      4) Confidentiality of both donor and recipient
      5) No cost to family for evaluation, maintenance, recovery procedures
      6) Noninterference with funeral arrangements
      7) Estimated timetable, extent of recovery procedure for both organs and tissues
      8) Postdonation letter to family if requested
   b. *Continual encouragement for family to express feelings and fears*
      1) Disfigurement
      2) Cost
      3) Funeral arrangements
      4) Time frame
      5) Inability of next of kin to make decision
   c. *Support decision, no matter what is decided*
   d. *Offer to make referral to social worker, chaplain, and/or crisis intervention nurse*
   e. *Make referral to appropriate community agency*

D. Expected outcomes/evaluation

1. After the potential donor is identified, consent is obtained, and all organs and tissues are matched with potential recipients, donor is taken to operating room, where the recovery process begins
2. Transplant surgeon at donor site, in consultation with associates at transplant center, will make final decision whether an organ can be transplanted at this time
3. Once that decision has been made, transplant surgeon recovers organ for recipient and returns to transplant center to begin transplant operation
4. When potential donor is a tissue-only donor, all tissues except bone will be recovered in morgue
5. Donor's family will receive a call from the donation coordinator once donor operation has been completed, if they wish; they should receive a letter 2 weeks after donation to follow up on any problems or concerns

(e.g., positive or negative experiences from the process, billing problems, recipient follow-up, if known)
6. Medical and nursing staff are also contacted within a 24- to 48-hour period to seek out their perceptions of process and any misconceptions associated with donation; they will then receive a letter from donation coordinator, who will give recipient follow-up information and thank them for assistance through long process of organ and tissue donation

III. POST-TRANSPLANTATION EMERGENCIES

Once the transplantation has been completed, the patient is monitored very closely for signs of rejection. Clinical organ transplantation incorporates five major immunosuppressive agents today: corticosteroids, azathioprine (Imuran), cyclosporine, antithymocyte preparations, and OKT3. The goal of immunosuppression is to suppress the immune response adequately to prevent rejection of the transplanted organ while maintaining sufficient immunity to prevent overwhelming infection.

The two major post-transplant emergencies that may have the patient seek treatment in an ED are rejection and infection. If patients suspect a problem with their transplant, they contact either their registered nurse transplant coordinator or the transplant surgeon. After speaking with either the surgeon or the nurse, these patients may present to the ED.

Post-transplant patients may also present in the ED for many other reasons that may or may not be transplant related. This section addresses other common reasons that these patients present in the ED.

A. Pathophysiology of transplant rejection

The immune system protects the host against invasion of foreign substances. Transplanted organs are seen as foreign by the body, and the immune system is activated to destroy, or reject, this invader. The more similar the transplanted organ is to the recipient's tissue, the less the immune system will respond. The goal of transplantation is to minimize the immune response by implanting a donor organ that is as similar to the recipient's tissue as possible and then suppressing the immune response through immunosuppressive therapy.

Rejection is the recognition and response to foreign donor antigens by the recipient's immune system. The antigens can be part of the ABO system, HLA antigens, or antigens to which humans are exposed in daily life. The three classifications of rejection are hyperacute, acute, and chronic.

1. **Hyperacute rejection**
   a. *Occurs within minutes to hours after graft transplantation*
   b. *Preformed antibodies react quickly to ABO or class I HLA (A, B, or C) antigens from donor tissue*
   c. *Antibodies more prevalent in recipients who have had multiple transfusions, multiple pregnancies, or prior transplant*
   d. *Kidney are at greatest risk*
      1) Antibodies attach to vascular endothelium
      2) Results in activation of the clotting mechanism and massive intravascular coagulation in glomerular vessels
      3) Causes tissue necrosis
   e. *No treatment, but improved cross-matching techniques and careful screening have helped reduce this complication*
2. **Acute rejection**
   a. *Usually seen 1 week to 1 year after transplantation*

    b. *Cellular immunity, the T-cell response, is thought to be primarily responsible for acute rejection, although antibody system also participates*

        1) Antigens from graft tissue are processed by the recipient's antigen processing cells (APCs)

        2) Presented to helper T cells

        3) Stimulates interleukin production and T-cell proliferation

        4) Interleukins recruit other inflammatory cells, such as macrophages

        5) Activate cytotoxic cells, which invade and destroy the graft if not checked

        6) Memory T cells are also produced, which would lead to accelerated rejection if recipient ever required another transplant and same antibodies were present in graft

        7) Both interleukin and helper T cells stimulate antibody production, increasing overall immune response against graft

        8) Immunosuppressive therapy depresses inflammatory and immune responses, preventing or minimizing rejection

    c. *Confirmation of rejection*

        1) Identified by laboratory studies that indicate deterioration in function, such as increased blood urea nitrogen (BUN), creatinine, liver enzyme levels

        2) Cardiac diagnosed by heart biopsy

        3) Symptoms do not appear until process is too advanced to treat effectively

        4) Regular follow-up will provide early diagnosis of rejection

        5) Extent of rejection is determined by recipient's response to immunosuppressive therapy

3. Chronic rejection

    a. *Occurs over months to years after transplantation*

    b. *Gradual decrease in organ function caused by progressive fibrotic changes in vascular supply of graft*

    c. *Actual cause unknown*

    d. *May be T-cell action and multitude of mediators such as interleukins and lymphokines that are part of immune system*

    e. *Only treatment is retransplantation, with exception of renal transplants, for which dialysis can be resumed*

    f. *Rejection process results in presence of infiltrates of inflammatory cells and vascular and tissue damage that lead to organ failure*

    g. *Nonspecific changes of inflammation*

        1) Fever

        2) Malaise

        3) Tenderness or swelling around graft site

    h. *Recognition of rejection is specific to graft type*

        1) Kidney and liver: decrease in function accompanied by altered laboratory studies

        2) Heart: recognized by development of atherosclerotic changes in coronary arteries; biopsy confirms diagnosis

B. Assessment

1. Subjective data collection

    a. *History of present illness*

        1) Transplant rejection

            a) Nausea

            b) Vomiting

            c) Weight gain: greater than 3 pounds

            d) Graft site tenderness

  e) Shortness of breath
  f) General malaise
  g) Burning on urination
  h) Medication compliance
  i) Current medications
   (1) Cyclosporine
   (2) Azathioprine (Imuran)
   (3) Prednisone
   (4) Antibiotics
   (5) Antacids
   (6) Hypertensive medications
 2) Chronic rejection
  a) Fever
  b) Malaise
  c) Tenderness or swelling around graft site
 3) Infection
  a) Bacterial: usually seen during first 6 months
   (1) Meningitis
   (2) Pneumonia
  b) Fungal
   (1) *Candida*
   (2) *Aspergillus*
  c) Viral: usually seen 6 months after transplantation
   (1) Cytomegalovirus
   (2) Herpes simplex or zoster
b. *Medical history*
 1) Disease process before transplantation
 2) Organ transplanted
 3) Hypertension

2. Objective data collection

a. *Physical examination*
 1) Increased respiratory rate
 2) Edema, either general or at graft site
 3) Hypertension
 4) Fever: usually low grade, to 99°F (37.2°C)
 5) Pain on palpation of graft site: transplanted kidney is located in lower pelvic bowl
 6) Change in volume of urine produced (seen only in kidney transplant patients)
 7) Decreased bile drainage (liver transplant patients continue to have biliary stent in place for up to 3 months)
 8) Jaundice
b. *Diagnostic data and procedures*
 1) CBC with differential
 2) Cultures
  a) Blood
  b) Urine
  c) Sputum
  d) Spinal fluid
 3) Urinalysis
 4) Kidney function tests (BUN, creatinine)
 5) Liver function tests (serum glutamic-oxaloacetic transaminase [SGOT]/aspartate aminotransferase [AST], serum glutamate pyruvate transaminase

[SGPT]/alanine aminotransferase [ALT], bilirubin, total and direct) will be elevated during rejection episodes

  6) Drug levels
    a) Cyclosporine
    b) Azathioprine (Imuran)
    c) Adrenocortical steroids
    d) Antibiotic levels (because these patients receive antibiotics for 3 to 4 months after transplantation)
  7) Pulmonary function tests
  8) Electrocardiogram (ECG)

C. Analysis: differential nursing diagnosis/collaborative problems

1. **Ineffective breathing pattern**
2. **Impaired gas exchange**
3. **Risk for altered tissue perfusion**
4. **Fluid volume excess**
5. **Pain**
6. **Fluid volume deficit related to vomiting and fever**
7. **Risk for infection related to immunosuppressive therapy**
8. **Knowledge deficit related to transplantation and self-care**

D. Planning/interventions

1. **Put patient in single room if possible**
2. **No benefit to strict isolation procedures over various simplified procedures, including hand washing only; differences among practitioners**
3. **Prepare patient for biopsy of transplanted organ to determine whether rejection has occurred**
   a. Biopsy of liver and kidney patients done in OR
   b. Biopsy of heart patients done in cardiac catheterization laboratory
4. **Admit patient for further observation**
   a. Change in drug regimen
   b. Possibility of retransplantation
5. **Institute pain relief measures (e.g., medications)**
6. **Administer oxygen therapy**
7. **Measure accurate weight**
8. **Measure accurate fluid intake and output**
9. **Administer antiemetics**
10. **Obtain infectious disease consultation**

E. Expected outcomes/evaluation

1. **Monitor laboratory results to determine whether infection or rejection**
2. **Monitor patient's response to**
   a. Pain; relief is demonstrated by
     1) Facial responses
     2) Relaxed posture
     3) Normalization of vital signs
     4) Verbalization of pain relief
   b. Antiemetics; patient verbalizes decreased nausea, no vomiting noted
   c. Oxygen therapy
     1) Normal breathing pattern returns

      2) Respiratory rate decreased

      3) Use of accessory muscles suspended

      4) Patient verbalizes relief

      5) Satisfactory oxygen saturation by pulse oximeter

  3. Monitor patient's fluid status through

    a. Accurate measurement of intake and output to determine

      1) Fluid retention

      2) Kidney function

    b. Accurate scale weight

  4. Admit for further evaluation

    a. Change in drug regimen

    b. Resolution of infectious process

F. Special considerations

  1. Trauma

    a. Kidney transplant patients

      1) Placement of organ in lower pelvic cavity

      2) Native kidneys not removed

    b. Kidney-pancreas combined

      1) Kidney with pancreas in lower iliac area

      2) Pancreas drains into bladder

  2. Myocardial infarctions: may be seen up to 5 years after transplantation

    a. Graft atherosclerosis: heart transplant patients have denervated transplanted organ; therefore, they do not have usual early symptoms associated with a myocardial infarction; usual new symptom is congestive heart failure or sudden death

    b. Kidney transplant patients: after transplantation, these patients return to more normal lifestyle and improved nutritional status without restrictions; their hearts may not have compensated for increased fluid volume or activity level

  3. Malignancies: a risk resulting from immunocompromised state

    a. Lymphomas

    b. Kaposi's sarcoma

    c. Squamous cell carcinoma

    d. Gynecological malignancies

  4. Drug toxicities and adverse effects

    a. Cyclosporine

      1) Nephrotoxicity

      2) Hepatotoxicity

    b. Azathioprine (Imuran)

      1) Bone marrow suppression

        a) Thrombocytopenia

        b) Leukopenia

      2) Hepatic dysfunction

        a) Adrenocortical steroids (prednisone)

      3) Avascular necrosis of hip

      4) Gastrointestinal effects

        a) Pancreatitis

        b) Ulcers

        c) Diverticulitis

      5) Cataracts

      6) Hyperglycemia

      7) Diabetes mellitus

BIBLIOGRAPHY

Ad Hoc Committee of the Harvard Medical School to Examine the Definition of Brain Death. (1968). A definition of irreversible coma. *Journal of the American Medical Association, 205,* 337–340.

Cecka, J. M., & Terasaki, P. I. (Eds.). (1996). *Clinical transplants.* Los Angeles: UCLA Tissue Typing Laboratory.

Davis, A. J., & Aroskar M. A. (1991). *Ethical dilemmas and nursing practice.* East Norwalk, CT: Appleton & Lange.

Emergency Nurse Association. (1992). *Role of the emergency nurse in tissue and organ procurement.* Park Ridge, IL: ENA.

Evans, R. W., Orians, C. E., & Ascher, N. L. (1992). The potential supply of organ donors: An assessment of the efficiency of organ procurement efforts in the United States. *JAMA, 267,* 239–246.

First, M. R. (1991). The dilemma of organ donation and distribution. *Journal of Transplant Coordination, 1*(2), 65–69.

Guidelines for the determination of death: Report of the medical consultants on the diagnosis of death to the President's Commission for the Study of Ethical Problems in Medicine and Biomedical and Behavioral Research. (1981). *Journal of the American Medical Association, 246,* 2184–2186.

Gurka, A. M. (1989). The immune system: Implications for critical care nursing. *Critical Care Nurse, 9,* 24–35.

Hawthorne, J. L. (1993). Immunocompromised patients. In J. M. Clochesy et al (Eds.), *Critical care nursing* (pp. 1116–1134). Philadelphia: W. B. Saunders

Kaufman, H., & Lynn, J. (1986). Brain death. *Neurosurgery, 19,* 850–855.

Schaeffer, M. J., & Alexander, D. C. (1992). U. S. system for organ procurement and transplantation. *American Journal of Hospital Pharmacy, 49,* 1733–1740.

United Network for Organ Sharing. (1996). *Annual report of the U.S. Scientific Registry for Organ Transplantation and The Organ Procurement and Transplantation Network.* Richmond, VA: Health and Resources and Services Administration and the Division of Organ Transplantation.

Joan Walker, RN, BScN

CHAPTER **16**

Orthopedic Emergencies

MAJOR TOPICS

I. GENERAL STRATEGY

The aim in caring for the patient with an orthopedic emergency is to restore and preserve function.

A. Assessment

1. **Primary survey/resuscitation** (see Chapter 1)
2. **Secondary survey** (see Chapter 1)
3. **Psychological, social, and environmental factors**
    a. For syndromes of overuse, history of
        1) Repetitive actions
        2) High forces
        3) Awkward joint posture
        4) Direct pressure (e.g., leaning on elbow, kneeling)
        5) Vibration (e.g., use of power tools)
        6) Prolonged constrained posture

    b. Recent unrelated illnesses
        1) Infections (e.g., as possible cause of septic arthritis or osteomyelitis in children)
            a) Streptococcal infections, including rheumatic fever
            b) Urinary tract infections
            c) Upper respiratory tract infections
            d) Ear infections
            e) Gastrointestinal disorders, infections
            f) Postpolio syndrome
            g) Temporal arteritis

4. Focused survey
    a. Subjective data
        1) History of present condition
            a) Trauma
                (1) Mechanism of injury, onset of symptoms, duration of symptoms
                (2) Precipitating factors: pre-existing injuries, associated symptoms, medical problems
                (3) Aggravating factors
                (4) Relieving factors, remedies attempted by patient to relieve symptoms
            b) Pain assessment using "PQRST"
                (1) Use patient's own words
                (2) Ask patient to describe severity of pain using scale ranging from 1 to 10
                (3) Region (location, radiation, referred)
                (4) Time (time and rate of onset, duration, rate of increase in swelling)
            c) Associated symptoms
                (1) Changes in neurovascular function
                (2) Ability to bear weight
                (3) Range of motion
                (4) Weakness versus pain as presenting symptom
            d) Mass or swollen areas
                (1) Onset
                (2) Size
                (3) Location
                (4) Symptoms: pain, tenderness, numbness, weakness
        2) Medical history
            a) Chronic illnesses
                (1) Anemia, bleeding, coagulation deficiency
                (2) Cardiovascular conditions (indication of peripheral vascular disease)
                (3) Diabetes mellitus (associated with peripheral neuropathies, decreased microcirculation)
                (4) Arthritis, degenerative or rheumatoid
                (5) Acute inflammatory diseases
                (6) Paget's disease (localized areas of bone destruction followed by replacement with overdeveloped, light, soft, porous bone and associated with deformities such as thickening of portions of the skull and bending of weight-bearing bones; cause unknown)
                (7) Use of medications that predispose to fractures (e.g., phenytoin sodium and corticosteroids)
                (8) Use of injectable neurotoxic medications (e.g., penicillin G, diazepam, hydrocortisone, chlorpromazine, tetanus toxoid, hydroxyzine)

(9) Disorders associated with peripheral nerve injury (e.g., alcoholism, sudden significant weight loss, carcinomatous neuropathy)

(10) Prior injury or surgery of affected extremity

(11) Pre-existing disabilities, metabolic disorders

b) Current health status

    (1) Recent injury or problem with affected extremity

    (2) Allergies

    (3) Current medications, therapies

    (4) Tetanus immunity status (if skin breaks present)

    (5) Pregnancy (swelling precipitates overuse syndromes; prone to falls with pelvic ligament laxity)

    (6) Vitamin deficiency

b. *Objective data*

    1) Physical examination

      a) Inspection

        (1) Both sides of body to visualize symmetry, contour, size, alignment

          (a) Valgus: deformity of distal portion of joint that is angulated away from midline of body (e.g., knock-knees, hallux valgus)

          (b) Varus: deformity of distal portion of joint that is angulated toward midline of body (e.g., bowleg and pigeon-toe)

        (2) Skin and soft tissue

          (a) Color changes and hair loss associated with peripheral vascular disease

          (b) Ecchymosis

          (c) Gross deformities (associated with arthritis, tumors, swelling)

          (d) Muscle mass (hypertrophy and atrophy)

          (e) Scars indicative of previous injury, surgery, invasive procedures, intravenous (IV) drug abuse

        (3) Joints

          (a) Deformity (e.g., nodules in fingers, toes, knees)

          (b) Swelling caused by inflammation, infection, trauma

          (c) Redness caused by inflammation associated with infection, cellulitis, gouty arthritis

          (d) Range of motion (passive and active)

          (e) Rotation: position of joint, extremity, ability to rotate internally or externally

      b) Palpation

        (1) Skin and soft tissue

          (a) Temperature (use back of fingers to assess)

          (b) Swelling and pitting edema

        (2) Muscle tone

          (a) Decreased as a result of musculoskeletal, neurological, metabolic, or infectious disorders; organophosphate poisoning; and/or fatigue

          (b) Increased as a result of spasms, injury, cramps, tremors (associated with electrolyte disorders, neurological conditions, infections [tetanus])

        (3) Muscle strength (assess range of motion before muscle strength, because muscular contraction may produce enough pain to inhibit further examination)

          (a) Ask patient to resist movement or move against resistance

          (b) Strength is subjectively graded by examiner on scale ranging from 1 to 5 scale; all findings are recorded and used as a baseline

0: paralysis, no muscular contraction detected

1: only slight contractility and no joint motion

2: active movement, full range of motion with gravity eliminated

3: active movement, full range of motion against gravity

4: active movement, full range of motion against gravity and some resistance

5: active movement, full range of motion against full resistance

  (4) Deep tendon reflexes
    (a) Assess major reflexes (biceps, brachioradialis, triceps, patellar knee jerk, Achilles tendon)
    (b) Grade: 0, none; +1, below normal; +2, average; +3, stronger than average; +4, intense (clonus)
  (5) Joints
    (a) Temperature
    (b) Pain or tenderness with palpation
    (c) Crepitation with movement
    (d) Passive range of motion (done by examiner)
    (e) Joint stability (varies with each joint)
  (6) Bones
    (a) Tenderness along length
    (b) Resistance to deforming force
    (c) Deformity, crepitus, tenderness
  (7) Gait: ask patient to walk, if tolerated, both away and toward examiner, assessing balance, control, posture, movement of arms and legs
c) Peripheral nerve assessment (Table 16–1)
d) Peripheral vascular assessment
  (1) Inspection
    (a) Skin for acute (pallor) and chronic (cyanosis, pigmentation) circulatory changes
    (b) Amount and distribution of hair
    (c) Skin texture
    (d) Skin ulcers
    (e) Inspection of veins for distention (unilateral vs. bilateral)
  (2) Palpation
    (a) Temperature of skin

Table 16–1 PERIPHERAL NERVE ASSESSMENT

Nerve	Motor	Sensory
Radial	Extend wrist or thumb	Feeling on dorsum of thumb
Median	Oppose thumb to base of small finger	Feeling on tip of index finger
Ulnar	Abduct (fan) fingers	Feeling on tip of small finger
Tibial	Plantar flex toes (curl down)	Feeling on bottom of foot
Superficial peroneal	Laterally evert foot	Feeling on lateral aspect of dorsum of foot
Deep peroneal	Dorsiflex toes (curl toes up)	Feeling in first toe web space (between first and second toes)

(b) Pitting edema

(c) Quality of arterial pulses (brachial, radial, ulna [overlying tissue may obscure, patency determined by Allen's test], femoral, popliteal, posterior tibial, and dorsalis pedis [may be congenitally absent or may branch higher in ankle]); presence of pulse does not rule out arterial injury

(d) Grading of pulse quality

0: no pulse
1: weak and easily obliterated with pressure
2: difficult to palpate but easy to feel once located
3: easily palpated and considered normal
4: strong and bounding

(3) Capillary blanch test

(a) Used when unable to palpate pulses because of casts, splints, dressings

(b) Is nonspecific measure of tissue perfusion, which can be affected by multiple factors

(c) Normal time for color to return after blanching is 2 seconds or less

(4) Doppler assessment of artery

2) Diagnostic procedures

a) Radiology

(1) Plain films provide data on bone and joint changes, useful for diagnosing open joint injuries (air visible in joint space); standard for acute fractures and dislocations; does not show soft tissue disorders, except swelling

(2) Computed tomography (CT) used for diagnosis

(a) Fractures involving articular surfaces (tibial plateau, calcaneus, talus)

(b) Fracture/dislocations that are difficult to visualize or too dangerous to manipulate (e.g., pelvis for complex fractures, sacrum, acetabulum)

(c) Fracture of scapula, carpal bones, tarsal bones; dislocations of humeral and femoral heads, radioulnar or sternoclavicular joints

(d) Stress fractures

(e) Bony changes, metastatic processes

(3) Angiography used to diagnose and treat vascular injuries, prevent hemorrhage, and relieve ischemia; useful for recognizing and selectively embolizing major bleeding vessels via an arterial catheter and injuries of extremities with suspected vascular involvement (e.g., knee dislocations or penetrating wounds)

(4) Magnetic resonance imaging (MRI) for soft tissue disorders such as ligament injury, meniscal damage, tendon ruptures, muscle tears, tumors and hematomas, spinal structures, tumor, infection, degenerative disorders

(5) Technetium bone scans for stress fractures and metastatic disease

(6) Arthroscopy used to evaluate injury to joint structures

b) Laboratory procedures (Table 16–2)

Table 16–2 LABORATORY PROCEDURES TO AID DIAGNOSIS OF ORTHOPEDIC CONDITIONS

Test	Examples
Alkaline phosphatase level	Increased with elevated metabolic bone activity
Calcium level	Increased with metastatic bone cancer, acute osteoporosis, multiple myeloma, and prolonged immobilization Decreased with hypoparathyroidism, osteomalacia, and rickets
Creatine kinase level	Increased in necrosis or atrophy of skeletal muscles, traumatic muscle injury, strenuous exercise, and progressive muscular dystrophy (obtain isoenzymes for diagnosis)
Lactate dehydrogenase level	Increased in muscular dystrophy and damage to skeletal muscles
Phosphorus level	Increased in fracture healing, osteoporosis, and hypoparathyroidism
Serum glutamic-oxaloacetic transaminase level	Increased in any muscle damage, muscular dystrophy, and liver disease
Serum glutamic-pyruvic transaminase level	Increased in skeletal muscle damage
Uric acid level	Increased in gout, multiple myeloma, arthritis, and hyperparathyroidism
C-reactive protein	Positive in acute inflammatory change, widespread metastasis, and rheumatoid arthritis
Antinuclear antibodies	Positive in rheumatoid arthritis, systemic lupus erythematosus, and inflammatory arthritis
Serum rheumatoid factor	Positive in rheumatoid arthritis and some chronic inflammatory diseases
Erythrocyte sedimentation rate	Increased with septic arthritis, osteomyelitis, and inflammatory arthritis

Adapted with permission from Schoen, D. C. (1986). *The nursing process in orthopedics.* Norwalk, CT: Appleton-Century-Crofts.

B. Analysis: differential nursing diagnosis/collaborative problems

1. **Activity intolerance**
2. **Anxiety/fear**
3. **Impaired physical mobility**
4. **Impaired skin integrity**
5. **Knowledge deficit**
6. **Pain**
7. **Risk for injury**
8. **Self-care deficit**
9. **Tissue perfusion, altered**

C. Planning/interventions

1. **Determine priorities of care**
   a. *Control and maintain airway (and cervical spine alignment), breathing, circulation*

b. Assess for other life-threatening conditions

c. Assess for limb-threatening conditions

d. Assess for hypovolemia

e. Ensure adequate urine output

f. Prevent infection

g. Control pain

h. Prevent complications

i. Prepare for operative procedures

j. Provide psychosocial support and necessary interventions

k. Educate patient/significant other

2. **Develop nursing care plan specific to patient's presenting emergency**
3. **Obtain and set up necessary equipment and supplies**
4. **Initiate appropriate interventions on basis of nursing care plans**
5. **Record data as appropriate**

D. Expected outcomes/evaluation

1. **Monitor patient's response and outcomes, adjusting nursing care plans as indicated**

   a. Specific interventions

   b. Disposition/discharge planning
2. **Record all pertinent data**
3. **If positive outcomes are not demonstrated, re-evaluate assessment and/ or plan of care**

E. Age-related considerations

1. **Pediatric**

   a. Growth and development related

   1) Child's bone structure different from adult's; children considered skeletally immature

   2) Skeleton of infant and young child is largely cartilaginous

      (a) Bones narrow and flexible

   3) Periosteum is thicker and resists disruption

      a) Provides circulation and nutrients to bone

      b) Allows bone to be more elastic and resists fracture

         (1) Greenstick: shaft of bone (diaphysis) fractured on one side, but cortex intact on other side

         (2) Torus: buckling of one side of cortex; involves metaphysis (area adjacent to growth plate); patient often presents with pain but no deformity

   4) Children have open epiphysis (growth plate) until after adolescence; this area is more susceptible to trauma; fractures to epiphysis constitute one third of all fractures and are described according to Salter-Harris classification system

      a) Type I: epiphysis separated from metaphysis

      b) Type II: epiphyseal plate slipped with metaphyseal fracture, producing triangular fragment in metaphysis (most common type of fracture)

      c) Type III: intra-articular fracture involving epiphysis, which is also slipped (surgery is required to maintain blood supply and prevent growth disturbance)

        d) Type IV: fracture that includes intra-articular space, epiphysis, epiphyseal plate, metaphysis (surgical repair is required)

        e) Type V: crush injury of epiphyseal plate, resulting in arrested growth; poor prognosis for normal growth

    5) Child's ligaments are more resistant than epiphysis to trauma

        a) Dislocations rare

        b) Fractures often accompany dislocation

        c) Sprains (ligaments tear) unusual in young children but do occur in adolescents

    6) General appearance

        a) Observe legs while child is walking

            (1) Infants have bowlegged (genu varum) appearance from birth to 2 or 3 years

            (2) Infants tend to evert feet and walk on inner aspects of feet

            (3) At 18 to 36 months, child may appear knock-kneed (genu valgum)

            (4) Normal leg configuration should be present at approximately 6 to 7 years

        b) Feet appear flatfooted

            (1) Medial longitudinal arch normally obscured by fat pads until approximately 2 years

            (2) Arch better visualized when child not weight bearing, such as when seated or on tiptoe

        c) Child may normally walk with in-toeing (pigeon-toed)

            (1) Rotational alignment of legs changes as skeleton matures, producing spontaneous correction

            (2) Pathological changes may be produced by disorders of feet, lower legs, hips

  b. *"Pearls"*

    1) Fractures result from significant force: history should be appropriate for pattern of injury

    2) Warning flags to watch for in children younger than 1 year: spiral fracture, unwitnessed or unexplained injury, fracture in healing stages, history of other fractures, fracture that does not fit mechanism of injury stated

    3) Approximately 25% of fractures in children younger than 3 years caused by nonaccidental trauma

    4) Produces fractures unique to children

    5) Limping in children uncommon; suspect hip disorder if found

    6) Unwillingness to bear weight requires further investigation

2. Geriatric

  a. *Aging related*

    1) Loss of bone minerals and mass

        a) Regeneration prolonged

        b) Bones become more brittle

        c) Loss of vertebral body height results from compression that occurs with normal aging, which leads to kyphosis

    2) Muscles lose ability to regenerate new fibers to replace ones lost because of age (atrophy)

        a) Decreased muscular strength and endurance, extremities with "flabby" appearance, shuffling gait

        b) Longer contraction time and tendency to fatigue more easily, which may cause muscle tremors, even at rest

  b. *"Pearls"*

    1) Joint stiffness and degenerative changes contribute to decreased mobility

2) Posture affected by age-related changes
3) Gait affected by posture, balance, strength, flexibility
4) Changes in feet common
    a) Foot size decreases because of loss of subcutaneous fat
    b) Skin is drier; corns and calluses form at pressure points; epidermis thins and loses natural moisture
    c) Decreased circulation from peripheral vascular disease may delay healing; venous stasis or arterial occlusion produces ulceration
    d) Toenails thicken, affecting shoe fit
    e) Bunion and toe overlapping or under-riding may occur
5) Osteoporosis promotes fractures, especially in vertebral bodies, ribs, proximal femur
6) Osteoarthritis (degeneration of movable joints) affects mostly weight-bearing joints of knees, vertebrae, small joints of hand and feet
7) Rheumatoid arthritis (systemic disease of connective tissue resulting in joint inflammation) produces swelling, stiffness, ankylosis, redness, warmth of joints
8) Pathological fracture may be due to other chronic changes
9) Paget's disease
    a) Metabolic disease that causes excessive bone resorption and deposits
    b) Middle-aged and elderly men primarily affected
    c) Affected bones tend to fracture easily

II. SPECIFIC SOFT TISSUE EMERGENCIES

The soft tissue of the extremities includes the skin, muscles, tendons, ligaments, nerves, and blood vessels. Injuries may occur with or without a bony injury, and in some cases it is difficult to make the diagnosis. A careful clinical examination along with radiological studies to rule out skeletal trauma is necessary to identify the problem. Certain disorders may result from chronic overuse and may not have an acute history of injury.

A. Contusions/Hematoma

A contusion is a closed wound in which a ruptured blood vessel has hemorrhaged into the surrounding tissues. The blood may form a hematoma if bleeding is sufficient and has been contained. This may result from blunt external forces or exertional stresses. Symptoms may include swelling, discoloration, and tenderness. Populations at risk are those involved in physical activities, sports, or abusive relationships, and patients who are on anticoagulant therapy or who have a history of clotting disorders.

1. Assessment
  a. Subjective data
    1) History of direct blow to affected area
      a) Object of contact
      b) Onset of swelling, discoloration
      c) Therapies initiated to relieve symptoms
    2) Medical history indicative of easy bruising
      a) Peripheral vascular disease
        (1) Medications (e.g., anticoagulants [warfarin or Coumadin])
        (2) Clotting factor deficiencies
  b. Objective data
    1) Physical examination

        a) Skin discoloration reflecting age of contusion
           (1) Twenty-four to 48 hours after injury: area tender and swollen; ecchymosis may not appear
           (2) Reddish blue or purple color may take up to several days to appear, depending on location of injury, distance of injured blood vessels from skin surface, and amount of bleeding
           (3) Five to 7 days: color begins changing on periphery, proceeding toward center; takes on green tint
           (4) Seven to 10 days: yellow tint
           (5) Ten to 14 days or longer: brown
           (6) Two to 4 weeks: clears
        b) Size
        c) Location
    2) Diagnostic procedures
        a) Radiographs to rule out associated fractures
        b) Clotting studies to rule out bleeding disorder
        c) Complete blood count (CBC) with platelet count to rule out significant blood loss and thrombocytopenia as possible cause of bleeding

2. Analysis: differential nursing diagnosis/collaborative problems
    a. Pain related to injury
    b. Risk for impaired skin integrity related to tissue injury
    c. Physical mobility, impaired related to injury location and pain
    d. Knowledge deficit related to therapeutic regimen

3. Planning/intervention
    a. Rest affected extremity with elevation to minimize bleeding and edema formation
    b. Splint extremity to protect from further injury or iatrogenic injury
    c. Apply cold packs to stimulate vasoconstriction
        1) Use for 20 minutes at a time, four times per day, for the first 48 to 72 hours
        2) Wrap cold pack to protect skin from cold and further injury
    d. Apply pressure dressing to decrease hemorrhage and swelling
    e. Administer analgesics as ordered
    f. Discharge planning and education
        1) Using cold packs
        2) Applying and removing compressive dressing
        3) Evaluating neurovascular function and report changes
        4) Using physical assistive devices (e.g., cane, crutches, walker)
        5) Indications/precautions for prescribed medications
    g. Arrange appropriate follow-up care

4. Expected outcomes/evaluation (see Appendix B)

B. Strains and sprains

    Injuries to the structures around a joint are usually due to excessive stretch or sudden force. This results in pulling on the structures, which causes tears in muscle and/or tendon. A sprain is the stretching, separation, or tear of a supporting ligament; and a strain is the separation or tear of a musculotendinous unit from a bone. Injury may result in pain, inability to weight bear fully, and swelling of the affected area. Sprains and strains are rare in small children whose epiphyseal plates are still open and more vulnerable to forces. Athletes and obese patients resuming physical fitness are at risk for these types of injuries. Both are classified as to the amount of damage.

- First degree: minor tear in the fibers, minimal swelling, minor discomfort, absent or minor ecchymosis
- Second degree: partial tear, joint intact, more severe swelling, visible ecchymosis
- Third degree: complete disruption of ligament; joint may be open; minimal to severe swelling; resultant separation of muscle from muscle, muscle from tendon, or tendon from bone

1. **Assessment**
   a. *Subjective data*
      1) History of present condition
         a) Sudden stretching, twisting, or excessive force to joint (popping sound may be heard or felt)
         b) Pain in joint (ranges from localized to severe and disabling; may be aggravated by movement, muscle tension, weight bearing)
      2) Medical history
         a) Injury, surgery, or problems with joint
         b) Rheumatoid arthritis predisposes to tendon rupture because of associated deformity changes
         c) Steroid injections are associated with tendon rupture; may result from injection within tendon sheath and excessive volume
         d) Current medication
   b. *Objective data*
      1) Physical examination of affected joint
         a) General survey
            (1) Inspection
               (a) General appearance: swelling, deformity, ecchymosis
            (2) Palpation
               (a) Tenderness over affected area
               (b) Swelling; may have associated muscle spasms
            (3) Loss of motor function, ranging from minor to severe
            (4) Alteration in sensation as a result of swelling
   c. *Diagnostic procedures*
      1) Radiograph of joint to rule out associated fracture or dislocation; stress view of joint may aid in detecting ligamentous injury
2. **Analysis: differential nursing diagnosis/collaborative problems**
   a. *Pain related to inflammation and tissue damage*
   b. *Physical mobility, impaired related to pain*
   c. *Tissue perfusion, altered peripheral related to tissue edema*
   d. *Knowledge deficit related to therapeutic regimen*
3. **Planning/interventions**
   The mnemonic RICE may be used to remember therapy for most soft tissue injuries: *R*est, *I*ce, *C*ompression, *E*levation
   a. *Rest affected joint*
      1) Non-weight bearing with crutches
      2) Protect from stress: avoid use
      3) Splint to decrease movement
   b. *Ice*
      1) Apply for 20 minutes at a time: perform range of motion four times per day as early as possible
      2) Repeat regimen four times a day for the first 24 hours
      3) Application of ice promotes vasoconstriction and reduces swelling
   c. *Compression: use elastic bandage to provide support and help reduce swelling*

    d. *Elevation: raise injured part to level of heart during the first 24 hours after injury to reduce swelling*

    e. *Medications as ordered*

       1) Analgesics

       2) Anti-inflammatory agents

    f. *Discharge planning and education*

       1) Resting extremity

       2) Applying cold packs

       3) Applying and removing compression dressing

       4) Elevating injured extremity

       5) Indications/precautions for prescribed medication

    g. *Arrange follow-up care*

4. Expected outcomes/evaluation (see Appendix B)

C. Low back pain

    Low back pain affects up to 60 to 80% of the population at some time. Intervertebral disk disease and disk herniation are common causes of back pain and are most prominent in otherwise healthy people between the ages of 30 and 40 years. Disk degeneration is a normal part of the aging process in all adults. Pain is the primary symptom, which may be localized or radiate. Symptoms vary depending on the specific structure involved. Risk factors include obesity, poor body mechanics, lifting or moving heavy objects, prolonged sitting, poor office furniture design, and floor surfaces. Ninety percent of low back pain is musculoskeletal in nature and yet it never receives a precise diagnosis. Most back pain is benign. The lumbar spinal column provides weight bearing, spinal cord protection, and trunk movement.

1. Assessment

    a. *Subjective data*

       1) History of present illness

          a) Pain (PQRST)

          b) Recent trauma or chronic injury

          c) Time of occurrence:

             (1) Acute, < 7 days

             (2) subacute, 7 days to 7 weeks

             (3) chronic, > 7 weeks

          d) Associated symptoms (e.g., paresthesia, radiation of pain, impaired function of bladder, bowel, or sexual function)

          e) Psychosocial stressors

          f) Success of past therapeutic measures

       2) Medical history

          a) Previous back injury or strain

          b) Obesity

          c) Occupation or profession

          d) Current pregnancy or other gynecological problems, LNMP

          e) Previous treatments, surgeries, medications

          f) Tobacco use; may relate to poor nutritional status and delayed healing

          g) IV drug abuse; may be related to nutritional status and other associated medical problems

          h) Infectious diseases (e.g., tuberculosis, also known as Pott's disease: begins as tuberculous osteomyelitis of the vertebrae and progresses to damage of intervertebral disks)

    b. *Objective data*

       1) Physical assessment

      a) Inspection
        (1) Gait and posture
          (a) Steppage gait (associated with footdrop, usually secondary to lower motor neuron disease)
          (b) Leans to hurt side with knee flexed on that side
          (c) Stiff, rigid trunk
        (2) Abnormal spinal curvature (lordosis, kyphosis, scoliosis)
      b) Palpation
        (1) Point tenderness or general area of tenderness
        (2) Mass (e.g., size, location, quality of firmness)
      c) Spinal range of motion
      d) Deep tendon reflexes (DTRs)
      e) Motor function
        (1) Weakness (toe-heel walk)
        (2) Footdrop (loss of full dorsiflexion)
          (a) Difficulty climbing stairs
      f) Sensory testing
        (1) Sharp-dull discrimination
      g) Rule out other causes
        (1) Rectal examination (e.g., prostate)
        (2) Pelvic examination (e.g., uterine or pelvic inflammatory disease)
        (3) Arterial pulses (i.e., vascular)
        (4) Hip rotation (i.e., orthopedic)
    2) Diagnostic procedures
      a) Radiographs: lumbar, sacral, pelvic films
      b) CT scan
      c) MRI
      d) Myelogram
    3) Laboratory studies
      a) CBC
      b) Erythrocyte sedimentation rate (ESR)
      c) Serum electrolytes
      d) Blood urea nitrogen (BUN)
      e) Urinalysis
      f) Pregnancy test
      g) Liver function tests (LFTs)

2. Analysis: differential nursing diagnosis/collaborative problems

  a. Pain related to muscle spasm and/or inflammation/injury
  b. Physical mobility impaired related to pain
  c. Knowledge deficit: pain management techniques and prevention of recurrence
  d. Anxiety/fear related to cause of back pain and prognosis

3. Planning/intervention

  a. Position of comfort (pelvic tilt may reduce pain)
  b. Application of cold pack for the first 48 to 72 hours
  c. Massage
  d. Maintain bed rest for up to 2 to 3 days
  e. Analgesics
  f. Nonsteroidal anti-inflammatory medications
  g. Instruct on use of physical assistive devices (e.g., walker, braces)
  h. Instruct on methods of proper body mechanics.
  i. Instruct on home safety: install railings; remove loose floor mats
  j. Arrange for appropriate follow-up care

4. Expected outcomes/evaluation (see Appendix B)

D. Overuse/cumulative trauma disorders

Symptoms of overuse are typically due to repetitive and forceful use of the extremities in a work setting or as part of leisure activities. Injuries can be attributed to a multitude of factors, including lack of conditioning, overuse, misuse, and trauma. The repetitive stress produces soft tissue microtears and inflammation. This can lead to tendon inflammation and synovitis, muscle tears (typically at musculotendinous junctions), ligamentous disorders, degenerative joint disease, bursitis, and nerve entrapment.

1. Bursitis

Bursitis is an inflammation of a bursa, or sac, that covers a bony prominence between bones, muscles, and tendons. The bursa contains only a small amount of viscous fluid. The inflammation is the result of trauma (e.g., a direct blow or a chronic injury associated with prolonged, repetitive use) or is due to infection (bacterial or fungal). The more common sites of bursitis are the shoulder, elbow, hip, knee, and heel of the foot. It is important to determine whether the bursitis is due to inflammation or infection, because definitive therapy differs.

a. Assessment

  1) Subjective data

    a) History of present condition

      (1) Recent acute injury

      (2) Recent localized infection

      (3) Repetitive use of area: e.g., participating in vigorous sports; leaning on elbows; kneeling; pressure from shoe rubbing on back of foot

      (4) Pain: may have sudden or gradual onset and may persist for several days and then diminish abruptly or gradually

      (5) Decreased joint range of motion

    b) Medical history: previous/current bursitis, infections, arthritis

  2) Objective data

    a) Inspection

      (1) Redness and warmth over area

      (2) Swelling

      (3) Limited range of motion of extremity

      (4) Increased pain with activity

      (5) Unusually severe pain suggestive of infection

      (6) Shoulder (subacromial): pain at upper humerus and in subacromial area; pain may radiate up to neck and down to fingertips

      (7) Elbow (olecranon): swollen area caused by acute trauma

      (8) Hip (trochanteric): tenderness over greater trochanter; best elicited with patient lying on side with affected hip uppermost and ipsilateral knee slightly flexed

      (9) Knee (prepatellar): does not involve knee joint: localized, fluctuant mass can usually be palpated over anterior aspect of knee; often referred to as "housemaid's knee"

      (10) Heel (posterior calcaneal): inflamed and thickened area at back of heel

    b) Palpation

      (1) Warmth

      (2) Soft or firm area

b. Analysis: differential nursing diagnosis/collaborative problems

  1) Pain related to inflammatory process

  2) Physical mobility, impaired related to increased pain with activity

  3) Anxiety/fear related to unknown diagnosis and/or prognosis

4) Knowledge deficit related to therapeutic regimen
   c. *Planning/interventions*
   1) Rest affected area
      a) Immobilize joint with splint
      b) Use moleskin over heel; wear properly fitting shoes
   2) Apply ice over affected areas during acute stage
   3) Administer medications as ordered
      a) Anti-inflammatory drugs
      b) Analgesics, usually non-narcotic
      c) Steroids
      d) Antibiotics if joint aspirated and infection noted
   4) Discharge planning and education
      a) Using immobilization device (e.g., sling, brace)
      b) Applying cold packs
      c) Applying and removing compressive dressing
      d) Elevating injured extremity
      e) Indications/precautions for prescribed medications
   5) Arrange follow-up care for orthopedic evaluation and possible need for
      a) Bursal injection
      b) Bursal aspiration and possible incision or drainage if infection present
      c) Physical therapy
   d. *Expected outcomes/evaluation* (see Appendix B)

2. **Tendinitis**

   Tendinitis is an inflammation of the tendons and tendon-muscle attachments. Inflammation is due to excessive, unaccustomed repetitive stress. The inflammation may be acute or chronic. Tendinitis commonly occurs in the shoulder (rotator cuff tendinitis), elbow (lateral or medial epicondylitis [also known as tennis elbow]), knee (patellar tendinitis [also known as jumper's knee]), and heel (Achilles tendinitis).
   a. *Assessment*
   1) Subjective data
      a) History of present condition
         (1) Repetitive motions with affected extremity
         (2) Prolonged use of area, such as leaning on elbow while seated at desk
         (3) Localized pain described as deep ache; typically becomes worse with motion
      b) Medical history of tendinitis
   2) Objective data
      a) Physical examination
         (1) Swelling
         (2) Tenderness with pressure applied in rolling motion over tendon
      b) Diagnostic procedures: radiographs to identify whether calcification has occurred; because tendons are less vascular than other structures, tendinitis can lead to calcific deposits
   b. *Analysis: differential nursing diagnosis/collaborative problems*
   1) Pain related to inflammatory process
   2) Physical mobility, impaired related to swelling and pain with movement
   3) Anxiety/fear related to pain and unknown diagnosis or prognosis
   4) Knowledge deficit related to therapeutic regimen
   c. *Planning/interventions*
   1) Rest by avoiding use
   2) Apply cold pack to relieve pain and swelling

  3) Apply compressive dressing to support joint
  4) Elevate to decrease swelling
  5) Administer medications, as ordered
     a) Non-narcotic analgesics
     b) Anti-inflammatory agents
  6) Provide discharge planning and education
     a) Using immobilization device to rest affected area
     b) Applying and removing compressive dressing twice daily
     c) Using and applying cold compress
     d) Elevating injured extremity
     e) Indications/precautions for prescribed medications
  7) Arrange for follow-up care
     a) Orthopedic evaluation
     b) Physical therapy
  d. *Expected outcomes/evaluation* (see Appendix B)

3. Nerve entrapment syndromes

The nerve entrapment syndromes result from compression of a peripheral nerve as it traverses a closed compartment. Other structures are contained within the compartment that can swell and compress nerve fibers. This tends to occur in the arm. The median nerve is involved in the pronator syndrome (entrapment at the forearm) and the carpal tunnel syndrome (entrapment at the wrist). The ulnar nerve is involved in the cubital tunnel syndrome (entrapment at the elbow). Tarsal tunnel syndrome involves compression of the medial tibial nerve at the medial malleolus. Greater than 80% of patients are older than 40 years at diagnosis. Nerve entrapment syndromes occur twice as frequently in women as men. Pregnant women are at risk for carpal tunnel syndrome. Patients involved in repetitive actions are prone to nerve entrapment syndromes.

  a. *Assessment*
  1) Subjective data
     a) History of present condition
        (1) Overuse risk factors
        (2) Pain in muscle group, joint, or tendon or along distribution of affected nerve
        (3) Paresthesia, tingling, numbness
        (4) Pregnancy
     b) Medical history
        (1) Rheumatoid arthritis
        (2) Arthritis (degenerative)
        (3) Growth hormone abnormality (acromegaly)
        (4) Metabolic disorders (e.g., hypothyroidism, gout, diabetes mellitus)
        (5) Alcoholism
        (6) Tumors
        (7) Connective tissue disorders (e.g., amyloidosis, hemochromatosis)
  2) Objective data
     a) Physical examination
        (1) Soft tissue swelling
        (2) Possible atrophy in surrounding muscles (thenar eminence)
        (3) Muscle weakness (musculus opponens pollicus, which opposes thumb to fifth finger)
     b) Diagnostic procedures
        (1) Tinel's sign (sensation of tingling felt in distal extremity when injured nerve is percussed)
        (2) Phalen's test (acute flexion of wrist for 1 minute causes exacerbation

of paresthesia along distribution of median nerve; diagnostic of carpal tunnel syndrome)

(3) Electromyography to identify muscle disease or defects in transmission of electrical impulses across anatomical areas

b. *Analysis: differential nursing diagnosis/collaborative problems*

1) Pain related to entrapment of nerves

2) Anxiety/fear related to symptoms and unknown diagnosis or prognosis

3) Knowledge deficit related to therapeutic regimen

c. *Planning/interventions*

1) Rest by immobilizing affected area (use of cock-up splint, especially at night)

2) Apply ice if swelling present

3) Elevate if swelling present

4) Administer anti-inflammatory medications as ordered

5) Provide discharge planning and education

a) Resting affected area with immobilization device

b) Applying cold packs

c) Applying and removing compressive dressing

d) Elevating affected area

e) Indications/precautions for prescribed medications

6) Arrange orthopedic referral for follow-up care

d. *Expected outcomes/evaluation* (see Appendix B)

III. SPECIFIC EMERGENCIES OF BONY SKELETON

Certain fractures and virtually all dislocations constitute an emergency in the sense that they are a threat to a person's life or limb.

A. Dislocations

A dislocation occurs when the articular surfaces of bones forming a joint are no longer in contact and lose their anatomical position. Bone ends may move because of congenital weakness, diseases that affect the articular and periarticular structures, and associated trauma. Dislocations are considered an emergency because of the danger of injury to adjacent nerves and blood vessels in the form of compression, stretching, or ischemia. Dislocations are described in terms of the distal segment in relation to the proximal segment (e.g., anterior or posterior dislocation). Joint subluxations occur when some articular surface contact remains but is not complete. A person with a suspected or known orthopedic injury should be carefully assessed for both fracture and dislocation. If either one is suspected, the limb should be splinted, a neurovascular examination performed, radiographic examination completed for confirmation of diagnosis, and then the injury reduced as soon as possible. Table 16–3 discusses specific findings and treatment of various dislocations.

1. **Assessment**

a. *Subjective data*

1) History of present condition

a) Report of significant force that corresponds to type of dislocation observed

(1) If absent, suspect pre-existing condition

(2) If caused by trauma, look for additional injuries

b) Symptoms since dislocation

(1) Intense pain

Table 16–3 COMMON DISLOCATIONS

Body Area	Typical Mechanism of Injury	Clinical Findings	Treatment
Shoulder			
Anterior	Fall on outstretched arm or direct impact on shoulder	Arm abducted, cannot bring elbow down to chest or touch opposite ear with hand	Splint in position of comfort; reduce as soon as possible
Posterior	Rare; strong blow in front of shoulder; with violent convulsions or seizures	Arm held at side, unable to externally rotate	As above
Elbow—radius and ulna	Fall on outstretched hand with elbow in extension	Loss of arm length, painful motion, and rapid swelling; nerve lesions may occur	As above Surgical repair if dislocation is associated with fracture to radial head or olecranon
Radius—head (children)	Pulled, or nursemaid's, elbow caused by sudden pull, jerk, or lift on child's wrist or hand	Pain, refusal to use arm; limited supination; can flex and extend at elbow; may have no deformity	Reduce, place in sling; advise parents that this may recur until age 5 years
Hip—usually posterior	Blow to knee while hip is flexed and adducted (sitting with crossed knees); common in passengers seated in front seat	Hip flexed, adducted, internally rotated, and shortened; may have associated fracture of femur; sciatic nerve injury (lies posterior)	Splint in position of comfort; reduce as soon as possible
Patella	May be spontaneous	Knee flexed; can palpate patella lateral to femoral condyle	Reduce (may occur spontaneously), immobilize with cast or splint
	Associated with other trauma	Excessive swelling, tenderness, and palpable soft tissue defect	Surgical repair of soft tissue injury or fractures
Knee (rare)	Direct severe blow to upper leg or forced hyperextension of knee	Ligamentous instability (requires disruption of structures); inability to straighten leg; peroneal nerve and popliteal artery injury common—must assess distal neurovascular function	Immediate neurovascular assessment; reduce
Ankle	Ankle is complex joint, with multiple ligaments providing stability; dislocation is usually associated with other injury such as fracture and soft tissue trauma	Swelling, tenderness, and loss of alignment and function	Splint; usually necessitates open reduction, because this joint has complex motion and must have accurate alignment

            (2) Neurovascular compromise: paresthesia, hypesthesia, numbness, inability to move because of paralysis or patient's resistance to use

        c) Initial treatment

            (1) Immobilization techniques

            (2) Attempts to reduce

            (3) Use of ice or compressive dressing

            (4) Medications used

    2) Medical history

        a) Previous injury or surgery, especially joint replacement, in affected joint

        b) Previous dislocation of affected joint, if any

  b. Objective data

    1) Physical examination

        a) Inspection

            (1) Obvious deformity in affected joint

                (a) Discrepancy in extremity lengths

                (b) Abnormal position: rotation (internal or external) or alignment (angulated)

                (c) Color

            (2) Loss of mobility as a result of

                (a) Dislocated bones

                (b) Paralysis

        b) Palpation

            (1) Tenderness

            (2) Deformity

            (3) Pulses

                (a) Arterial compromise: local pulses may be difficult to palpate because of swelling; Doppler pulses may be present; arterial flow should return after reduction is completed; if insufficiency remains, vascular injury must be ruled out

                (b) Venous obstruction

                (c) Delayed capillary refill time ($<$ 2 seconds is normal)

                (d) Temperature

            (4) Range of motion: active and passive testing

            (5) Motor strength testing using scale ranging from 1 to 5

            (6) Neurological exam: paresthesia, numbness, paralysis

    2) Diagnostic procedures

        a) Immediate radiographs to verify dislocation and identify associated fractures

        b) Vascular studies, as indicated by physical examination findings and history

2. Analysis: differential nursing diagnosis/collaborative problems

  a. Pain related to neurovascular compressive forces and dislocation

  b. Physical mobility, impaired related to dislocation and pain

  c. Risk for injury: peripheral neurovascular dysfunction related to dislocation, nerve injury, or vascular injury or swelling

  d. Anxiety related to pain, treatment methods, and lifestyle implications

  e. Knowledge deficit related to therapeutic regimen and self-care

3. Planning/intervention

  a. Determine distal neurovascular function

  b. Immobilize joint to prevent further injury and help relieve pain. Reassess neurovascular status

  c. Elevate joint

  d. Apply ice to reduce swelling

    e. Prepare for immediate reduction
       1) Informed consent, as necessary
       2) Analgesia and sedation (e.g., conscious sedation)
       3) Needed equipment and personnel
       4) Postreduction immobilization devices
       5) Documentation of distal neurovascular function before and after reduction
       6) Radiographs before and after reduction
    f. Provide discharge planning and education
       1) Maintaining immobilization for prescribed time frame
       2) Applying cold packs
       3) Performing neurovascular assessment and reporting changes
       4) Indications/precautions for prescribed medications
    g. Arrange for follow-up care or admission to hospital for pain management, surgical intervention, physical assistive device training
  4. Expected outcomes/evaluation (see Appendix B)

B. Fractures

    A fracture is defined as a break in the continuity of a bone. The break may result from application of repetitive action or a significant force to the bone or may occur as a consequence of an everyday force being applied to a bone that has been weakened by a pre-existing pathological process (i.e., pathological fracture). Fractures may be classified as closed or open (also known as compound). Trauma constitutes the major cause of fractures. Mechanisms of injury include motor vehicle crashes, motor pedestrian collisions, motorcycle collisions, falls, and sports. Open fractures place the patient at risk for wound contamination, infection, and periosteal stripping, which may lead to devascularization of the bone. Crush injuries are of special concern because of the extensive damage to surrounding soft tissues and degree of fracture comminution. Children are at less risk for fractures because of the elasticity of their skeletal structure. The elderly are more prone to fractures because of bone structure changes associated with the natural aging process and metastatic diseases. The goal in treating fractures is to restore bone alignment and function and reduce disability. Table 16–4 provides a description of fractures.

  1. General considerations
    a. Appearance or angulation of break on radiograph (Fig. 16–1)
       1) Transverse
       2) Oblique
       3) Spiral
       4) Comminuted (multiple splintered bone fragments)
       5) Avulsion (fragment of bone connected to ligament breaks off from rest of bone)
       6) Impacted (fracture involves bone end driven firmly into another bone end)
       7) Torus (usually seen in children; a buckling of bone surface)
       8) Compression (bone deformed by compression, usually vertebrae)
       9) Greenstick (usually seen in children; involves partial thickness of bone)
       10) Epiphyseal fracture (described according to Salter-Harris classification)
    b. Soft tissue disruption
       1) Closed fracture (simple fracture) does not have skin disruption
       2) Open fracture (compound) with skin disruption caused by
          a) Force that produces fracture also causes skin laceration (e.g., gunshot wound)
          b) Fracture segments puncture skin

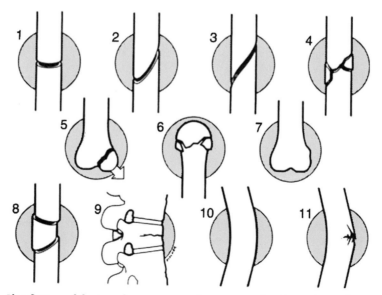

FIGURE 16–1. Classification of fractures by appearance: *1,* transverse; *2,* oblique; *3,* spiral; *4,* comminuted; *5,* avulsion; *6,* impacted; *7,* torus; *8,* segmented; *9,* compression; *10,* bending; *11,* greenstick. (With permission from American College of Surgeons, Committee on Trauma. [1982]. *Early care of the injured patient* [3rd ed., p. 283]. Philadelphia: W. B. Saunders.)

      c) External objects involved in trauma cause skin disruption

2. **Assessment**

   a. *Subjective data*

     1) History of present condition

       a) Mechanism of injury and estimate of force (e.g., distance of fall, how patient fell, landing surface)

       b) Direction in which force was applied

       c) Position in which patient was found

       d) Pain; may be referred, usually distal

       e) Associated injuries (e.g., head, chest, abdomen)

       f) Limited range of motion of affected extremity

       g) Alcohol or drug use

     2) Medical history

       a) Previous injury or surgery in affected extremity

       b) Current medications

       c) Chronic diseases or conditions (e.g., diabetes mellitus, immunosuppressive disorders)

       d) Nutritional status

       e) Use of tobacco products, especially in calcaneal fractures

       f) Tetanus immunization status, if break in skin integrity

       g) Corticosteroid use will cause delay in healing and mask symptoms

   b. *Objective data*

     1) Physical examination: general trauma assessment should be performed after primary and secondary surveys to identify all injuries and implement necessary interventions; examination of fracture or most painful area should follow assessment of rest of body because muscle spasms and pain may obscure other findings; repeated physical assessments should be completed after fracture pain has been relieved to be sure that complications or other injuries have not been overlooked

       a) Inspection

Table 16–4 COMMON FRACTURES

Bone	Typical Mechanism of Injury	Clinical Findings*	Treatment*
Humerus			
Neck	Fall on outstretched arm (may occur with dislocated shoulder)	Ecchymosis of shoulder, upper arm, and chest wall	Immobilize with sling, may splint or internally reduce if severe
Shaft	Direct trauma, twisting of arm	Radial nerve injury often occurs with fracture of lower third of bone	Immobilize with sling, use hanging arm cast if able to be mobile
Supracondylar	Fall on extended, outstretched arm (usually occurs in children)	Rapid swelling of elbow; pain	Admit to hospital for close neurovascular observation and definitive care
Radius			
Head	Fall on outstretched arm	Swelling; pain on lateral side of elbow; decreased range of motion in elbow; may have associated wrist injury	Immobilize; treatment varies according to range of motion and association with dislocated elbow
Shaft	Usually occurs with falls, altercations, and motor vehicle crash	Pain along bone (bones are mostly subcutaneous, therefore easy to palpate)	Splint for comfort (tight muscular compartments and interosseous membrane provide stabilization against movement)
Distal	Colles' fracture (angulated dorsally)—fall on outstretched hand	Distal fragment is deviated dorsally ("silver fork")	Immobilize with splint; reduce if displaced, cast
	Smith's fracture (angulated toward volar surface)—fall onto dorsum of hand	Reverse of Colles' fracture	
Radius—Galeazzi's fracture	Oblique fracture at junction of middle and distal thirds of radius with disruption of distal radioulnar joint—fall or blow on dorsal and lateral side of wrist and distal radius (commonly occurs in adults)	Wrist and radial shaft tenderness and shortening	Usually unstable; needs open reduction
Ulnar			
Monteggia's fracture	Fracture of proximal third of ulna with anterior dislocation of radial head	Pain and swelling around elbow, pain worse with attempts at rotation; radial dislocation may be missed if elbow not included in radiograph	Immobilize for comfort; closed reduction for children, open for adults
Nightstick fracture	Isolated fracture of midshaft of ulna as result of sharp blow	If ulna is angulated, injury to radius is also present	Immobilize; these fractures require 8 to 16 weeks to heal
Wrist—carpus (navicular)	Usually occurs with falls on outstretched hand or direct blow; common in young men whose strong muscles prevent injury to lower radius (navicular is longest of carpal bones)	Pain in wrist, most severe in anatomical snuff-box; swelling; radiographs should include oblique view	Immobilize; cast for at least 3 months to be sure fracture has reunited

Site	Cause/Mechanism	Clinical Findings	Treatment
Pelvis	Low velocity—elderly people; high velocity—all age groups (motor vehicle crashes, falls, and crushing forces)	Hypovolemia—retroperitoneal space can hold 4 L of blood; associated with multisystem trauma, especially genitourinary; tenderness with ilial wing compression or palpation of symphysis; ecchymosis (late sign) in flank and peritoneal area	Splint to immobilize; begin fluid resuscitation, using caution as needed (e.g., if urinary catheter is part of routine care, must assess for further injury); admit for observation and care
Femur			
Head or neck (intracapsular)	Caused by fall or spontaneous break (osteoporosis)	Pain in hip or referred to knee; leg shortened and externally rotated	Splint for comfort; surgical repair
Trochanter (extracapsular)	As above	Has greater blood supply; therefore, blood loss is heavier	As above
Shaft	Associated with high force	Powerful muscle groups cause angulation and over-riding to produce deformity; severe pain; blood loss into tissue and from intravascular volume	Traction splint; admit for definitive care
Tibia			
Plateau (extends into knee joint)	Fall on extended leg, direct blow; rotation stress on extended leg (in pedestrians)	If radiographs are questionable or normal, may aspirate joint; usually associated with soft tissue injuries	Splint for comfort, compressive dressing; refer to orthopedist for definitive care
Shaft	Direct trauma—its position at distal end of leg exposes it to more trauma (e.g., car bumper); or rotation and leverage strain (as with stepping into deep hole while running) Open fractures more common because bone is subcutaneous on its anterior or medial surfaces	Associated with fractures in rest of body (ipsilateral extremity or elsewhere); must determine whether fibula is also fractured, because it acts as splint if intact Prone to complications: 1. Increased incidence of compartment syndrome (tibia borders three of four myofascial compartments of lower leg) 2. Arterial injuries common with fractures of upper third	Splint for comfort; refer to specialist for evaluation and definitive care
Fibula			
Proximal	Direct blow to side of leg	May have concomitant peroneal nerve injury	Splint, until diagnosis made, then crutches
Distal 2 inches	As above	Associated with ankle injuries	As above
Shaft	As above	Considered minor	As above, symptomatic care
Ankle	See discussion of ankle dislocations (Table 16–3)	Sprained ankles in children are uncommon—should be evaluated for Salter-Harris I fracture	See Table 16–3.

*Clinical findings and treatments listed here are in addition to general ones.

(1) Deformity, angulation of bony structures; compare with opposite extremity
(2) Swelling, pallor
(3) Pain with palpation
(4) Muscle spasm may be felt or seen
(5) Integrity of skin (e.g., abrasions, contusions, open wounds)
(6) Open fractures
    (a) Obvious skin wound with or without bone fragment present
    (b) Size of wound opening
    (c) Presence of contamination
    (d) Drainage from wound
  b) Palpation
    (1) Abnormal mobility at or between joints
    (2) Crepitus (grating sensation occurring as broken bone ends rub together); should never be deliberately produced
    (3) Joints above and below painful area should be assessed because referral of pain may mislead examiner
    (4) Vascular examination: assess pulses proximal and distal to fracture and compare with opposite extremity
    (5) Neurological examination: assess for sensation, motor strength
  c) Immobilization devices should be checked to be sure they are adequate and have not caused constriction or excessive pressure
  d) Neurovascular status should be checked before and after each intervention and at regular intervals after care has been completed
2) Diagnostic procedures
  a) General principles of radiography
    (1) Should use at least two views 90 degrees to each other
    (2) Joints above and below fracture must be seen, preferably on same film
    (3) Children should have comparison views with opposite extremity to evaluate epiphyseal configuration
    (4) Pelvis should be included if major lower limb injuries are present
    (5) Gas (air) may be evident with open fractures in soft tissue planes
  b) Special studies may be needed to view fracture or diagnose complication
    (1) Stress views
    (2) CT scan
    (3) Angiography
    (4) MRI

3. **Analysis: differential nursing diagnosis/collaborative problems**
  a. Tissue perfusion, altered peripheral related to edema and possible vascular injury
  b. Fluid volume deficit related to blood loss
  c. Pain related to injury, swelling, possible nerve injury, or ischemia
  d. Risk for injury: peripheral neurovascular function related to fracture, nerve injury, or blood vessel involvement or swelling
  e. Skin integrity, impaired related to soft tissue injury or open fracture
  f. Risk for infection related to open fracture and impaired skin integrity
  g. Physical mobility, impaired related to pain and therapeutic plan
  h. Anxiety/fear related to pain, injury, and lifestyle implications

4. **Planning/intervention**
  a. Immobilization: early use of splints, especially traction, can significantly reduce pain and swelling

b. *Splint fracture in position found unless circumstances warrant movement (e.g., inability to transport patient "as is" and pulseless distal extremity)*

c. *Military antishock trousers (MAST) suit may be used to immobilize fractures, but they need to be monitored closely for circulatory compromise*

d. *Immobilize joints above and below injury when possible to prevent further injury*

e. *Splints should be rigid and well padded and allow radiographical penetration*

f. *Establish IV access to provide volume replacement to maintain hemodynamic stability and for administration of analgesics and sedation*

g. *Elevate to decrease swelling*

h. *Apply cold packs to decrease swelling*

i. *If open fracture is present, goal is to prevent infection*

    1) Administer IV antibiotics, as ordered

    2) Cover wound with sterile saline dressings

    3) Administer tetanus prophylaxis as indicated

    4) Prepare for surgical debridement

    5) If surgical debridement is delayed, wound usually flushed with 1 to 2 L normal saline and dry, sterile dressing is applied

    6) Avoid use of bacteriostatic cleaning solutions in wound (inhibits wound healing)

j. *If closed reduction is performed in emergency department*

    1) Obtain special procedure permit if needed

    2) Administer anesthetic as ordered (e.g., conscious sedation)

    3) Monitor patient carefully during and after procedure, because patient may require large dose of medication for reduction and then become obtunded after pain is relieved

    4) If IV regional anesthesia is used, monitor tourniquet time and effectiveness every 5 minutes

    5) Assemble needed equipment and personnel

    6) Immobilize after reduction

k. *Administer pain medications as ordered; report if analgesia not reducing pain level*

l. *Provide discharge planning and education*

    1) Performing cast care

    2) Performing neurovascular assessment and changes to report

    3) Applying cold packs

    4) Elevating affected extremity

    5) Training with physical assistive devices (walker, crutches, three-dimensional boot)

    6) Using support devices (e.g., sling, knee immobilization device)

m. *Arrange follow-up orthopedic care*

5. Expected outcomes/evaluation (see Appendix B)

C. Traumatic amputations

The loss of a body part presents a serious challenge to all involved in the patient's care. It is important to remain focused on the identification of life-threatening injuries and not to be distracted on the limb-threatening injuries during all phases of the resuscitation. The injury may occur alone or may be combined with other trauma as a result of tearing, crushing, or lacerating forces. The amputated part may or may not be reimplantable. The eventual outcome of the case depends on multiple factors. Factors decreasing the success of the outcome include excessive bacterial contamination, prolonged period of time between the injury and the institution of cooling (> 6 hours in the proximal arm or leg or > 12 hours in distal extremities), and severe degloving or avulsing. Children tend to have better success with replantation than adults.

1. **Assessment**
   a. *Subjective data*
      1) History of amputating force
         a) Mechanism of injury: object or agent causing amputation
            (1) Laceration that produces a straight-edged ("guillotine") cut has greatest potential for successful replantation
            (2) Crush injuries are associated with extensive soft tissue damage, which decreases chances for successful replantation
            (3) Avulsion injuries are associated with forceful stretching and tearing of tissue, making soft tissue damage more widespread, both distally and proximally
         b) Time of injury
      2) Patient's overall condition and needs
         a) Age: patients older than 50 years generally have more advanced vascular degenerative changes, which interfere with healing
         b) Occupation
            (1) Type of occupational protective devices normally used or worn during work
            (2) Body part is evaluated to determine whether, after replantation, it will be functional or a hindrance (especially if it has limited motor or sensory function)
            (3) Replantation involves lengthy hospitalization and rehabilitation; person's ability to be away from work or home is considered in overall decision making about replantation
         c) Emotional status
            (1) Ability to cooperate and tolerate long recovery and rehabilitation
            (2) Ability to withstand degree of pain and disability with replanted part
      3) Medical history
         a) Cigarette smoking: nicotine is potent vasoconstrictor and decreases healing; patient is generally advised to abstain from smoking
         b) Chronic illnesses that influence outcome
            (1) Peripheral vascular health
            (2) Bleeding disorders
            (3) Patient's general health and ability to withstand prolonged use of anesthesia
         c) Allergies
         d) Tetanus immunization status
         e) Hand dominance, when applicable
   b. *Objective data*
      1) Physical examination
         a) Patient
            (1) General survey: if patient has sustained multiple injuries, replantation may not be considered because of potential or actual hemodynamic instability and inability to withstand lengthy surgical procedure
            (2) Stump: viability of blood vessels, nerves, other tissue
            (3) Amount and type of contamination
            (4) Estimate of blood loss
         b) Amputated part

        (1) Absolute contraindications for replantation

           (a) Significant life-threatening injuries

           (b) Extensive damage to soft tissue injury (e.g., degloving, crush, or mangled part)

           (c) Inappropriate handling (e.g., storage in formalin, preservative)

        (2) Relative contraindications for replantation

           (a) Avulsion injury

           (b) Ischemia time (time from injury) greater than 4 to 6 hours if not cooled (warm ischemia time) and greater than 18 hours if cooled (cool ischemia time)

           (c) Amount and type of contaminants (difficult to debride and susceptibility to life-threatening infections)

           (d) Previous surgery or injury to part that complicates healing

        (3) Thumb and multiple digits are carefully evaluated because they are high priority for replantation

    2) Diagnostic procedures: radiograph of stump and amputated part

2. Analysis: differential nursing diagnosis/collaborative problems

    a. Peripheral tissue, altered peripheral related to injury and amputation

    b. Pain related to laceration and tissue damage

    c. Impaired skin integrity related to effects of injury

    d. Risk for infection related to open wound, interrupted perfusion, and possible contamination

    e. Anxiety/fear related to loss of productiveness, change in lifestyle

3. Planning/intervention

    a. For patient

    1) Control hemorrhage without causing further tissue damage

        a) Apply direct pressure and pressure dressing

        b) Do not use tourniquet and clamps unless bleeding absolutely cannot be controlled; blood pressure cuff can be applied approximately 30 mm Hg higher than systolic pressure

    2) Splint and slightly elevate injured extremity

    3) Do not manipulate distal part if partially attached because this may potentiate injury

    4) Patient should have nothing by mouth in preparation for impending surgery

    5) Clean skin around stump with copious amounts of saline to remove contaminants; do not use other solutions because they may cause cellular damage

    6) Administer medications as directed

        a) Tetanus prophylaxis

        b) Antibiotics

        c) Medications recommended by replantation center

    7) Keep patient informed and include in decision making

    8) Allow or encourage patient and family to verbalize feelings and fears; provide psychosocial support

    b. For amputated part

    1) Gently lift off contaminants; do not rub or clean with soap, water, or antiseptic solution

    2) Wrap in sterile gauze

    3) Moisten wrap with sterile normal saline or lactated Ringer's solution: do not soak, wrap in, or use any type of water

        a) Place wrapped part in plastic bag, and seal securely to prevent entry of water from ice bath used during transportation

      b) Place sealed bag in ice; do not allow uncovered part to come in direct contact with ice; do not freeze, which causes further cellular damage

4. Expected outcomes/evaluation (see Appendix B)

D. Joint effusions

      Joint effusions involve the collection of fluid in a joint as a result of an inflammatory process, previous surgery, or trauma. Effusions commonly occur in the knee joint. An extreme stretching of the knee ligaments may result in microscopic tears of the meniscus, resulting in synovial fluid collection. Patients with prior knee surgery and traumatic injuries to the area are at risk for joint effusions. Patients with hemophilia who sustain minimal blunt force to the knees are at risk for hemarthrosis (blood collection in the joint space).

1. Assessment
    a. *Subjective data*
      1) History of present condition
        a) History of recent or past trauma
        b) Joint involved, isolated or multiple
        c) Recent surgical procedure
        d) Recent infection
        e) Substance abuse, risk of septic arthritis
        f) Medication usage (e.g., diuretics are associated with hyperuricemia, which may lead to gouty arthritis)
        g) Repetitive use of joint
        h) Onset and speed of fluid accumulation
        i) Inability to weight bear fully
        j) Fevers, chills
      2) Medical history
        a) Arthritis
        b) Gout
        c) Knee surgery
        d) Infectious processes
        e) Sexually transmitted disease
        f) Bleeding disorders
    b. *Objective data*
      1) Physical examination
        a) Inspection
          (1) Pain
          (2) Swelling
          (3) Redness
          (4) Skin changes
        b) Palpation
          (1) Tenderness
          (2) Limited range of motion
      2) Diagnostic procedures
        a) Radiographs of joint; comparison to other extremity
        b) Joint aspiration
        c) Laboratory tests: CBC, ESR, urine analysis, Venereal Disease Research Laboratories (VDRL), hepatitis B-, C-reactive protein

2. Analysis: differential nursing diagnosis/collaborative problems
    a. *Pain related to inflammatory process*
    b. *Alteration in physical mobility related to pain and swelling*
    c. *Knowledge deficit related to treatment regimen*

3. **Planning/interventions**
   a. *Immobilize affected joint*
   b. *Administer medications as ordered*
      1) Analgesics
      2) Steroids
      3) Anti-inflammatory drugs
      4) Antibiotics
   c. *Prepare and assist patient with radiographs*
   d. *Prepare and assist with arthrocentesis*
      1) Differentiates between hemarthrosis, and infectious/inflammatory processes
      2) White blood cell count: 20,000 to 60,000 associated with inflammatory process, 100,000 associated with infection
   e. *Instruct on self-care measures at home*
   f. *Instruct on specific signs and symptoms indicating a need for medical re-evaluation*
   g. *Facilitate completion of paperwork for employment release*
4. **Expected outcomes/evaluation** (see Appendix B)

E. Costochondritis

Costochondritis is an acute, self-limiting inflammation of the rib and sternal junction and may involve one or several junctions. Inflammation may be due to physical exertion or repetitive movements. Pain in this region is similar to that of a rib fracture or myocardial infarction. A patient presenting with chest pain who is at risk for myocardial ischemia must have a thorough cardiac evaluation before assuming the symptoms are musculoskeletal in origin. Costochondritis is most commonly seen in people older than 20 years.

1. **Assessment**
   a. *Subjective data*
      1) History of presenting condition
         a) Pain: onset, location, duration, radiation or referred
         b) Characteristics: described as sharp, pleuritic, unilateral, peristernal
         c) Factors that worsen or alleviate symptoms (e.g., movement, deep inspiration)
         d) Medications
      2) Medical history
         a) Injury, surgery
         b) Medical history: cardiac, inflammatory processes
         c) Infections: recent upper respiratory tract infection
   b. *Objective data*
      1) Physical examination of chest
         a) Inspect skin for swelling, ecchymosis, deformity
         b) Pain that is reproducible (e.g., point tenderness to palpation, pain on deep inspiration, movement of upper extremities, coughing)
      2) Diagnostic procedures
         a) Radiographs to rule out other chest trauma
         b) Laboratory studies: infection indexes (ESR, C-reactive protein, white blood cell)
         c) ECG to rule out cardiac pathology
2. **Analysis: differential nursing diagnosis/collaborative problems**
   a. *Pain related to inflammatory process*
   b. *Ineffective breathing pattern related to pain*

> *c. Anxiety/fear related to unknown origin of chest pain*

3. **Planning/intervention**

   a. Rest

   b. Encourage deep breathing to prevent respiratory complications

   c. Medications as ordered

   d. Analgesics

   e. Anti-inflammatory medications

   f. Instruct patient to avoid exertional activities that exacerbate symptoms

   g. Instruct patient to report any increased symptoms

   h. Follow-up care arrangements/instructions

4. **Expected outcomes/evaluation** (see Appendix B)

IV. SPECIFIC LIFE-THREATENING COMPLICATIONS ASSOCIATED WITH ORTHOPEDIC INJURIES

A. Hemorrhage from fractures

The blood loss associated with fractures ranges from mild to severe or life threatening. It may be visible (e.g., in open fractures) or concealed, except for signs of soft tissue swelling, and may continue for 24 to 72 hours after injury. Table 16–5 lists approximate blood loss associated with each type of fracture. If the patient is already hypovolemic from other causes or prone to bleeding because of clotting dysfunction, the magnitude of the blood loss may be greater.

1. **Assessment**

   a. Subjective data

   1) History of fracture

   2) Medical history: potential for increased blood loss

      a) Bleeding disorders

      b) Anemia

      c) Alcohol use, acute or chronic

      d) Medications, steroid use, anticoagulants

   3) Hypothermia, environmental factors

   b. Objective data

   1) Physical examination

      a) Length and circumference of injured extremity can be compared with those of uninjured side to estimate volume lost into soft tissue (Fig. 16–2)

Table 16–5   ESTIMATED LOCAL BLOOD LOSS IN FRACTURES

Body Area	Volume Loss (L)
Humerus	1.0–2.0
Elbow	0.5–1.5
Forearm	0.5–1.0
Pelvis	1.5–4.5
Hip	1.5–2.5
Femur	1.0–2.0
Knee	1.0–1.5
Tibia	0.5–1.5
Ankle	0.5–1.5

With permission from American College of Surgeons, Committee on Trauma. (1982). *Early care of the injured patient* (3rd ed., p. 284). Philadelphia, W. B. Saunders.

FIGURE 16–2. Injured thigh considered as a cylinder for computational purposes: change in volume (= blood loss) corresponding to changes in radius. (With permission from Trunkey, D. D., Sheldon G. F., & Collins, J. A. [1985]. The treatment of shock. In G. D. Zuidema, R. B. Rutherford, & W. F. Ballinger [Eds.], *The management of trauma* [4th ed., p. 106]. Philadelphia: W. B. Saunders.)

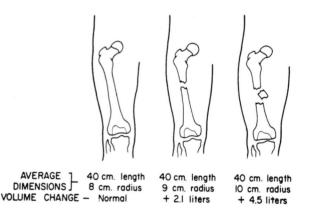

AVERAGE DIMENSIONS	40 cm. length 8 cm. radius	40 cm. length 9 cm. radius	40 cm. length 10 cm. radius
VOLUME CHANGE —	Normal	+ 2.1 liters	+ 4.5 liters

b) Vascular examination of extremity and comparison to unaffected extremity

   2) Diagnostic procedures (see Chapter 17)

2. Analysis: differential diagnosis/collaborative problems (see Chapter 19)

3. Planning/interventions (see Chapter 17)

  a. Maintain airway, breathing, circulation

  b. Supplemental oxygen

  c. Initiate IV

  d. Immobilize to decrease blood loss

  e. Application of pneumatic antishock garment in cases of severe pelvic fractures, although use of device remains controversial

  f. Elevate to decrease blood loss

  g. Apply ice to encourage vasospasm and constriction

4. Expected outcomes/evaluation (see Appendix B)

B. Fat embolism syndrome

After a fracture or bone surgery, small fat globules may appear in the blood. The origin of the fat is unknown, but it is theorized to result either from the fracture site or from an alteration of lipid stability associated with the stress of trauma. The fat globules can circulate, causing occlusion of blood vessels to the brain, kidney, lungs, or other organs. Patients who have long bone fractures and pelvic fractures are at risk for fat embolism syndrome, which commonly occurs within 24 to 48 hours after injury. The incidence of fat emboli in long bone fractures is approximately 0.5 to 2%, and up to 5 to 10% in multiple fractures associated with pelvic injury. Fat embolism syndrome is a major cause of morbidity and mortality after musculoskeletal trauma.

1. Assessment

  a. Subjective data

    1) History of present condition

      a) Fracture or surgery of long bone 24 to 72 hours before onset of symptoms (usually lower extremity fracture and pelvis)

      b) Most common in patients with multiple injuries and those with long bone fractures

    2) Chief complaint

      a) Tachypnea

      b) Tachycardia

      c) Hypoxemia

      d) Fever (38 to 40°C or 101.4 to 104°F)

e) Petechiae (occur in 50–60% of patients; found over chest, axillae, conjunctiva)

f) Alteration in mental status (lethargy, restlessness, confusion, seizures, coma)

  b. *Objective data*

   1) Physical examination

    a) Respiratory system

     (1) Tachypnea

     (2) Hemoptysis

     (3) Cough

     (4) Crackles

     (5) Cyanosis

    b) Cerebral function

     (1) Unusual behavior (e.g., restlessness, disorientation, delirium, abusiveness)

     (2) Syncope

     (3) Altered level of consciousness

    c) Renal function

     (1) Hematuria

     (2) Oliguria

    d) Fever (100.4–104°F [38–40°C])

    e) Petechiae in buccal membranes, conjunctival sac; over chest, neck, shoulders; in anterior axillary folds

   2) Diagnostic procedures

    a) Chest radiograph

     (1) Initially appears normal

     (2) Progresses to bilateral diffuse haziness and interstitial edema (inflammatory response to fat microemboli)

     (3) Changes occur late and in only approximately one third of patients with fat embolism syndrome

    b) Electrocardiogram reveals right-sided heart strain

    c) Arterial blood gas values

     (1) Hypoxemia (arterial partial pressure of oxygen [PaO_2] <60 mm Hg)

     (2) Increased carbon dioxide retention as fat embolism syndrome develops

    d) Pulse oximetry monitoring reveals decreased oxygen saturation

    e) Fat globules in urine (not always found)

    f) Thrombocytopenia (platelets as low as 50,000/mm³)

     (1) Consumed by injury and/or clotting process

     (2) Diluted with banked blood and/or intravenous fluids

     (3) Aggregated around fat globules

2. Analysis: differential nursing diagnosis/collaborative problems

  a. *Tissue perfusion, altered cardiopulmonary, cerebral, and renal related to location of emboli*

  b. *Impaired gas exchanged related to occlusion of blood vessels*

  c. *Ineffective breathing pattern related to impaired gas exchange*

  d. *Anxiety/fear related to severity of symptoms and prognosis*

3. Planning/interventions

  a. *Administration of high-flow oxygen*

  b. *Mechanical ventilation with positive end-expiratory pressure or continuous airway pressure if unable to maintain PaO_2 above 60 mm Hg*

  c. *IV fluid replacement to maintain cardiac function and maintain urinary output*

    d. Vasopressor/inotropic support
    e. IV corticosteroids
    f. Encourage family and patient to ask questions and discuss feelings
    g. Need for admission to hospital and close monitoring
    h. Need for surgical stabilization of fractures
4. **Expected outcomes/evaluation** (see Appendix B)

C. Compartment syndrome

    The extremities have multiple compartments that encase the muscles, nerves, and blood vessels. They are enveloped by fascia, which is a tough and nonelastic membrane. Compartment syndrome occurs when compartmental pressures increase from an internal or an external force. Increased internal pressures result from bleeding into the compartment and soft tissue swelling. External forces include rigid casts, splints, air splints, pneumatic antishock pants. As intracompartmental pressures rise, the vascular and neurological structures become compromised. Initially, the low-flow microcirculation is obstructed, producing edema, which further increases the intracompartmental pressures. High-flow arteries remain patent until pressure exceeds the systolic blood pressure.

    Compartment syndrome tends to occur most often in the lower arm, hand, lower leg, and foot. It is rare in the upper arm and upper leg because of the larger size of the compartments, which can accommodate a greater volume. When it does occur in the upper extremity, it is usually associated with prolonged compression. These findings need to be monitored closely and documented because the patient may need an emergent fasciotomy.

1. **Assessment**
    a. Subjective data
        1) History of present condition
            a) Injury to extremity
                (1) Fracture, usually closed although compartment syndrome can occur with open fracture
                (2) Crushing force
                (3) Prolonged compression
                (4) Vascular injury, especially after repair when edema is greatest
                (5) High-pressure injections of foreign substance into deep compartment
                (6) Burns
                    (a) Circumferential electrical
                (7) Hypothermia or frostbite
                (8) Venomous snake or spider bites
                (9) Cannulation of artery
            b) Prolonged overuse of extremity may present as chronic compartment syndrome
                (1) During forced march
                (2) In long-distance runners
            c) Recent surgery in extremity
            d) Use of casts, wraps, splints, circumferential tape, pneumatic antishock garments
            e) Hydration status; patients with decreased volume may be less prone to compartment syndrome
        2) Medical history
            a) Hemophilia (increased tendency to bleed)

b) Nephrotic syndrome (edema resulting from increased capillary filtration)

c) Pre-existing nerve dysfunction

   b. Objective data

     1) Physical examination (five *P*'s)

       a) *Pain* (sensory fibers of nerves tend to be affected by pressure first)

         (1) Out of proportion to injury

         (2) Progressive

         (3) Intense

         (4) Increased with palpation over compartment

         (5) Increased with passive flexion motion of affected compartment muscles

       b) *Paresthesia* (or hypothesia) along nerve that traverses affected compartment

       c) *Paralysis* (or weakness) resulting from ischemia or pressure of motor fibers in affected nerve

       d) *Pallor* resulting from obstructed microcirculation

       e) *Pulse* usually present

       f) *Tenseness* over palpated compartment

   c. Diagnostic procedures

     1) Compartment pressure measurement

       a) Pressure up to 10 mm Hg considered normal

       b) Pressure above 30 to 40 mm Hg should be monitored for trends and clinical symptoms

     2) Laboratory studies to identify muscle injury

       a) Urine for myoglobinuria

       b) Blood for enzyme levels: creatine kinase, lactate dehydrogenase, serum glutamic-oxaloacetic transaminase

2. Analysis: differential nursing diagnosis/collaborative problems

   a. Tissue perfusion, altered related to increased intracompartment pressure

   b. Pain related to increased compartment pressure and tissue ischemia

   c. Anxiety/fear related to unknown procedures and hospitalization

3. Planning/interventions

   a. Remove all forms of external compression

   b. Avoid interventions that impede circulation

   c. Avoid application of ice because this promotes further vasoconstriction

   d. Avoid excessive elevation of limb; may impair arterial flow

   e. Prepare and assist with fracture reduction if indicated

   f. Administer analgesics as ordered

   g. Prepare for operative fasciotomy to restore neurovascular function

   h. Provide patient and family education

4. Expected outcomes/evaluation (see Appendix B)

BIBLIOGRAPHY

Bigos, S, Bowyer, O, Braen, G., et al. (1994). *Acute low back problems in adults* (Clinical Practice Guideline No. 14, AHCPR Publication No. 95-0642. Rockville, MD: Agency for Health Care Policy and Research, Public Health Service, U.S. Department of Health and Human Services.

Blue, C. (1996). Preventing back injury among nurses. *Orthopaedic Nursing, 15*(6), 9–20.

Brown, D. E., & Neuman, R. D. (1995). *Orthopaedic secrets.* Philadelphia: Hanley & Belfus.

Childs, S. (1996). Osteoarticular *Mycobacterium tuberculosis. Orthopaedic Nursing, 15,* 29–33.

Epps, C. H., Jr. (1994). *Complications in orthopaedic surgery* (3rd ed.). Philadelphia: J. B. Lippincott.

Halpern, J. (1994). Orthopedic emergencies. In A. R. Klein, G. Lee, A. Manton, & J. G. Parker (Eds.), *Emergency nursing core curriculum* (4th ed., pp. 405–434). Philadelphia: W. B. Saunders.

Jones, A. L. (1994). Complications of musculoskeletal trauma. In M. A. Lopez-Viego (Ed.), *The Parkland trauma handbook.* (pp. 425–429). St. Louis, MO: Mosby–Year Book.

Jones, A. L. (1994). Principles of fractures and dislocations. In M. A. Lopez-Viego (Ed.), *The Parkland trauma handbook* (pp. 415–418). St. Louis, MO: Mosby-Year Book.

Krug, B. (1997). Rheumatoid arthritis and osteoarthritis: A basic comparison. *Orthopaedic Nursing, 16*(5), 73–75.

Mabee, J., & Bostwick, T. (1993). Pathophysiology and mechanism of compartment syndrome. *Physician Assistant, 6,* 59–66.

McCullen, G. M., & Yuan, H. A. (1997). Low back pain. In R. E. Rakel (Ed.), *Conn's current therapy* (pp. 43–45). Philadelphia: W. B. Saunders.

Mims, B. (1989). Fat embolism syndrome: A variant of ARDS. *Orthopaedic Nursing, 8*(3), 22–26.

Paletta, J. (1997). Nursing care of sports-related injuries. *Orthopaedic Nursing, 16*(6), 43–46.

Papapoulos, S. E. (1997). Paget's disease of bone: Clinical, pathogenic and therapeutic aspects. *Baillières Clinical Endocrinology Metabolism, 11*(1), 117–143.

Patel, P., & Lauerman, W. (1997). The use of magnetic resonance imaging in the diagnosis of lumbar disc disease. *Orthopaedic Nursing, 16*(1), 59–65.

Patterson, M. (1998). Child abuse: Assessment and intervention. *Orthopaedic Nursing, 17*(1), 49–54.

Ross, D. (1996). Chronic compartment syndrome. *Orthopaedic Nursing, 15*(3), 23–27.

Sheon, R. P. (1997). Repetitive strain injury. *Postgraduate Medicine, 102*(4), 72–85.

Stuart, M. J., & Karaharju, T. (1994). Acute compartment syndrome: Recognizing the progressive signs and symptoms. *The Physician and Sportsmedicine 22,* 91–95.

Waeckerle, J. F., & Steele, M. T. (1996). Fractures and dislocations. In J. E. Tintinalli, E. Ruiz, & R. L. Krome (Eds.), *Emergency medicine, a comprehensive study guide* (4th ed., pp. 1258–1262). New York: McGraw-Hill.

Williamson, J. B., & Jones, A. L. (1994). Pediatric fractures. In M. A. Lopez-Viego (Ed.), *The Parkland trauma handbook* (pp. 547–566). St. Louis, MO: Mosby–Year Book.

Susan Albrecht, PhD, RN, MPM
Lisa Marie Bernardo, RN, PhD

CHAPTER **17**

Pain Management

MAJOR TOPICS

Overview of Pain

Definitions of Pain

Pain Response

Acute and Chronic Pain

Theories of Pain

Ethical Issues in Pain Management

Physiology of Pain

Nursing Process

I. OVERVIEW OF PAIN

Pain is a common human experience and is a frequent reason for seeking emergency treatment. Emergency nurses must be astute to the presence of pain in their patients. Knowledge of pain behaviors and coping strategies help the nurse recognize the effects of pain or the potential for pain. An understanding of basic pharmacological and nonpharmacological strategies assists emergency nurses in preparing a plan of care and subsequent interventions to alleviate or ameliorate pain. Proper evaluation techniques allow the nurse to determine the success of interventions. Emergency nurses should participate in activities to strengthen their knowledge in relation to pain, its meaning, and its treatment. Educational efforts should be designed to increase nurses' knowledge of advances in pain management and to debunk negative attitudes and beliefs about pain.

II. DEFINITIONS OF PAIN

A. Pain is a sensory experience associated with actual and potential tissue damage as well as a physiological response to this damage

B. Pain is whatever the person experiencing it describes it to be; it exists when the person says it does, as manifested in verbal and nonverbal behavior

III. PAIN RESPONSE

A. The person's response to pain is a learned response influenced by

1. **Age**
2. **Socioeconomic status**
3. **Gender**
4. **Ethnicity**
5. **Religion**
6. **Culture**
7. **Values**

B. Individual pain behavior is adaptive and directed toward modifying pain with relation to pain threshold and pain tolerance

1. **Pain threshold**
   a. "The point at which a stimulus is perceived as pain" (Ludwig-Beymer, Huether, & Schoessler, 1994, p. 439)
   b. Does not vary significantly in an individual or among people over time; increase of pain in one location may increase pain threshold in another; that is, a person with injured knee may complain more about knee pain than about chronic hip pain
2. **Pain tolerance**
   a. "The amount of pain a person is willing to tolerate before outwardly responding to it" (Ludwig-Beymer et al., 1994, p. 439).
   b. Can be decreased with repeated exposure to pain, fatigue, anger, boredom, apprehension, and sleep deprivation

IV. ACUTE AND CHRONIC PAIN

A. Pain is subdivided into acute and chronic; Table 17-1 compares their characteristics.

Table 17-1 COMPARISON OF ACUTE AND CHRONIC PAIN

Characteristic	Acute Pain	Chronic Pain
Definition	Protective mechanism that alerts patient to condition or situation that is harmful to body	Persistent pain over time
Onset	Sudden	Sudden or insidious, leading to suffering
Duration	Short term	Six months or greater
Source	Infection, trauma, procedure, or treatment related	Unknown; if known, treatment may be prolonged or ineffective; cancer related; low back; neuralgia; myofascial; phantom limb; AIDS-related
Significance of pain	Pain is significant	Patient looks for significance/meaning of pain
Behaviors/feelings	Hope that pain will diminish; anxiety related to pain and its pathology	Hopelessness, helplessness, meaninglessness, depression
Prognosis	Great likelihood that pain will be relieved	Complete relief not possible

AIDS, acquired immunodeficiency syndrome.
Adapted from Ludwig-Beymer, P., Huether, S., & Schoessler, M. (1994). Pain, temperature regulation, sleep, and sensory function. In K. McCance & S. Huether (Eds.), *Pathophysiology: The biologic basis for disease in adults and children* (pp. 437–476). St. Louis, MO: Mosby–Year Book. Used with permission.

V. THEORIES OF PAIN

A. Gate control theory

1. "Gate" in spinal cord processes ascending and descending pain impulses
2. With stronger ascending impulses
   a. Gate opens
   b. Impulse ascends to brain
   c. Pain is experienced
3. With stronger descending impulses
   a. Gate closes
   b. Pain is decreased

B. Pattern theory

1. Pattern of noxious stimulation is coded by central nervous system (CNS), which results in perception of pain
2. Pain is produced by spatiotemporal patterns of neuronal impulses (as opposed to stimulation of specific pain receptors)
3. Theory ignores evidence of receptor fiber specialization and complex nature of pain experience

VI. ETHICAL ISSUES IN PAIN MANAGEMENT

A. Use of placebos

1. Placebos are not justified as a means of diagnosis or treatment and offer no benefits to offset any associated risks, such as undermining the adult's or child's trust in health care professionals

B. Withholding of narcotics for fear of addiction

1. No data correlate administration of narcotics to pediatric patients with subsequent drug addiction
2. Addiction should not manifest if appropriate medications are prescribed and administered for appropriate pain and appropriate monitoring is conducted

C. Withholding of narcotics for fear of respiratory depression

1. Infants and children safely can receive opioids without fear of respiratory depression when they are administered at recommended guidelines, especially for calculating initial dose and when patients are monitored at appropriate intervals
2. No evidence suggests that opioid-induced respiratory depression is more likely to occur in children compared with adults

VII. PHYSIOLOGY OF PAIN

Current emergency nursing practices require a basic understanding of the pathophysiology of pain to assess a patient's pain, intervene effectively, and evaluate patient outcomes. The pathophysiology of pain involves the CNS, afferent pathways, and efferent pathways.

A. CNS

1. Composed of thalamus, hypothalamus, medulla, cortex, reticular formation system, and limbic system
2. Perceives, describes, and localizes pain; controls emotional and affective response to pain

B. Afferent pathways

1. Composed of nociceptors, A and C fibers, dorsal horn of spinal column, and afferent neurons in spinothalamic tract
2. Carries pain messages to spinal cord
3. Spinal cord transfers pain message to brain
4. Terminates in dorsal horn of spinal cord
5. Nerve endings do not adapt to repeated painful stimuli; repeated stimuli heighten their sensitivity
6. When hypersensitive (also known as hyperalgesia), slightest painful stimulus is interpreted as very painful
7. Secondary neurons transmit pain through the spinothalamic tract to brain
8. A fibers
   a. *Carry well-localized, sharp pain sensations*
   b. *Myelinated*
9. C fibers
   a. *Carry diffuse burning or aching sensations*
   b. *Unmyelinated*

C. Efferent pathways

1. Run from periaqueductal gray (gray matter that surrounds cerebral aqueduct in midbrain) to periphery
2. Responsible for modulation or inhibition of afferent pain signals

VIII. NURSING PROCESS

A. Assessment

1. **Primary survey/resuscitation** (see Chapter 1)
2. **Secondary survey** (see Chapter 1)
3. **Psychological, social, and environmental factors**
   a. *Recognize ethnic, cultural, special needs, age, and other factors when assessing pain*
4. **Focused survey**
   a. *Subjective data*
      1) Vocal/verbal response (Table 17–2)
      2) History of pain in relation to current injury or illness
         a) Provoking factors (acute or chronic)
            (1) Is pain provoked by something specific (e.g., movement, food)?
            (2) Are there any interventions that make pain or discomfort worse or better (e.g., lying still)?
            (3) What activities was patient performing when pain began?
         b) Quality of pain

Table 17–2   BEHAVIORAL RESPONSES TO PAIN

Age Group	Vocalizations	Facial Expressions	Body Movements	Coping Strategies
Infants	Crying Fussy Irritable	Lowered brows Drawn together Eyes closed (young infant) Eyes open (older infant) Mouth open	Generalized body responses; rigid or thrashing (young infant) Localized body response; withdraws stimulated area (older infant)	Oral simulation (sucking) Crying Fetal position
Toddlers/ preschoolers	Crying Screaming Verbalizes "boo-boo," "It hurts" Asks to stop painful stimulus Points to area of pain	Eyes closed or open Furrowed brow	Physical resistance Uncooperative Restless Clinging	Oral stimulation Crying while sleeping (toddlers) Rocking Closing eyes/turning away Lying still or being active (preschoolers)
School age	Crying Verbalizing pain quality, location, duration	Withdrawn facial expression Furrowed brow	Muscle rigidity Gritted teeth Clenched fists Splinting/guarding Lying still	Verbal stalling Being active or lying still Talking about the pain Using distraction techniques Sleeping Playing or watching television
Adolescents	Verbalizing pain Crying	Withdrawn Eyes closed Furrowed brow	Muscle tension and body control Splinting/guarding Lying still	Verbalizing pain Taking medication or initiating actions to relieve pain Sleeping
Adults	Groaning Moaning Sobbing Grunting Shouting Praying Crying out for help	Frowning Staring Furrowed brow Teeth clenching	Thrashing Tossing Rocking Muscle rigidity	Lying still Protective behaviors Posturing Massaging
Elderly	Sighing Moaning Grunting Chanting Praying Crying for help	Eyes squeezed closed Withdrawn look Furrowed brow Staring	Rocking Clutching side rails Muscle rigidity	Wandering Rubbing Guarding

Adapted from Bernardo, L., & Conway, A. (1998). Pain assessment and management. In T. Sond & J. Rogers (Eds.), *Manual of pediatric emergency nursing* (pp. 686–711). St. Louis, MO: Mosby–Year Book; Katz, E., Kellerman, K., & Siegel, S. (1980). Behavioral distress in children with cancer undergoing medical procedures: Developmental considerations. *Journal of Consulting and Clinical Psychology*, 48(3), 356–365. Copyright © (1980) by the American Psychological Association. Adapted with permission.

(1) Description of pain in patient's own words (e.g., burning, stabbing, dull, aching, throbbing)

3. Region/radiation of pain
   a) Have patient point with one finger to area of pain or discomfort, such as abdomen, chest, extremity, head
   b) Ask patient whether there is pain anywhere else in body

4. Severity of pain
   a) Offer a pain-rating scale
   b) Ask patient to describe the severity of pain (e.g., minor/minimal to "worst pain I ever had")

5. Time pain began
   a) When did pain begin?
      (1) Acute (hours, days)
      (2) Chronic (months, years)
   b) Has discomfort remained the same since its onset, or has it improved or worsened? Ask patient to describe progression of pain

6. Pain rating
   a) Examples of pediatric scales
      (1) FACES Pain Rating Scale (Nix, Clutter, & Wong, 1994; Wong & Baker, 1988): for use in children 3 years of age or older
      (2) Numeric scale: for use in children as young as 5 years of age if they count and understand numbering
      (3) Poker chip scale: for use in children as young as 4 years of age if they can count and understand numbering
   b) Examples of adult scales
      (1) Visual analogue scales
      (2) Numeric pain scales

7. Patient/family initiated measures to relieve pain
   a) Administration of prescribed or over-the-counter analgesics
      (1) Dose: Correct pediatric dose based on milligram per kilogram amount (e.g., parent may be administering infant dose of acetaminophen to toddler, and pain is persisting). Time of last dose
   b) Administration of other medications (nonanalgesics) taken by the patient
      (1) Names of medications
      (2) Dosage
      (3) Potential for synergistic reactions/effects
   c) Home remedies administered by patient or family
   d) Foods
      (1) Type of food
      (2) Amount eaten
      (3) Time of last meal
   e) Herbs, natural or homeopathic preparations
      (1) Type of preparation
      (2) Amount ingested, topically applied (i.e., cream), or inhaled
      (3) Time of last preparation intake
   f) Physical interventions
      (1) Massage
      (2) Application of ice or heat
      (3) Splinting
      (4) Wrapping (elastic bandages)

8. Patient's and family's past experiences with acute or chronic pain

9. Patient's and family's report of effectiveness of previous pharmacological and nonpharmacological pain management

b. *Objective data*

1. Physical examination

a) General survey for pain-specific findings

(1) Inspection

(a) Presence of traumatic wounds

(b) Diaphoresis

(c) Palmar sweating

(d) Dilated pupils

(e) Pallor

(f) Decreased oxygen saturation

(2) Auscultation

(a) Heart and lung sounds: tachycardia, tachypnea, increased blood pressure

(3) Palpation (specific areas of pain)

(a) Abdomen

(b) Joints

(c) Chest

(d) Extremities

2. Behavioral response to pain (see Table 17–2)

B. Analysis: differential nursing diagnosis/collaborative problems

1. **Pain**
2. **Pain, chronic**

C. Planning/interventions

1. **Determine priorities**

a. *Treat underlying disease or injury process*

b. *Consider patient's and family's physical, social, cultural, and psychological needs, beliefs, and experiences*

c. *Use therapeutic communication strategies to acknowledge patient's pain experience and to convey acceptance of patient's response to pain*

d. *Encourage patient and family to participate in patient's pain management*

2. **Develop nursing care plan specific to patient's presenting pain-related emergency**

a. *Check prescribed medication for dose and frequency*

b. *Check patient's history for drug allergies*

c. *Involve patient and family in selection of pain management strategies*

d. *Monitor vital signs before, during, and after initiation of narcotic analgesic to assess patient's reactions*

e. *Administer adjuvant analgesics and/or medications as needed to potentiate analgesia*

f. *Teach patient and family about safety of narcotic administration, especially if there is fear of addiction, which leads to patient's and family's refusal of narcotics*

g. *Apply patient's previously successful pain management strategies*

3. **Initiate pain management interventions based on nursing plan of care**

a. *Initiate pharmacological interventions*

1) Administer non-narcotic analgesics

a) Acetaminophen

(1) Indications: temporary relief of minor aches and pains associated with common cold, headache, toothache, muscular aches, backache, minor pain of arthritis, menstrual pain, fever reduction

(2) Contraindications: active liver disease or severe dysfunction; cachexia; chronic alcoholism

(3) Side effects: acceptably safe in usual dosage except in patients with hepatic dysfunction; also unsafe in those who use substances that increase hepatic enzymes (e.g., ethanol, phenobarbital, isoniazid)

(4) Routes: oral and rectal

b) Salicylates

(1) Indications: temporary relief of headache, pain, fever, muscle aches and pains, menstrual pain, toothache pain, minor aches and pains of arthritis

(2) Contraindications: hypersensitivity to salicylates; bleeding disorders, vitamin K deficiency; asthma; peptic ulceration; coagulopathies; administration to children of all ages with varicella or flulike illness because of its association with Reye's syndrome

(3) Side effects: irritation and damage to gastrointestinal (GI) mucosa; increase in bleeding caused by inhibition of platelet aggregation (low doses); prolongation of prothrombin time (high doses); unwanted CNS effects with intensive treatment

(4) Routes: oral and rectal

c) Nonsteroidal anti-inflammatory agents (NSAIDs) (e.g., ibuprofen)

(1) Indications: temporary relief of minor aches and pains associated with the common cold, headache, toothache, muscular aches, backache, minor arthritis pain, menstrual pain, fever reduction

(2) Contraindications: hypersensitivity, asthma, severe renal disease, severe hepatic disease

(3) Side effects: GI effects: nausea, anorexia, vomiting, dyspepsia, heartburn, abdominal discomfort, bleeding, hematemesis, heartburn, abdominal discomfort, bleeding, peptic ulcer activation; CNS effects: headache, dizziness; blood dyscrasia: thrombocytopenia, granulocytopenia, agranulocytosis, fatal pancytopenia

(4) Routes: oral, intramuscular (IM), intravenous (IV)

2) Administer narcotic analgesics

a) Morphine sulfate

(1) Indications: potent analgesic for relief of moderate to severe pain

(a) Immediate-release oral forms: moderate to severe pain

(b) Suppositories: moderate to severe chronic pain and severe acute pain

(2) Contraindications: convulsive states (status epilepticus, tetanus, strychnine poisoning); hypersensitivity to morphine; respiratory depression in absence of resuscitative equipment; acute or severe bronchial asthma; suspected paralytic ileus

(3) Side effects: constipation, lightheadedness, dizziness, drowsiness, sedation, nausea, vomiting, diaphoresis, dysphoria, euphoria

(4) Routes: IV, IM, oral, rectal, topical (patch)

b) Meperidine hydrochloride

(1) Indications: relief of moderate to severe pain

(2) Contraindications: hypersensitivity to meperidine; monoamine oxidase inhibitor use within previous 14 days

      c) Side effects: lightheadedness, dizziness, sedation, nausea, vomiting, diaphoresis

      d) Routes: IV, IM, subcutaneous, oral

   3) Administer sedative agents

      a) Midazolam

         (1) Indications: sedation to impair memory of events, induction of sleepiness or drowsiness, relief of apprehension

         (2) Contraindications: known hypersensitivity to midazolam, acute narrow glaucoma, pregnancy, existing CNS depression, shock

         (3) Side effects—IM route: headache, pain, induration, redness/muscle stiffness at injection site; IV route: hiccups, nausea, vomiting, coughing, oversedation, headache, drowsiness, tenderness, pain, redness, irritation, phlebitis at injection site

         (4) Routes: intravascular, IM, intranasal, oral

      b) Diazepam

         (1) Indications: antianxiolytic; status epilepticus, severe recurrent convulsive seizures, skeletal muscle spasms; symptomatic relief of alcohol withdrawal

         (2) Contraindications: drowsiness; reduce dosage by at least one third and administer in small increments when using with narcotic analgesic

         (3) Side effects: when administered IV, hypotension, muscular weakness, thrombosis, phlebitis at site

         (4) Routes: IV, oral

   4) Administer anesthetic agents (per institution policy)

      a) Local anesthetic (e.g., lidocaine hydrochloride)

         (1) Indications: local anesthetic for infiltration and nerve block; topical anesthesia for procedures or relief of dermatological conditions; used in combination with other medications for topical relief of pain (Table 17–3)

         (2) Contraindications: decreased dose requirements in heart and liver disease because half-life is longer in patients with liver disease

         (3) Side effects: inadvertent intravascular injection, CNS toxicity (lightheadedness, tinnitus, coma)

Table 17–3 OTHER TOPICAL ANESTHETICS

Name	Ingredients	Indications	Special Considerations
TAC	Tetracaine Adrenaline Cocaine	Topical anesthetic for minor wounds not involving fingers, toes, penis, nose	Wear a glove when preparing TAC; hold TAC in place on wound; observe for blanching of skin; additional lidocaine filtration may be needed
LET	Lidocaine Epinephrine Tetracaine	Topical anesthetic for minor wounds not involving fingers, toes, penis, nose; may be safer than TAC (does not contain cocaine)	Wear a glove when preparing LET; hold LET in place on wound; observe for blanching of skin; additional lidocaine infiltration may be needed
Emla cream	Lidocaine	Topical anesthetic (cream based) that is applied to body area before procedure to decrease pain (venous cannulation site, lumbar puncture site)	Requires at least 30 to 60 minutes to work; may require reapplication if first procedure attempt is unsuccessful

        (4) Routes: topical, oral, injectable

    5) Inhaled anesthetics (nitrous oxide)

       a) Indications: analgesia

       b) Contraindications: pneumothorax; recent middle ear surgery, bowel obstruction

       c) Side effects: generalized depression of CNS function, mild respiratory depression, nausea, vomiting

       d) Route: inhalation

    6) Administer other pharmacological strategies

       a) Patient-controlled analgesia (PCA)

          (1) Indicated for patients with sickle cell crisis, cancer pain, renal colic, or pain from other chronic illnesses who are able to communicate, comprehend explanations, and follow directions

          (2) Can be used with children as young as 5 or 6 years

          (3) Assess whether patient has any allergies or adverse reactions to prescribed medication

          (4) Explain the use of PCA pump to patient and family

          (5) Collaborate with physician, patient, and family on adjustment of lockout interval, basal rate, and demand dosage

          (6) Obtain venous access

          (7) Obtain baseline vital signs, oxygen saturation, and pain scale response

          (8) Assist patient in using PCA device

          (9) Reassess patient's pain response

          (10) Document patient's pain response and amount and frequency of drug dosing

    7) Conscious sedation

       a) Indicated for procedures (e.g., suturing, fracture reduction) and performed by qualified emergency physician and emergency nurse

       b) Assess time of patient's last oral intake

       c) Assess whether patient has any allergies or adverse reactions to prescribed medications

       d) Explain procedure to patient and family

       e) Obtain proper equipment, including cardiopulmonary monitor, blood pressure monitor, pulse oximeter, suction equipment, endotracheal intubation equipment, narcotic reversal agents

       f) Obtain venous access

       g) Secure monitoring equipment to patient

       h) Obtain baseline set of vital signs and level of consciousness

       i) Assist physician in administering sedative

       j) Assist physician in administering analgesic

       k) Titrate sedative and analgesic to desired response

       l) Monitor patient's vital signs, cardiac rate and rhythm, oxygen saturation, level of consciousness, and pain response throughout procedure

       m) Continue to monitor patient after procedure for changes in vital signs, oxygen saturation, level of consciousness, pain response

       n) Determine whether patient is eligible for discharge (awake, able to ambulate, able to drink and swallow)

  b. Initiate nonpharmacological interventions to enhance patient's coping strategies

    1) Support family presence during procedures and treatments

       a) Rehearse with patient and family, if time permits, what will be expected of them during procedure or treatment

      b) Demonstrate to family how they can support patient before, during, and after procedures or treatments

      c) Prepare family for what will occur during procedure or treatment

      d) Offer family respite care as needed

  2) Position patient for comfort

      a) Apply splint, sling, or swathe for extremity injuries

      b) Position patient in fetal position (side lying with knees drawn up) for abdominal or back pain

      c) Use pillows or towel rolls to keep patient positioned properly

  3) Initiate cutaneous stimulation

      a) Apply ice for fractures or sprains

      b) Apply heat/warm compresses for infiltrated IV infusions or muscle spasms/cramps; avoid heat to abdomen if surgical process is suspected

      c) Massage painful area

         (1) Helpful for tense muscles

         (2) Avoid if inflammatory process is present

  4) Use distraction techniques, which work by increasing patient's pain tolerance

      a) Music

         (1) Provide headsets with audio cassette tapes to young children, adolescents, adults, elderly patients

         (2) Encourage patients of all ages to use their own cassette recorder or radio

      b) Storytelling/imagery

         (1) Engage children and adolescents in conversation: "What is your favorite subject in school?"

         (2) Engage adult and elderly patients in reminiscing or descriptions: "What was it like to live during the depression?"

      c) "Treasure chests"

         (1) Supply treasure chest for young and school-age children that includes magic wands, soap bubbles, dolls, soft balls to squeeze, Slinkys, soft hammer, storybooks, "good luck" charms that helped other children, puzzles, hand games, coloring books

         (2) Supply treasure chest for adolescents, adults, and elderly patients that includes age-appropriate magazines, audio and video tapes, games, puzzles

  c. Use relaxation/breathing techniques

    1) Young children

      a) Provide pinwheels for deep breathing and relaxation; allow child to take them home

      b) Sing familiar songs with child

    2) Older children and adolescents

      a) Use progressive relaxation, in which child tightens and releases various body muscles

      b) Offer thinking games, such as riddles, word games, or counting games

    3) Adults

      a) Use progressive relaxation

      b) Use guided imagery

      c) Use deep-breathing techniques

      d) Engage in conversation as distraction technique

    4) Elderly

       a) Use progressive relaxation

       b) Use deep-breathing techniques

       c) Engage in conversation as distraction technique

    d. *Promote positive self-talk*

       1) Reinforce to patients of all ages how well they are managing with their pain during procedure or treatment

       2) Verbally encourage patients of all ages: "You can make it"; "You are doing great!"

    e. *Use pressure with or without massage*

D. Expected outcomes/evaluation

    1. Monitor patient responses and outcomes, adjusting nursing care plan as indicated

      a. *Pharmacological interventions*

       1) Subjective data

       2) Objective data

         a) Readminister pain scale

         b) Reported pain is decreased

           (1) Continue with present pain management regimen

         c) Reported pain is same or increased

           (1) Reassess amount of medication administered; consider increasing dose while keeping within recommended dosage

           (2) Reassess route of medication delivery; consider using same medication by different route

           (3) Consider administering different medication

E. Record all pertinent data

    1. Vital signs and oxygen saturation readings

    2. Pain scale ratings

    3. Physical and behavioral response to analgesics

    4. Disposition

      a. *Hospitalization*

       1) Report successful and unsuccessful pain management techniques to inpatient nursing staff

       2) Continue pharmacological and nonpharmacological interventions

      b. *Home*

       1) Ensure patient's and family's understanding of home pharmacological pain regimen

       2) Provide emergency department's telephone number for questions or concerns

       3) Provide information on what to do if pain returns or is not controlled

       4) For patients with chronic pain, consider referral to pain clinic or pain specialist

BIBLIOGRAPHY

American Academy of Pediatrics. (1992). Guidelines for monitoring and management of pediatric patients during and after sedation for diagnostic and therapeutic procedures. *Pediatrics, 89,* 1110–1115.

American College of Emergency Physicians. (1993). The use of pediatric sedation and analgesia. *Annals of Emergency Medicine, 22,* 626–627.

Bernardo, L., & Conway, A. (1998). Pain assessment and management. In T. Soud & J. Rogers (Eds.), *Manual of pediatric emergency nursing* (pp. 686–711). St. Louis, MO: Mosby–Year Book.

Carroll, D., & Bowsher, D. (1993). *Pain management in nursing care.* Oxford, England: Butterworth-Heinemann, Linacer House.

Cornock, M. (1996). Psychological approaches to cardiac pain. *Nursing Standard, 11*(2), 34–38.

Dukes, M. (1996). *Meyler's side effects of drugs* (13th ed.). Amsterdam, the Netherlands: Elsevier.

Duthie, B. (1998). *Mudell's drugs in current use and new drugs* (44th ed.). New York: Springer.

French, G., Painter, E., & Coury, D. (1994). Blowing away shot pain: A technique for pain management during immunization. *Pediatrics, 93*(3), 384–388.

Gaukroger, P. (1993). Patient-controlled analgesia in children. In N. Schechter, C. Berde, & M. Yaster (Eds.), *Pain in infants, children and adolescents.* Baltimore, MD: Williams & Wilkins.

Katz, E., Kellerman, K., & Siegel, S. (1980). Behavioral distress in children with cancer undergoing medical procedures: Developmental considerations. *Journal of Consulting and Clinical Psychology, 48,* 356–365.

Lebovits, A., Florence, B., Hunko, V., Fax, M., & Bramble, C. (1997). Pain knowledge and attitudes of health care providers: Practice characteristics differences. *Clinical Journal of Pain, 13,* 237–243.

Ludwig-Beymer, P., Huether, S., & Schoessler, M. (1994). Pain, temperature regulation, sleep, and sensory function. In K. McCance & S. Huether (Eds.), *Pathophysiology: The biologic basis for disease in adults and children* (pp. 437–476). St. Louis, MO: Mosby–Year Book.

McCaffery, M. (1979). *Nursing management of the patient with pain* (2nd ed). Philadelphia: J. B. Lippincott.

McCaffery, M., & Wong, D. (1993). Nursing interventions for pain control in children. In N. Schechter, C. Berde, & M. Yaster (Eds.), *Pain in infants, children, and adolescents* (pp. 295–316). Baltimore, MD: Williams & Wilkins.

McCloskey, J., & Bulechek, G. (Eds.). (1993). *Nursing interventions classification (NIC)* (2nd ed., pp. 101, 183, 412, 420). St. Louis, MO: Mosby–Year Book.

Mosby–Year Book. (1998). *Mosby's genRX: The complete reference for generic and brand drugs.* (8th ed.). St. Louis, MO: Mosby–Year Book.

Nix, K., Clutter, L., & Wong, D. (1994). *The influence of the type of instructions in measuring pain intensity in young children using the FACES Pain Rating Scale.* Unpublished manuscript.

Nolan, K. (1993). Ethical issues in pediatric pain management. In N. Schechter, C. Berde, & M. Yaster (Eds.), *Pain in infants, children, and adolescents* (pp. 123–132). Baltimore, MD: Williams & Wilkins.

Medical Economics Co. (1998). *PDR for non-prescription drugs* (19th ed.). Montvale, NJ: Author.

Puntillo, K. (1991). Physiology of pain and its consequences in critically ill patients. In K. Puntillo (Ed.), *Pain in the critically ill: Assessment and management.* Gaithersburg, MD: Aspen.

Sullivan, R. (1989). Triage: A sub-specialty of emergency nursing. *Nursing, 3,* 26–33.

Thelan, L., Urden, L., Lough, M., & Stacy, K. (1998). Pain and sedation. In L. Thelan, L. Urden, M. Lough, & K. Stacy (Eds.), *Critical care nursing: Diagnosis and management* (pp. 169–201). St. Louis, MO: Mosby–Year Book.

Trautman, D. (1998). Pain management. In L. Newberry (Ed.), *Sheehy's emergency nursing principles and practice* (4th ed., pp. 175–181). St. Louis, MO: Mosby–Year Book.

Tusek, D., Church, J., & Fazio, V. (1997). Guided imagery as a coping strategy for perioperative patients. *AORN Journal, 66,* 644–649.

Wall, P., & Melzack, R. (1989). *Textbook of pain.* New York: Churchill Livingstone.

White, P. (1996). *Anesthesia drug manual.* Philadelphia: W. B. Saunders.

Wong, D., & Baker, C. (1988). Pain in children: A comparison of assessment scales. *Pediatric Nursing, 14*(1), 9–17.

Charose James, RN, BSN, CEN

CHAPTER **18**

Respiratory Emergencies

MAJOR TOPICS

General Strategy

Specific Medical Emergencies

Adult Respiratory Distress Syndrome

Asthma

Acute Bronchitis

Bronchiolitis

Chronic Obstructive Pulmonary Disease

Croup (Laryngotracheobronchitis)

Acute Epiglottitis

Hyperventilation

Pleural Effusion

Pneumonia

Pulmonary Embolus

Specific Surgical Respiratory Emergencies

Rib Fractures

Flail Chest

Pneumothorax

Tension Pneumothorax

Hemothorax

Open Pneumothorax

Pulmonary Contusion

Esophageal Disruption

Ruptured Bronchus and Trachea

Ruptured Diaphragm

I. GENERAL STRATEGIES

A. Assessment

1. **Primary survey/resuscitation** (see Chapter 1)
2. **Secondary survey** (see Chapter 1)
3. **Physiological, psychosocial, and environmental factors**
   a. *Blunt or penetrating trauma to thorax or any other area of body: from burns, fractures, motor vehicle crashes, assaults, falls*
   b. *Shock of any type, sepsis*
   c. *Multiple blood transfusions, fluid resuscitation*
   d. *Disseminated intravascular coagulation (DIC)*

  e. *Postsurgical recovery or immobility*
  f. *Drug overdose*
  g. *Medications, including oral contraceptives (could lead to pulmonary thromboembolus)*
  h. *Allergies*
  i. *Pulmonary disorders, pulmonary-vascular disease*
  j. *Metabolic disorders*
  k. *Neuromuscular disorders*
  l. *Heredity: tendency to develop certain respiratory diseases, such as asthma, appears to be familial in nature*
  m. *Immunodeficiency status: human immunodeficiency virus (HIV) infection, therapeutic immunosuppression, underlying disease impairing pulmonary defense system*
  n. *Respiratory infections: recent respiratory infections may increase susceptibility to other respiratory infections*
  o. *Aspiration*
  p. *Obesity*
  q. *Atrial fibrillation: may precipitate thrombus*
  r. *Smoking*
  s. *Inhalation of toxic or caustic substances such as gases, animal products, chemicals, metals, wood dusts, pharmaceuticals, and other dusts, sprays, and plant substances*
  t. *Environmental pollution*
  u. *Occupational exposure (e.g., among firefighters, coal miners, cotton mill workers)*
  v. *Changes in weather to extremes of hot or cold; humidity changes*
  w. *Exercise induced*
  x. *Emotional distress: may precipitate asthma attack*
  y. *Recent travel*

4. Focused survey
  a. *Subjective data*
   1) History of present illness
    a) Chief complaint
     (1) Dyspnea, shortness of breath
     (2) Pain: provocation, quality, region, radiation, severity, timing
     (3) Coughing, choking
     (4) Hemoptysis
     (5) Sputum production
     (6) Pallor, cyanosis
     (7) Diaphoresis
     (8) Hoarseness
     (9) Dysphagia
     (10) Hematemesis
     (11) Abnormal respiratory sounds (e.g., wheezing, rhonchi)
     (12) Anxiety/restlessness
     (13) Injury: mechanism and time
     (14) Time of onset of symptoms
     (15) Association with exertion
     (16) Association with chest pain
     (17) Fever, chills
     (18) Nausea, vomiting, diarrhea
     (19) Anorexia, weight loss
     (20) Current medications and allergies

        (21) Current immunization status

    2) Medical history

        a) Pulmonary diseases

        b) Cardiac diseases

        c) Renal disease

        d) Autoimmune disorders

        e) Allergies to substances or materials, atopy

b. *Objective data*

    1) Physical examination

        a) General survey

            (1) Respiratory rate, rhythm, depth, effort

            (2) Pulse: rate, rhythm, amplitude

            (3) Blood pressure, pulsus paradoxus

            (4) Capillary refill

            (5) Skin and mucosa: color, temperature, moisture

            (6) Temperature

            (7) Level of consciousness

            (8) Pupillary size and reactivity

            (9) Carpopedal spasms: spasms of hands and feet sometimes seen in hyperventilation syndrome, possible tingling around mouth

        b) Inspection

            (1) Nose: nasal flaring

            (2) Trachea

            (3) Neck veins

            (4) Pharynx

            (5) Thorax

                (a) Shape of chest: deformities, symmetry, anteroposterior (AP) diameter; barrel chest may be present in chronic obstructive pulmonary disease (COPD)

                (b) Wounds: open or closed; surgical wounds

                (c) Posture

                (d) Respiratory excursion

                (e) Paradoxical chest motion

                (f) Use of accessory muscles

                (g) Abnormal retraction or bulging of interspaces

        c) Palpation

            (1) Areas of tenderness, crepitus, deformity

            (2) Respiratory excursion

            (3) Vocal or tactile fremitus

            (4) Subcutaneous emphysema

            (5) Tracheal position, movement

        d) Percussion

            (1) Note distribution of sound

            (2) Diaphragmatic level

        e) Auscultation

            (1) Breath sounds

                (a) Presence or absence

                (b) Increase or decrease

                (c) Distribution

            (2) Adventitious sounds, always abnormal

                (a) Wheezing: musical sound

                (b) Crackles or rales: small popping sounds produced by passage of air through secretions or lightly closed airways

Table 18–1   BLOOD GAS: NORMAL VALUES

Variable	Arterial	Capillary	Venous
pH	7.35–7.45	7.35–7.45	7.31–7.41
Pao_2	80–100	40–60	35–40
$Paco_2$	35–45	35–45	41–51
HCO_3	22–26	22–26	22–26
BE	±2	±2	±2
Acid/base	pH 7.35–7.45	Increased pH = alkalosis > 7.45	
		Decreased pH = acidosis < 7.35	
Metabolic component	Bicarbonate HCO_3 22–26 mEq	Increased HCO_3 = metabolic alkalosis > 26 mEq	
		Decreased HCO_3 = metabolic acidosis < 22 mEq	
Respiratory component	$Paco_2$ 35–40 mm Hg	Increased $Paco_2$ = respiratory acidosis > 40 mm Hg	
		Decreased $Paco_2$ = respiratory alkalosis < 35 mm Hg	

Pao_2, partial pressure of arterial oxygen; $Paco_2$, partial pressure of arterial carbon dioxide; HCO_3, bicarbonate radical; BE, base excess.

From Tipsord-Klinkhammer, B., Andreoni, C. P. (1998). *Quick reference for emergency nursing*. Philadelphia: W.B. Saunders. Used with permission.

      (c) Rhonchi: snoring, low-pitched sounds similar to wheezes, produced by air passing through narrowed air passages

      (d) Pleural friction rub: grating heard with inspiration and expiration due to inflammation of the pleural surfaces

    (3) Voice sounds: sound of a spoken word may be increased or decreased when modified by disease

  2) Diagnostic procedures

    a) Cardiac monitor/electrocardiogram (ECG)

    b) Pulse oximetry to monitor oxygen saturation levels

    c) Laboratory studies

      (1) Complete blood count (CBC)

      (2) Serum electrolytes

      (3) Arterial blood gases (ABGs) (Tables 18–1 and 18–2); capillary gases, venous gases

      (4) Type and screen, type and cross-match blood

      (5) Urinalysis (U/A)

Table 18–2   INTERPRETATION OF ARTERIAL BLOOD GAS VALUES

Variable	pH	Pco_2	$HCO_3{}^-$
Respiratory acidosis	↓	↑	Normal
Respiratory acidosis with metabolic compensation	↓	↑	↑
Metabolic acidosis	↓	Normal	↓
Metabolic and respiratory acidosis	↓	↑	↓
Metabolic alkalosis	↑	Normal	↑
Metabolic alkalosis with respiratory compensation	↑	↑	↑
Respiratory alkalosis	↑	↓	Normal
Metabolic and respiratory alkalosis	↑	↓	↑

      (6) Blood alcohol level: ethanol [ETOH])—elevations may lead to respiratory depression, possible aspiration

      (7) Drug levels (urine, serum): may explain cause of increased or decreased respiratory rate or depth

      (8) Coagulation studies (prothrombin time [PT], partial thromboplastin time [PTT])

      (9) Thoracentesis fluid analysis

  e) Radiology

      (1) Chest radiograph, rib films

      (2) Computed tomography (CT) scan

      (3) Esophagogram

      (4) Lung scan (ventilation-perfusion scan)

  f) Other procedures

      (1) Esophagoscopy

      (2) Bronchoscopy

      (3) Simple spirometry: to estimate patient's ability to exhale (significant in asthma)

      (4) Peak flow rate is measurement of choice in asthma; a decreasing peak flow should raise suspicion of narrowed airways

      (5) Forced expiratory volume (FEV_1) is amount of air that can be forced from lungs in 1 second. FEV_1 of less than 80% of predicted tidal volume is indicative of obstructive lung disease

  g) Preparation of patient for diagnostic procedures

      (1) Physical preparation

      (2) Emotional support

      (3) Teaching of patient and significant others

      (4) Written consent, as appropriate

B. Analysis: differential nursing diagnosis/collaborative problems

1. **Anxiety/fear**
2. **Cardiac output, decreased**
3. **Fluid volume excess or deficit**
4. **Impaired gas exchange**
5. **Ineffective airway clearance**
6. **Ineffective breathing pattern**
7. **Knowledge deficit**
8. **Pain**
9. **Risk for infection**
10. **Noncompliance**
11. **Tissue perfusion, altered cardiopulmonary function**

C. Planning/interventions

1. **Determine priorities**
   - a. *Control and maintain airway, breathing, circulation*
   - b. *Prevent complications*
   - c. *Control pain*
   - d. *Relieve anxiety and emotional distress*
   - e. *Educate patient/significant others*
2. **Develop nursing care plan specific to patient's emergency**
3. **Obtain and set up necessary equipment and supplies**

D. Evaluation

1. **Monitor responses and outcomes of patient and/or significant others; if positive outcomes are not demonstrated, re-evaluate assessment and/or plan of care**
   a. *Specific interventions*
   b. *Disposition/discharge planning*
2. **Record data as appropriate**

E. Age-related considerations

1. **Pediatric**
   a. *Growth and development related*
      1) Ribs are more compliant; adult-level compliance reached by age 20 years
      2) Mediastinum thinner, more mobile
      3) Infants are obligate nose breathers; children depend on diaphragm for adequate chest expansion; may exhibit grunting or head bobbing with respiratory distress
      4) Airways are small in size and easily obstructed by edema or mucus
      5) Children's metabolic rate and oxygen consumption much higher than those of adults
   b. *"Pearls"*
      1) Increased thoracic compliance may result in internal injury without visual external evidence of trauma
      2) Airway resistance in infants is 15 times greater than in adults
      3) Accessory muscles of inspiration tire quickly owing to less reserve muscle glycogen
      4) Greater body surface area and increased respiratory rate lead to rapid heat and water loss with infection and fever
2. **Geriatric**
   a. *Aging related*
      1) Decreased vital capacity, forced expiratory volume, maximum midexpiratory flow
      2) Increased residual volume and functional residual capacity
      3) Decreased static muscle strength and elastic lung recoil
      4) Increased work of breathing
      5) Decreased diffusion capacity and arterial oxygenation
      6) Increased ventilation-perfusion inequality, alveolar-arterial oxygen gradient
   b. *"Pearls"*
      1) Pulmonary defense mechanisms are reduced, making elderly more susceptible to infections
      2) Diminished ventilatory response to hypoxic and hypercapnic challenge
      3) Elderly report dyspnea as breathlessness
      4) Causes of dyspnea in elderly include
         a) Functional impairment of pulmonary or cardiopulmonary system
         b) Impaired oxygen delivery secondary to hematological dysfunction
      5) ECG is mandatory because acute myocardial infarction (AMI) can present with dyspnea
      6) Aspiration mortality rate 40 to 70%; also significant cause of pulmonary morbidity
      7) Pneumonia is leading infectious disease cause of death in elderly; first sign may be deterioration in general health; nonpulmonary complaints, such as malaise and lethargy, are common

8) Normal patients older than 60 years can expire 75% of vital capacity in 1 second
   a) 65 to 75% = mild obstruction
   b) 50 to 65% = moderate obstruction
   c) Less than 50% = severe obstruction

II. SPECIFIC MEDICAL EMERGENCIES

A. Adult respiratory distress syndrome

Adult respiratory distress syndrome (ARDS) is a sudden, progressive, severe pulmonary disorder characterized by dyspnea, hypoxemia, and diffuse bilateral infiltrates. The syndrome is caused by direct pulmonary injury or results from systemic illness or trauma. Specific pulmonary insult occurs from pneumonia, embolism, aspiration, inhalation of smoke or toxins, prolonged exposure to oxygen, high-altitude pulmonary edema, and lung contusions. Indirect pulmonary assaults causing ARDS include sepsis, DIC, pancreatitis, uremia, anaphylaxis, drug overdose, eclampsia, radiation therapy, shock, multisystem trauma, and massive blood transfusions. The lung tissue responds to the assault with a diffuse inflammatory reaction in the microvasculature of the lungs. The release of chemical mediators, alveolar macrophages, and vasoactive substances cause increased permeability of the capillary and alveolar membranes with resultant pulmonary edema. Damage to the alveolar epithelium causes decreased surfactant, and the alveolar and interstitial edema contributes to the decreased lung compliance. The resultant atelectasis causes severe respiratory distress, leading to failure. The lungs are typically scarred if the patient survives. ARDS is also known as adult hyaline membrane disease, wet lung, post-traumatic pulmonary insufficiency, Da Nang lung, shock lung, acute lung injury (ALI), and pulmonary contusion. It affects approximately 150,000 adults per year, with a mortality risk of 40 to 70%, even though often it occurs in adults in the absence of chronic illness or lung disease. Investigational treatment modalities include pharmacological therapies to inhibit the destructive activity of the chemical mediators and alternative ventilation procedures.

1. **Assessment**
   a. *Subjective data*
      1) History of present illness
         a) Sudden marked respiratory distress
         b) Trauma
         c) Shock
         d) Multiple transfusions
         e) Fluid overload
         f) Embolism
         g) Drug overdose
         h) Near-drowning incident
         i) Inhalation of caustic toxic materials
         j) Pulmonary contusion
         k) Burns
         l) Aspiration
         m) Radiation
         n) Uremia
         o) Eclampsia
      2) Medical history
         a) Heart disease
         b) Lung disease

    c) Past surgeries

    d) Pancreatic disease

    e) Central nervous system (CNS) disease

    f) Allergies

    g) Smoking

  b. Objective data

    1) Physical examination

      a) Tachypnea: usually first sign

      b) Hypoxia, hyperventilation, respiratory distress

      c) Cyanosis

      d) Hypotension, tachycardia

      e) Restless, anxious behaviors

      f) Auscultation of fine to coarse crackles, possible adventitious sounds

    2) Diagnostic procedures

      a) ABGs

      b) Chest radiograph: white infiltrates are usually present; pulmonary edema without cardiomegaly

      c) Respiratory function measures (FEV_1, forced vital capacity [FVC])

      d) Shunting studies

      e) Electrolytes, CBC

2. Analysis: differential nursing diagnosis/collaborative problems

  a. Ineffective airway clearance related to possible injury and increased secretions

  b. Impaired gas exchange related to noncompliant lungs and impaired pulmonary-capillary permeability

  c. Tissue perfusion, altered related to impaired gas exchange

  d. Cardiac output, decreased related to high end expiratory pulmonary pressure (if a high positive end-expiratory pressure (PEEP) is set on ventilator)

  e. Fluid volume excess related to overhydration

  f. Anxiety/fear related to dyspnea, hypoxemia, and illness

3. Planning/interventions

  a. Maintain airway, breathing, circulation; initiate humidified oxygen therapy; prepare for probable intubation and ventilator support (tidal volume decreases as lungs lose compliance); obtain ABGs, and observe for changes

  b. Place patient in high-Fowler's or side-lying position whenever possible

  c. Assist with secretion removal: have patient cough and deep breathe; use incentive spirometry to help loosen secretions and facilitate coughing, suction as indicated

  d. Initiate at least one intravenous (IV) catheter, and carefully monitor fluid administration and urine output (more than 30 mL/hr urine output desirable)

  e. Administer medications as indicated

    1) Analgesics, sedation, and corticosteroids are commonly used to facilitate intubation and ventilation

    2) Paralytic agents may be necessary as lung compliance continues to deteriorate and PEEP levels are increased to maintain gas exchange

  f. Continuously monitor airway, breathing, circulation; level of consciousness, and vital signs of patient; assessment of respiratory and cardiac function should be ongoing

  g. Prepare for advanced hemodynamic monitoring: arterial and central venous catheters, Swan-Ganz catheter

  h. Actively communicate with patient and significant others to educate them about patient's status, procedures, plan of care

i. Allow calm significant others to accompany hemodynamically stable patient in treatment area

4. **Expected outcomes/evaluation** (see Appendix B)

B. Asthma

Asthma is a chronic, reversible obstructive pulmonary disease that is caused by airway inflammation and increased airway responsiveness (bronchospasm) to stimuli. The typical presentation is dyspnea, wheezing, and a cough. Multiple factors may be involved in an attack, including biochemical, immunological, endocrine, infectious, autonomic, and psychological precipitators. Typically, environmental factors trigger the response in those individuals with an inherited predisposition to the disease. An allergen or stimulant causes B lymphocytes to produce immunoglobulin E (IgE), which attaches to mast cells and basophils in the bronchial walls. These cells then release their chemical mediators: histamine, prostaglandins, bradykinins, slow-reacting substances of anaphylaxis (SRS-A), and leukotrienes. Steroids interrupt the release of the chemical mediators. These mediators cause mucus secretion, inflammation, and bronchospasm. Chronic inflammation causes hyperresponsiveness of the airways, which can be stimulated by exercise or cold air.

Status asthmaticus is a life-threatening emergency: the bronchospasm does not respond to conventional therapy. This leads to worsening hypoxemia, acid-base balance disturbance, and eventual respiratory arrest if uninterrupted. Ten to 15 million Americans have asthma, it affects more males than females, and it is the most common chronic childhood illness. Asthma affects approximately 5 to 10% of children and is more prevalent among lower income, inner city black children, children with low birth weight or of young mothers, and those with genetic atopic disease. Two thirds of patients with asthma are diagnosed by the age of 40 years. The morbidity and mortality of asthma are increasing, causing approximately 5000 deaths per year. The death rate of asthma is greater for females and for African-Americans.

1. **Assessment**
   a. *Subjective data*
      1) History of present illness
         a) Dyspnea, cough, wheezing
         b) Restlessness resulting from increased hypoxia
         c) Tightness in chest
         d) Symptoms of infection: productive cough, fever, general "cold" symptoms such as malaise, sore throat, "stuffy nose"
         e) Exposure to known allergens
         f) Emotional factors
         g) Environmental factors: exposure to extremes of heat/cold, humidity, dust, mold, smoke, pets
         h) Current medications/combinations, over-the-counter medications, inhalers, and steroids
         i) Time of onset of symptoms
      2) Medical history
         a) Previous asthma problems, including last emergency department (ED) visit or admission for asthma
         b) Hereditary asthma/allergy problems
         c) Lung disease
   b. *Objective data*
      1) Physical examination

a) Wheezing on inspiration and/or expiration: not always present as in significantly decreased air movement
b) Prolonged expiratory phase of respiratory cycle
c) Dyspnea
d) Use of accessory muscles
e) Tachypnea
f) Cough: dry or productive
g) Tachycardia
h) Pulsus paradoxus: present in some patients
i) Hyperresonance
j) Pallor and/or cyanosis
k) Diaphoresis
l) Physical exhaustion
m) Restlessness
n) Orthopneic posturing
o) Children with significant hypoxemia may demonstrate somnolence, decreased respiratory effort, decreased heart rate, possible periodic apnea

2) Diagnostic procedures
   a) Laboratory studies
      (1) CBC: leukocytosis, eosinophilia, increased hematocrit (if possible, obtain specimen before bronchodilator therapy and steroids)
      (2) Electrolytes: potassium and chloride may be decreased in long-standing respiratory acidosis
      (3) ABGs: may be normal initially, then reflective of hypoxemia, hypercarbia (an ominous sign), and resulting respiratory acidosis
      (4) Sputum studies
      (5) Theophylline level
   b) Chest radiograph
   c) Objective measurement of airflow obstruction: spirometry, peak flow meter
   d) Pulse oximetry

2. Analysis: differential nursing diagnosis/collaborative problems

a. *Ineffective airway clearance related to bronchospasm, edema, and increased mucus production in airways*
b. *Impaired gas exchange: hypoxemia, related to increased mucous production and obstruction of airflow*
c. *Ineffective breathing pattern resulting from impaired exhalation and anxiety*
d. *Anxiety/fear related to shortness of breath and prognosis*
e. *Knowledge deficit related to diagnosis and therapeutic regimen for asthma*

3. Planning/interventions

a. *Use critical pathway, standard orders, or protocols if available*
b. *Position patient to facilitate breathing*
c. *Provide humidification via mask or open face tent, and provide oxygen as indicated; monitor oxygen saturation*
d. *Establish and maintain IV catheter for medications and fluids*
e. *Administer medications as indicated: usually includes bronchodilators and corticosteroids; possible use of magnesium or Heliox (helium-oxygen mixtures) for status asthmaticus*
f. *Assist patient in removal of secretions: coughing/deep-breathing exercises, suction as necessary*
g. *Continuously monitor ECG for cardiac dysrhythmias secondary to hypoxia or acidosis; respiratory status effects of medications, pulse oximetry, and ABGs*

h. *Push fluids to liquefy secretions using oral (PO) and/or IV routes as tolerated*
i. *Prepare for more aggressive ventilatory support*
j. *Protect patient from environmental, pharmaceutical, and emotional irritants that may exacerbate asthma attacks*
k. *Communicate frequently with patient, family, significant others*
l. *Explain all procedures*
m. *Allow calm significant other to remain with patient in treatment area when possible*
n. *Educate patient, family, and significant others regarding discharge instructions and follow-up treatment and evaluation; provide instructions related to disease process, aggravating allergens, precipitating factors, medications (purpose, route, dose, and side effects); stress that corticosteroid therapy should never be stopped abruptly but instead should be tapered off as prescribed; information about importance of hydration, use of home nebulizers and peak flow meters, relaxation techniques, and controlled breathing should also be given*
o. *Provide discharge instruction sheet in large print to reinforce verbal teaching*
p. *Arrange follow-up schedule*
4. **Expected outcomes/evaluation** (see Appendix B)

C. Acute bronchitis

Bronchitis is an inflammation of the bronchi and/or trachea that is believed to result from irritation of the bronchial mucosa by such elements as pollen, smoking, and inhalation of irritating substances. Acute bronchitis is commonly seen at the time of, or shortly after, an upper respiratory tract infection (URI) and is generally caused by influenza, parainfluenza, adenovirus, or rhinovirus. A secondary infection may also occur, but the acute episode generally clears without treatment unless a chronic disease is present. As a precursor to COPD, acute bronchitis is commonly found in middle-aged persons, is more common in men than in women, and occurs most frequently during the winter. This condition may be referred to as chronic bronchitis if it is characterized by persistent production of excess bronchial mucus.

1. **Assessment**
   a. *Subjective data*
      1) History of present illness
         a) Dyspnea, wheezing
         b) Cough: initially dry, then productive
         c) Fever
         d) Chest/back pains
         e) Malaise
         f) Repeated respiratory infections
         g) Environmental history: smoking, occupational factors (e.g., in coal miners, chemical workers)
      2) Medical history
         a) Recent URI
         b) Pulmonary disease
         c) Allergies
   b. *Objective data*
      1) Physical examination
         a) Respiratory rate: normal or slightly increased
         b) Use of accessory muscles for breathing
         c) Prolonged expiratory phase
         d) Rhonchi, wet lungs at bases

e) Chest resonant to percussion

f) Sputum: thin and clear to thick and purulent

g) Neck vein distention in chronic bronchitis secondary to cor pulmonale

2) Diagnostic procedures

a) Laboratory

(1) CBC

(2) Serum electrolytes

(3) Sputum examination: Gram's stain culture and sensitivity

b) Chest radiograph

c) Pulmonary function tests (PFTs)

2. Analysis: differential nursing diagnosis/collaborative problems

a. *Ineffective airway clearance related to irritation and inflammation of bronchial mucosa*

b. *Impaired gas exchange related to ventilation-perfusion imbalance*

c. *Anxiety/fear related to symptomatology and need to seek medical intervention*

d. *Knowledge deficit related to diagnosis, therapeutic regimen, and follow-up procedures*

3. Planning/interventions

a. *Position patient to facilitate breathing*

b. *Provide heated aerosol treatments and/or oxygen*

c. *Remove environmental irritants (including smoking)*

d. *Perform postural drainage as indicated*

e. *Increase oral fluids to liquefy secretions*

f. *Administer medications as prescribed (may include bronchodilators, corticosteroids, antianxiety drugs)*

g. *Reassure patient, family, and significant others*

h. *Explain all procedures*

i. *Educate patient, family, and significant others about disease process, impact of irritating substances, importance of fluids, signs of superimposed infection*

j. *Provide written discharge instructions*

k. *Arrange for follow-up care*

4. Expected outcomes/evaluation (see Appendix B)

D. Bronchiolitis

Bronchiolitis is a lower respiratory tract infection characterized by an inflammatory obstruction of the airway. This infection primarily affects children younger than 2 years, typically infants younger than 1 year old. When it does affect adults, the symptoms are generally mild. Respiratory syncytial virus (RSV) causes 90% of bronchiolitis infections and occurs primarily during the winter months. The other causes include parainfluenza virus, influenza, adenovirus (causing very severe illness), rhinovirus, enterovirus, herpes simplex, and mycoplasma pneumonia. The causative virus initiates an inflammatory response with profuse respiratory secretions and a necrotic response producing cellular debris and fibrin, creating obstruction of the bronchi and bronchioles (smaller airways), which contribute to upper airway reactivity. The airway obstruction leads to air trapping, high resistance, and atelectasis (patchy infiltrate on chest x-ray film). This results in a ventilation-perfusion defect, hypoxemia, and eventual fatigue. At risk for serious illness or complications are very young children or premature infants and children with chronic lung disease or hemodynamically significant congenital heart disease, immunodeficiency, or previous mechanical ventilation. Bronchiolitis/RSV is an important risk factor for the subsequent development of asthma.

1. **Assessment**
   a. *Subjective data*
      1) History of present illness
         a) Several days of mild/moderate URI symptoms of rhinorrhea, cough, and low-grade fever, progressing to increased dyspnea
         b) Increased cough
         c) Poor feeding, vomiting
         d) Irritability
         e) Decreased sleep
      2) Medical history
         a) Chronic lung disease
         b) Congenital heart disease with significant hemodynamic compromise
         c) Immunodeficiency
   b. *Objective data*
      1) Physical examination
         a) General survey
         b) Tachypnea, apnea possible in infants
         c) Tachycardia
         d) Decreased oxygen saturation
         e) Possible wheezing
         f) Signs of respiratory distress: grunting, nasal flaring, intercostal and suprasternal retractions
         g) Change in level of consciousness, lethargy
         h) Cyanosis
         i) Depressed fontanelle if dehydrated
      2) Diagnostic procedures
         a) Capillary blood gases or ABGs if acutely ill
         b) CBC
         c) Electrolytes to rule out dehydration
         d) Chest x-ray film to rule out pneumonia, pneumothorax, or foreign body, to show areas of atelectasis
         e) Rapid viral nasopharyngeal swab or aspirate for RSV/viral culture
2. **Analysis: differential nursing diagnosis/collaborative problems**
   a. *Ineffective airway clearance related to edema and secretions*
   b. *Ineffective breathing pattern related to paroxysmal coughing, fatigue*
   c. *Impaired gas exchange related to secretions, atelectasis, edema*
   d. *Activity intolerance related to increased work of breathing, hypoxemia*
   e. *Knowledge deficit of caregiver related to disease process*
   f. *Anxiety/fear of caregiver related to illness of child and hospital environment*
3. **Planning/interventions**
   a. *Maintain airway, breathing, circulation: frequent reassessment for early signs of fatigue/respiratory failure (in infants respirations consistently greater than 80, heart rate greater than 200); continuous pulse oximetry*
   b. *Oxygen therapy: mask, cannula, "blow-by," humidification*
   c. *Nebulizer treatments for wheezing*
   d. *Hydration: oral, if possible, or IV*
   e. *Prepare for admission for respiratory distress: persistent oxygen saturations less than 92%, respirations consistently above 70, fatigue, and apnea spells; may be given ribavirin for RSV if hospitalized*
   f. *Avoid stress of child, provide position of comfort with parents*
   g. *Suction as necessary*
   h. *Prepare for possible intubation for respiratory failure*
   i. *Provide discharge instructions*

1) Home nebulizer treatments
2) Fever management
3) Small, frequent feedings
4) Signs of increasing respiratory distress
5) Physician follow-up

4. Expected outcomes/evaluation (see Appendix B)

E. Chronic obstructive pulmonary disease

COPD is characterized by chronic or recurrent airflow obstruction. Smoking, environmental pollution, occupational exposure to chemicals, tuberculosis, aging, and heredity are causative factors in the development of COPD. These irritants, diseases, and genetic factors cause bronchial mucosal edema and smooth muscle contraction (resulting in increased airway resistance) and decreased elastic recoil. The physiological changes cause difficulty exhaling and impaired alveolar gas exchange. The disease entities that comprise COPD include asthma (airway reaction), chronic obstructive bronchitis (airway inflammation), and emphysema (airway collapse). Individuals generally have all three components present, but one type usually predominates. COPD affects approximately 1 of 10 people, and it is second only to heart disease in morbidity and mortality, causing more than 100,000 deaths per year. It typically affects men older than 45 years, but more women are developing the disease secondary to smoking.

Chronic obstructive bronchitis is characterized by inflammation of the bronchi, leading to increased mucus production and chronic cough. It is diagnosed by the presence of the symptoms for at least 3 months of the year for 2 consecutive years. Chronic irritation causes an increase in the number and size of mucous cells leading to increased mucus production and impaired ciliary function. These physiological changes also inhibit the normal defense mechanisms against infection. Because of the airway obstruction, airway collapse occurs, causing air trapping and chronic hypoxia with possible hypercapnia. Under normal physiological circumstances, the respiratory drive is triggered by high partial pressure of arterial carbon dioxide ($PaCO_2$). However, the patient with chronic obstructive bronchitis may have a chronically elevated $PaCO_2$ and lose this drive for a respiratory stimulus. Therefore, hypoxia becomes the respiratory stimulus, and excessive oxygen administration may obliterate that drive. Polycythemia and potential pulmonary hypertension leading to cor pulmonale may develop. Cor pulmonale is visibly evident in the classic "blue bloater" with symptoms of peripheral edema, anasarca, and chronic neck vein distention.

Emphysema is the disorder of impeded expiration caused by permanent overdistention of air spaces, alveolar wall destruction, partial airway collapse, and loss of elastic recoil of the lungs. Pockets of air form between the alveoli and within the lung parenchyma, causing increased ventilatory dead space and decreased functional lung tissue. This leads to a resultant increased work of breathing. In addition, the pulmonary capillary bed is essentially obliterated by enzymatic activity, causing decreased oxygen perfusion and ventilation. Protease and elastase are two enzymes that appear to be involved in this tissue-destructive component of emphysema because of the breakdown in the lung's normal defense mechanism involving α_1-antitrypsin. Symptoms of emphysema begin with dyspnea on exertion deteriorating to dyspnea at rest and accompanied by tachypnea. A cough is not typical, but respiratory infections are common because of alterations in normal respiratory defenses and immunity and may precipitate respiratory failure.

1. Assessment (refer to Table 18–3)

   a. Subjective data

Table 18–3 COMPARISON OF SYMPTOMS OF CHRONIC OBSTRUCTIVE BRONCHITIS AND EMPHYSEMA

Chronic Obstructive Bronchitis	Emphysema
"Blue bloater"	"Pink puffer"
Productive cough	Cough uncommon
Stocky build	Thin
Onset 40–50 years	Onset 50–75 years
Normal respiratory rate	Tachypnea
Hypoxemia	PaO_2 normal or slightly decreased
Increased $PaCO_2$	$PaCO_2$ usually low or normal until end stage
Cyanosis	
Polycythemia	Barrel chest
Cor pulmonale	Accessory muscle use
Peripheral edema	Leans forward while sitting
Risk for PE	Pursed-lip breathing
	Hyperresonance on percussion
X-ray film shows enlarged heart	Lung overinflation, diaphragm low

$PaCO_2$, partial pressure of arterial carbon dioxide; PE, pulmonary embolism; PaO_2, partial pressure of arterial oxygen.

1) History of present illness
    a) Dyspnea
    b) Current URI
    c) Air pollution
2) Medical history
    a) Lung disease
    b) Recent URI
    c) Cigarette smoking or exposure
    d) Cardiac disease
    e) Medications (and compliance), home oxygen, and allergies
  b. *Objective data*
    1) Physical exam
      a) Crackles, rhonchi, expiratory wheezes
      b) Inability to speak in complete sentences without taking a breath
      c) Tachycardia, cardiac dysrhythmias
      d) Decreased oxygen saturation
      e) Pulsus paradoxus
    2) Diagnostic procedures
      a) Laboratory studies
        (1) ABGs: hypoxemia, hypercarbia
        (2) CBC: polycythemia, eosinophilia, increased white cell count
        (3) Sputum: culture and sensitivity (C&S)
        (4) Enzymes: α_1-antitrypsin (deficiency indicative of emphysema)
      b) Chest radiograph
      c) Pulmonary function
        (1) Spirometry
        (2) Peak flow meter
      d) Pulse oximetry
2. Analysis: differential nursing diagnosis/collaborative problems
  a. *Ineffective airway clearance related to loss of elasticity of lung tissue and structural damage or irritation and inflammation of bronchial mucosa*
  b. *Impaired gas exchange: hypoxemia, hypercarbia, related to physiological damage at alveolar level or excess mucus*

     c. *Anxiety/fear related to dyspnea, need to seek medical attention, and prognosis*

     d. *Knowledge deficit related to diagnosis, therapeutic regimen, and follow-up*

3. Planning/interventions

     a. *Position patient to facilitate breathing*

     b. *Assist with removal of secretions*

     c. *Provide humidified breathing treatments and/or low-flow oxygen*

     d. *Obtain/monitor ABGs, monitor oximetry*

     e. *Prepare for more aggressive ventilatory support*

     f. *Maintain IV catheter for fluids and medications*

     g. *Administer prescribed medications: bronchodilators, steroids, antibiotics as indicated*

     h. *Hydrate patient via PO or IV route to liquefy secretions*

     i. *Monitor for cardiac dysrhythmias secondary to hypoxemia and medications*

     j. *Reassure patient and significant others*

     k. *Allow calm significant others to remain with patient when possible*

     l. *Explain all procedures*

     m. *Educate patient on how to use pursed-lip breathing and diaphragmatic breathing techniques properly*

     n. *Educate patient and significant others about body positioning for optimal air exchange; eating small, frequent meals as opposed to heavy traditional meals; importance of exercise; coughing and deep-breathing exercises; and adequate hydration*

     o. *Educate patient about medications, inhalers, nebulizers, possible need for pneumococcal and viral immunizations*

     p. *Provide a written discharge sheet to support learning*

     q. *Arrange follow-up care*

4. Expected outcomes/evaluation (see Appendix B)

F. Croup (laryngotracheobronchitis)

Croup is an acute viral clinical syndrome characterized by barking cough, hoarse voice, inspiratory stridor, and variable degrees of respiratory distress. This most commonly affects children ages 6 to 36 months (more often males), peaking in late fall and early winter. The most common causative agent is the parainfluenza virus type I, which causes the yearly winter epidemic. Other causes include the parainfluenza type III, adenovirus, RSV, and influenza A (which may produce very severe cases). The initial portal of entry is the nasopharynx, and it then spreads to the larynx and trachea, causing erythema and edema of the tracheal walls. An inflammatory exudate is produced and the vocal cords swell, causing the typical stridor, hoarseness, and barking cough. Symptoms typically occur or recur at night and usually resolve with humidified air. Total obstruction rarely occurs.

1. Assessment

     a. *Subjective data*

        1) History of present illness

            a) "Barking" cough

            b) Evidence of URI for 1 to 2 days

            c) Low-grade to moderate fever, rarely exceeds 102.2°F (39°C)

            d) Current medications

            e) Physical exhaustion

        2) Medical history: recent infections of measles, adenovirus, influenza A and B, rhinovirus, parainfluenza

     b. *Objective data*

        1) Physical examination

a) Croup cough: harsh, barking cough
b) Absent to minimal drooling
c) Stridor: inspiratory and expiratory
d) Normal epiglottis, inflamed pharynx
e) Bilateral diminished breath sounds
f) Suprasternal retractions
g) Tachypnea
h) Tachycardia
i) Low to moderate fever
j) Restlessness
k) Hoarse voice
l) Lethargy

2) Diagnostic studies
a) Radiology
(1) Neck: soft tissue radiograph (to rule out epiglottiditis)
(2) Chest radiograph
b) Laboratory studies
(1) CBC
(2) ABGs or capillary gases if indicated
(3) Direct or indirect laryngoscopy
c) Pulse oximetry

2. **Analysis: differential nursing diagnosis/collaborative problems**
   a. *Risk for ineffective airway clearance related to laryngeal edema and obstruction*
   b. *Anxiety/fear, parental related to symptomatology and need to seek medical attention*
   c. *Knowledge deficit related to diagnosis, therapeutic regimen, follow-up procedures*

3. **Planning/interventions**
   a. *Position patient to facilitate breathing*
   b. *Administer cool, humidified air, supplemented with oxygen as indicated by pulse oximetry*
   c. *Administer medications as prescribed*
      1) Racemic epinephrine for respiratory distress: requires period of observation (patient may rebound in 1–1½ hours)
      2) Corticosteroids: usually intramuscularly (IM)
   d. *Hydration: oral or IV*
   e. *Reassure patient and significant others*
   f. *Explain all procedures*
   g. *Allow calm significant other to remain with patient in treatment area*
   h. *Educate patient and significant others about signs of respiratory distress, disease process, use of cool, humidified air, increased fluids, and follow-up*
   i. *Provide parent with written instructions for clarification and reference*

4. **Expected outcomes/evaluation** (see Appendix B)

G. Acute epiglottitis

Acute epiglottitis is a life-threatening condition characterized by edema of the epiglottis and epiglottic folds not extending below the vocal cords. The onset of symptoms is usually rapid with a high temperature (usually > 101.3°F [38.5°C]), lethargy, anorexia, and a severe sore throat. These patients do not have the harsh cough symptomatic of croup. A "tripod" or "sniffing" position is often apparent, with mouth breathing, drooling, and an ominous, exhausted facial appearance displayed.

Epiglottitis is typically not seasonal and is more common in children (most often males), but may affect adults as well. In adults, the illness is most common among 20- to 40-year-olds and is reported to occur in 10 to 40 persons per million population. The incidence of childhood epiglottitis has dramatically decreased as a result of the *Haemophilus* influenza (HIB) vaccine, which has eliminated the most common cause of infection. When epiglottitis does occur, a child is at great risk for airway obstruction and should immediately be transferred via an ambulance to an accepting hospital with appropriate pediatric facilities. Airway access is best obtained in an operating room with the patient under anesthesia and an ear, nose, and throat (ENT) surgeon present if a surgical airway is required. The patients who die usually do so before they reach appropriate treatment facilities.

1. **Assessment**
   a. *Subjective data*
      1) History of present illness
         a) Dyspnea
         b) Fever (usually > 101.3°F [38.5°C]
         c) Severe sore throat
         d) Drooling
         e) Abrupt onset
      2) Medical history: Recent upper airway infection, immunizations
   b. *Objective data*
      1) Physical examination
         a) Do not examine pharynx, attempt IV access, draw blood, or obtain radiographs until emergency airway equipment and most skilled pediatric intubator are present
         b) Ill appearance of patient
         c) "Tripod" or "sniffing" position assumed
         d) Dysphagia, dysphonia, or aphonia
         e) Drooling
         f) Inspiratory stridor, expiratory snore
         g) Substernal and supraclavicular retractions
         h) High temperature: greater than 101.3°F (38.5°C)
         i) Adult may have tenderness to palpation of anterior neck/hyoid region
      2) Diagnostic procedures
         a) Radiology
            (1) Lateral neck: done first with as little disruption as possible to avoid laryngospasm
            (2) Chest radiograph
         b) Laboratory studies
            (1) CBC
            (2) ABGs
         c) Direct or indirect laryngoscopy
         d) Pulse oximetry if tolerated
2. **Analysis: differential nursing diagnosis/collaborative problems**
   a. *Ineffective airway clearance related to laryngospasm and edema*
   b. *Impaired gas exchange related to impeded airflow*
   c. *Anxiety related to difficulty in breathing and need to seek medical attention*
3. **Planning/interventions**
   a. *Allow significant others to stay with patient; encourage them to hold child if this is reassuring to child; it is of utmost importance not to upset patient with epiglottitis because this could precipitate life-threatening laryngospasm*
   b. *Provide calm, quiet atmosphere*
   c. *Position patient to facilitate breathing*

    d. Provide humidified "blow-by" oxygen held by parent or significant other when possible

    e. Assist with gentle removal of secretions as necessary

    f. Prepare for emergency endotracheal intubation, cricothyroidotomy, or tracheostomy

    g. Prepare for aggressive ventilatory support with bag-valve mask followed by ventilator when airway is secured

    h. Delay diagnostic procedures, except lateral neck radiograph, until epiglottitis is ruled out or patent airway is secured

    i. Maintain IV catheter for medications (not done until airway is secured)

    j. Administer prescribed medications: antibiotics, sedation

    k. Obtain and monitor ABGs, pulse oximetry

    l. Monitor for cardiac dysrhythmias secondary to alterations in ABGs

    m. Explain all ongoing procedures to parent, significant others, and patient when appropriate

  4. Expected outcomes/evaluation (see Appendix B)

H. Hyperventilation

    Hyperventilation is a manifestation of rapid breathing that increases the amount of carbon dioxide (CO_2) blown off in ventilation. Anxiety is a common precipitating factor; however, hyperventilation may be caused by a disease process, such as myocardial infarction (MI), intracerebral bleeding, ketoacidosis, or salicylate overdose. The cause must be determined before treatment is initiated. Hyperventilation is accompanied by a fall in the partial pressure of carbon dioxide (PCO_2), which causes constriction of cerebral vasculature, respiratory alkalosis, and tetany.

  1. Assessment

    a. Subjective data

      1) History of present illness

        a) Shortness of breath or feeling of air hunger

        b) Tingling sensation of extremities, lips

        c) Lightheadedness

        d) Diaphoresis

        e) Headache

        f) Chest discomfort

        g) Patient has experienced anxiety-producing situation

        h) Pregnancy

        i) Exercise

        j) Fever

        k) Pulmonary-related problems

        l) Cardiac history

        m) Time of onset

        n) Current medications, including over-the-counter drugs

      2) Medical history: panic attacks

    b. Objective data

      1) Physical examination

        a) Anxious or panicky appearance

        b) Jaw pain

        c) Carpopedal spasms (spasms of hands and feet sometimes seen in hyperventilation syndrome)

        d) Tachypnea

        e) Diffuse chest pain

        f) Confusion

2) Diagnostic procedures
    a) ABGs: increased partial pressure of oxygen (Po_2); decreased Pco_2
    b) Consider chest radiograph to determine other causes

2. **Analysis: differential nursing diagnosis/collaborative problems**
    a. *Impaired gas exchange related to hyperventilation*
    b. *Anxiety/fear related to precipitating event, perception of dyspnea, need to seek medical attention*
    c. *Knowledge deficit related to diagnosis, therapeutic regimen, follow-up procedure*

3. **Planning/interventions**
    a. *Place patient in comfortable position to facilitate breathing*
    b. *After ruling out medical causes, place paper bag over patient's nose and mouth to allow for rebreathing of CO_2; demonstrate procedure; use counting with inspiration/expiration to slow rate*
    c. *Stay with patient during rebreathing process*
    d. *Obtain and monitor ABGs, pulse oximetry*
    e. *Explain all procedures*
    f. *Provide verbal and written discharge instructions related to pathophysiology of hyperventilation, early recognition of predisposing situations, rebreathing exercises*

4. **Expected outcomes/evaluation** (see Appendix B)

I. Pleural effusion

Pleural effusion is the collection of excess fluid ($>$ normal of 15 mL) in the pleural space. Under normal physiological conditions, this fluid is formed by the parietal pleura and absorbed by the visceral pleura. Increased fluid accumulation may be due to (1) increased subpleural capillary pressure as in congestive heart failure (CHF), (2) decreased capillary oncotic pressure as in liver and renal failure, (3) inflammatory conditions such as infections, or (4) impairment/obstruction of lymphatic flow. In descending order of frequency, the most common causes of pleural effusion are CHF, pneumonia, malignancy, and pulmonary embolism. Dyspnea and pain or dull ache may or may not be present. Dyspnea is caused by fluid that inhibits lung expansion. If this amount is excessive, it can cause a mediastinal shift. The patient may be asymptomatic if the fluid is a relatively small amount (250 mL), and it may be detected only by x-ray film. Thoracentesis may be therapeutically performed to remove excess fluid but may be done for diagnostic fluid analysis as well. The appearance of the fluid may be hemorrhagic, chylous (white/thick), or purulent (empyema). An empyema must be drained and treated, or it will solidify and become fibrous and constricted, requiring surgical intervention and possibly causing permanent lung damage. An effusion may be recurrent, requiring repeated drainage, and may even require therapeutic adhesion formation of the parietal and visceral pleura.

1. **Assessment**
    a. *Subjective data*
        1) History of present illness
            a) Shortness of breath
            b) Cough
            c) Hemoptysis
            d) Pleuritic pain
        2) Medical history
            a) Congestive heart failure

b) Pulmonary embolus

c) Bacterial pneumonia

d) Malignancy, especially lung or breast

e) Tuberculosis

f) Pancreatitis

g) Abdominal surgery, subphrenic or hepatic abscess

b. *Objective data*

1) Physical examination

a) General survey

b) Tachypnea

c) Use of accessory muscles

d) Decreased movement of chest wall

e) Increased fremitus above effusion, absent fremitus over effusion

f) Dull to percussion

g) Auscultation diminished or absent over effusion, egophony present over effusion

2) Diagnostic procedures

a) Chest x-ray film, possible decubitus view

b) Ultrasonogram to identify area for thoracentesis

c) CT scan

d) Thoracentesis for fluid analysis: amount, protein, lactate dehydrogenase (LDH), amylase, glucose, differential, pH, Gram's stain with culture, cytology

2. **Analysis: differential nursing diagnosis/collaborative problems**

a. *Impaired gas exchange related to decreased lung space for ventilation*

b. *Pain related to effusion, dyspnea*

c. *Anxiety/fear related to difficulty in breathing*

d. *Knowledge deficit related to disease, therapeutic regimen*

3. **Planning/intervention**

a. *Maintain airway, breathing, and circulation; provide constant monitoring and assessment of respiratory rate, rhythm, depth, and effort, vital signs, pulse oximetry*

b. *Administer supplemental oxygen as needed*

c. *Set up and assist with thoracentesis; anticipate possible chest tube insertion; order postprocedure chest x-ray film*

d. *Administer pain medications as ordered*

e. *Minimize respiratory effort related to physical work*

f. *Allow family members to accompany patient*

g. *Educate about disease, treatments*

h. *Prepare for possible admission, other diagnostic tests*

i. *Treatment modalities for underlying problem: CHF, pneumonia*

4. **Expected outcome/evaluation** (see Appendix B)

J. Pneumonia

Pneumonia is an inflammation of the pulmonary parenchyma resulting from tissue invasion by inhaled, aspirated, or bloodborne pathogens causing an illness ranging in severity from mild to life threatening. The most common pneumonias are viral (60–90%), bacterial (cause the majority of deaths), or mycoplasmal. The other causes are fungi, rickettsiae, and parasites (or occasionally a noninfectious insult). Table 18–4 describes the most typical bacterial infections; additional agents include Legionella and *Chlamydia*. Viral causes include RSV, influenza, cytomegalovirus (CMV), herpes simplex, varicella, and Epstein-Barr virus. When a pathogen

Table 18–4   PNEUMONIAS

Streptococcus pneumoniae (Pneumococcal)
Organism:
Streptococcus pneumoniae: Gram-positive, lancet-shaped diplococcus; aerobe.
Risk Factors:
Young, elderly, immunosuppressed, alcoholic, COPD, cardiovascular disease, diabetes mellitus, hyposplenia. Highest risk in winter months.
Pathophysiology:
Bacteria is normal inhabitant of upper respiratory tract. Aspiration, inhalation, or hematogenous seeding are routes of entry. Damage occurs from overwhelming growth, which impairs gas exchange.
Clinical Manifestations:
Malaise, sore throat, rhinorrhea, chills, fever, rust-colored sputum, pleuritic chest pain, nausea, vomiting, abdominal pain, tachycardia, tachypnea, dyspnea, decreased breath sounds, dullness, rales, pleural friction rub. In the elderly, presentation may be a change in mental status or congestive heart failure.
Diagnostic Findings:
Leukocytes up to 40,000/mL with left shift.
Leukopenia.
Liver function tests abnormal.
CXR: Homogenous lobar or sublobular infiltrates.
Treatment:
Penicillin. In presence of meningitis, another drug should be added.
Staphylococcus aureus
Organism:
Staphylococcus aureus pneumoniae: Gram-positive, nonmotile, spherical organism.
Risk Factors:
IV drug abuse, immunocompromised patients, and as complication of influenza epidemic.
Pathophysiology:
Aspiration from upper respiratory tract leads to infections. Growth occurs rapidly in the debilitated host. Hematogenous seeding occurs in the dialysis patient or with IV drug use.
Clinical Manifestations:
Abrupt-onset fever, chills, cough, dyspnea, pleuritic chest pain. Purulent sputum ranging from yellow to pink. Frank hemoptysis is not uncommon. Patient looks toxic. Tachypnea, tachycardia, rales, rhonchi.
Diagnostic Findings:
WBC > 15000/mL.
+ blood cultures in 20% cases.
CXR: Bilateral lower lobe bronchopneumonia; early abscess formation or pleural effusion possible.
Treatment:
Hospitalization and treatment with penicillinase-resistant penicillin.
Nafcillin, methicillin, or oxacillin.
Treatment period 2 weeks unless bacteremia or emphysema occur, then 6 weeks.
Klebsiella pneumoniae
Organism:
Klebsiella pneumoniae: Gram-negative, nonmotile, encapsulated rods.
Risk Factors:
Men, over 50 years of age; alcoholism, heart disease, diabetes mellitus, COPD, aspiration.
Pathophysiology:
Causes necrosis of alveolar walls, multiple abscesses, loss of lung volume, and friable blood vessels.
Clinical Manifestations:
Fever, rigors, dyspnea, productive cough, hemoptysis, copious purulent sputum that is green or blood-streaked.
Diagnostic Findings:
Leukopenia or leukocytosis.
CXR: Lobar consolidation, typically of right upper lobe; rapid appearance of lung abscesses; pleural effusion common; bronchopneumonia in lower lobes.
Treatment:
Aminoglycoside and third-generation cephalosporin (cefotaxime, ceftriaxone, ceftizoxime).

Table 18–4   PNEUMONIAS (Continued)

Pseudomonas aeruginosa
Organism:
Pseudomonas aeruginosa: Gram-negative, motile rod, not encapsulated.
Risk Factors:
Second most common nosocomial infection; decreased host defenses or antimicrobial therapy;
   alcoholism, diabetes mellitus.
Pathophysiology:
Aspiration, necrosis of alveolar walls, multiple abscesses, loss of lung volume, and friable blood
   vessels.
Clinical Manifestations:
Same as *Klebsiella.*
Diagnostic Findings:
Leukocytosis with left shift.
Arterial hypoxemia.
Pseudomonas aeruginosa
Hypocapnia.
+ blood cultures in 33–50% of cases.
CXR: Patchy infiltrates in lower lobes; cavitation, empyema.
Treatment:
Antipseudomonas penicillin (azlocillin, piperacillin, ticarcillin) combined with aminoglycoside
   (tobramycin, amikacin).
Haemophilus influenzae
Organism:
Haemophilus influenzae: Gram-negative, pleomorphic motile rod; encapsulated and
   nonencapsulated strains.
Risk factors:
50 years of age; >50% have alcoholism, COPD; URI 2–6 weeks previously.
Encapsulated strain: Alcoholism, diabetes mellitus, COPD, impaired immune system.
Nonencapsulated strain: Exacerbation of bronchitis; nonbacteremic pneumonia.
Pathophysiology:
Bacterial infection that produces inflammation.
Clinical Manifestations:
Minimal elevations in TPR, dyspnea, rales, rhonchi, pleuritic chest pain, nausea, vomiting.
Diagnostic Findings:
Leukocytosis.
CXR: Bronchopneumonia, lower lobe and multilobular pleural effusions.
Treatment:
Ampicillin. If organism is ampicillin-resistant, chloramphenicol.

With permission from Lee, G., & Bristol, C. S. (1991). *Flight nursing: principles and practice* (pp. 315–329). St. Louis, MO: Mosby–Year Book. Data from Carden, D. L., & Smith, J. K. (1989). Pneumonias. Emergency Medical Clinics of North America, 7(2), 255–278.

COPD, chronic obstructive pulmonary disease; CXR, chest x-ray; IV, intravenous; URI, upper respiratory infection; TPR, temperature, pulse, respiration.

reaches the alveoli and starts replicating, fluids and anti-inflammatory cells enter the alveolar spaces to attack the infection, causing symptoms and radiographic signs of pneumonia. Differentiating between viral and bacterial pneumonia can be difficult. Viral infections are most common in winter and usually run their course in about 2 weeks. Bacterial pneumonia typically develops rather abruptly, with high temperature, coughing, and chest pain. In children, signs and symptoms of pneumonia depend on the age of the patient, specific pathogen, and severity of disease. Infants have less characteristic symptoms and are at greater risk for infection and complications. RSV and influenza are the most common viral causes in children younger than 1 year. In older children, pneumonia is usually subacute, with a nonproductive cough, moderate fever, headache, sore throat, and general fatigue. Bacteremia and complications such as empyema and meningitis may develop in elderly patients with pneumonia. An estimated 2 to 4 million cases of pneumonia occur annually. Pneumonia is the sixth leading cause of death in the United States (approximately 80,000 deaths annually) and the leading cause of death in the geriatric population. Those at greatest risk include patients with chronic illness, congenital anomalies, pulmonary disease, and immunosuppression.

1. **Assessment**
    a. *Subjective data*
        1) History of present illness
            a) Dyspnea
            b) Productive cough
            c) Pleuritic chest pain
            d) Fever/chills
            e) Changes in sensorium: may be presenting symptom in elderly patients
            f) Recent URI or flu
            g) Diarrhea: mycoplasma, legionella
            h) Abdominal pain: more common in children
            i) Allergies
            j) Current medications, including over-the-counter brands
        2) Medical history
            a) History of cigarette smoking
            b) Cardiac diseases (e.g., CHF)
            c) Pulmonary diseases
            d) COPD (pneumonia poses an immediate life-threatening situation to these patients)
            e) Immunosuppression
            f) High-risk category for HIV infection or known HIV infection or acquired immunodeficiency syndrome (AIDS)
            g) Congenital abnormalities
            h) Chronic illness: cystic fibrosis, cerebral palsy
            i) Previous pneumonia
            j) Immunizations: HIB, pneumococcal
    b. *Objective data*
        1) Physical examination
            a) Patient may appear acutely ill
            b) Possible fever, possible hypothermia in infants
            c) Possible cyanosis
            d) Lungs
                (1) Tachypnea: best single indicator and sometimes only sign in infant
                (2) Dullness on percussion
                (3) Increased tactile fremitus
                (4) Coarse crackles
                (5) Bronchial breath sounds over affected lobe
                (6) Possible pleural friction rub
                (7) Decreased respiratory excursion secondary to pain
            e) Tachycardia
            f) Infant: retractions, grunting, lethargy, vomiting, poor feeding, dehydration
        2) Diagnostic procedures
            a) Chest radiograph: pulmonary infiltrates
            b) Laboratory studies
                (1) CBC
                (2) Gram's stain and culture of sputum
                (3) Blood cultures: before antibiotics

(4) Cold hemagglutination (especially useful in mycoplasmal infection)

(5) ABGs

c) Pulse oximetry

2. **Analysis: differential nursing diagnosis/collaborative problems**

   a. *Risk for ineffective airway clearance related to increased mucus production and possible airway alteration*

   b. *Impaired gas exchange related to inflammation of lung parenchyma and increased secretions*

   c. *Anxiety related to symptomatology and need to seek medical attention*

3. **Planning/interventions**

   a. *Critical pathway or standard guidelines: prompt initiation of antibiotics for serious illness*

   b. *Position patient to facilitate breathing*

   c. *Provide humidified treatments and/or oxygen*

   d. *Assist with removal of secretions as necessary*

   e. *Obtain and monitor ABGs and respiratory status*

   f. *Initiate and maintain IV access for fluids and medications*

   g. *Provide fluid replacement (PO or IV) to liquefy secretions: observe intake and output status to ensure that fluid overload does not occur*

   h. *Administer prescribed medications: antibiotics, bronchodilators, antipyretics*

   i. *Monitor for cardiac dysrhythmias (secondary to hypoxemia and acidosis)*

   j. *Prepare for possible aggressive ventilatory support*

   k. *Reassure patient and significant others*

   l. *Explain all procedures*

   m. *Educate patient and significant others about pneumonia plan of care*

   n. *Isolation precautions if signs of possible tuberculosis*

4. **Expected outcomes/evaluation** (see Appendix B)

K. Pulmonary embolus

Pulmonary embolus (PE) is caused by a free-floating thrombus from the venous system of the legs, pelvis, or right side of the heart. A PE may consist of fat, bone, or amniotic fluid but is most often clotted blood. The thrombus lodges in a branch of the pulmonary artery, causing total or partial occlusion and potential infarct. This results in the affected area of the lung being ventilated but inadequately perfused. The embolus also releases histamine and prostaglandin, causing bronchoconstriction and pulmonary vasoconstriction and resulting in alveolar hypoventilation and intrapulmonary shunting. The decreased perfusion reduces surfactant, contributing to additional atelectasis. Pulmonary embolus is the third most common cardiovascular cause of death after ischemic heart disease and stroke in the United States (approximately 50,000 deaths per year), but it is difficult to specifically diagnose because of vague symptoms and specificity of the noninvasive diagnostic tests. On autopsy, 80 to 100% of patients with PE have deep venous thrombosis (DVT), whereas only 40% had clinical signs of DVT. Ten percent of patients with acute PE die within the first hour, those who survive are at risk for recurrent PE, and up to 70% develop pulmonary hypertension. PE may develop in any patient population (although it is rare in children), but the risk increases with age. PE should always be considered in the geriatric patient with shortness of breath. At autopsy, 70 to 90% of elderly patients who died during hospitalization were found to have PE. The highest incidence of recognized PE occurs in hospitalized patients.

1. **Assessment**

   a. *Subjective data*

1) History of present illness
   a) Dyspnea
   b) Chest pain
   c) Cough, hemoptysis
2) Medical history
   a) Trauma
   b) Long bone fracture/surgery
   c) Use of oral contraceptives
   d) History of thrombosis
   e) Immobility
   f) Obesity
   g) Pregnancy
   h) Classic factors for venous thrombus: venous stasis, hypercoagulability, altered vascular integrity
   b. *Objective data*
      1) Physical examination
         a) Small PE
            (1) No signs or symptoms
            (2) Tachypnea
            (3) Tachycardia
            (4) Localized crackles
            (5) Pleural friction rub
            (6) Pleuritic chest pain
            (7) Hemoptysis
            (8) Restlessness or confusion
         b) Massive PE
            (1) Same as for small PE
            (2) Hypotension
            (3) Signs of right-sided heart failure
            (4) Abnormal heart sounds
            (5) Cyanosis
            (6) Petechiae (particular to a fat embolus)
      2) Diagnostic procedures
         a) Chest radiograph
         b) Laboratory studies
            (1) Sedimentation rate: elevated
            (2) CBC: increased leukocytes
            (3) Fibrin split products: increased fibrin degradation products
            (4) ABGs
            (5) D-dimer: more specific test for fibrin split products
         c) ECG
         d) Pulse oximetry
         e) Venous: Doppler studies
         f) Ventilation-perfusion studies
         g) Pulmonary angiography
         h) Possible spiral CT with transesophageal echocardiogram (TEE) or magnetic resonance imaging (MRI)

2. **Analysis: differential nursing diagnosis/collaborative problems**
   a. *Impaired gas exchange related to occlusion of pulmonary artery*
   b. *Tissue perfusion, altered cardiopulmonary related to occlusion of vessel (pulmonary artery)*
   c. *Anxiety/fear related to sudden onset of symptoms, need to seek medical attention, and unknown prognosis*

3. **Planning/interventions**
   a. *Maintain airway, breathing, circulation*
   b. *Obtain and monitor ABGs*
   c. *Administer oxygen at high-flow rate (use caution in patients with known COPD)*
   d. *Continuously monitor: respiratory status, cardiac status, vital signs, skin color*
   e. *Initiate and maintain IV catheter*
   f. *Arrange for diagnostic procedures*
   g. *Insert urinary catheter to monitor kidney function*
   h. *Administer prescribed medications: anticoagulants, bronchodilators, analgesics, cardiotonic agents as necessary to maintain blood pressure and cardiac output, possible thrombolytic therapy*
   i. *Provide patient with reassurance*
   j. *Allow calm significant other to remain with patient when possible*
   k. *Explain all procedures*
   l. *Educate patient and significant others about condition and course of treatment*
4. **Expected outcomes/evaluation** (see Appendix B)

III. SURGICAL RESPIRATORY EMERGENCIES

A. Rib fractures

Rib fractures usually result from blunt force or crush injuries, most commonly motor vehicle crashes (MVCs). They are not by themselves considered life threatening, but are especially significant in that they may be associated with more serious concomitant injuries. Fractures of the first and second ribs rarely occur except as a result of severe trauma and are commonly associated with injury to the lungs, aortic arch, or vertebral column. First rib fractures have a 40% mortality rate because of the frequently associated laceration of the subclavicular artery or vein. Left lower rib fractures are associated with splenic injury in 20% of patients. Right lower rib injury is associated with hepatic injury in 10% of patients. Sternal fractures are associated with an increased incidence of cardiac contusion. Children have very flexible rib cages and sternums, making rib fractures less common in children than in adults but conversely not providing the same protection to underlying structures. It is possible for serious underlying thoracic injury to be present in a child with an intact rib cage and sternum. The treatment for all age groups with rib fractures is very similar.

1. **Assessment**
   a. *Subjective data*
      1) History of present illness
         a) Localized pain aggravated by movement, respiration, coughing
         b) Onset may be associated with severe coughing
         c) Trauma, mechanism of injury
         d) Allergies
         e) Current medications
      2) Medical history
         a) COPD
         b) Osteodegenerative processes
   b. *Objective data*
      1) Physical examination
         a) Point tenderness on palpation
         b) Possible crepitus as ribs grate against one another

            c) Possible subcutaneous emphysema

            d) Hypoventilation, splinting secondary to pain

        2) Diagnostic procedures

            a) Radiology

                (1) Rib series: only 70% accurate

                (2) Chest radiograph

            b) ECG

            c) ABGs

            d) Pulse oximetry

2. Analysis: differential nursing diagnosis/collaborative problems

    a. Ineffective breathing pattern related to pain

    b. Pain related to fracture

    c. Knowledge deficit related to diagnosis, therapeutic regimen, follow-up procedures

3. Planning/interventions

    a. Place patient in high Fowler's position to facilitate gas exchange and breathing

    b. Monitor respiratory rate, rhythm, depth, and effort

    c. Administer medications as prescribed: analgesics

    d. Have patient cough and deep breathe to mobilize secretions while splinting to decrease pain

    e. Consider incentive spirometry: to assess tidal volume and help prevent atelectasis during course of recovery

    f. Prepare patient for hospitalization if any of following conditions exists: fractures of more than three ribs, fracture of first or second rib, suspected visceral injury, sternal injury or fracture, history of COPD, displaced fracture or fracture with jagged edges, flail chest

    g. Set up for and assist with intercostal nerve block for pain control

    h. Discourage circumferential taping of chest or use of rib binders to reduce pain because this may predispose to atelectasis

    i. Allow calm significant other to remain with patient when possible

    j. Educate patient and significant others about breathing exercises (including incentive spirometry), appropriate splinting techniques, nutrition, and hydration

    k. Provide verbal and written discharge instructions

4. Expected outcomes/evaluation (see Appendix B)

B. Flail chest

    Flail chest is an injury of the thorax that is usually the result of serious crush injury or high-speed MVC. Flail chest occurs when two or more adjacent ribs are fractured in two or more locations or when the sternum is detached. The result is a free-floating segment of the chest wall that is drawn inward with inspiration and outward with expiration, thus causing a paradoxical motion during respiration. The flail segment may not be evident initially because of muscle contraction and splinting. The end results are impaired ventilation and pain. Inefficient ventilation is caused by the loss of the bellows effect (less negative intrapleural pressure to expand the lung) and associated pulmonary contusion, dead space, and atelectasis. The patient has increased respiratory effort, decreased tidal volume, impaired cough, and hypoxia. Potential complications include hemothorax, pneumothorax, and associated myocardial or pulmonary contusion/ARDS.

1. Assessment

    a. Subjective data

   1) History of present illness
    a) Pleuritic chest pain
    b) Dyspnea
    c) Blunt chest trauma
    d) Allergies to medications and other substances
    e) Current medications
    f) Tetanus immunization status
   2) Medical history
    a) Cigarette smoking
    b) COPD
    c) Cardiac disease
    d) Pulmonary disease
    e) Recent thoracic surgery
  b. *Objective data*
   1) Physical examination
    a) Paradoxical chest wall motion
    b) Hyperventilation initially (as a compensatory mechanism) followed by hypoventilation
    c) Pallor and cyanosis
    d) Diaphoresis
    e) Confusion
    f) Ecchymoses over chest
    g) Signs of rib fracture
    h) Signs of pneumothorax or tension pneumothorax if present
    i) Hypotension
    j) Hyperresonance on injured side with decreased or absent breath sounds
   2) Diagnostic procedures
    a) Cardiac monitor/ECG
    b) Chest radiograph, rib series
    c) ABGs
    d) CBC
    e) Pulse oximetry

2. **Analysis: differential nursing diagnosis/collaborative problems**
  a. *Impaired gas exchange related to pain and paradoxical chest motion*
  b. *Pain related to fracture*
  c. *Anxiety/fear related to cause of flail chest, respiratory difficulty, fear of treatment, and outcome*

3. **Planning/interventions**
  a. *Maintain airway, breathing, and circulation; observe for dysrhythmias secondary to hypoxemia and acidosis; C-spine precautions, if indicated*
  b. *Administer supplemental, high-flow oxygen*
  c. *Stabilize chest wall: placing patient on injured side in semi-Fowler's position may assist in stabilization (sandbags may further impede respiratory effort and increase hypoxic state and should* not *be used)*
  d. *Establish two large-bore IV catheters for Ringer's lactate or normal saline (NS); limit fluids if hypovolemic shock is not present*
  e. *Possible diuretics (to prevent ARDS secondary to fluid overload)*
  f. *Obtain and monitor ABGs*
  g. *Set up for and assist with possible needle thoracostomy or chest tube insertion on injured side*
  h. *Prepare for and assist with intubation and mechanical ventilation (internal stabilization of flail segment via PEEP settings)*

      i. Continuously monitor and assess respiratory rate, rhythm, depth, and effort; cardiac rhythm; vital signs; degree of paradoxical chest motion; ABGs; and tissue perfusion (skin color, temperature, capillary refill)

      j. Administer analgesics as ordered; use small quantities so that respiratory rate and depth are not decreased

      k. Keep patient warm using blankets or heat lamps (use caution not to overheat or burn skin)

      l. Be prepared for possible surgery for internal fixation

      m. Handle patient gently; change patient's position gradually

      n. Minimize unnecessary environmental stimuli

      o. Reassure patient and significant others

      p. Explain all procedures

      q. Allow calm significant other to accompany stable patient to treatment area

   4. Expected outcomes/evaluation (see Appendix B)

C. Pneumothorax

    Pneumothorax results when air enters the pleural space, causing loss of negative intrapleural pressure and consequent partial or total collapse of the lung on the affected side. A pneumothorax may occur as a result of blunt or penetrating chest trauma. Blunt trauma is most frequently caused by a MVC that causes a laceration to the lung from a fractured rib. Mechanical ventilation or iatrogenic procedures may precipitate a pneumothorax, or it may also occur spontaneously. Spontaneous causes are designated as primary (which typically occurs in young, slender males between the ages of 20 and 40 years who smoke) or secondary from the rupture of a bleb in a patient with COPD, cystic fibrosis, or abscess from AIDS-related *Pneumocystis carinii* pneumonia. The incidence of identified pneumothorax is 2.5 to 18 per 100,000 population; many more cases resolve spontaneously without identification or diagnosis. Various invasive therapies may be used to prevent recurrent pneumothorax.

   1. Assessment

      a. Subjective data

        1) History of present illness

          a) Patient may be asymptomatic if pneumothorax is small

          b) Dyspnea, inability to catch breath

          c) Pleuritic pain (usually of sudden onset, may radiate to shoulders)

          d) Patient may be asymptomatic if pneumothorax is small

          e) Trauma

          f) Current medications

          g) Allergies

          h) Cigarette smoking

          i) Pneumonia, particularly *P. carinii*

        2) Medical history

          a) History of pneumothorax

          b) Pulmonary disease

          c) Cardiac disease

          d) Chronic illness: AIDS, cystic fibrosis

      b. Objective data

        1) Physical examination

          a) Tachypnea, possible tachycardia

          b) Tracheal deviation toward uninjured side if tension pneumothorax

          c) Hyperresonance on injured side

          d) Decreased tactile and vocal fremitus on injured side

e) Decreased or absent breath sounds on injured side

f) Subcutaneous emphysema may or may not be present

2) Diagnostic procedures

a) Chest radiograph

b) ABGs

c) Pulse oximetry

d) CBC

e) ECG

2. Analysis: differential nursing diagnosis/collaborative problems

a. *Impaired gas exchange related to ventilation-perfusion mismatch*

b. *Pain related to pneumothorax*

c. *Anxiety/fear related to difficulty in breathing*

d. *Knowledge deficit related to diagnosis, therapeutic regimen, follow-up procedures*

3. Planning/interventions

a. *Maintain airway, breathing, and circulation; C-spine precautions if indicated*

b. *Administer supplemental oxygen*

c. *Provide continuous monitoring and assessment of respiratory rate, rhythm, depth, and effort; vital signs, pulse oximetry; ABGs*

d. *Administer analgesics as ordered*

e. *Set up for and assist with chest tube insertion and post-procedure chest x-ray film*

f. *Anticipate use of Heimlich valve: one-way flutter valve that allows easier transport of patient or for possible discharge to home*

g. *Assist patient into sitting position after chest tube placement*

h. *Allow calm significant other to accompany patient in treatment area when possible*

i. *Educate patient and significant other about signs and symptoms of exacerbations of pneumothorax, activity restrictions, appropriate breathing exercises, plan of care*

4. Expected outcomes/evaluation (see Appendix B)

D. Tension pneumothorax

Tension pneumothorax occurs when a perforating injury to the chest allows air to enter the pleural space on inspiration but does not allow the air to escape on expiration. A tension pneumothorax may rapidly be fatal because rising intrathoracic pressure causes a mediastinal shift, which collapses the lung and compresses the heart, great vessels, and trachea to the unaffected side of the chest. As venous return is impeded, hypotension and shock follow.

1. Assessment

a. *Subjective data*

1) History of present illness

a) Sudden chest pain that is referred to shoulder

b) Dyspnea, patient unable to catch breath

c) Trauma

d) Allergies

e) Current medications

f) Tetanus immunization status

2) Medical history

a) Pulmonary disease

b. *Objective data*

1) Physical examination

a) Sudden onset of chest pain that is referred to shoulder
b) Cyanosis, severe dyspnea, patient unable to catch breath
c) Distended neck veins
d) Tracheal deviation to uninjured side
e) Hyperresonance on injured side
f) Decreased or absent breath sounds on affected side
g) Hypotension, signs of shock

2) Diagnostic procedures
a) Needle thoracostomy
b) Cardiac monitor/ECG
c) Chest radiograph: reveals mediastinal shift, lung collapse
d) ABGs, CBC
e) Pulse oximetry

2. **Analysis: differential nursing diagnosis/collaborative problems**
a. *Impaired gas exchange related to ventilation-perfusion mismatch*
b. *Cardiac output, decreased related to decreased venous return secondary to compression of great vessels*
c. *Anxiety/fear related to respiratory compromise*

3. **Planning/interventions**
a. *Maintain airway, breathing, and circulation; C-spine precautions, if indicated*
b. *Perform or assist with needle thoracostomy using a 14- to 16-gauge needle inserted into the second intercostal space/midclavicular line or fifth intercostal space/midaxillary line on the injured side to relieve tension; anticipate chest tube insertion and use of Heimlich valve or underwater seal chest drainage system*
c. *Administer supplemental oxygen*
d. *Insert two large-bore IV catheters (14 or 16 gauge) with LR or NS*
e. *Perform continuous monitoring and assessment of respiratory rate, rhythm, depth, effort; tracheal position; vital signs; neck vein distention; signs and symptoms of shock; ABGs; oximetry*
f. *Explain all procedures*
g. *Encourage calm significant other to accompany patient in treatment area when possible*
h. *Educate patient and significant other about plan of care and hospital stay*
i. *Prepare patient for hospitalization*

4. **Expected outcomes/evaluation** (see Appendix B)

E. Hemothorax

Bleeding and accumulation of blood in the pleural space may result from injury to the chest wall, great vessels, or lung from penetrating or blunt trauma. Accumulation of blood in the pleural space may cause a mediastinal shift, resulting in impairment of venous return or lung compression with a significant blood loss (which may exceed 2500 mL). Hypotension or shock may develop. Emergency thoracotomy may be necessary to identify and repair the bleeding source if there is 1000 mL of blood in the chest or blood drainage greater than 200 mL/hr for 3 to 4 hours.

1. **Assessment**
a. *Subjective data*
1) History of present illness
a) Patient may be asymptomatic if hemothorax is small
b) Dyspnea

   c) Chest pain

   d) Trauma

   e) Allergies

   f) Current medications

   g) Tetanus immunization status

  2) Medical history

   a) Pulmonary disease

   b) Cardiac disease

 b. Objective data

  1) Physical examination

   a) If patient has major hemothorax, signs of shock may be present

   b) Dullness on injured side on percussion

   c) Decreased breath sounds on injured side

   d) Possible mediastinal shift

   e) Respiratory distress

  2) Diagnostic procedures

   a) Cardiac monitor/ECG

   b) Pulse oximetry

   c) Chest radiograph (upright if possible)

   d) ABGs, CBC, coagulation studies

2. Analysis: differential nursing diagnosis/collaborative problems

 a. *Impaired gas exchange related to ventilation-perfusion mismatch*

 b. *Fluid volume deficit related to fluid shift from intravascular space to intrapleural space*

 c. *Pain related to thoracic trauma*

 d. *Anxiety/fear related to dyspnea, cause of hemothorax, treatment modalities, need to seek medical attention*

 e. *Knowledge deficit related to diagnosis, therapeutic regimen, follow-up procedures*

3. Planning/interventions

 a. *Maintain airway, breathing, and circulation; C-spine precautions, if indicated*

 b. *Administer supplemental oxygen*

 c. *Set up for and assist with chest tube insertion and drainage system; autotransfusion and/or emergency thoracotomy may be performed as life-saving intervention*

 d. *Prepare for possible intubation and ventilator support*

 e. *Establish two large-bore 14- or 16-gauge IV catheters for LR or NS with blood tubing*

 f. *Administer blood or blood products as ordered*

 g. *Provide continuous monitoring and assessment of respiratory rate, rhythm, depth, effort; vital signs; ABGs; cardiac rhythm; tissue perfusion/capillary refill; pulse oximetry*

 h. *Monitor intake and output of fluids, including chest drainage, urine output*

 i. *Keep patient warm with blankets or heat lamp; observe for overheating*

 j. *Administer analgesics as prescribed*

 k. *Position patient comfortably and change patient position gradually to avoid hypotensive episode*

 l. *Explain all procedures*

 m. *Permit calm significant others to accompany patient in treatment area if patient is stable*

 n. *Educate patient and significant others about plan of care*

      o. Prepare patient for hospital admission
4. **Expected outcomes/evaluation** (see Appendix B)

F. Open pneumothorax

Open pneumothorax is a life-threatening condition in which an opening (at least two thirds the size of diameter of the trachea) from the outside of the body penetrates into the chest wall. Air passes from the atmosphere, through the chest wall, into the pleural space, and out again, often producing a sucking sound. With smaller wounds, a valvelike effect may allow entry of air on inspiration, but prevent exit of air on expiration. The result is a rapidly progressive tension pneumothorax. A hemothorax is commonly associated with traumatic open pneumothorax.

1. **Assessment**
   a. *Subjective data*
      1) History of present illness
         a) Dyspnea
         b) Chest pain
         c) Trauma
         d) Allergies
         e) Current medications
         f) Tetanus immunization status
      2) Medical history
         a) Pulmonary disease
         b) Cardiac disease
   b. *Objective data*
      1) Physical examination
         a) Tachypnea
         b) Penetrating wound to chest
         c) Sucking sound from wound site on inspiration
         d) Bubbling at wound on expiration
         e) Decreased or absent breath sounds on injured side
         f) Hyperresonance on affected side on percussion
         g) Signs of shock, if present
         h) Signs of tension pneumothorax, if present
         i) Dyspnea, chest pain
      2) Diagnostic procedures
         a) Cardiac monitor/ECG
         b) Pulse oximetry
         c) Chest radiograph
         d) CBC, ABGs
2. **Analysis: differential nursing diagnosis/collaborative problems**
   a. *Impaired gas exchange related to inflow of atmospheric air to intrapleural space and lung collapse*
   b. *Pain related to cause of injury*
   c. *Anxiety/fear related to respiratory difficulty, treatment modalities, need to seek medical attention, and prognosis*
3. **Planning/interventions**
   a. *Maintain airway, breathing, and circulation; C-spine precautions*
   b. *Fully inspect anterior and posterior chest*
   c. *Cover chest wound with occlusive dressing taped on three sides (observe for signs of developing tension pneumothorax such as tracheal deviation/distended neck veins: remove occlusive dressing to decompress if necessary and then replace and continue to monitor)*

    d. *Administer supplemental high-flow oxygen*

    e. *Prepare for potential medical interventions as indicated; chest tube insertion, emergency thoracotomy, and/or autotransfusion if associated with massive hemothorax*

    f. *Establish two large-bore IV catheters (14 or 16 gauge) for LR or NS*

    g. *Administer blood or plasma expanders as indicated*

    h. *Perform continuous monitoring of respiratory rate, rhythm, depth, and effort (observe for signs of developing tension pneumothorax); vital signs; ABGs; pulse oximetry; cardiac rhythm; tissue perfusion; level of consciousness; fluid intake and output (including chest tube drainage if applicable)*

    i. *Keep patient warm with blankets or heat lamps*

    j. *Change patient's position gradually*

    k. *Administer analgesics as indicated*

    l. *Explain all procedures*

    m. *Reassure patient and family/significant others*

    n. *Permit calm significant others to accompany patient in treatment area*

    o. *Educate patient and significant others about plan of care*

4. Expected outcomes/evaluation (see Appendix B)

G. Pulmonary contusion

    Pulmonary contusion is a "bruise" of the lung as a result of a blunt chest trauma that usually occurs as the result of a rapid deceleration injury. It may be either localized or generalized and is usually associated with other chest injuries, such as rib fractures and flail chest. In pulmonary contusion, blood extravasates into the lung parenchyma, causing alveolar and interstitial edema, leading to tissue anoxia and a change in tissue permeability. This can result in decreased compliance, increased pulmonary vascular resistance, and decreased pulmonary blood flow. The signs and symptoms may not be immediately apparent; therefore, diagnosis is often made only by suspecting the condition. Symptoms usually do not develop for 12 to 48 hours and may develop into ARDS. Treatment may include unconventional modes of ventilation (e.g., synchronous independent lung ventilation or high-frequency jet ventilation). Pulmonary contusion occurs in almost 75% of patients with blunt chest trauma and has a 40% mortality.

1. Assessment

    a. *Subjective data*

      1) History of present illness

        a) Chest pain, possible chest wall contusions, or abrasions

        b) Dyspnea, hyperpnea

        c) Development of nonproductive cough

        d) Hemoptysis

        e) Trauma

        f) Allergies

        g) Current medications

      2) Medical history

        a) Pulmonary disease

        b) Cardiac disease

    b. *Objective data*

      1) Physical examination (50% have no physical findings)

        a) Increasing tachypnea

        b) Local or generalized crackles, wheezing

        c) Possible chest contusions or abrasions

        d) Tachycardia

    e) Hemoptysis

    f) Dyspnea

  2) Diagnostic procedures

    a) Cardiac monitor/ECG

    b) Pulse oximetry

    c) Chest radiograph: reveals pulmonary infiltrates, (usually not evident until 12 hours after injury), hemothorax

    d) Chest CT

    e) ABGs, CBC

2. Analysis: differential nursing diagnosis/collaborative problems

  a. Impaired gas exchange: hypoxia related to ventilation-perfusion mismatch

  b. Pain related to injury and chest movement with breathing

3. Planning/interventions

  a. Maintain airway, breathing, and circulation, C-spine precautions, if indicated

  b. Position patient to facilitate breathing (may be positioned with injured side up)

  c. Provide supplemental humidified oxygen

  d. Assist with removal of secretions as needed (aggressive pulmonary hygiene)

  e. Provide humidified breathing treatments as needed

  f. Insert two large-bore IV catheters for LR or NS; restrict fluid administration if no signs of hypovolemic shock are present to prevent pulmonary fluid overload and ARDS

  g. Perform continuous monitoring and assessment of respiratory rate, rhythm, depth, effort; breath sounds; vital signs; pulse oximetry; ABGs; cardiac monitor; fluid intake and output

  h. Set up for and assist with intubation and mechanical ventilation, as indicated

  i. Administer medications as ordered: analgesics, diuretics for fluid overload, corticosteroids for inflammation

  j. Encourage deep breathing and turning in semi-Fowler's position (if no cervical spine injury) to prevent atelectasis

  k. Assist patient into position of comfort

  l. Allow calm significant other to remain with patient when possible

  m. Educate patient and significant other about plan of care

  n. Prepare patient for admission

4. Expected outcomes/evaluation (see Appendix B)

H. Esophageal disruption

Because the esophagus is well protected by both its position and surrounding structures, it is rarely affected by penetrating trauma and even less often by blunt trauma. When injury does occur, it is frequently overlooked because of the presence of other injuries and initial lack of apparent clinical findings. It may be associated with a pneumothorax. Failure to detect this injury, however, may result in life-threatening complications resulting from neck or mediastinal corrosion from digestive chemicals, contamination of bacteria, and loss of fluids, leading to shock and respiratory failure.

1. Assessment

  a. Subjective data

    1) History of present illness

      a) Coughing, choking

      b) Chest pain, sudden onset: possible perforation of intrathoracic esophagus

      c) Epigastric pain, sudden onset: possible perforation of intraperitoneal or lower esophageal segment

      d) Neck pain, sudden onset: possible perforation of cervical esophageal portion

      e) Hematemesis, blood in nasogastric (NG) tube

      f) Hoarseness

      g) Dyspnea, respiratory distress

      h) Dysphagia

      i) Trauma (penetrating or blunt)

      j) Allergies

      k) Current medications

      l) Tetanus immunization status

    2) Medical history

      a) Esophageal varices

      b) Esophageal hernias

  b. *Objective data*

    1) Physical examination

      a) Possible subcutaneous or mediastinal emphysema

      b) Increased respiratory rate

      c) Signs of pneumothorax, if present

      d) Signs of shock, if present

    2) Diagnostic procedures

      a) Cardiac monitor/ECG

      b) Chest radiograph: findings may include

        (1) Mediastinal widening

        (2) Pneumomediastinum

        (3) Pulmonary contusions

        (4) Subcutaneous emphysema

        (5) Pneumothorax

        (6) Pleural effusion

      c) Lateral cervical spine films

      d) Nasogastric intubation

      e) Esophagogram

      f) Esophagoscopy (performed if esophagogram is negative)

      g) Pleural fluid evaluation (may contain gastric contents, bile)

      h) CBC, ABGs

2. Analysis: differential nursing diagnosis/collaborative problems

  a. *Risk for fluid volume deficit related to fluid shifts*

  b. *Risk for infection related to disruption of integrity of esophagus with contents emptied into thoracic cavity*

  c. *Pain related to tissue irritation/inflammation*

  d. *Anxiety/fear related to dyspnea, pain, need to seek medical attention, diagnosis, and prognosis*

3. Planning/interventions

  a. *Maintain airway, breathing, and circulation, C-spine precautions, if indicated*

  b. *Administer supplemental high-flow oxygen*

  c. *Establish two large-bore IV catheters for LR or NS with blood tubing*

  d. *Set up for and assist with potential medical interventions, as indicated: chest tube insertion; esophagogram/esophagoscopy*

  e. *Perform continuous monitoring and assessment: vital signs; tissue perfusion: skin color, temperature, capillary refill; sensorium; fluid intake and output; chest drainage (e.g., amount and character) if applicable*

  f. *Perform careful continuous NG suctioning*

g. *Obtain blood cultures, as indicated*
h. *Administer medications as ordered: analgesics, antibiotics*
i. *Prepare patient for surgery/hospitalization*
j. *Position patient comfortably; change patient's position gradually*
k. *Maintain calm, efficient manner and calm environment*
l. *Reassure patient and significant others*
m. *Explain all procedures*
n. *Permit calm significant other to remain with patient when possible*
o. *Educate patient and significant others about plan of care*

4. **Expected outcomes/evaluation** (see Appendix B)

I. Ruptured bronchus and trachea

These injuries, which occur most commonly at the distal trachea or proximal main stem bronchi, result from compressive shear forces generated by severe blunt trauma (causing suddenly increased pressure within the airway against a closed glottis) or, less often, by penetrating trauma. It may also rarely result from intubation. The severity of clinical signs and symptoms is dependent on the size of the wound, injury level, degree of injury to the lung, and resulting airflow changes. Airway continuity may be maintained by the fascia that surrounds the trachea and bronchi. Symptoms may be delayed for 3 to 4 days; conversely, this injury may have immediate symptoms and may be fatal. Because these injuries are uncommon, a high index of suspician must be maintained.

1. **Assessment**
   a. *Subjective data*
      1) History of present illness
         a) Respiratory distress
         b) Cough
         c) Violent trauma, fracture of first five ribs
         d) Allergies
         e) Current medications
         f) Tetanus immunization status
      2) Medical history: pulmonary disease
   b. *Objective data*
      1) Physical examination
         a) Respiratory distress
         b) Hemoptysis
         c) Intercostal retractions
         d) Progressive mediastinal/subcutaneous emphysema
         e) Signs of pneumothorax
         f) Persistent air leak after chest tube insertion
         g) Airway obstruction
      2) Diagnostic procedures
         a) Cardiac monitor/ECG
         b) Pulse oximetry
         c) Chest radiograph: reveals pneumomediastinum
         d) Bronchoscopy, fiberoptic endoscopy
         e) CBC, ABGs
2. **Analysis: differential nursing diagnosis/collaborative problems**
   a. *Ineffective airway clearance related to disruption of integrity of airway structures*
   b. *Anxiety/fear related to respiratory distress*
3. **Planning/interventions**

a. *Establish and maintain airway, breathing, and circulation*
b. *Suction airway to maintain patency*
c. *Administer supplemental high-flow oxygen*
d. *Place patient in semi-Fowler's position*
e. *Insert two large-bore IV catheters (14 or 16 gauge) for LR or NS*
f. *Set up for and assist with chest tube insertion*
g. *Set up for and assist with intubation and mechanical ventilation; if major leak persists after chest tube insertion, endotracheal tube may be inserted distal to rupture*
h. *Set up for and assist with tracheobronchoscopy, as indicated*
i. *Provide continuous monitoring and assessment of vital signs; respiratory status; ABGs; tissue perfusion; monitor for air embolism (sudden cardiovascular deterioration)*
j. *Reassure patient and significant others*
k. *Explain all procedures*
l. *Permit calm significant others to accompany stable patient in treatment area*
m. *Prepare patient for surgery/hospitalization; immediate surgery indicated in presence of massive air leak that prevents adequate air intake; small tear may be treated conservatively with airway management*
n. *Educate patient and significant others about plan of care*
4. **Expected outcomes/evaluation** (see Appendix B)

J. Ruptured diaphragm

Although a ruptured diaphragm is generally due to a deceleration injury (e.g., compression of the thorax against a steering wheel causing a rapid rise in intra-abdominal pressure), it should be considered in all patients who have sustained chest or abdominal trauma. The left side of the diaphragm is more likely to be ruptured, because the right side is somewhat protected by the liver. Because of the ruptured diaphragm, the abdominal contents herniate into the chest and cause compression of the lungs and mediastinum, with resultant decreased venous return to the heart. This is a potentially life-threatening injury.

1. **Assessment**
    a. *Subjective data*
        1) History of present illness (initially patient may be asymptomatic)
            a) Dyspnea
            b) Dysphagia
            c) Sharp shoulder pain
            d) Abdominal tenderness
            e) Trauma: blunt or penetrating
            f) Allergies
            g) Current medications
            h) Tetanus immunization status
        2) Medical history
    b. *Objective data*
        1) Physical examination
            a) Bowel sounds in lower to middle chest
            b) Decreased breath sounds or unilateral breath sounds
            c) Heart sounds shifted to opposite side of rupture
            d) Hyperresonance on percussion
            e) Signs and symptoms of shock (e.g., tachycardia, hypotension)
            f) Dyspnea
            g) Dysphagia

2) Diagnostic procedures
   a) Chest radiograph: may be normal 25% of time; may show tip of NG tube above diaphragm, unilaterally elevated hemidiaphragm, hollow or solid mass above the diaphragm, and shift of mediastinum away from affected side
   b) Peritoneal lavage fluid in chest tube

2. Analysis: differential nursing diagnosis/collaborative problems
  a. *Ineffective airway clearance related to increased intrathoracic pressure*
  b. *Impaired gas exchange related to ventilation-perfusion mismatch*
  c. *Cardiac output, decreased related to compression of great vessels and mediastinum by abdominal contents*
  d. *Pain related to injury and increased intrathoracic pressure*

3. Planning/interventions
  a. *Position patient to facilitate breathing*
  b. *Provide humidification treatment and/or supplemental oxygen*
  c. *Assist with removal of secretions, as necessary*
  d. *Initiate two large-bore IV catheters (14 or 16 gauge) for LR or NS*
  e. *Prepare for potential intubation and mechanical ventilation*
  f. *Continuously monitor: respiratory status, cardiac rate and rhythm, vital signs, ABGs, fluid intake and output*
  g. *Insert NG tube*
  h. *Prepare for chest tube insertion*
  i. *Prepare for definitive surgical intervention*
  j. *Assist patient into position of comfort*
  k. *Administer analgesics as ordered*
  l. *Explain all procedures*
  m. *Allow calm significant others to accompany patient in treatment area when possible*
  n. *Educate patient and significant others about plan of care*

4. Expected outcomes/evaluation (see Appendix B)

BIBLIOGRAPHY

Bastnagel-Mason, P. (1994). Abdominal injuries. In V. Cardona, P. Hurn, P. Mason, A. Scanlon, & S. Veise-Berry (Eds.), *Trauma nursing: From resuscitation through rehabilitation* (2nd ed., p. 526). Philadelphia: W. B. Saunders.

Cronin, S. (1997). Nursing care of clients with disorders of the lower airways and pulmonary vessels. In J. Black & E. Matassarin-Jacobs (Eds.), *Medical-surgical nursing, clinical management for continuity of care* (5th ed., pp. 1105–1122). Philadelphia: W. B. Saunders.

Darr, C. (1998). Asthma and bronchiolitis. In B. Barber & P. Rosen (Eds.), *Emergency medicine, concepts and clinical practice, vol. II* (4th ed., pp. 1137–1147). St. Louis, MO: C. V. Mosby.

Emergency Nurses Association. (1993). Respiratory emergencies. In *Emergency nursing pediatric course* (pp. 51–71). Chicago: Author.

Emergency Nurses Association. (1995). Thoracic and neck trauma. In *Trauma nursing core course* (4th ed., pp. 137–169). Chicago: Author.

Emergency Nurses Association. (In press). Respiratory medical emergencies. In *Orientation module* (2nd ed.). Chicago: Author.

Eitzen, E. (1998). Croup, epiglottitis, and bacterial tracheitis. In B. Barber & P. Rosen (Eds.), *Emergency medicine, concepts and clinical practice, vol. II* (4th ed., pp. 1123–1135). St. Louis, MO: C. V. Mosby.

Feied, C. (1998). Pulmonary embolism. In B. Barber & P. Rosen (Eds.), *Emergency medicine, concepts and clinical practice, vol. II* (4th ed., pp. 1770–1800). St. Louis, MO: C. V. Mosby.

Frakes, M. (1996). An overview of magnesium in the emergency department. *Journal of Emergency Nursing, 22*(3), 213–220.

Frakes, M. (1997). Asthma in the emergency department. *Journal of Emergency Nursing, 23*(5), 429–435.

Georgitis, J. (1997). Asthma therapy: What's new and is it necessarily better? *Chest, 112*(1), 3–4.

Glow, D. (1987). *RSV. Pediatric hints #52.* Omaha, NB: Children's Hospital.

Harn, P., & Hartsock, R. (1994). Thoracic injuries. In V. Cardona, P. Hurn, P. Mason, A. Scanlon, & S. Veise-Berry (Eds.), *Trauma nursing from resuscitation through rehabilitation* (2nd ed., pp. 481–489). Philadelphia: W. B. Saunders.

Kaloud, H., Smolle-Juettner, F., Prause, G., & List, W. (1997). Iatrogenic ruptures of the tracheobronchial tree. *Chest, 112*(3), 774–778.

Kearney, K. (1998). Thoracic trauma. In L. Newberry (Ed.), *Sheehy's emergency nursing principles and practice (4th ed., pp. 291–306).* St. Louis, MO: C. V. Mosby.

Kirelik, S., Russell, S., Schutzman, S., & Caputo, G. (1998). Pneumonia. In B. Barber & P. Rosen (Eds.), *Emergency medicine, concepts and clinical practice, vol. II* (4th ed., pp. 1150–1157). St. Louis, MO: C. V. Mosby.

Klein, A. R., Lee, G., Manton, A., & Parker, J. G. (Eds.). (1994). Respiratory emergencies. In *Emergency nursing core curriculum* (4th ed., pp. 479–515). Chicago: Emergency Nurses Association.

Koran, Z., Kunz-Howard, P., & Baxter, C. (1998). Respiratory emergencies. In L. Newberry (Ed.), *Sheehy's emergency nursing principles and practice* (4th ed., pp. 431–457). St. Louis, MO: C. V. Mosby.

Lanros, N., & Barber, J. (1997). Pulmonary and respiratory emergencies. In *Emergency nursing with certification preparation and review* (4th ed., pp. 351–363). Stanford, CT: Appleton & Lange.

Letourneau, M., Schuh, S., & Gausche, M. (1997). Respiratory disorders. In R. Barkin (Ed.), *Pediatric emergency medicine concepts and clinical practice* (2nd ed., pp. 1056–1126). St. Louis, MO: C. V. Mosby-Year Book.

Mandavia, D., & Daily, R. (1998). Chronic obstructive pulmonary disease. In B. Barber & P. Rosen (Eds.), *Emergency medicine, concepts and clinical practice, vol. II* (4th ed., pp. 1494–1508). St. Louis, MO: C. V. Mosby.

Manifold, S. (1995). Case history: Traumatic adult respiratory distress syndrome—A multisystem approach. *International Journal of Trauma, 1*(3), 74–80.

McEwen, J. (1998). Pleural disease. In R. Barkin & P. Rosen (Eds.), *Emergency medicine, concepts and clinical practice, vol. II* (4th ed., pp. 1521–1525). St. Louis, MO: C. V. Mosby.

McGillis, H. (1996). Comprehensive program to improve care leads to reduced ED use by patients with asthma: One hospital's experience. *Journal of Emergency Nursing, 22*(1), 18–23.

Melio, F., & Holmes, D. (1998). Upper respiratory tract infections. In B. Baber & P. Rosen (Eds.), *Emergency medicine, concepts and clinical practice, vol. II* (4th ed., pp. 1529–1531). St. Louis, MO: C. V. Mosby.

Moran, G., & Talan, D. (1998). Pneumonia. In B. Barber & P. Rosen (Eds.), *Emergency medicine, concepts and clinical practice, vol. II* (pp. 1553–1568). St. Louis, MO: C. V. Mosby.

National Heart, Lung, and Blood Institute. (1997). *National asthma education and prevention program. Expert panel report 2: Guidelines for the diagnosis and management of asthma.* Bethesda, MD: Author.

Nowak, R., & Tokarski, G. (1998). Adult acute asthma. In B. Barber & P. Rosen (Eds.), *Emergency medicine, concepts and clinical practice, vol. II* (4th ed., pp. 1470–1478). St. Louis, MO: C. V. Mosby.

Pike-Amato, T. (1996). Thrombolytic therapy in a 79 year old man with massive pulmonary embolism and unstable hemodynamic status. *Journal of Emergency Nursing, 22*(1), 14–17.

Pruszczyk, P., Torbicki, A., Pacho, R., Chlebus, M., Kuch-Wocial, A., Pruszynski, B., & Hubert, G. (1997). Noninvasive diagnosis of suspected severe pulmonary embolism. *Chest, 112*(3), 722–728.

Stein, P., & Henry, J. (1997). Clinical characteristics of patients with acute pulmonary embolism stratified according to their presenting syndromes. *Chest, 112*(4), 974–978.

Tapson, V. (1997). Pulmonary embolism: The diagnostic repertoire. *Chest, 112*(3), 578–580 (editorial).

Thelan, L., Urden, L., Lough, M., & Stacy, K. (1998a). Pulmonary disorders. In *Critical care nursing, diagnosis and management* (3rd ed., pp. 660–673). St. Louis, MO: C. V. Mosby.

Thelan, L., Urden, L., Lough, M., & Stacy, K. (1998b). Trauma. In *Critical care nursing, diagnosis and management* (3rd ed., pp. 1074–1077). St. Louis, MO: C. V. Mosby.

Thomas, C. (Ed.). (1993). *Taber's cyclopedic medical dictionary* (17th ed.). Philadelphia: F. A. Davis.

Williams, J., Hutson, H., & Spears, K. (1998). Dyspnea. In B. Barber & P. Rosen (Eds.), *Emergency medicine, concepts and clinical practice vol. II* (4th ed., p. 1465).

Cynthia A. Horvath, BSN, MSN, CEN

CHAPTER **19**

Shock Emergencies

MAJOR TOPICS

General Strategy

Specific Shock Emergencies

Hypovolemic Shock

Cardiogenic Shock

Distributive Shock

I. GENERAL STRATEGY

Shock is defined as a complex clinical syndrome that develops when there is inadequate tissue (cellular) perfusion. The cell is deprived of, and often unable to use, oxygen and nutrients essential for survival. Metabolic waste products cannot be removed, thereby compounding the problem. The sequelae of inadequate perfusion and cellular oxygen debt that continue unabated are cellular death, organ and system failure, and ultimate death of the individual. Because of the varying causes, a clinically useful classification defines three major categories: hypovolemic, cardiogenic, and distributive or vasogenic shock (Table 19–1).

The physiological alterations and pathological changes that occur during shock may be roughly divided into three stages: compensated, uncompensated, and irreversible. The clinical findings manifested by the patient in each stage are presented with each

Table 19–1 THREE MAJOR CATEGORIES OF SHOCK

Category	Physiological Alteration
Hypovolemic	Decreased intravascular volume
	Redistribution of intravascular volume
Cardiogenic	Decreased contractility
	Impaired ventricular filling
	Impaired ventricular outflow
Distributive	Decreased vascular tone and/or redistribution of intravascular volume

specific category of shock as it applies. Familiarity with the pathophysiological changes in each stage and resulting physical findings should assist the clinician in determining the severity of the shock state as well as the effectiveness of resuscitation efforts.

- **Compensated (nonprogressive) stage:** various receptors sense the drop in systemic pressure, causing a cascade of physiological changes. Homeostatic compensatory mechanisms mediated by the sympathetic nervous system are activated to restore adequate tissue perfusion and preserve vital organ function: the brain and heart. Oxygen delivery ($\dot{D}o_2$) to nonvital organs is insufficient to meet cellular demands (measured as oxygen consumption [$\dot{V}o_2$]. To remain viable, the cells convert from aerobic to anaerobic metabolism. Although beneficial at this time, this conversion results in a drastic reduction in energy production and accumulation of lactic acid, the by-product of anaerobic metabolism. The resulting lactic acidemia begins to cause cellular damage.
- **Uncompensated (progressive) stage:** compensatory mechanisms begin to fail to maintain adequate tissue perfusion to vital organs. Mechanisms that were initially helpful become ineffective and damaging. Cellular derangement and death within all organ systems begin to occur at this point. Additional pathological responses to the shock state (i.e., severe lactic acidemia and inflammatory/immune system activation) may lead to multiple-system deterioration or failure. Even if $\dot{D}o_2$ is sufficient, a number of cells may not be able to use the oxygen as a result of cellular damage.
- **Irreversible (refractory) stage:** the final stage of shock is the critical point at which no treatment can reverse the process. Cellular destruction is so severe that death is inevitable. At this stage, specific types of shock are clinically indistinguishable. Currently, there are no clinical or diagnostic indicators to predict the point at which the patient has progressed to the irreversible stage.

Each patient's shock state is unique, and manifestations are highly individualized. The actual progression varies and may be altered by several factors, such as the specific type of shock, patient age, severity and duration of hypoperfusion, and presence of underlying disease. More than one form of shock may be occurring simultaneously (e.g., hemorrhagic and cardiogenic). Appropriate identification of the types of shock and point of progression assists in the institution of correct, timely therapy. Each form of shock is described separately in the following sections of this chapter.

A. Assessment

1. **Primary survey/resuscitation (see Chapter 1)**
2. **Secondary survey (see Chapter 1)**
3. **Psychological, social, and environmental factors**
   a. *Chronic diseases*
   b. *Extremes of age (< 1 year and > 65 years)*
   c. *Familial factors*
   d. *Noncompliance with medical regimen*
   e. *Substance abuse*
   f. *Lack of knowledge, absence of injury prevention or control, and/or failure to take or understand use of prescribed medications*
   g. *Immobility*
   h. *General debilitation*
   i. *Malnutrition*
   j. *Recent surgery or instrumentation*
   k. *Splenectomy*
   l. *Exposure of immunocompromised patient to others with viral or infectious illnesses not considered virulent (e.g., common cold)*
   m. *Abuse or neglect*
   n. *Exposure to allergens or new items in environment*
4. **Focused survey**
   a. *Subjective data*

1) History of present illness
    a) Pain: PQRST
        (1) Provoked
        (2) Quality
        (3) Radiation/region
        (4) Severity
        (5) Time
    b) Injury: mechanism, time, force, weapon, protective devices
    c) Fatigue and generalized weakness
    d) Syncope and orthostatic dizziness
    e) Dyspnea and orthopnea
    f) Palpitations
    g) Vomiting and hematemesis
    h) Diarrhea, melena, hematochezia
    i) Altered mentation, decreased level of consciousness, headache, behavioral changes
    j) Sense of impending doom, apprehension, anxiety
    k) Vaginal bleeding
    l) Abdominal cramping or pain
    m) Epistaxis or hemoptysis
    n) Polyuria
    o) Thirst
    p) Sensation of feeling cold
    q) Fever and chills
    r) Erythematous, macular rash
    s) Inflamed mucous membranes
    t) Edema: location, type
    u) Alteration in motor and sensory function (paraplegia or quadriplegia)
    v) Urticaria
    w) Pruritus
2) Medical history
    a) Current and significant findings: knowledge of presence of one or more of the following may assist in identifying type of shock (direct or indirect factors), anticipating potential altered physiological responses to shock if underlying chronic disease is present, and recognizing possible abnormalities in patient's response to therapy or need to modify standard therapy for shock state
        (1) Endocrine disorder
        (2) Liver/pancreatic disease
        (3) Gastrointestinal disorder or disease
        (4) Renal disease
        (5) Vascular disease
        (6) Cardiac disorder/atherosclerotic heart disease
        (7) Pulmonary disease
        (8) Hematological disorder
        (9) Substance abuse
        (10) Allergies and asthma
        (11) Previous surgical procedure or instrumentation
        (12) Immunocompromised conditions such as neoplastic disease, post-organ transplant, acquired immunodeficiency syndrome (AIDS)
        (13) Prolonged immobility
    b) Current medications: knowledge of proper or improper use of one or more of following may assist in identifying type of shock (direct or

indirect factors), anticipating potential altered physiological responses to shock with certain medications, and recognizing possible abnormalities in patient's response to therapy or need to modify standard therapy for shock state

    (1) Cardiotonic agents

    (2) Antihypertensives

    (3) Diuretics

    (4) Anticoagulants

    (5) Antidysrhythmics

    (6) Corticosteroids

    (7) Aspirin

    (8) Insulin

    (9) Specific pulmonary drugs

    (10) Chemotherapeutic drugs

    (11) Immunosuppressants

  c) Allergies

    (1) Medications

    (2) Environmental agents

    (3) Food

3) Record data as appropriate

b. *Objective data*

1) Physical examination

  a) General survey

    (1) Level of consciousness and mental status; includes Glasgow Coma Score (GCS) or AVPU scale (*a*lert, responds to *v*erbal stimuli, responds to *p*ainful stimuli, *u*nresponsive)

    (2) Posture and motor activity

    (3) General development and appearance

    (4) Skin: color, temperature, moisture, turgor, cyanosis (peripheral and central)

    (5) Vital signs: temperature, pulse (rate and quality), respirations (rate and rhythm), blood pressure

    (6) Orthostatic blood pressure and heart rate (when feasible)

    (7) Odors: breath and body

  b) Inspection

    (1) Surface trauma

    (2) Neck veins

    (3) Mucous membranes

    (4) Rash and urticaria

    (5) Ecchymosis

    (6) Areas of erythema

    (7) Abnormal use of accessory muscles

    (8) Symmetry of chest movement

    (9) Sunken eyes and fontanelles (young child or infant)

  c) Auscultation

    (1) Breath sounds: depth, quality, location of normal and abnormal breath sounds, presence of adventitious sounds (crackles, wheezes, pleural friction rub)

    (2) Heart sounds: rate and rhythm (apical), S_1 and S_2, S_3 and S_4, other sounds (e.g., murmurs)

    (3) Bowel sounds: hyperactive, hypoactive, absent

    (4) Fetal heart tones (gravid uterus)

  d) Palpation

(1) Areas of pain, tenderness, or crepitus

(2) Areas of edema: dependent and pitting

(3) Skin turgor

(4) Peripheral perfusion: quality of peripheral pulses, equality of pulses, capillary refill (may be an insensitive and unreliable indicator), temperature of skin and moisture

2) Diagnostic procedures

a) Laboratory: the following diagnostic procedures may assist in identifying the type of shock, assessing physiological responses, guiding management, and evaluating responses to therapeutic interventions

(1) Complete blood count (CBC)

(2) Serum electrolytes

(3) Creatinine and blood urea nitrogen (BUN)

(4) Arterial blood gas (ABG) values

(5) Serum glucose

(6) Serum lactate

(7) Urinalysis

(8) Ethanol level

(9) Drug screen

(10) Cardiac enzymes, isoenzymes, myoglobin, troponin

(11) Coagulation studies

(12) Blood type and cross-match

(13) Cultures

(14) Serum drug levels, as indicated (e.g., digoxin)

b) Radiology

(1) Chest radiograph

(2) Skull and cervical spine radiographs

(3) Computed tomography (CT) scan

(4) Other studies as indicated by specific injury or underlying disease process

c) Invasive and noninvasive procedures or devices

(1) Invasive: peritoneal lavage, thoracostomy, culdocentesis, lumbar puncture, nasogastric tube, urinary catheter, central venous pressure (CVP) catheter, pulmonary artery catheter (with or without venous oxygen saturation capability), intra-arterial catheter, and others as necessary

(2) Noninvasive: 12- to 15-lead electrocardiogram (ECG), pulse oximetry (SpO_2 values may be inaccurate because of vasoconstriction/shunting of blood from the skin), in-line end-tidal carbon dioxide, transcutaneous oxygen (PtO_2) and carbon dioxide ($PtCO_2$), and bioimpedance cardiac output

B. Analysis: differential nursing diagnosis

1. **Impaired gas exchange**
2. **Fluid volume deficit**
3. **Decreased cardiac output**
4. **Altered tissue perfusion**

C. Planning/interventions

1. **Determine priorities**
   a. *Control and maintain airway and breathing*

    b. *Identify and correct circulation deficits*

    c. *Maintain and support circulation*

    d. *Prevent complications*

    e. *Control pain*

    f. *Relieve anxiety and apprehension*

    g. *Educate patient/significant others*

2. **Develop nursing care plan specific to patient's presenting emergency**
3. **Obtain and set up necessary equipment and supplies**
4. **Institute appropriate interventions on basis of nursing care plan**
5. **Record data as appropriate**

D. Age-related considerations

1. **Pediatric**
   a. *Growth/development related*
      1) Infants have relatively fixed stroke volume and are able to increase cardiac output only by increasing heart rate
      2) Children have relatively small blood volume, 80 to 85 mL/kg (greater in infants)
      3) Large percentage of body weight in infants is fluid, making them susceptible to dehydration
      4) Core temperature regulation is more difficult in infant and young child because of high body surface area–body mass ratio, small glycogen stores in liver, and lack of substantial subcutaneous tissue in presence of thin skin
   b. *"Pearls"*
      1) Children may have subtle signs if hypovolemia is present; a child can lose up to 25% of circulating volume before recognizable changes occur
      2) Hypotension should be considered a late sign indicating severe shock
      3) *Early indicators* of hypovolemic shock in a child are pallor with cool and clammy skin and tachycardia (> 160 in infant, > 140 in preschool-age child, > 120 in school-age child to puberty); *bradycardia* should be considered an ominous sign
      4) Major extremity fractures in pediatric population rarely result in hypovolemic shock unless major vessel is lacerated and actively bleeding externally
      5) Lacerations rarely result in significant blood loss, although scalp lacerations may be the exception
      6) As in adult population, closed head injuries do not cause hypovolemic shock; other sources of volume loss should be sought
      7) Infusion volumes depend on size of child and estimated volume loss; amount is roughly equal to one fourth of normal blood volume, or approximately 20 mL/kg
      8) Accidental hypothermia during resuscitation is significant problem for infant and young child; preventive measures are essential
2. **Geriatric**
   a. *Aging-related physiological changes begin at about age 30 years*
      1) Cardiac function
         a) Cardiac output decreases by almost 50%
         b) Increased rigidity of valves and loss of vessel elasticity
         c) Decrease in baroreceptor sensitivity and response to endogenous catecholamines (receptor response rather than production)
         d) High percentage of elderly with coronary artery disease
         e) Diminished perfusion to all major organs
         f) Increased irritability of cardiac muscle

2) Pulmonary function
   a) Reduced vital capacity
   b) Decreased elasticity and expiratory muscle strength
   c) Diminished blood flow through pulmonary circulation
   d) Diminished cough reflex and effectiveness of ciliary mechanism
b. *"Pearls"*
   1) Because of reduction in physical reserve, any form of shock is poorly tolerated, resulting in rapid progression
   2) Because of physiological changes, reduced compensatory responses, and presence of one or more pre-existing diseases, elderly may not have classic signs and symptoms of shock; responses may be absent, delayed, or altered
   3) Normal physical assessment findings used to assess severity of shock and response to therapy may be misleading; poor preshock baseline status (e.g., diminished peripheral perfusion, mental status, blood pressure, heart rate) may be due to intrinsic disease or altered by medications; consider and be alert to use of medications such as beta blockers, presence of pacemaker, or hypertension (a baseline drop of 30% from known normal indicates impaired perfusion despite what appears to be a "normal blood pressure")
   4) Because of pulmonary changes, partial pressure of arterial oxygen (PO_2) equal to or greater than 80 mm Hg at 80 years of age should be considered within normal limits; 1 mm Hg may be subtracted for each subsequent year up to the age of 90 to determine normal
   5) Early hemodynamic measuring devices, such as central venous, intra-arterial, and pulmonary artery catheters, can assist in proper fluid and pharmacological management as well as continual monitoring
   6) Obtain baseline medical and physical activity levels as soon as possible from family or significant others
   7) Hypothermia is more likely in elderly during hypovolemic resuscitation; this condition is poorly tolerated and may have deleterious results (e.g., cardiac irritability and increased acidosis); measures to prevent hypothermia or to warm patient should be instituted as soon as possible
   8) Elderly patients in septic shock may exhibit hypothermia rather than more common fever and chills; rectal temperatures are generally more accurate in elderly with suspected infection
   9) Pre-existing renal and liver disease may necessitate adjustment of medication dosages

E. Obstetrical considerations (also see Chapter 13)

1. **"Pearls"**
   a. *Approach to pregnant patient is almost identical to that of nonpregnant patient*
   b. *Resuscitation priorities are also same for pregnant patient; resuscitation of mother supersedes that of fetus*
   c. *Physiological hypervolemia may mask extent of bleeding by mother; hypotension may not occur until a loss of 1500 mL has occurred*
   d. *Normal physiological response to shock (endogenous release of catecholamines) causes profound placental vasoconstriction, resulting in inadequate perfusion to fetus, although mother appears stable; vigorous and prompt volume replacement in hypovolemic shock is mandatory to avoid fetal demise*
   e. *Fetus normally has a low oxygen content; however, persistent maternal hypoxemia compromises fetus; therefore, adequacy of mother's airway and breathing should be ensured*
   f. *Inferior vena cava compression (vena cava syndrome) by gravid uterus can*

reduce venous return by 30%; proper position for pregnant patient is on her left side; right hip elevation and manual displacement of uterus may also be used if turning is contraindicated (e.g., spinal cord injury); if patient is immobilized on backboard, board may be tipped to place patient on her left side

g. *Inflation of abdominal portion of pneumatic antishock garment (PASG) is contraindicated because of possibility of fetal damage and compromise of venous return*

h. *Because of delay in gastric emptying and decreased motility, patient is at extreme risk for aspiration, and nasogastric tube should be passed as soon as possible*

i. *If non-cross-matched blood replacement is urgently needed, type O, Rh-negative blood is preferred to prevent sensitization and future complications with subsequent pregnancies*

II. SPECIFIC SHOCK EMERGENCIES

A. Hypovolemic shock

Hypovolemic shock is the most commonly seen form of shock, and is characterized by inadequate intravascular volume resulting from the loss or redistribution of whole blood, plasma, or other body fluid. Absolute hypovolemia refers to an actual loss of volume. A relative hypovolemic state exists when the normal blood volume fails to fill the available intravascular space (i.e., redistributed to third spaces).

The pathophysiological changes, decreased venous return, diminished stroke volume, and reduced cardiac output ultimately lead to inadequate perfusion and cellular oxygenation. If the loss of volume continues, arterial pressure eventually drops and tissue perfusion to vital organs becomes inadequate. Loss may be classified as internal or external as well as hemorrhagic or nonhemorrhagic. The loss of whole blood, or hemorrhage, is the most common cause of hypovolemic shock. A variety of causes and names exist for both types (Table 19–2).

If hypovolemic shock is identified early and therapy is instituted, the chances of survival are good. However, the mortality rate increases dramatically if decompensation and significant loss of organ perfusion develop and remain for any length of time.

1. Assessment
  a. *Subjective data*
    1) History of present illness
      a) Injury: mechanism, time, force, weapon, protective devices
      b) Hematemesis
      c) Melena or hematochezia

Table 19–2 CAUSES AND ALTERATIONS IN HYPOVOLEMIC SHOCK

Etiologies/Types	Alterations
Traumatic shock (blunt or penetrating injury)	Decreased intravascular volume
Gastrointestinal bleeding	
Hemorrhagic pancreatitis	
Aortic dissection	
Dehydration (hyperglycemia, excessive diuresis, vomiting, diarrhea)	
Burn shock	Redistribution of intravascular volume
Intestinal obstruction	
Cirrhosis	

        d) Hematuria
        e) External bleeding
           (1) Vaginal bleeding
           (2) Epistaxis or hemoptysis
           (3) Surgical incision
           (4) Open wounds
        f) Pain
        g) Orthostatic dizziness
        h) Fatigue and generalized weakness
        i) Thirst (occurs secondary to cellular dehydration)
        j) Nausea
        k) Protracted vomiting
        l) Protracted diarrhea
        m) Polyuria
        n) Excessive perspiration (environmental exposure)
        o) Excessive drainage from fistula or ostomy
        p) Cutaneous disruption (burns and extensive dermatitis)
        q) Lack of appropriate fluid intake (inadequate ingestion, abuse, neglect)
        r) Pregnancy
    2) Medical history
        a) Significant medical illnesses and surgical procedures: see Section A.4.a.2)a)
        b) Current medications (prescription and nonprescription): see Section A.4.a.2)b)
        c) Allergies
        d) Time of last meal (potential aspiration)
        e) Alcohol/drug use
  b. *Objective data*
    1) Physical examination: clinical manifestations will depend on degree and severity of shock; *earliest indicators* of shock usually include tachycardia, cutaneous changes, and increased respiratory rate. A four-tiered classification of hypovolemic shock is illustrated in Table 19–3, which summarizes most common signs, symptoms, and treatment based on percentage of blood/fluid loss; stages through which hypovolemic shock may progress are outlined next.

Table 19–3 ESTIMATED FLUID AND BLOOD LOSSES (BASED ON 70-KG MAN)

Variable	Class I	Class II	Class III	Class IV
Blood loss (mL)	Up to 750	750–1500	1500–2000	>2000
Blood loss (% blood volume)	Up to 15%	15–30%	30–40%	>40%
Pulse rate	<100	>100	>120	>140
Blood pressure	Normal	Normal	Decreased	Decreased
Pulse pressure (mm Hg)	Normal or increased	Decreased	Decreased	Decreased
Respiratory rate	14–20	20–30	30–40	>35
Urine output (mL/hr)	>30	20–30	5–15	Negligible
CNS/mental status	Slightly anxious	Mildly anxious	Anxious, confused	Confused, lethargic
Fluid replacement (3:1 Rule)	Crystalloid	Crystalloid	Crystalloid and blood	Crystalloid and blood

CNS, central nervous system.
(Adapted from American College of Surgeons Committee on Trauma. (1997). *Advanced trauma life support instructor manual* (6th ed., p. 108). Chicago, IL.)

a) **Compensated stage:** loss of circulating volume of 15 to 30%; equivalent to Class II (there are minimal clinical symptoms in Class I volume loss in otherwise healthy patient; blood volume is restored within 24 hours via compensatory mechanisms; therefore, volume replacement is often unnecessary)

(1) Altered mentation or behavior: anxiety (may be expressed as fright or hostility); restlessness or tremulousness; possible reports of thirst and weakness

(2) Altered peripheral perfusion: cool, pale skin; clammy or moist skin; weak, thready peripheral pulses; normal or delayed capillary refill (not always valid predictor); flat neck and peripheral veins

(3) Altered hemodynamic variables: mild tachycardia; narrowed pulse pressure (rise in diastolic pressure with minimal or no change in systolic); orthostatic changes: increase in pulse rate of 20 bpm and drop in systolic pressure of 10 to 20 mm Hg; normal or mildly decreased CVP, pulmonary artery pressure (PAP), and pulmonary capillary wedge pressure (PCWP)

(4) Hyperpnea; tidal volume one to two times normal

(5) Normal or mild decrease in urine output (normal: adults, 0.5–1 mL/kg/hr; pediatric patients, 1–2 mL/kg/hr)

(6) Mildly dry mucosa and decreased skin turgor (most notable in nonhemorrhagic fluid losses)

(7) Sunken eyes and fontanelles (young child or infant)

(8) External wound (assess source and determine whether arterial or venous)

b) **Uncompensated stage:** loss of circulating volume of 30 to 40%; equivalent to Class III hemorrhage

(1) Altered mentation or behavior: lethargic, apathetic

(2) Altered peripheral perfusion: cool, pale, mottled skin with mild peripheral cyanosis; diaphoresis; extremely weak, thready peripheral pulses (pulses may be absent); delayed capillary refill

(3) Altered hemodynamic variables: significant tachycardia and possible dysrhythmias or abnormal heart sounds; hypotension (systolic pressure < 30 mm Hg of known normal) and decreased pulse pressure (avoid orthostatic maneuvers in hypotensive patients); decreased CVP, PAP, and pulmonary capillary wedge pressure (PCWP)

(4) Increased respiratory rate with decrease in tidal volume; abnormal breath sounds (scattered crackles) may be present

(5) Decreased urine output

(6) Dry mucosa; decreased skin turgor

(7) Mild hypothermia may be present

c) **Irreversible stage:** loss of more than 40% of circulating volume; equivalent to Class IV hemorrhage

(1) Altered mentation or behavior: extremely obtunded and/or comatose

(2) Altered peripheral perfusion: cold, pale or mottled, cyanotic (central and peripheral) skin; marked diaphoresis; absent peripheral pulses; prolonged capillary refill

(3) Altered hemodynamic variables: marked tachycardia, dysrhythmias, and abnormal heart sounds; bradycardia (preterminal event); severe hypotension; markedly decreased CVP, PAP, PCWP

      (4) Rapid and shallow respirations, agonal respiration (preterminal event), and abnormal breath sounds

      (5) Oliguria progressing to anuria

      (6) Hypothermia usually present

  2) Diagnostic procedures: the following diagnostic procedures may assist in identifying type of (hypovolemic) shock, assessing physiological responses, guiding management, and evaluating responses to therapeutic interventions.

    a) Peritoneal lavage

    b) Thoracostomy

    c) Pericardiocentesis

    d) Culdocentesis

    e) ECG (continuous bedside monitoring)

    f) Nasogastric tube insertion

    g) Urinary catheter

    h) Radiology

      (1) Radiographs as indicated

      (2) Arteriogram

      (3) Intravenous (IV) pyelogram

      (4) Ultrasonogram

      (5) CT Scan

    i) Laboratory

      (1) CBC (caution must be used when interpreting the initial hematocrit; it may not drop immediately with blood loss, and is usually elevated if hypovolemia is a result of sequestration of fluid or selectively lost (as seen in burns)

      (2) Electrolytes, BUN, and creatinine and glucose

      (3) Coagulation profile

      (4) Type and cross-match

      (5) Amylase

      (6) Lactate

      (7) ABGs

      (8) Guaiac testing (stool and gastric secretions)

      (9) Urinalysis

      (10) Peritoneal lavage fluid analysis

    j) Hemodynamic devices (as needed when available)

      (1) CVP catheter

      (2) Pulmonary artery catheter

      (3) Arterial catheter

    k) Pulse oximeter or similar device

    l) Fetal monitoring devices (when available); otherwise auscultate fetal heart rate with assessment of maternal vital signs

  3) Calculate revised trauma score and pediatric trauma score if shock is result of traumatic injury

2. Analysis: differential nursing diagnosis

  a) Impaired gas exchange related to decreased tissue perfusion

  b) Fluid volume deficit related to hemorrhage or fluid shifts

  c) Decreased cardiac output related to altered preload or afterload

  d) Altered tissue perfusion related to fluid volume deficit and decreased cardiac output

  e) Anxiety/fear related to shock state symptoms

3. Planning/interventions

  a. Maintain patent airway; C-spine precautions if indicated b. Anticipate use of airway adjuncts or artificial airway

    c. Anticipate use of manual ventilation via bag-valve-mask device if ventilatory efforts are inadequate

    d. Prepare for mechanical ventilation (with or without positive end-expiratory pressure [PEEP]) after placement of artificial airway

    e. If respirations adequate, administer high-flow oxygen

    f. If no pulse present, initiate basic and advanced life support measures

    g. Control volume loss (institute universal precautions)

        1) External: hemorrhagic

            a) Apply direct pressure to bleeding site

            b) Use pressure points if direct pressure unsuccessful

            c) Use of PASG remains controversial; some application of device in presence of lower extremity and pelvic fractures for splinting may be useful; contraindications to their use: pulmonary edema, suspected ruptured diaphragm, left ventricular dysfunction; several other relative contraindications exist, including compression of abdomen in pregnant patient and abdominal evisceration.

            d) *Last resort* measures: apply tourniquet, or clamp and ligate vessels; avoid if possible

            e) Surgical intervention

        2) Internal: hemorrhagic

            a) PASG: see section II.A.3.g.1)c)

            b) Surgical intervention

            c) Saline lavage (for upper gastrointestinal tract bleeds); use of ice in saline remains controversial

        3) External: nonhemorrhagic (e.g., major burns or extensive dermatitis)

            a) Cover injured areas with dressings and sheet

            b) Increase ambient temperature

        4) Internal: nonhemorrhagic: administer specific pharmacological agents to stop or correct underlying cause of volume loss (e.g., insulin, vasopressin, antiemetics, antidiarrheal agents)

    h. Establish IV access

        1) Two percutaneous IV catheters: preferably upper extremities; obtain blood samples for laboratory analysis and type and cross-match

        2) Large-bore catheters: 14 to 16 gauge for adults; 22 or larger gauge for pediatric patients

        3) Central venous catheter when indicated

        4) If unable to obtain access in pediatric patient, attempt

            a) Cutdown (may occur in adults as well)

            b) Intraosseous cannulation in children younger than 6 years

   i. Provide intravascular volume replacement with specific fluid loss (some controversy exists about best suited fluid)

        1) Select appropriate fluid or combination

            a) Balanced salt solutions (crystalloids): lactated Ringer's solution (most commonly accepted resuscitation fluid) and normal saline

            b) Hypertonic saline solutions

            c) Colloids: plasma, albumin, dextran, and hetastarch (hydroxyethyl starch [Hespan])

        2) Estimate resuscitation fluid requirements: initial amount, type, and speed at which fluids are infused dictated by patient's clinical manifestations and severity of volume deficit (see Chapter 5 for burn resuscitation formula)

            a) Adults: 1 to 2 L of lactated Ringer's solution as initial bolus; initial bolus may be guided by weight at 10 to 20 mL/kg; 3:1 rule may also be used as rough guide in determining total crystalloid volume if hemorrhage present; for each 1 mL of blood lost, 3 mL of fluid is administered; if colloid used, bolus at 5 to 10 mL/kg or 1:1 ratio (also see Chapter 5 for calculated fluid requirements of major burn patient)

    b) Pediatric patients: 20 mL/kg lactated Ringer's or normal saline bolus as quickly as possible; repeat a second and third time (increasing up to 50–60 mL/kg) if no improvement after each bolus; if no improvement and the patient has received 50 to 60 mL/kg, blood should be administered

  3) Prepare for infusion of blood or blood components when indicated

    a) If blood is needed immediately, it is possible to use universal donor type O blood (Rh-negative cells are preferable to avoid sensitization and future complications, particularly for women of childbearing age); type-specific and typed and cross-matched blood (most preferred) should be used as soon as available and administered in a 1:1 ratio; blood substitutes are currently under investigation

    b) Blood components (i.e., fresh frozen plasma, platelets, and cryoprecipitate) may be needed under unusual circumstances for clotting factor replacement

    c) Autologous blood from noncontaminated penetrating thoracic injury (autotransfusion) may be considered

  4) Mechanical and manual pressure infusion devices should be used as indicated

  5) Titrate further volume replacement on basis of patient's hemodynamic response and diagnostic findings

  6) All fluids and blood should be warmed (trauma patients especially) and blood filtered

  7) Potential for fluid overload during fluid resuscitation of geriatric patient should be considered

  8) Although not commonly seen in emergency setting, anticipate complications of blood administration: hypothermia, hypocalcemia, coagulopathies, decreased platelets, antigen-antibody reaction

  9) Elevate patient's legs (modified Trendelenburg's position if feasible)

  10) Turn pregnant patient onto left side; elevate right hip if turning contraindicated and displace uterus manually

j. Obtain specimen for ABG determination

  1) Correct acid-base imbalances: respiratory alkalosis is expected in compensated stage, no treatment is necessary; expect significant metabolic acidosis in severe or long-standing shock: sodium bicarbonate ($NaHCO_3$) should not be used routinely to raise pH (correction of metabolic acidosis comes as result of improving perfusion and tissue oxygenation)

  2) Treat hypoxemia

k. Insert urinary catheter

l. Insert nasogastric tube when indicated to prevent aspiration or assess for presence of blood

m. Prevent or limit heat loss (particularly trauma, pediatric, and geriatric populations)

  1) Increase ambient temperature

  2) Remove wet clothing

  3) Cover exposed skin with blanket as soon as possible (wrap pediatric patient's head as well)

  4) Warm administered oxygen: not to exceed 104°F (40°C) if hypothermic

  5) Warm, administered IV fluids or blood not to exceed 38°C (100.4°F)

6) Use heat lamps
n. *Pharmacological therapy*
1) Administer appropriate antiarrhythmics as necessary if unable to treat underlying cause
2) Steroid administration is rare; patients with Addison's disease and adrenalectomized patients are exceptions
3) Administer medications IV or intraosseous unless contraindicated
4) Inotropic and vasopressor support is *contraindicated* as sole treatment of hypovolemic shock; specific pharmacological support of cardiovascular function may be indicated after volume replacement and based on preexisting disease or coexisting nonhypovolemic shock
o. *Maintain calm, efficient manner*
p. *Minimize environmental stimuli*
q. *Explain all procedures and events*
r. *Encourage questions and verbalization of fears*
s. *Remain with patient as much as possible*
t. *Allow calm significant other to accompany hemodynamically stable patient into treatment area*
u. *Continually monitor and assess patient's responses*
1) Fluid intake and output every 30 to 60 minutes; *urine output is reasonably sensitive indicator of adequate volume resuscitation and should be monitored closely*
4. **Expected outcomes/collaborative problems** (see Appendix B)

B. Cardiogenic shock

The hallmark of this shock category is impaired ability of the heart's pumping mechanism. Ventricular ischemia, structural variations, and dysrhythmias are the primary abnormalities that lead to cardiogenic shock. It is most commonly seen as a complication of acute myocardial infarction (AMI) in those with muscle compromise greater than 40%. Although the incidence has dropped over the past several years (owing to sophisticated monitoring and new therapies), the mortality of cardiogenic shock remains high: 65 to 90%. Failure of the left ventricle to eject the circulating volume ultimately results in decreased cardiac output and inadequate tissue perfusion. The intrinsic compensatory mechanisms activated by a reduced cardiac output are usually inadequate in this form of shock and may, in fact, be detrimental to the patient.

Other causes include cardiomyopathies, valvular dysfunction, rupture of papillary muscle or ventricular septum, and direct myocardial injury from trauma. Additional causes not discussed in this chapter are referred to as obstructive, or restrictive, types of cardiogenic shock. Causes include cardiac tamponade, tension pneumothorax, pulmonary embolus, and aortic stenosis. (Refer to discussions in Chapters 3 and 11).

1. **Assessment**
a. *Subjective data*
1) History of present illness
a) Pain or discomfort in chest
b) Blunt chest injury (mechanism, time, force, protective devices) or electrical burn
c) Nausea
d) Dyspnea or orthopnea
e) Diaphoresis
f) Sense of impending doom and apprehension

g) Thirst

h) Sensation of feeling "cold"

2) Medical history

   a) Congenital cardiac anomaly

   b) Previous myocardial infarction

   c) Other cardiac diseases

   d) Surgery (general and/or cardiovascular)

   e) Thromboembolic phenomenon

   f) Current medications (prescription and nonprescription)

   g) Allergies

   h) Alcohol and/or drug use

b. *Objective data*

1) Physical examination: clinical manifestations depend on degree of shock

   a) Compensated stage

     (1) Altered mentation or behavior: anxiety and apprehension; restlessness; fear; weakness and fatigue

     (2) Normal or mild decrease in urine output (normal: adults, 0.5–1 mL/kg/hr; pediatric patients, 1–2 mL/kg/hr)

     (3) Altered peripheral perfusion: pale or chalky skin; diaphoresis; weak, thready peripheral pulses; normal or delayed capillary refill; flat neck and peripheral veins; jugular vein distension (indicating right ventricular failure)

     (4) Altered hemodynamic variables: tachycardia (mild); S_3 may be present; narrowed pulse pressure (rise in diastolic pressure); normal or mild drop in systolic blood pressure; CVP, PAP, and PCWP may be normal or slightly elevated

     (5) Altered pulmonary function: hyperpnea; orthopnea; mild basilar crackles

     (6) Geriatric patients may progress rapidly through this stage

     (7) Normal physiological changes occurring in pregnant patient may mask important vital signs in this stage

   b) Uncompensated stage

     (1) Altered mentation: lethargic, apathetic

     (2) Oliguria

     (3) Altered peripheral perfusion: pale or mottled skin with mild peripheral cyanosis; diaphoresis; extremely weak, thready pulses (peripheral pulses may be absent); delayed capillary refill

     (4) Altered hemodynamic parameters: tachycardia (significant) and possible dysrhythmias and S_3; hypotension, decrease in systolic blood pressure of more than 30 mm Hg from known normal ($<$ 90 mm Hg in nonhypertensive patient), and decreased pulse pressure; elevated CVP, PAP, PCWP, decreased cardiac output

     (5) Altered pulmonary function: tachypnea with decrease in tidal volume; increasing pulmonary congestion and crackles; central cyanosis

   c) Irreversible shock

     (1) Altered mentation: extremely obtunded or comatose

     (2) Altered peripheral perfusion: cold, pale or mottled, and cyanotic skin; clammy or moist skin; absent peripheral pulses; prolonged capillary refill

     (3) Altered hemodynamic variables: marked tachycardia and dysrhythmias; bradycardia (usually preterminal if tachycardia is present

initially); severe hypotension (systolic blood pressure < 60 mm Hg); CVP, PAP, PCWP markedly elevated

    (4) Altered pulmonary function: respirations rapid and shallow, progressing to agonal (preterminal event); marked diffuse crackles and wheezes; marked central cyanosis

    (5) Anuric or oliguric

  2) Diagnostic procedures: see section I.A.4.b.2)a)

2. Analysis: differential nursing diagnosis

  a. Impaired gas exchange related to decreased tissue perfusion

  b. Decreased cardiac output related to myocardial pump failure

  c. Altered tissue perfusion related to myocardial pump failure

  d. Anxiety/fear related to shock state, symptoms, and prognosis

3. Planning/interventions

  a. Maintain patent airway

  b. Anticipate use of airway adjuncts or artificial airways

  c. Anticipate use of manual ventilation via bag-valve-mask device if ventilatory efforts are inadequate

  d. Prepare for mechanical ventilation (with or without PEEP) after placement of artificial airway

  e. Administer high-flow oxygen if respiration adequate

  f. If no pulse present, initiate basic and advanced life support

  g. Obtain IV access, draw blood for laboratory analysis, and administer normal saline at "keep open" rate; if AMI patient is candidate for thrombolytic therapy, multiple sticks (e.g., for ABGs and IV catheters) should be avoided

  h. If unable to obtain access in pediatric patient, attempt

    1) Cutdown (may occur in adult as well)

    2) Intraosseous cannulation: children younger than 6 years

  i. Obtain 12- to 15-lead ECG and correct symptomatic dysrhythmias (e.g., bradycardias and premature ventricular contractions; see Chapter 3)

  j. Turn pregnant patient onto left side

  k. Correct pre-existing volume deficit or enhance preload (right ventricular infarct) cautiously; this is contraindicated in patients with evidence of pulmonary congestion

    1) Infuse small boluses of fluid: normal saline, lactated Ringer's solution, blood products (if laboratory data support administration), or colloid

    2) Closely monitor hemodynamic status; patient's response dictates total amount to be infused

  l. Obtain specimen for ABG determination

    1) Correct acid-base imbalances: respiratory alkalosis expected in compensated stage, no treatment necessary; expect metabolic acidosis in uncompensated and irreversible stages: sodium bicarbonate should not be used routinely to raise pH (correction of the metabolic acidosis comes as result of improving perfusion and tissue oxygenation)

    2) Treat hypoxemia

  m. Insert urinary catheter

  n. Insert nasogastric tube when indicated to prevent aspiration

  o. Administer the following pharmacological agents alone or in combination (additional agents are available and may be used according to physician's preference)

    1) Decrease preload

      a) Furosemide (Lasix)

      b) Nitrates (nitroglycerin)

   c) Morphine sulfate (used for pain relief; reduction in preload is secondary effect)

  2) Increase contractility

   a) Dopamine hydrochloride (Intropin)

   b) Dobutamine hydrochloride (Dobutrex)

   c) Amrinone lactate (Inocor)

   d) Milrinone (Primacor)

  3) Decrease afterload

   a) Nitroprusside sodium (Nipride)

   b) Nitrates (nitroglycerin)

   c) Angiotensin-converting enzyme (ACE) inhibitors e.g., captoril (Capoten), enapril (Vasotec)

  4) Increase afterload

   a) Norepinephrine bitartrate (Levophed)

   b) Epinephrine

 p. Administer pharmacological agents via IV or intraosseous route unless contraindicated

 q. Prepare patient for reperfusion therapy or assist devices (i.e., percutaneous transluminal coronary angioplasty [PTCA], intra-aortic balloon pump [IAPB], as necessary)

 r. Maintain calm, efficient manner

 s. Minimize environmental stimuli

 t. Explain all procedures and events

 u. Encourage questions and verbalization of fears

 v. Remain with patient as much as possible

 w. Allow calm significant other to accompany hemodynamically stable patient into treatment area

 x. Continually monitor and assess patient's responses

4. Expected outcomes/collaborative problems (see Appendix B)

C. Distributive shock

Distributive, or vasogenic, shock is characterized by an abnormal placement of the intravascular volume. Initially, cardiac function and blood volume may be normal. However, widespread alterations in the systemic vasculature and the vessels themselves result in a maldistribution of the intravascular volume within the circulatory network and tissue. The three major types discussed are septic, neurogenic, and anaphylactic.

Septic shock is thought to be a widespread systemic response to sepsis, which, if left untreated, eventually leads to circulatory shock. Sepsis has been linked to more than 100,000 deaths per year in the United States. The estimated annual incidence is 400,000, a significant increase compared with incidence a decade ago. The increasing incidence has been attributed to the aging of the population, longevity of patients with chronic diseases, and high frequency among those with AIDS. The most common infecting organisms are gram-negative bacilli, but yeast, fungi, and gram-positive bacteria are also known to be causative agents. *Staphylococcus aureus* is the organism most often identified with toxic shock syndrome, a form of septic shock.

The pathophysiological characteristics of septic shock are believed to be initiated by toxins released by the specific organism. Cellular, humoral, and immunological systems activate a complex series of reactions resulting in the release of mediators such as cytokines and tumor necrosis factor. These substances and others—more than 30 have been identified—are the modulators of the multisystem derangement.

Massive vasodilation and increased capillary permeability are the major factors related to the maldistribution of intravascular volume and subsequent relative hypovolemic state. Inadequate perfusion secondary to peripheral pooling and third-space shifting, in addition to alterations in cellular metabolism, have a profound effect on every organ system.

The changes evolve so that the patient progresses through two phases. The initial, or hyperdynamic, state is characterized by a significant fall in systemic vascular resistance (SVR) and high cardiac output. The second phase is referred to as the hypodynamic phase. This phase of decreased cardiac output and extreme vasoconstriction conforms to the classic shock picture.

Although the understanding of the molecular events in septic shock have grown significantly in the last decade, bedside management remains primarily supportive. The mortality attributed to septic shock has been estimated to be as high as 60%. Fortunately, a number of therapies (e.g., endotoxin and cytokine antagonists and nitric oxide inhibitors) have been developed and are currently being tested in animal and clinical trials.

1. **Assessment**
   a. *Subjective data*
      1) History of present illness
         a) Hyperthermia
         b) Hypothermia (noted more often in very old or very young)
         c) Shaking chills
         d) Purulent drainage or discharge
         e) General malaise and weakness or fatigue
      2) Medical history
         a) Recent surgery or invasive procedure or instrumentation
         b) Recent obstetrical procedure or abortion
         c) Recent traumatic wound or thermal injury
         d) Chronic illnesses, particularly those that result in immunosuppression (e.g., cancer and AIDS)
         e) Presence of long-term invasive devices: indwelling urinary catheter, tracheostomy, external vascular access devices
         f) Splenectomy
         g) Current medications
            (1) Prolonged or inappropriate antibiotic use
            (2) Immunosuppressive drug therapy (corticosteroids, cytotoxic drugs, antirejection drugs [for organ transplant recipient])
            (3) Illicit drug injections
            (4) Immunization status
         h) Allergies
         i) Last menstrual period: if toxic shock syndrome is suspected, ask about tampon use
   b. *Objective data*
      1) Physical examination: clinical manifestations depend on phase of shock, patient's overall health, and volume status
         a) **Hyperdynamic phase:** moderate alteration in sensorium (early indicator); peripheral perfusion—skin warm, dry, and flushed, peripheral pulses easily palpable (may be bounding), capillary refill normal; altered hemodynamic parameters—moderate tachycardia, normal blood pressure or mild hypotension, widened pulse pressure (decreased diastolic pressure), decreased CVP, PAP, and PCWP, decreased SVR, and elevated cardiac output; tachypnea and increased minute ventilation—adventitious breath sounds (crackles and wheezes) may be pres-

ent (tachypnea is early indicator); urine output within normal limits; septic foci may be identified—purulent exudate, cellulitis, expectora, discharge, and necrotic tissue; hyperthermia (seen most often) or hypothermia, presence of skin rash (toxic shock syndrome or meningococcal organism); normal physiological changes occurring in pregnant patient may cause confusion in interpreting vital signs in this stage

    b) **Hypodynamic phase** (similar to uncompensated and irreversible stages of hypovolemic and cardiogenic shock): altered mentation—lethargy and apathy progressing to coma; oliguria progressing to anuria; peripheral perfusion—skin clammy and pale or mottled with moderate to severe cyanosis, weak and thready pulses (which may be absent), and prolonged capillary refill; altered hemodynamic parameters—significant tachycardia and dysrhythmias may occur, bradycardia (preterminal event), profound hypotension, decreased pulse pressure, elevated CVP, PAP and PCWP, and altered pulmonary function—respirations rapid and shallow progressing to agonal (preterminal event), increasing pulmonary congestion (crackles and wheezes), and central cyanosis

2) Diagnostic procedures

    a) Chest and abdominal radiographs, if appropriate

    b) Laboratory: CBC with differential leukocyte count; urinalysis; coagulation profile; ABGs; electrolytes, glucose, BUN and creatinine; serum lactate; culture and sensitivity testing—blood, urine, sputum, wound drainage, stool, cerebrospinal fluid

    c) Lumbar puncture

    d) Abdominal paracentesis

    e) Culdocentesis

    f) Twelve- to 15-lead ECG and continuous bedside monitoring

    g) Use of hemodynamic devices: central venous catheter, pulmonary artery catheter, arterial catheter

    h) Pulse oximetry

    i) Fetal monitoring device (when available); otherwise auscultate fetal heart tones with assessment of maternal vital signs

3) Analysis: differential nursing diagnosis

    a) Impaired gas exchange related to decreased tissue perfusion

    b) Decreased cardiac output related to alteration in preload and afterload

    c) Altered tissue perfusion related to alteration in venous capacity secondary to cause

    d) Anxiety/fear related to shock state

4. Planning/interventions

    a) Maintain patent airway

    b) Anticipate use of airway adjuncts or artificial airways

    c) Anticipate use of manual ventilation via bag-valve-mask device if ventilatory efforts are inadequate

    d) Prepare for mechanical ventilation (with or without PEEP) after placement of artificial airway

    e) Administer high-flow oxygen if respirations adequate

    f) If pulse is absent, initiate basic and advanced life support measures.

    g) Establish IV access

        (1) Two percutaneous IV catheters: obtain blood for laboratory analysis, including blood cultures

        (2) Large-bore catheters: 14 to 16 gauge in adult, 22 gauge or larger in pediatric patient

      (3) Central venous and pulmonary artery catheters as indicated

      (4) Intraosseous cannulation if percutaneous route unsuccessful (age < 6 years)

h) Correct pre-existing or present relative intravascular volume deficit (significant volume may be needed in hyperdynamic stage)

    (1) Select appropriate fluid or combination (controversy exists over which fluid is best suited)

      a. Balanced salt solutions (crystalloids): lactated Ringer's solution and normal saline

      b. Colloids: plasma, albumin, dextran, and hetastarch (hydroxyethyl starch [Hespan])

    (2) Rate of administration and amount of fluid infused are based on physical findings and patient's response

    (3) Fluids should be warmed if patient is hypothermic

i) Obtain specimen for ABG determination

    (1) Correct acid-base imbalances: respiratory alkalosis is expected in hyperdynamic stage, but no treatment is necessary (early indicator); expect severe metabolic acidosis in hypodynamic stage; sodium bicarbonate should not be used routinely to raise pH (correction of metabolic acidosis comes as result of improving perfusion and tissue oxygenation/utilization)

    (2) Treat hypoxemia

j) Anticipate and prepare for insertion of nasogastric tube for decompression and emptying of stomach to prevent potential aspiration

k) Insert urinary catheter

l) Elevate lower extremities (modified Trendelenburg's position) if feasible

m) Place pregnant patient on left side

n) Administer the following pharmacological agents alone or in combination (other agents may be used according to physician's preference)

    (1) Increase afterload: vasopressors

      a. Phenylephrine hydrochloride (Neo-Synephrine)

      b. Epinephrine hydrochloride (Adrenaline Chloride)

      c. Norepinephrine (Levophed)

    (2) Increase contractility: cardiotonic agents

      a. Dopamine hydrochloride (Intropin)

      b. Dobutamine hydrochloride (Dobutrex)

      c. Amrinone lactate (Inocor)

    (3) Decrease afterload: vasodilators

      a. Nitroprusside sodium (Nipride)

      b. Nitrate (nitroglycerin)

o) Identify and remove septic foci if possible

    (1) Invasive devices (e.g., Foley catheter and external vascular access devices)

    (2) Debride or drain wounds and necrotic tissue

    (3) Remove tampon

p) Administer additional pharmacological agents

    (1) Broad-spectrum antibiotics according to suspected organisms (may administer combination, e.g., aminoglycosides, cephalosporins)

    (2) Corticosteroids (controversial)

    (3) Antipyretics for temperature above 101°F (38.3°C); no aspirin for children younger than 12 years

q) If hypothermia is present, initiate measures to rewarm and prevent further heat loss

      r) Administer pharmacological agents IV or intraosseous unless contrain-
dicated

      s) Explain all procedures and events

      t) Encourage questions and verbalization of fears

      u) Remain with patient as much as possible

      v) Allow calm significant other to accompany hemodynamically stable
patient into treatment area

      w) Continually monitor and assess patient's response

    5) Expected outcomes/collaborative problems (see Appendix B)

    Neurogenic shock is characterized by loss of sympathetic vasomotor function. The loss of sympathetic tone and uninhibited parasympathetic responses causes extreme vasodilation in the systemic vasculature, producing a maldistribution of the circulating volume. Blood pools in the periphery cause a decrease in venous return and a reduction in cardiac output. These physiological changes create a relative hypovolemic state. The decrease in cardiac output and circulatory flow results in inadequate tissue perfusion and cellular oxygenation. Two clinical manifestations of note are bradycardia and warm, flushed skin in the presence of hypotension, the opposite response seen in most forms of shock. The most commonly associated cause of neurogenic shock is spinal cord injury (SCI), or "spinal shock." Additional causes that inhibit or depress outflow from the vasomotor center in the medulla include brain injury, spinal anesthesia, depressant action of drugs (narcotics and barbiturates), hypoxia, and lack of glucose or excessive insulin (insulin shock).

1. **Assessment**
   a. *Subjective data*
      1) History of present illness
         a) Injury to brain stem or spinal cord (high thoracic or low cervical): mechanism, time, force, weapon, protective devices
         b) Pain at injury site immediately above level of lesion
         c) Neuromuscular function at scene and trend of status; may have to obtain from prehospital providers or family members
         d) If related to inappropriate or inadvertent insulin dosage, reports of fatigue and weakness should be explored (insulin shock)
      2) Medical history
         a) Current medications
         b) Allergies
         c) Time of last meal
         d) Alcohol/drug and tobacco use
   b. *Objective data*
      1) Physical examination
         a) Surface trauma
         b) Altered mentation: confusion progressing to apathy and lethargy; if injury to brain stem (medulla) is present, patient may be comatose; level of consciousness in SCI without concomitant injuries is usually normal
         c) Peripheral perfusion: skin warm, dry, and flushed below level of lesion; skin may be cool and clammy above lesion; peripheral pulses easily palpable; capillary refill normal
         d) Altered hemodynamic parameters: bradycardia; hypotension and decreased pulse pressure; normal or slightly decreased CVP, PAP, PCWP
         e) Tachypnea may be present (depending on level of injury)
         f) Urine output usually within normal limits; may progress to oliguria
         g) Neuromuscular function (paraplegia or quadriplegia): areflexia; loss of motor ability below level of lesion; loss of sensation below lesion;

poikilothermy; loss of sphincter tone (bladder and rectal); possible priapism; piloerection

    2) Diagnostic procedures

        a) Radiology: spinal films (lateral and oblique); skull films; CT scan

        b) Laboratory: CBC; electrolytes, glucose, BUN and creatinine; ABGs; urinalysis; serum lactate; alcohol level; drug screen

        c) Use of hemodynamic devices as indicated: central venous catheter pulmonary artery catheter, arterial catheter

        d) Pulse oximetry

        e) ECG and continuous bedside monitoring

        f) Fetal monitoring devices (when available): otherwise auscultate fetal heart tones with assessment of maternal vital signs

2. Analysis: differential nursing diagnosis

    a. *Impaired gas exchange related to decreased tissue perfusion*

    b. *Decreased cardiac output related to alteration in preload and afterload*

    c. *Altered tissue perfusion related to increased vascular capacity*

    d. *Potential for injury related to presence of SCI*

3. Planning/interventions

    a. *Maintain patent airway without hyperextension or rotation of neck if SCI is present; stabilize cervical spine throughout resuscitation until cervical spine injury is ruled out*

    b. *Anticipate use of airway adjuncts or artificial airways (usually nasotracheal intubation to prevent hyperextension of neck)*

    c. *Anticipate use of manual ventilation via bag-valve-mask device if ventilatory efforts are inadequate*

    d. *Prepare for mechanical ventilation after placement of artificial airway*

    e. *If pulse absent, initiate basic and advanced life support measures*

    f. *Administer high-flow oxygen if respirations adequate*

    g. *Obtain IV access*

        1) Two percutaneous catheters: obtain blood sample for laboratory analysis

        2) Intraosseous cannulation if percutaneous route is unsuccessful (age < 6 years)

        3) Central venous and pulmonary artery catheters, as indicated

    h. *Correct pre-existing or current relative intravascular volume deficit with appropriate fluid or combination (physician preference and patient condition will dictate administration of additional fluids; vasopressor therapy may be used alone)*

        1) Balanced salt solutions: lactated Ringer's solution (most common) and normal saline

        2) Colloids: plasma, albumin, dextran, and hetastarch (hydroxyethyl starch [Hespan])

        3) Blood and blood components if indicated

    i. *Estimate fluid requirements*

        1) Initial amount and speed at which fluids are infused are dictated by patient's clinical manifestations indicating severity of volume deficit; care should be taken not to overhydrate

        2) Titrate further volume replacement on basis of patient's response and diagnostic findings

        3) If temperature regulation is impaired, fluids should be warmed

    j. *Turn pregnant patient onto left side; if contraindicated, elevate right hip and displace uterus manually*

    k. *Analyze ABG results and correct*

        1) Acid-base imbalance: respiratory alkalosis is expected if patient is hyper-

pneic, no treatment is necessary; metabolic acidosis may be present: sodium bicarbonate should not be used routinely to increase pH (improvement will occur by increasing perfusion and cellular oxygenation)

   2) Treat hypoxemia

   l. Assist with removal of pulmonary secretions if injury inhibits effective cough

   m. Insert urinary catheter

   n. Insert nasogastric tube for decompression and emptying of stomach to prevent potential aspiration

   o. Elevate lower extremities (modified Trendelenburg's position) if feasible

   p. Administer the following pharmacological agents alone or in combination if patient has symptoms of hypotension and/or bradycardia

   1) Vasopressors: phenylephrine hydrochloride, epinephrine hydrochloride, norepinephrine, ephedrine

   2) Dysrhythmic agents (bradycardia): atropine sulfate

   3) Dextrose (50% dextrose): if related to hypoglycemia

   4) Corticosteroids, if indicated

   5) Naloxone hydrochloride (Narcan) if narcotic ingestion or injection is suggested

   q. Reduce severity of poikilothermy by, for example, increasing ambient temperature, using blankets

   r. Administer pharmacological agents via IV or intraosseous route

   s. If SCI present, prepare for and assist with realignment of spine (tong insertion/halo vest)

   t. Explain all procedures and events

   u. Encourage questions and verbalization of fears

   v. Remain with patient as much as possible

   w. Allow calm significant other to accompany hemodynamically stable patient into treatment area

   x. Continuously monitor and assess patient's response

4. **Expected outcomes/collaborative problems** (see Appendix B)

Anaphylactic shock is usually of sudden onset, resulting from a systemic antigen-antibody response or hypersensitivity reaction. The mechanism may be one of several: immunoglobulin E mediated, complement activation (C3a and C5a), direct activation, cyclo-oxyenase inhibitors, or idiopathic (no known cause). When anaphylactic shock occurs, vasoactive mediators such as histamine and leukotrienes are released into the blood by the mast cells and basophils, causing massive vasodilation and changes in capillary permeability.

A state of relative hypovolemia exists secondary to pooling of blood in the peripheral circulation and the massive fluid shift from the intravascular to the extravascular space. This results in numerous physiological alterations, including decreased venous return, reduced cardiac output, subsequent decrease in tissue perfusion, and inadequate cellular oxygenation. Unlike other forms of shock, a concomitant threat to life often occurs in the form of airway and ventilatory compromise.

The mediators target specific organs, most notably the smooth muscle of the bronchopulmonary tree and tissue in the upper airway (in addition to the vascular alterations causing the hypoperfusion). Edema formation in the mucosa of the upper airway may be so severe as to obstruct the airway completely. In the absence of complete airway obstruction, bronchospasms may prevent adequate ventilation. If the airway and breathing are severely compromised, treatment of the "shock" process becomes secondary. Fortunately, with rapid identification, both conditions can be identified and treated promptly to prevent sudden death.

Common causes include various types of food (shellfish), hormones, drugs (iodine, antibiotics, nonsteroidal anti-inflammatory drugs [NSAIDs]), environmental substances (latex, pollen), and insect stings. The degree of reaction usually varies according to the route and amount of exposure. If the onset of symptoms are slow, in most cases the reaction is less severe. Although uncommon, there have also been documented cases of recurrent symptoms occurring after apparent resolution of the initial reaction. These subsequent reactions, termed biphasic or multiphasic anaphylaxis, have been estimated to occur in 6 to 20% of this population. Onset of additional occurrences have been anywhere from 1 to 72 hours after resolution of the initial symptoms.

1. **Assessment**
   a. *Subjective data*
      1) History of present illness
         a) Onset: relationship between exposure to substance and reaction (minutes to days)
         b) Route and length of exposure
         c) Sense of impending doom
         d) Pruritus
         e) Urticaria and rash
         f) Sudden headache
         g) Abdominal pain, vomiting, diarrhea
         h) Dyspnea
         i) Shortness of breath
         j) Syncope
      2) Medical history
         a) Allergies: foods, medications, hay fever, asthma
         b) Family history of allergies
         c) Current medications (prescription and nonprescription); specific drugs that may alter effectiveness or response to treatment: beta blockers, tricyclic antidepressants, thyroid hormones, some antihistamines
         d) Time of last meal
   b. *Objective data*
      1) Physical examination
         a) Altered mentation: anxiety and restlessness progressing to lethargy and coma
         b) Cutaneous and mucosal alterations: uticaria; pruritus; angioedema (orbits, mouth, pharynx, uvula, neck, trachea, larynx)
         c) Peripheral perfusion: skin warm and flushed, progressing to cool and clammy; palpable peripheral pulses progressing to weak and thready or absent pulses; normal capillary refill progressing to delayed
         d) Altered hemodynamic parameters and cardiac function: tachycardia; dysrhythmias; angina; hypotension; progression to cardiac arrest
         e) Altered respiratory function: tachypnea; adventitious breath sounds, stridor, and wheezing; use of accessory muscles and nasal flaring; possible rapid progression to respiratory arrest
         f) Oliguria progressing to anuria
      2) Diagnostic procedures
         a) Laboratory: ABGs; electrolytes, glucose, BUN and creatinine; serum lactate; urinalysis
         b) Chest radiograph
         c) Twelve-lead ECG
         d) Use of hemodynamic devices as indicated: central venous catheter, pulmonary artery catheter, arterial catheter (generally not necessary)

e) Pulse oximeter or similar device

f) Fetal monitoring device (when available): otherwise auscultate fetal heart tones with assessment of maternal vital signs

2. **Analysis: differential nursing diagnosis**

a. *Impaired gas exchange related to decreased tissue perfusion and bronchospasm*

b. *Decreased cardiac output related to alteration in preload and afterload*

c. *Altered tissue perfusion related to alteration in venous capacitance and decreased cardiac output*

d. *Anxiety/fear related to manifestations of allergic or anaphylactic reaction*

e. *Knowledge deficit related to therapeutic regimen and avoidance of allergens*

3. **Planning/interventions**

a. *Maintain patent airway*

b. *Anticipate rapid deterioration. Prepare airway adjuncts or artificial airways*

c. *Anticipate use of manual ventilation via bag-valve-mask device if ventilatory efforts are inadequate (this method may not be effective owing to upper and lower airway edema and spasms)*

d. *Prepare for mechanical ventilation (with or without PEEP) after placement of artificial airway*

e. *In no pulse, initiate basic and advanced life support measures*

f. *Administer high-flow oxygen if respirations adequate*

g. *Establish IV access*

1) One or two percutaneous catheters: obtain blood sample for laboratory analysis

2) Intraosseous cannulation if percutaneous route is unsuccessful (age < 6 years)

h. *Administer one or a combination of the following pharmacological agents*

1) Epinephrine (first-line therapy)

a) May be administered subcutaneously if patient is mildly hypotensive or has mild compromise of airway and breathing (1:1000 solution)

b) Administer IV if life is threatened by obstructed airway and/or severe hypotension (1:10,000 solution); administer in small, controlled doses to prevent cardiac ischemia and dysrhythmias, especially in pregnant or geriatric patient and patient with history of coronary artery disease, hypertension, tachydysrhythmias

c) Doses may need to be repeated until condition stabilizes

2) Antihistamines

a) Diphenhydramine (Benadryl)

b) Cimetidine (Tagamet)

3) Bronchodilators (if bronchoconstriction remains)

a) Theophylline (aminophylline)

b) Aerosolized albuterol (Proventil)

4) Corticosteroid (for prolonged urticaria or late-phase response)

5) Glucagon (for refractory anaphylaxis in patients receiving beta-blocker therapy)

i. *Central venous catheter, as indicated*

j. *Turn pregnant patient onto left side*

k. *Volume replacement is not usually necessary after vasopressor administration; however, if intravascular volume deficit is suspected, replace with appropriate fluid or combination*

1) Balanced salt solution: lactated Ringer's solution or normal saline

2) Colloids: plasma, albumin, and hetastarch (hydroxyethyl starch [Hespan])

l. *Estimate fluid requirements*

1) Initial amount and speed at which fluids are infused dictated by patient's clinical manifestations indicating severity of volume deficit; care should be taken not to overhydrate

2) Titrate further volume replacement on basis of patient's response and diagnostic findings

   m. *If ABGs are obtained, analyze results and correct*

1) Acid-base imbalance: expect metabolic acidosis if shock state is prolonged, and possible respiratory acidosis if airway/ventilatory status compromised (carbon dioxide retention); sodium bicarbonate should not be used routinely to treat metabolic acidosis—the problem will resolve with correction of shock; respiratory acidosis is corrected by adequate ventilation

2) Treat hypoxemia

   n. *Insert urinary catheter if indicated*

   o. *Explain all procedures and events*

   p. *Encourage questions and verbalization of fears*

   q. *Remain with patient as much as possible*

   r. *Allow calm significant other to accompany hemodynamically stable patient into treatment area*

   s. *Continuously monitor and assess patient's response*

4. **Expected outcomes/collaborative problems** (see Appendix B)

BIBLIOGRAPHY

American College of Chest Physicians/Society of Critical Care Medicine Consensus Conference Committee. (1992). Definitions for sepsis and organ failure and guidelines for the use of innovative therapies in sepsis. *Critical Care Medicine, 20*(6), 864–874.

American College of Surgeons, Committee on Trauma. (1997) Shock. In *Advanced trauma life support course: Instructors manual* (6th ed., pp. 97–117). Chicago, IL: Author.

Anderson, M. R., & Blumer, J. L. (1997). Advances in the therapy for sepsis in children. *Pediatric Clinics of North America, 44*(1), 179–205.

Asensio, J. A., Demetriades, D., Berne, T. V., & Shoemaker, W. C. (1996). Invasive and noninvasive monitoring for early recognition and treatment of shock in high-risk trauma and surgical patients. *Surgical Clinics of North America, 76*(4), 985–997.

Baker, C. C., & Huynh, T. (1995). Sepsis in the critically ill. *Current Problems in Surgery, 32*(12), 1018–1083.

Bone, R. C. (1991). Let's agree on terminology: Definitions of sepsis. *Critical Care Medicine, 19,* 973–976.

Brady, W. J., Jr., Luber, S., Carter, C. T., Guertler, A., & Lindbeck, G. (1997). Multiphasic anaphylaxis: an uncommon event in the emergency department. *Academy of Emergency Medicine, 4*(3), 193–197.

Brady, W. J., Jr., Luber, S., & Joyce, T. P. (1997). Multiphasic anaphylaxis: Report of a case with prehospital and emergency department considerations. *Journal of Emergency Medicine, 15*(4), 477–481.

Britt, L. D., Weireter, L. J., Riblet, J. L., Asensio, J. A., & Maull, K. (1996). Priorities in the management of profound shock. *Surgical Clinics of North America, 76*(4), 645–660.

Carcillo, J. A., & Cunnion, R. E. (1997). Septic shock. *Critical Care Clinics, 13*(3), 553–574.

Chapman, C. A. (1998). Shock emergencies. In L. Newberry (Ed.), *Sheehy's emergency nursing: Principles and practice* (4th ed., pp. 515–523). St. Louis, MO: Mosby-Year Book.

Crowley, S. R. (1996). The pathogenesis of septic shock. *Heart & Lung, 25*(2), 124–134.

Hollenberg, S. M., & Parrillo, J. E. (1998). Shock. In A. S. Fauci, E. Braunwald, K. Isselbacer, J. D. Wilson, J. B. Martin, D. L. Kaspir, S. L. Hauser, & D. L. Longo (Eds.), *Harrison's principles of internal medicine* (14th ed., pp. 214–222). New York: McGraw-Hill.

Hudak, C. M., Gallo, B. M., & Morton, P. G. (1998). *Critical care nursing: A holistic approach* (7th ed.). Philadelphia: Lippincott-Raven.

Jones, K. (1996). Shock. In J. M. Clochesy, C. Breu, S. Cardin, A. A. Whittaker, & E. B. Rudy (Eds.), *Critical care nursing* (2nd ed., pp. 1371–1380). Philadelphia: W. B. Saunders.

Kline, J. A. (1998). Shock. In P. Rosen & R. Barkin (Eds.), *Emergency medicine: Concepts and clinical practice* (4th ed., pp. 86–106). St. Louis, MO: Mosby Year Book.

Martinot, A., Leclerc, F., Cremer, R., Leteurtre, S., Fourier, C., & Hue, V. (1997). Sepsis in neonates and children: Definitions, epidemiology, and outcome. *Pediatric Emergency Care, 13*(4), 277–281.

Mattox, K. L., Bickell, W., Pepe, P. E., Burch, J., & Feliciano, D. (1989). Prospective MAST study in 911 patients. *Journal of Trauma, 29*(8), 1104–1112.

Munford, R. S. (1998). Sepsis and septic shock. In A. S. Fauci, E. Braunwald, K. Isselbacher, J. D. Wilson, J. B. Martin, D. L. Kaspir, S. L. Hauser, & D. L. Longo (Eds.), *Harrison's principles of internal medicine* (14th ed., pp. 776–780). New York: McGraw-Hill.

Ognibene, F. P. (1997). Pathogenesis and innovative treatment of septic shock. *Advances in Internal Medicine, 42,* 313–338.

Tuite, P. K. (1997). Recognition and management of shock in the pediatric patient. *Critical Care Nursing Quarterly, 20*(1), 52–61.

Cathy McDeed-Breault, RN, MSN, CEN, CANP

CHAPTER **20**

Toxicological Emergencies

MAJOR TOPICS

I. GENERAL STRATEGY

Toxicological emergencies include acute poisonings and intake of substances of abuse. These situations pose a unique challenge to the emergency department (ED) nurse. The American Association of Poison Control Center's annual report states that 90.4% of cases occur in the home and 39% involved children younger than 3 years. In addition, they found that 94% of toxin exposures were acute and 85.7% were unintentional (Litovitz et al., 1995). Ingesting over-the-counter (OTC) drugs such as antihistamines, antidiarrheal medications, and indigestion remedies in conjunction with other medications may cloud or mask the true symptoms of an acute poisoning. Consider the possibility of OTC drug ingestion or coingestion with all potential poisoning situations. Drugs of abuse may include prescription and nonprescription drugs, inhalants, and illicit drugs. Patients may also use more than one drug in combination, resulting in polysubstance abuse, or may ingest a substance in combination with alcohol, leading to fatalities. When dealing with an altered level of consciousness (LOC), consider organic causes in your differential diagnosis—thyroid disease, hypoglycemia, and hypoxia—and always consider the purposeful or accidental exposure to a toxin or chemical.

A. Assessment

1. **Primary survey/resuscitation (see Chapter 1)**
2. **Secondary survey (see Chapter 1)**
3. **Psychological, social, and environmental factors: initial attention must always focus on life-saving measures**
   a. *Psychological factors*
      1) Patient may seek care not for treatment of addiction or overdose but for related symptoms
      2) Behavior may not match age of patient because addiction/overdose changes developmental stages
      3) Substance abuse leads to failure to fulfill obligations at home, work, school
      4) Assess personality traits; increased stress/guilt may lead to emergency
      5) Assess suicidal ideation/intent and prior attempts
      6) Age of patient
   b. *Social factors*
      1) Support network
         a) Family, significant others, friends
         b) Social agencies: check for agency involvement (e.g., legal system, protective services)
         c) Parental supervision: may be lacking if pediatric/adolescent case
      2) Occupational exposure
      3) Fiscal status: insurance may determine aftercare availability
      4) Religious beliefs
   c. *Environmental factors*
      1) Primary residence: homeless, apartment, home
      2) Who lives with patient
      3) Availability of substances/medications/alcohol
      4) Storage of substances: original containers, child-proof caps
   d. *Risk factors*
      1) Family history of substance abuse/poisoning
      2) Adolescent use of gateway substances or those drugs used before addiction
         a) Alcohol
         b) Marijuana
         c) Cigarettes
         d) Inhalants
      3) Peer group abuse of substances or peer pressure
      4) Psychiatric disorders, especially depression
      5) Decreased/inappropriate supervision of young children
4. **Focused survey**
   a. *Subjective data*
      1) History of present illness
         a) Obtain basic information regarding abuse/ingestion from patient, family, friends
            (1) Name and amount of substance
            (2) Time of use
            (3) Acute versus chronic use
            (4) First aid measures instituted before ED arrival/prehospital care

          (5) Symptoms experienced

          (6) Current life situation: medical or psychiatric illness, traumatic event

          (7) Chemicals used to cut/lace drug: e.g., talc, strychnine

          (8) Location of patient when poisoning occurred: home, work, recreation

          (9) Type of tablets ingested: enteric-coated tablets slow absorption time

          (10) Emesis occurrence

  2) Type of exposure

    a) Inhalation: snorting

    b) Oral ingestion

    c) Dermal contact

    d) Smoked

    e) Injected

  3) Reason for exposure

    a) Accidental

    b) Intentional: suicide attempt, substance abuse

    c) Recreational

    d) Occupational

      (1) Chemical exposure

      (2) Pesticide use

      (3) Stain glass worker: lead exposure

      (4) Paint stripper: carbon monoxide (CO)

  4) Polysubstance use: may lead to masking of symptoms

    a) Prescription drugs

    b) OTC medications

    c) Substance abuse treatment medications: e.g., disulfiram, methadone

    d) Alcohol use

    e) Illicit drug use

  5) Infection history

    a) Hepatitis

    b) Human immunodeficiency virus (HIV)

    c) Syphilis

    d) Endocarditis

    e) Tuberculosis

  6) Medical history

    a) Allergies

    b) Previous trauma, medical/surgical history, including falls, head injuries

    c) Previous hospitalizations

    d) Tetanus status

    e) Withdrawal history

    f) History of blackouts, tremors, mood swings

b. *Objective data*

  1) Physical exam: remove all clothing items

    a) General survey

      (1) LOC

      (2) Vital signs, including temperature

      (3) Mental status exam

      (4) Seizure activity

    b) Inspection

      (1) Skin

      (2) Tremors/tics

        (3) Gait: ataxia

        (4) Pupils: size, nystagmus, reactivity

        (5) Odors: alcohol, ketones, almonds

        (6) Nares: epistaxis, perforation of septum

    c) Auscultation

        (1) Heart: murmurs, dysrhythmias

        (2) Lungs: crackles, wheezing

    d) Palpation: use universal precautions because drug paraphernalia/used needles may be hidden in clothing

        (1) Abdomen: size, pain, tenderness, ascites

        (2) Bruising, fractures, deformity

  2) Diagnostic procedures

    a) Lab

        (1) Therapeutic blood levels

        (2) Fingerstick glucose (FSG)

        (3) Serum/urine drug screen

        (4) Serum alcohol/breathalyzer

        (5) Complete blood count (CBC)

        (6) Electrolytes

        (7) Other: Arterial blood gas (ABG), liver function tests (LFTs), coagulation panel (prothrombin time [PT], partial thromboplastin time [PTT]), urinalysis (UA), renal panel, thyroid studies, rapid plasma reagin (RPR), Venereal Disease Research Laboratories (VDRL)

    b) Twelve- to 15-lead electrocardiogram (ECG), cardiac monitor, and pulse oximetry

    c) Radiology

        (1) Chest radiograph (CXR)

        (2) Abdominal radiograph

        (3) Cervical spine radiograph: if trauma is suspected

        (4) Other: computed tomographic (CT) scan, magnetic resonance imaging (MRI) based on history

B. Analysis: differential nursing diagnosis/collaborative problems

1. **Anxiety/fear**
2. **Decreased cardiac output**
3. **Impaired gas exchange**
4. **Ineffective airway clearance**
5. **Ineffective coping**
6. **Risk for injury**
7. **Risk for poisoning**
8. **Sensory/perceptual alteration: visual, auditory, and kinesthetic**
9. **Tissue perfusion, altered cardiopulmonary**

C. Planning/interventions

1. **Determine patient care priorities**
   a. *Primary life-saving measures: airway, breathing, circulation per advanced cardiac life support guidelines*
   b. *Secondary life-saving measures*
      1) Prevent aspiration
      2) Control seizure activity
      3) Control behavior and prevent injury to self and others

a) Consider pharmacotherapy
b) Use restraints per institutional policy
c) Decrease anxiety through education, family involvement, and sedation
d) For all cases of coma or suspected poisoning, consider use of oxygen, dextrose, and naloxone as initial therapy

c. *Provide gastrointestinal (GI) decontamination as appropriate*
   1) Prevent absorption
      a) Induce emesis
         (1) Administer syrup of ipecac to pediatric patients or adults within 30 minutes of ingestion if substance does not induce seizure activity/ respiratory depression
         (2) Ipecac may be repeated once if emesis does not occur
         (3) Contraindications to ipecac
             (a) Central nervous system (CNS) depression
             (b) Ingesting substances that may induce seizures, such as tricyclics
             (c) Corrosive ingestion
             (d) Coingestion of sharp objects
             (e) Children younger than 6 months and the elderly
             (f) Nontoxic ingestions
             (g) Prior vomiting
             (h) When it delays administration of antidote
         (4) Note: charcoal may be better in absorbing toxin than syrup of ipecac
      b) Gastric lavage
         (1) Use large-bore tube such as 36- to 40-gauge orogastric tube
         (2) Consider intubation if patient requires airway protection secondary to respiratory depression
         (3) Continue lavage until contents return clear
         (4) Contraindications to lavage
             (a) Ingestion of caustics
             (b) Coingestion of sharp objects
             (c) Nontoxic ingestions
      c) Charcoal administration
         (1) Dose depends on patient size and weight
         (2) Administer orally or via lavage tube
         (3) Specific overdoses may require multiple dose charcoal (e.g., phenobarbital)
         (4) Contraindications to charcoal
             (a) Corrosive ingestion
             (b) Decreased or absent bowel sounds
             (c) Toxins not bound by charcoal such as metals, iron

d. *Promote ocular decontamination*
   1) Irrigate for 15 to 30 minutes or longer for alkali solutions with lukewarm warm water or saline
   2) Ensure that pH of eye is neutral before discontinuing flushing
   3) Assess for corneal burns
   4) Refer to ophthalmology for continued discomfort

e. *Promote dermal decontamination*
   1) Ensure that provider protective gear is used
   2) Remove all contaminated clothes
   3) Immediately flush area with water/saline, particularly for caustic exposures, including hair and under nails
   4) Indications for use
      a) Organophosphates

      b) Gasoline hydrocarbons

      c) Acids/alkalis

      d) Any chemical that may burn skin

   f. Promote excretion

     1) Cathartic administration

      a) Mix and administer with charcoal orally or via lavage tube

        (1) Magnesium sulfate

        (2) Magnesium citrate

      b) Use single doses of cathartics; do not repeat

      c) Contraindications to cathartics: use with caution with absent bowel sounds, especially in pediatric and elderly patients

        (1) Avoid use in patients with pre-existing renal failure and heart failure

     2) Whole bowel irrigation (controversial)

      a) Administer nonabsorbable bowel evacuant solution orally or via lavage tube (GoLYTELY, Colyte)

      b) Administer every 4 to 6 hours until stools are clear

      c) Patient may experience nausea, vomiting, abdominal cramping

      d) Note: procedure is controversial because of risk of electrolyte imbalance

      e) Contraindications to whole gut lavage

        (1) Pre-existing GI disease

        (2) Ileus, perforation, or obstruction

     3) Urine alkalinization using sodium bicarbonate

      a) Contraindications

        (1) Pulmonary edema

        (2) Renal failure

     4) Hemodialysis

     5) Hemoperfusion

   g. Administer antidote therapy (see specific toxicological agent)

     1) Oxygen: carbon monoxide (CO)

     2) Naloxone: opiates

     3) Atropine/pralidoxime: organophosphates

     4) Cyanide antidote kit: cyanide

     5) Flumazenil: benzodiazepines

   h. Administer chelation therapy for heavy metal poisoning

     1) Edetate calcium disodium (EDTA): lead

     2) BAL (dimercaprol, British antilewisite): mercury, arsenic, gold

     3) Deferoxamine: iron

     4) d-Penicillamine: mercury

2. Record data as appropriate

3. Disposition

   a. Assess need for inpatient treatment versus continued care with primary provider

     1) Assess for suicidal ideation and make appropriate referrals before discharge

   b. Involve family members/significant others in disposition plan

   c. Consider patient and family support group referral

   d. Contact regional poison control center for information, treatment modalities, and poison prevention information

   e. Use other drug resources such as Physician's Desk Reference (PDR) and Poisondex

D. Expected outcomes

1. Monitor patient response to treatment and outcomes of interventions

   a. If positive outcomes are not achieved, re-evaluate plan of care and modify

2. **Educate patient regarding disease process and its effects on body**
3. **Educate patient regarding medications, their use, and storage to prevent accidental poisoning**

E. Age-related considerations

1. **Pediatrics**
   a. *Growth and development related*
      1) Children: most poisonings occur in children younger than 6 years and in home
         a) Most pediatric poisonings are accidental ingestions
      2) Adolescents: risks for drug use include
         a) Membership in a socially deviant group
         b) Peer group use of drugs
         c) Use of drugs by significant adults
         d) Family use of drugs
         e) Warning signs of potential substance abuse
            (1) Sudden change in behavior
            (2) Drop in school performance
            (3) Change in clothing style or peer group attachment
         f) Most drug abuse in teens is self-inflicted; gestures are rarely intended to end in death
2. **Geriatrics: always consider polypharmacy use**
   a. *Aging related*
      1) Evaluate for mental illness or depression
      2) Consider chronic salicylism in confused elderly patients

II. SPECIFIC TOXICOLOGICAL EMERGENCIES

A. Alcohol abuse

Alcohol is one of the most commonly abused drugs in the United States. It is a component of roughly 70% of overdose cases in an ED. Alcoholism is a chronic illness characterized by impaired control over drinking, causing physiological, psychological, and/or social dysfunction. Alcohol affects all socioeconomic levels and affects slightly more males than females. Alcohol affects all body systems, including the CNS, GI, and cardiovascular systems. It is metabolized in the liver.

Alcohol, although it causes a state of euphoria, is actually a depressant. Its use depresses thought processes and the CNS. Alcohol may be the primary drug of abuse or may be concomitant to another drug ingestion. It is contained in beverages, perfumes, mouthwashes, and many OTC preparations (e.g., NyQuil).

1. **Assessment**
   a. *Subjective data*
      1) History of present illness
         a) Symptoms may or may not be related to alcohol intoxication
         b) Assess patient for signs of trauma from falls/head injury
         c) Describe drinking episode: how much consumed, time, percentage of alcohol content
      2) Medical history
         a) Associated medical illness
            (1) Seizures/epilepsy

        (2) Liver disease

        (3) GI bleeding or varices

        (4) Traumatic injury or recent fractures

        (5) Suicide gestures, anxiety, or depression history

     b) Concurrent medication use

        (1) Prescription and/or OTC drug

        (2) Lithium or disulfiram use

        (3) Seizure medications

     c) Patterns of alcohol abuse

        (1) Consumption pattern and type of alcohol

        (2) Time since last drink

        (3) Blackout history, detoxification history

        (4) Change in tolerance

     d) Allergies

   3) Risk factors

     a) Family history of alcoholism

     b) Heavy drinking: more than five drinks in one sitting

     c) Use of other drugs

 a. Objective data

   1) Physical exam

     a) General survey

        (1) LOC

        (2) Vital signs

        (3) Appearance

        (4) Odors: alcohol, breath mints, mouthwash

     b) Inspection

        (1) Assess intoxication signs: ataxia, nystagmus, slurred speech, hypothermia

        (2) Assess withdrawal status: tremors, hyperthermia, hypovolemia, hallucinations, diaphoresis, nausea/vomiting

        (3) Assess skin: spider angiomas, scars from falls, unexplained bruises/burns, gynecomastia, hygiene

     c) Palpation

        (1) Abdominal tenderness, ascites

   2) Diagnostic procedures

     a) Cardiac: monitor, 12- to 15-lead ECG

     b) Laboratory

        (1) Serum blood alcohol and/or breathalyzer

        (2) CBC, serum electrolytes

        (3) Serum/urine drug screens

        (4) Liver function tests (LFTs)

        (5) Coagulation panel

     c) Radiology: rule out trauma

        (1) Radiographs: cervical spine, CXR

        (2) CT scan and/or MRI

     d) Other

        (1) Pulse oximetry

        (2) UA

2. Analysis: differential nursing diagnosis/collaborative problems

  a. Ineffective airway clearance related to altered LOC

  b. Impaired gas exchange related to ineffective breathing pattern

  c. Risk for fluid volume deficit related to dehydrating effects of alcohol

    d. *Risk for injury related to falls, seizure potential*

    e. *Anxiety/fear related to altered LOC*

    f. *Sensory/perceptual alteration related to CNS effects of alcohol*

3. Planning/interventions

    a. *Promote airway maintenance and gas exchange*

      1) Maintain airway, breathing, circulation

      2) Position patient on side to prevent aspiration

      3) Maintain suction and airway devices at bedside

      4) Monitor oxygen saturation

      5) Monitor ABGs

    b. *Maintain normovolemia and nutritional support*

      1) Initiate intravenous (IV) therapy with normal saline (NS) or 5% dextrose in NS (D5NS)

      2) Monitor intake and output (I&O)

      3) Administer glucose 50% (D50W) if patient is hypoglycemic

      4) Offer well-balanced diet if not contraindicated

      5) Administer thiamine and multivitamins to combat Wernicke-Korsakoff syndrome and malnutrition

      6) Replace depleted electrolytes as ordered: potassium, magnesium

    c. *Prevent injury*

      1) Limit patient ambulation to prevent falls

      2) Monitor for seizure activity

      3) Monitor behavior to prevent self-harm or harm to others

    d. *Provide emotional support to decrease anxiety*

      1) Continually orient to time, place, events

      2) Explain all procedures

      3) Use nonjudgmental attitude

      4) Encourage family/significant other to remain at bedside to decrease anxiety

      5) Encourage patient participation in problem solving to increase coping mechanisms

    e. *Minimize stimulation to decrease sensory alteration*

      1) Use quiet environment

      2) Keep lights on to decrease shadows and visual hallucinations

    f. *Minimize behavior escalation to decrease violence potential*

      1) Decrease stimulation and noise as needed

      2) Closely monitor patient behavior to prevent escalation

      3) Use restraints per institutional policy: chemical, soft, leather

      4) Administer pharmacological agents as ordered: orally (PO), IV, or intramuscularly (IM)

        a) Benzodiazepines: chlordiazepoxide, lorazepam, diazepam

        b) Antipsychotics: haloperidol

    g. *Promote patient and family support and education*

      1) Assess knowledge of disease process and its effects on body

      2) Assess present and past coping mechanisms

      3) Assess patient and family readiness to learn

      4) Encourage participation in referral process: social agencies, Al-Anon

    h. *Discharge planning*

      1) Initiate social service consult or psychiatric evaluation as needed

      2) Review discharge medications with patient and family

      3) Refer to Alcoholics Anonymous/other support group as appropriate

      4) Encourage consistent primary care follow-up to encourage sobriety

4. Expected outcomes (see Appendix B)

B. Opiate abuse

Opiates are narcotics, substances derived from the opium poppy. They include morphine sulfate, heroin, and semisynthetic derivatives such as hydrocodone. Opiates are prescribed to decrease severe pain. They blunt the perception of pain and are used for preoperative sedation and a supplement to anesthesia. Opiates usually produce a brief euphoria followed by a pleasant dreamlike state. Frequent use of opioids may lead to addiction and tolerance. Death occurs from the side effects of the drugs, most notably respiratory arrest and pulmonary edema.

1. **Assessment**
    a. *Subjective*
        1) History of present illness
            a) Substance ingested and amount
            b) Route of ingestion: PO, IV, nasal inhalation, smoked, skin popping
            c) Time of ingestion: acute versus chronic use, tolerance
            d) Polysubstance abuse, including chemicals used to "cut" the drug or dilute it: e.g., quinine, sugar, starch
            e) Symptoms: classic triad: pinpoint pupils, decreased respirations, and coma
                (1) Decreased LOC/coma
                (2) Respiratory depression/arrest: slow, deep respirations of three to four per minute
                (3) Hypotension/bradycardia
                (4) Seizures (associated with meperidine)
                (5) Nausea/vomiting, constipation
        2) Medical history
            a) Chronic infection status: HIV, hepatitis, endocarditis
            b) Suicidal ideation/gesture
            c) Detoxification history
            d) Medical, surgical, and trauma history: history of chronic conditions/pain
    b. *Objective*
        1) Physical exam
            a) General survey
                (1) LOC: apathy, drowsiness, lethargy
                (2) Respiratory status: apnea; depression; labored; pink, frothy sputum
                (3) Seizure activity
            b) Vital signs: hypotension, bradycardia
            c) Pupils: miosis is hallmark of narcotic abuse
            d) Skin: track marks, lesions secondary to skin popping, abscesses, cyanosis
            e) Lung auscultation: crackles
        2) Diagnostic procedures
            a) Serum/urine toxicology screen
            b) Positive reversal of symptoms with naloxone
            c) Other: cardiac monitor, ABGs, CXR
2. **Analysis: differential nursing diagnosis/collaborative problems**
    a. *Ineffective airway clearance related to altered LOC*
    b. *Impaired gas exchange related to respiratory depression*
    c. *Altered tissue perfusion, cardiopulmonary related to decreased cardiac output/ peripheral vascular resistance*
    d. *Risk for poisoning, opiate toxicity related to ingestion*
3. **Planning/interventions**
    a. *Airway maintenance and improved gas exchange: maintain airway, breathing, circulation*

1) Suction as needed
2) Assist ventilations if apneic after administering naloxone: intubation, bag-valve mask (BVM)
3) Monitor oxygen saturation (pulse oximetry)
4) Note: do not administer ipecac because of respiratory depression and seizure potential

b. *Continuous monitoring to assess perfusion*
1) Monitor vital signs, respiratory effort, and cardiac rhythm
2) Maintain urine output
3) Check lung sounds to assess for development of pulmonary edema
4) Initiate IV access

c. *Decrease risk of poisoning*
1) Administer antidotal therapy: naloxone (short-acting narcotic antagonist)
   a) Actions: opioid antagonist and will precipitate withdrawal
   b) Administer IM, IV, via endotracheal tube; may need to repeat doses (especially with propoxyphene [Darvon]) secondary to its short length of action
   c) Prepare for potentially violent patient on awakening

d. *Disposition*
1) Assess respiratory status before discharge
2) Consider repeated naloxone therapy before disposition
3) Refer to support services or Narcotics Anonymous
4) Provide information on detoxification procedures

e. *Assist patient with identifying coping strategies*
1) Encourage patient to ventilate feelings
2) Use nonjudgmental approach; assess need for psychiatric consult
3) Assist patient with problem solving
4) Encourage family/other support
5) Discuss effects of addiction on body and resulting medical complications

4. Expected outcomes (see Appendix B)
5. Age-related considerations
a. *Pediatrics*
1) Children and neonates should receive naloxone if suspected overdose or maternal addiction

C. Cocaine abuse

Cocaine is one of the most popular drugs of abuse. "Snorting" or intranasal use is the most common route of administration; however, it can be smoked or injected. "Crack" or free-based smokable cocaine is more purified and gives the user a "rush" similar to IV use. It has a higher addiction potential. Cocaine stimulates the CNS and autonomic nervous system to increase the release of catecholamines from the adrenergic nerve terminals, and it blocks the reuptake of dopamine and norepinephrine in the CNS. This causes the symptomatology of abuse such as increased motor activity and euphoria. Medicinally, cocaine is used as an anesthetic and vasoconstrictor in nasal surgery.

1. Assessment
a. *Subjective*
1) History of present illness
   a) Route of ingestion
   b) Time of ingestion: cocaine's effects are short lived compared with other amphetamines

c) Polysubstance abuse: alcohol, downers (sedatives), speedballs (heroin and cocaine combination)

d) Body packing: ingestion of large amounts of cocaine-filled balloons/condoms to avoid law enforcement detection

e) Symptoms

    (1) Mood changes: euphoria, decreased fatigue, increased energy, agitation, aggression

    (2) Cardiac: tachycardia, palpitations, hypertension, chest pain, angina

    (3) Pupils: dilated pupils are hallmark

    (4) Seizures

    (5) Other: restless, jittery, anxious, weight loss, drug craving for more cocaine, tactile hallucinations with chronic use such as "cocaine bugs" (feeling insects crawling under skin)

  2) Medical history

    a) Cardiac or neurological history: cerebrovascular accident (CVA), seizures, myocardial infarction

    b) Psychiatric history: suicidal ideation, substance abuse history

    c) Antibody status: HIV, hepatitis, tuberculosis (TB)

    d) Family history of substance abuse

    e) Pregnancy: cocaine causes increased incidence of spontaneous abortions

b. *Objective*

  1) Physical exam

    a) LOC: may range from hypomania to euphoria to depressed

    b) Seizure activity

    c) Vital signs: tachycardia with increased incidence of dysrhythmias, hypertension, hyperthermia

    d) Pupillary response: mydriasis, photophobia

    e) Skin: perforated nasal septum from snorting, skin infections/abscesses

  2) Diagnostic procedures

    a) Lab: serum/urine toxicology screen, UA

    b) Cardiac: monitor, 12- to 15-lead ECG, monitor for dysrhythmias

    c) Radiography: to detect body packing and rule out pulmonary edema

      (1) CT/MRI to rule out CVA, head trauma, intracranial hemorrhage

      (2) CXR

2. Analysis: differential nursing diagnosis/collaborative problems

a. *Ineffective airway clearance related to altered LOC*

b. *Tissue perfusion, altered cardiac related to coronary arterial vasoconstriction*

c. *Tissue perfusion, altered cerebral related to cocaine-induced vasoconstriction*

d. *Knowledge deficit related to cocaine addiction process*

3. Planning/interventions

Note: Most patients are seen in the ED for management of complications secondary to cocaine use. Treatment is aimed at supportive, corrective measures.

a. *Maintain airway, breathing, circulation*

  1) Suction and position patient to maintain airway as needed

  2) Monitor pulse oximetry and provide supplemental oxygen if needed

  3) Assist with intubation as required

b. *Monitor cardiac output*

  1) Assess for dysrhythmias and treat per protocol

  2) Monitor vital signs: treat hypertension and hyperthermia; avoid vasopressors because patient is already sympathetically stimulated

  3) Monitor urine output and check for myoglobin secondary to increased muscular activity

c. *Support tissue perfusion*

1) Establish IV access and administer fluids per symptoms
2) Assess LOC and pupil changes
3) Treat seizures per protocol and prevent patient injury
4) Treat delirium or psychosis with haloperidol as ordered

d. *Enhance knowledge deficit*
1) Assess patient/family knowledge of effects of cocaine on body
2) Educate regarding cocaine addiction/dependence
3) Encourage patient to verbalize fears and anxiety

e. *Discharge planning*
1) Assess suicidal risk and refer for psychiatric evaluation as indicated
2) Provide referral information for patient follow-up
3) Provide family referral to support services/counseling

4. **Expected outcomes** (see Appendix B)

D. Amphetamine abuse

Amphetamines are synthetic sympathomimetic drugs that stimulate the CNS, producing a feeling of super energy. They are commonly used to suppress appetite, elevate mood, and stay awake. Amphetamines are available in oral, intranasal, or parenteral forms. Crystalline rock forms such as "ice" are smoked. Common amphetamines include caffeine, crystal methamphetamine, dextroamphetamine, and methylphenidate (Ritalin). Most recently, the weight reduction medication, fenfluramine (Redux) was withdrawn from the market because of its side effects, which included pulmonary hypertension and valvular heart disease.

1. **Assessment**
a. *Subjective*
1) History of present illness
a) Type of drug ingested
b) Route: PO, smoked, snorted, IV, body packing
c) Time of ingestion and quantity: if a body pack ruptures, a large quantity will be absorbed into system at one time
d) Reason for use: suicidal, recreational, intentional, weight loss
e) Presenting symptoms: same as cocaine but longer duration
(1) Fenfluramine: amnesia, depression, confusion
2) Medical history
a) Previous substance abuse
b) Medical, surgical, traumatic, and psychiatric history
c) History of obesity, attention deficit disorder (ADD) (treated by Ritalin), hyperactivity and narcolepsy

b. *Objective*
1) Physical exam
a) LOC: anxious, restless, decreased fatigue, paranoia/delusions
b) Vitals: tachycardia, hypertension, hyperthermia
c) Pupillary response: mydriasis
d) Neurological: seizure activity, tremors
e) Cardiac: murmurs, shortness of breath, cardiomyopathy
2) Diagnostic procedures
a) Lab: serum/urine tox screen
b) Cardiac: 12- to 15-lead ECG, echocardiogram (fenfluramine users)
c) Radiography: abdominal film to assess body packing

2. **Analysis: differential nursing diagnosis/collaborative problems**
a. *Ineffective airway clearance related to altered LOC*

  b. *Decreased cardiac output related to hypertension, heart failure, and tachycardia*

  c. *Risk for poisoning: amphetamine toxicity related to ingestion*

  d. *Risk for injury: violence related to effects of amphetamines*

 3. Planning/interventions

  a. *Maintain airway, breathing, circulation*

   1) Suction and position patient to maintain airway as needed

   2) Monitor pulse oximetry and provide supplemental oxygen if needed

   3) Assist with intubation as required

   4) Monitor and treat hyperthermia with external cooling measures

  b. *Maintain cardiac output*

   1) Cardiac monitoring and treat arrhythmias per protocol

   2) Treat hypertension as indicated

  c. *Decrease risk of poisoning*

   1) Perform GI decontamination as indicated; do not induce emesis, which may lead to aspiration

    a) Perform gastric lavage

    b) Activated charcoal prevents systemic absorption

  d. *Decrease risk for violence*

   1) Decrease sensory stimulation by placing patient in a quiet area

   2) Use consistent nonjudgmental caregivers and set appropriate limits on behavior

   3) If other measures fail, consider restraints to prevent staff and patient injury: soft, leather, or chemical

    a) Monitor restrained patients per institutional policy

    b) Consider haloperidol for psychotic symptoms

  e. *Discharge planning*

   1) Assist patient in developing coping mechanisms, especially if a chronic user

    a) Depression and suicidal ideation may be seen in withdrawal

   2) Assess family support system

   3) Refer patient/family to detoxification center and/or to support services

   4) Educate patient regarding effects of amphetamines on body

   5) Encourage follow-up with primary care provider, if patient used fenfluramine, to have cardiac and pulmonary workup

 4. Expected outcomes (see Appendix B)

E. Lysergic acid (LSD) abuse

  Psychedelic drugs such as LSD cause changes in thought, mood, and perception and consciousness. The hallucinogenic effects last 6 to 12 hours and may cause visual illusions and alteration in both sound and color intensity. LSD is known to flood the user with stimuli. LSD is colorless, odorless, and tasteless and comes in liquid or tablet form. It may also be absorbed via the skin. Initial symptoms are sympathomimetic. LSD may be "laced" with phencyclidine (PCP), strychnine, or cocaine. Unlike most substances, there is no withdrawal syndrome to LSD, nor is there physical dependence.

 1. Assessment

  a. *Subjective*

   1) History of present illness

    a) Route of ingestion

    b) Time of use

    c) Reason for use: accidental, recreational

    d) Substance used to lace or cut drug

e) Polysubstance use

f) Symptoms

(1) Paranoia

(2) Hallucinations, especially visual changes such as intense colors, "flowing objects"

(3) Mood changes: poor judgment, short attention span

2) Medical history

a) Previous LSD use, which may cause flashback or bad "trip"

b) Psychiatric history

b. *Objective*

1) Physical exam

a) LOC: ranges from euphoria to fear, anxiety and panic

b) Vital signs: tachycardia, hypertension, hyperthermia

c) Pupil response: mydriasis

d) Mental status changes: hallucinations, paranoia, psychosis

2) Diagnostic procedures

a) Serum/urine toxicology screen

2. **Analysis: differential nursing diagnosis/collaborative problems**

a. *Altered thought process related to the mood-altering effects of LSD*

b. *Risk for injury: violence related to the mood-altering effects of LSD*

c. *Sensory perceptual alteration: visual, kinesthetic related to hallucinating effects of LSD*

d. *Potential for poisoning: LSD toxicity related to ingestion*

3. **Planning/interventions**

a. *Maintain orientation to environment*

1) Frequently orient patient to time, place, and events

2) Move patient to calm, quiet environment if possible

3) Encourage family to stay with patient and provide reassurance

4) Explain effects of drug to patient/family

b. *Decrease risk for violence*

1) Attempt to "talk down" an agitated and anxious patient

2) Maintain calm, nonjudgmental attitude and offer calm reassurance

3) Consider use of soft, leather, or chemical restraints if all measures to provide patient and staff safety fail, per institutional protocol

a) Chemical restraints include diazepam, haloperidol

c. *Minimize sensory-perceptual alteration*

1) Reinforce to patient that effects of drug are time limited

2) Assist patient in separating hallucinations from real life events

3) When effects of drug are diminished, educate patient regarding effects of LSD on body

d. *Decreased potential for LSD toxicity*

1) Advise patient of potential for recurring flashbacks

2) Discuss possibility of bad "trip"

4. **Expected outcomes** (see Appendix B)

5. **Age-related considerations**

a. *Pediatrics: mood changes range from agitation to withdrawal to catatonia*

1) LSD making comeback among high school students

F. Phencyclidine (PCP) abuse

PCP is a widely used street drug known as a dissociative anesthetic, which decreases awareness of one's surroundings. PCP was initially used as an IV surgical anesthetic in veterinary and human medicine. Its use was discontinued when patients experienced terrifying "emergence reactions," such as delusions and paranoia, when its effects wore off. PCP is consumed by dusting it on a cigarette and smoking it, in pill form, snorting, and through skin contact. It is rapidly absorbed in the blood-stream and quickly distributes to tissues with a high lipid content. Effects of PCP include muscular rigidity, thought disorganization and violent, agitated behavior. PCP affects the CNS, causing stimulation or depression and cholinergic-like symptoms. Common street names include angel dust, cadillac, CJ, killer weed, magic mist, and cyclones. Acute complications resulting from the increased rigidity include rhabdomyolysis and renal failure. Other complications include respiratory depression/apnea, cerebral hemorrhage, and psychosis.

1. **Assessment**
   a. *Subjective*
      1) History of present illness
         a) Route of exposure
         b) Circumstances of use: accidental versus recreational deliberate use
         c) Concomitant drug use
         d) Symptoms
            (1) Violent combative behavior, increased strength, lack of pain sensation
            (2) Pupil changes: bidirectional nystagmus in awake patient is classic, miosis
            (3) Tremors/increased strength: "superhuman" as result of decreased pain feedback mechanism
      2) Medical history
         a) Previous PCP use
         b) History of recent trauma: death usually occurs from associated trauma/injury
         c) Antibody status (e.g., HIV)
         d) Medical and psychiatric history
   b. *Objective*
      1) Physical exam
         a) LOC: varies from drowsiness to irritability, euphoria and extreme agitation
         b) Vital signs: tachycardia, hypertension
         c) Neurological findings
            (1) Nystagmus: bidirectional (horizontal, vertical, rotary)
            (2) Tremors and hyperactivity, dizziness/ataxia
            (3) Anesthesia to painful stimuli
            (4) Seizures, myoclonus
            (5) Drowsiness, drooling
         d) Mental status: bizarre, combative behavior with altered thought process and paranoia
         e) Urine output: measure amount and check for myoglobinuria
         f) GI: nausea/vomiting, abdominal pain
      2) Diagnostic procedures
         a) Urine and serum toxicology screen
         b) Urine to check for myoglobinuria
         c) Creatinine kinase (CK) level
         d) Glucose level: hypoglycemia
2. **Analysis: differential nursing diagnosis/collaborative problems**
   a. *Sensory–perceptual alteration: kinesthetic related to the effects of PCP ingestion*

b. Risk for injury, violence related to the hallucinatory and mood- and anesthetic-altering effects of PCP

c. Anxiety/fear related to thought disorganization

3. Planning/interventions

a. Maintain support of vital functions

1) Maintain airway patency

a) Intubation may be required because of apnea

2) Monitor vitals and treat hypertension and hyperthermia

3) Treat seizure activity as ordered

4) Monitor urine output for rhabdomyolysis

b. Decrease sensory perceptual alteration

1) Use quiet, nonstimulating room if possible

2) Do not leave patient unattended; consider security standby if needed

3) Use consistent caregivers as much as possible

4) Keep side rails up to prevent falls

5) Consider pharmacological interventions to decrease hallucinations: diazepam, haloperidol, lorazepam

c. Maintain environmental orientation to decrease anxiety

1) Explain all procedures before initiation

2) Continually reorient to time and place

3) Encourage family to remain at bedside to increase familiarity with surroundings

4) Consider psychiatric consult for anxiety/depression after acute therapy

5) Discharge in care of family/friend

d. Maintain violence protection for staff, patients, visitors; PCP patients have increased strength and do not feel pain because of anesthetic effects of drug; therefore, they may be strong enough to break leather restraints

1) Do not try to "talk patient down" because patients become quickly agitated and forceful

2) Use restraints if violence begins to escalate to ensure safety of others: chemical (haloperidol); short-term paralysis (ensure airway and ventilatory maintenance); avoid phenothiazines, which may increase seizures

a) Leather (soft restraints are generally ineffective)

b) Handcuffs: police application

c) Monitor restrained patient per institutional policy

3) Contact law enforcement for security backup as needed

4) Monitor and assess patient for injuries: patient may be unaware of any injuries

5) Wear gloves when approaching patient because PCP may be absorbed through skin

4. Expected outcomes (see Appendix B)

G. Inhalant abuse

Inhaling vapors from volatile substances such as solvents and hydrocarbons is a common practice, particularly among adolescents. They offer a cheap high because they are easily obtained and are uncontrolled. Toluene-containing products are the most commonly abused and include metallic spray paint, glues, and aerosols from spray cans. Metallic gold spray paint produces the most desired effect. Other commonly sniffed substances include cleaning fluids, paints, lacquer, and White Out, or typewriter correction fluid. Hydrocarbons produce a floating or numbing sensation and euphoria when inhaled and induce a pleasurable sensation. The substances are generally poured into a paper or plastic bag and inhaled (bagging), poured on a rag and held over the nose (huffing), or inhaled from the container (sniffing). Inhaled vapors are readily absorbed into the bloodstream and cross the blood-brain barrier, reaching the brain in high concentrations.

1. **Assessment**
   a. *Subjective*
      1) History of present illness
         a) Age of patient
         b) Type of substance inhaled/empty solvent cans
         c) Method of inhalation: sniffing, huffing, bagging
         d) Polysubstance abuse
         e) Symptoms
            (1) GI: nausea
            (2) Muscle weakness/paralysis, seizure activity
            (3) Neurological: headache, altered LOC, coma
            (4) Intoxication: euphoria, incoordination, confusion, disorientation
      2) Medical history
         a) Head trauma or neurological findings
         b) Psychiatric history
   b. *Objective*
      1) Physical exam
         a) LOC: ranges from euphoria to intoxicated appearance to comatose
         b) Odor: check breath and clothing for odor of solvent
         c) Mouth and nose: check for circumoral red spots if using spray paint, correction fluid; nose bleeds, sores in the nose
         d) Neurological findings: ataxia, wide base gait, memory loss
         e) Polyneuropathy: decreased sensation, motor loss, decreased reflexes peripherally
         f) Cardiac: decreased potassium level, dysrhythmias causing sudden death (sudden sniffing death)
         g) Other: paint/glue on hands/face, bloodshot eyes
      2) Diagnostic procedures
         a) Laboratory analysis
            (1) UA: check for hematuria, proteinuria, myoglobinuria
            (2) Serum electrolytes, calcium, phosphorus
            (3) LFTs and renal panel
         b) Cardiac: monitor, 12- to 15-lead ECG, ABGs to determine if acidotic
2. **Analysis: differential nursing diagnosis/collaborative problems**
   a. *Risk for poisoning: hydrocarbon abuse related to ingestion*
   b. *Decreased cardiac output related to cardiac dysrhythmias*
   c. *Altered tissue perfusion, cerebral related to decreased cerebral blood flow*
3. **Planning/interventions**
   a. *Decrease risk of poisoning*
      1) Airway maintenance: no specific antidote exists
      2) Maintain metabolic processes
         a) IV access
         b) Replace diminished electrolytes, especially potassium
         c) Consider sodium bicarbonate therapy for metabolic acidosis
         d) Maintain urine output to prevent renal failure secondary to myoglobinuria
   b. *Improve cardiac output*
      1) Monitor for dysrhythmias and treat per protocol
      2) Continually monitor for sudden cardiac arrest (seen with toluene abuse)
   c. *Maintain neurological function*

1) Treat seizures per protocol
2) Assess for hemi/quadriparesis and monitor progress

4. Expected outcomes (see Appendix B)

H. Carbon monoxide (CO) poisoning

CO is a colorless, odorless, and tasteless gas that binds with hemoglobin to form carboxyhemoglobin (COHb). This combination decreases the ability of the blood to carry oxygen, leading to severe hypoxia. CO is produced by the combustion of organic materials in the setting of an enclosed space or poor ventilation. Common sources of CO include auto exhaust systems, smoke from wood fires, propane heaters, hibachi and sterno (canned heat) stoves, and faulty furnaces. Length of exposure to the gas contributes to the poisoning. Symptoms rarely correlate with the serum COHb levels, although values less than 20% rarely become symptomatic. Death is usually the result of dysrhythmias.

1. Assessment

a. *Subjective*

1) History of present illness
   a) Ventilation: enclosed space
   b) Degree of exposure: time, mechanism (e.g., fire)
   c) Occupational/purposeful exposure (e.g., suicidal)
   d) Symptoms
      (1) Headache: most common
      (2) Nausea and vomiting, dizziness
      (3) LOC: may present awake, sleepy, or comatose
      (4) Seizures: seen at higher COHb levels
2) Medical history
   a) Cardiac disease, especially dysrhythmias
   b) Respiratory problems
   c) Suicidal tendencies
   d) Recent crisis/trauma resulting in ineffective coping mechanisms

b. *Objective*

1) Physical exam
   a) Skin signs: "cherry red" skin and mucous membranes are classically noted but are considered terminal finding
   b) Cardiac: dysrhythmias, hypotension, increased episodes of angina, ST- and T-wave changes indicating ischemia or infarction
2) Diagnostic procedures
   a) ABG
   b) COHb: half-life is 4 hours
   c) UA to assess myoglobin
   d) Cardiac: monitor, 12- to 15-lead ECG, pulse oximetry, serial cardiac enzymes
   e) Radiography
      (1) CXR to rule out pulmonary edema, acute respiratory distress syndrome (ARDS)
      (2) CT scan/MRI

2. Analysis: differential nursing diagnosis/collaborative problems

a. *Impaired gas exchange related to CO inhalation*
b. *Risk for poisoning: CO toxicity related to inhalation*
c. *Decreased cardiac output related to dysrhythmias*

3. Planning/interventions

a. *Improve gas exchange*

1) Remove from poorly ventilated area
2) Maintain airway, breathing, circulation
3) Provide 100% oxygen via mask: mainstay of therapy to decrease the half-life of COHb
4) Consider hyperbaric oxygen therapy (HBO) to increase oxygen delivery to tissues under pressure

b. *Decrease poisoning risk*
1) Educate patient regarding sources of CO poisoning
2) Review symptoms of poisoning
3) Advise patient to keep areas with combustible products well ventilated
4) Advise regarding use of CO detectors in home/work environment
5) Yearly maintenance of stoves/furnaces

c. *Enhance cardiac output*
1) Treat seizure activity as needed
2) Monitor for arrhythmias and hypotension per protocol
3) Monitor serial cardiac enzymes

d. *Encourage effective coping strategies*
1) Consider psychiatric consult as needed
2) Provide referral to social support service to assist with decreasing crisis/trauma

4. **Expected outcomes** (see Appendix B)

I. Salicylate poisoning

Salicylates are very common antipyretic, analgesic, and anti-inflammatory OTC products. There are more than 200 products that contain aspirin. Toxicity may result from acute or chronic exposure, particularly in children and the elderly. Poisoning affects the GI mucosa, coagulation, and acid-base status. Metabolic acidosis is common in children, and respiratory alkalosis with stimulation of the CNS respiratory center is common in adults. Peak serum levels of salicylate occur 2 to 4 hours after acute ingestion, but this may vary depending on the type of pill ingested (i.e., enteric-coated tablets have a longer absorption time). A toxic dose to produce symptoms is 200 to 300 mg/kg and more than 500 mg/kg is considered lethal. Common salicylate-containing products include Pepto-Bismol, Dristan, Excedrin, Alka-Seltzer, and Midol.

1. **Assessment**
   a. *Subjective*
      1) History of present illness
         a) Chronic versus acute exposure: chronic use may be common in elderly
         b) Reason for use: suicide attempt, accidental exposure, child neglect
         c) Dosage form: effervescent, noncoated tablet, enteric coated
            (1) Enteric-coated tabs disintegrate in intestines and decrease gastric mucosal effects
            (2) Serum salicylate peak levels after enteric-coated use at 6 to 9 hours
         d) Symptoms
            (1) Tinnitus
            (2) Nausea and vomiting, dehydration
            (3) Change in vital signs: increase in depth and rate of respirations (classic sign), increased temperature and heart rate
            (4) CNS effects: dizziness, lethargy, stupor, seizures
            (5) Pulmonary edema: noncardiogenic
      2) Medical history
         a) Age of patient

        b) Psychiatric history, especially depression

        c) Chronic pain

        d) Breast-feeding mothers using salicylate products

        e) Infants using teething gels

    b. *Objective*

      1) Physical exam

        a) Vital signs: tachypnea, hyperthermia, tachycardia

        b) Neurological: seizure activity, coma/stupor (ominous sign)

        c) Respiratory: assess lungs for pulmonary edema, tachypnea

        d) GI: occult bleeding/hemorrhage

      2) Diagnostic procedures

        a) Laboratory

          (1) Serum salicylate level: on arrival and 6 hours after ingestion; compare level to nomogram for toxicity

          (2) CBC, electrolytes, glucose level

          (3) ABGs to assess for acidosis

          (4) Coagulation studies

        b) Radiographs: CXR (assess pulmonary edema)

        c) Other: UA, fecal occult blood, pulse oximetry

        d) Cardiac: monitor, 12- to 15-lead ECG

2. Analysis: differential nursing diagnosis/collaborative problems

    a. *Ineffective breathing pattern related to respiratory stimulation*

    b. *Impaired gas exchange related to ineffective breathing pattern*

    c. *Risk for poisoning: salicylate toxicity related to ingestion*

3. Planning/interventions

    a. *Maintain airway, breathing, circulation*

    b. *Prevent absorption*

      1) Induce emesis or lavage

      2) Administer charcoal with or without cathartic (rule out GI bleed before administration)

    c. *Maintain hydration*

      1) IV initiation with isotonic saline or dextrose if hypoglycemic

      2) Monitor urine output and assess for hematuria/myoglobinuria

      3) Monitor hypoglycemia: treat with D50W

      4) Replenish depleted electrolytes, especially potassium

    d. *Enhance excretion*

      1) Consider urine alkalinization

      2) Peritoneal lavage or hemodialysis for severe acute ingestion

    e. *Maintain effective gas exchange*

      1) Monitor ABG results and correct acidosis with hyperventilation and sodium bicarbonate

      2) Monitor respiratory rate and lung sounds for development of pulmonary edema

    f. *Decrease temperature with external cooling measures*

    g. *Decrease poisoning risk*

      1) Educate patient on effects of acute and chronic aspirin use

      2) Educate caregivers/parents on use of aspirin in children

      3) Provide primary care provider contact to family for follow-up

4. Expected outcomes (see Appendix B)

5. Age-related considerations

    a. *Pediatrics: poisoning usually related to accidental ingestion or incorrect dosing*

      1) Less common than in the past because of increased use of acetaminophen

      2) Teething gels may contain salicylates

3) Life-threatening complication of salicylate use after viral infection: Reye's syndrome; do not use salicylates after viral infection

4) Oil of wintergreen topical agent is most toxic preparation because of its high salicylate content

5) Educate parents to keep ipecac at home in case of ingestion

b. *Geriatric*

1) Increased risk of chronic toxicity as result of decreased renal function

2) Patients may chronically use aspirin for all medical problems

3) Assess patient's skin for chronic/easy bruising

4) Patients may be exposed to increased risk of bleeding and ulcer disease

J. Acetaminophen poisoning

A common analgesic with antipyretic properties, acetaminophen is seen in many OTC products and in combination with narcotics. It is rapidly absorbed from the GI tract and is metabolized by the liver. It is widely used because it has few side effects and drug interactions. Toxicity produces delayed hepatic necrosis and LFTs. Common products containing acetaminophen include Comtrex, NyQuil, Percogesic, Sine-Aid, and Darvocet-N.

1. **Assessment**

a. *Subjective*

1) History of present illness

a) Acute versus chronic exposure

b) Concomitant use of alcohol or other drugs

c) Reason for exposure: e.g., suicide, chronic pain

d) Dose form: regular or extended-release product; affects absorption

e) Symptoms: four phases

(1) Phase 1: within 24 hours of ingestion—malaise, nausea and emesis, diaphoresis

(2) Phase 2: 24 to 28 hours—right upper quadrant pain, decreased urine output, nausea abates, LFTs rise

(3) Phase 3: 72 to 96 hours—nausea and emesis, malaise, jaundice, hypoglycemia, enlarged liver, coma may result; coagulopathies are common, including disseminated intravascular coagulopathy (DIC)

(4) Phase 4: 7 to 8 days after ingestion—"recovery," resolution of symptoms, LFTs return to normal

2) Medical history

a) Age

b) Psychiatric history

c) Alcohol abuse history

d) Pre-existing liver disease

b. *Objective*

1) Physical exam

a) Abdominal pain: right upper quadrant

b) Hepatomegaly

c) Skin: jaundice

2) Diagnostic procedures

a) Laboratory

(1) Serum acetaminophen level 4 hours after ingestion: important indicator of eventual hepatotoxicity; compare to nomogram for acetaminophen toxicity

(2) LFTs

(3) CBC, electrolytes, coagulation panel

(4) Serum/urine toxicology screen

2. **Analysis: differential nursing diagnosis/collaborative problems**
   a. *Potential for poisoning: acetaminophen toxicity related to ingestion*
   b. *Anxiety/fear related to prognosis*
3. **Planning/interventions**
   a. *Maintain airway, breathing, circulation*
   b. *Decrease poisoning potential*
      1) Prevent absorption
         a) Lavage
         b) Charcoal
         c) Cathartics
   c. *Maintain hydration*
      1) IV access initiated
   d. *Administer antidote:* N-acetylcysteine (NAC, Mucomyst)
      1) Give orally or via lavage tube
      2) Oral dose may cause vomiting as result of foul taste; mix with soft drink
      3) NAC in IV form available on an experimental basis
      4) Monitor LFTs for return to baseline
   e. *Decrease anxiety*
      1) Explain all procedures before initiation
      2) Discuss effects of acetaminophen toxicity on body
      3) Consider psychiatric consult before disposition if appropriate
      4) Educate patient/caregivers regarding difference in acetaminophen dosage preparations for different age groups
4. **Expected outcomes** (see Appendix B)
5. **Age-related considerations**
   a. *Pediatric*
      1) Children tend to suffer less hepatotoxicity than adults possibly because of tendency to vomit earlier
      2) Children should be offered same treatment as adults, including Mucomyst
      3) Parents/caregivers need to read dosing on products! Infant Tylenol drops are more concentrated than liquid children's Tylenol and cannot be used interchangeably
      4) Consider abuse/neglect in poisoning situations
   b. *Elderly*
      1) Hepatic damage may be severe especially if patient is taking other hepatotoxic medications regularly
      2) Patients with history of chronic alcohol abuse need to use caution when using Tylenol because use may cause severe hepatotoxicity

K. Tricyclic antidepressant poisoning

Tricyclic antidepressant (TCA) medication overdoses can be extremely lethal and should be managed aggressively. Their lethality is related to their very narrow therapeutic index. They are analogs of the phenothiazines and share anticholinergic and alpha-adrenergic blocking properties. These actions produce cardiotoxic effects and CNS depression, resulting in fatalities. TCAs are absorbed from the GI tract and are rapidly distributed. Once absorbed, they become highly bound to plasma proteins, making them difficult to remove from the body. Death results from cardiotoxic effects. Examples of TCAs include amitriptyline, desipramine, doxepin, trazodone, and nortriptyline.

1. **Assessment**
   a. *Subjective*

1) History of present illness
   a) Amount of drug ingested and time
   b) Type of medication
   c) Accidental versus intentional ingestion
   d) Symptoms
      (1) LOC: ranges from alert to disoriented, lethargic to comatose; progression may be rapid!
      (2) Neurological: twitching, seizures
      (3) Vital signs: tachycardia, hypotension, hyperthermia, decreased respirations
      (4) Pupils: mydriasis
      (5) Anticholinergic: dry mouth, urinary retention
2) Medical history
   a) Cardiac: dysrhythmias
   b) Neurological: seizures
   c) Psychiatric: depression, prior suicide attempt, nocturnal enuresis
  b. *Objective*
   1) Physical exam
      a) Cardiac depressant effects: prolonged PR, wide QRS, QT prolongation, ST depression, atrioventricular (AV) conduction disturbance, cardiac arrest
      b) Dysrhythmias: premature ventricular contractions (PVCs), supraventricular tachycardia (SVT), ventricular tachycardia (VT) (sinus tachycardia is sensitive early indicator of toxic doses)
      c) Mental status: disoriented, lethargic, slurred speech
      d) Neurological: seizure activity, fine tremors
   2) Diagnostic procedures
      a) Cardiac: monitor, 12- to 15-lead ECG
      b) Laboratory: serum/urine toxicology screen
         (1) Cardiac enzymes
         (2) Electrolytes
         (3) UA: check for myoglobin
      c) Other: ABGs, pulse oximetry
2. **Analysis: differential nursing diagnosis/collaborative problems**
  a. *Ineffective breathing pattern related to CNS depression*
  b. *Decreased cardiac output related to dysrhythmias*
  c. *Potential for poisoning: tricyclic toxicity related to ingestion*
3. **Planning/interventions**
  a. *Maintain airway, breathing, circulation*
   1) Provide adequate oxygenation; intubate if needed
  b. *Initiate IV access*
  c. *GI decontamination: never administer ipecac due to seizure potential*
   1) Prevent absorption
      a) Lavage, charcoal
      b) Multidose charcoal every 2 hours may be more effective than one dose
  d. *Control cardiotoxicity and improve cardiac output*
   1) Monitor for dysrhythmias a minimum of 6 hours after ingestion and treat per order
   2) Obtain and monitor ABGs and correct acidosis: mainstay of therapy
      a) Serum alkalinization with sodium bicarbonate and hyperventilation: *Sodium Bicarbonate* is treatment of choice with wide QRS because it enhances protein binding of drug and should be repeated until QRS reaches normal parameters

3) Correct hypotension: fluid bolus
   a) Use catecholamine pressors as needed to supplement: epinephrine, norepinephrine
 e. *Decrease poisoning risk*
   1) Control seizure activity
      a) IV diazepam or lorazepam, phenytoin
      b) Prevent patient injury
   2) Educate patient regarding effects of TCAs on body
4. Expected outcomes (see Appendix B)

L. Sedative-hypnotic poisoning

Sedative-hypnotics are CNS depressants whose chief effect is respiratory depression. These effects are increased by the ingestion of alcohol or other depressant medications, and their addiction potential is high. These medications are commonly prescribed to induce sleep and to allay anxiety. They are known to relax inhibitions and act as mood elevators. They may also be used as anticonvulsants. They include the barbiturates (phenobarbital, methohexital [Brevital], and thiopental [Pentothal]); nonbarbiturates such as benzodiazepines (diazepam, oxazepam (Serax), flurazepam [Dalmane], chlordiazepoxide [Librium]); and antihistamines (hydroxyzine [Atarax, Vistaril]). The benzodiazepines have a low order of toxicity when ingested alone and rarely cause death, whereas others may cause hypotension and deep coma. The barbiturates are highly toxic with a high abuse potential because of their euphoric effects (see barbiturate poisoning).

1. Assessment
 a. *Subjective*
   1) History of present illness
      a) Type of drug and age of patient
      b) Amount and route (PO, IM, IV)
      c) Use of alcohol or other drugs: combining alcohol and benzodiazepines can be lethal
      d) Symptoms of tolerance or withdrawal, especially with barbiturates
      e) Reason for use
      f) Symptoms
         (1) Antihistamine abuse: CNS excitation (children), CNS depression (adults)
         (2) Meprobamate: CNS depression, coma, hypotension
         (3) Benzodiazepines: drowsiness, stupor, slurred speech
   2) Medical history
      a) Psychiatric: anxiety, panic attacks, depression, suicidal ideation
      b) Substance abuse history: alcohol, heroin, LSD
      c) Seizure history
 b. *Objective*
   1) Physical exam
      a) Neurological: LOC, slurred speech, lethargy, ataxia
      b) Cardiac: hypotension, tachycardia
      c) Head, ears, eyes, nose, and throat (HEENT)
         (1) Pupillary changes: dilation or constriction
         (2) Oral: dry mouth
         (3) Respiratory: respiratory depression
   2) Diagnostic procedures
      a) Laboratory: serum/urine drug screen
      b) Blood alcohol/breathalyzer as appropriate

     c) Cardiac: 12- to 15-lead ECG, pulse oximetry

     d) Radiographs

       (1) CXR

       (2) CT scan/MRI

2. Analysis: differential nursing diagnosis/collaborative problems

   a. Ineffective breathing pattern related to CNS depression

   b. Risk for poisoning: sedative-hypnotic toxicity related to ingestion

3. Planning/interventions

   a. Maintain airway, breathing, circulation and effective breathing pattern

     1) Prevent absorption: do not administer ipecac because of seizure potential and respiratory depression

     2) Administer benzodiazepine antidote (flumazenil) as directed

   b. Improve breathing pattern and tissue perfusion

     1) Initiate IV access to treat hypotension

       a) Administer fluid challenge

       b) Vasopressors as needed

     2) Monitor respiratory status closely

       a) Pulse oximetry, ABGs, carbon dioxide detector if intubated

   c. Prevent toxicity

     1) Refer for psychiatric evaluation as needed

     2) Provide education on toxic effects of drug and addiction potential

     3) Refer for social support services to decrease anxiety and stress: stress management classes, biofeedback, group therapy, exercise

4. Expected outcomes (see Appendix B)

5. Age-related considerations

   a. Pediatrics

     1) Overdose in children tends to cause excitation rather than CNS depression; tonic-clonic seizures may also ensue

     2) Investigate reason for toxicity: misreading dosing labels, accidental, purposeful use to calm an "active" child

     3) Suspect abuse and neglect if history warrants

M. Barbiturate poisoning

    Barbiturates are highly toxic agents that depress the CNS. They have anticonvulsant properties and decrease GI and bladder motility. Barbiturates are classified according to their duration of action: short (methohexital [Brevital], thiopental [Pentothal]), intermediate (pentobarbital [Nembutal]), and long (phenobarbital) acting. They are highly concentrated in adipose tissue and have a high abuse potential. Poisoning may be mild or excessive, leading to profound shock and coma. Because of its euphoric "well-being" state, abstinence from chronic barbiturate use causes a severe withdrawal syndrome. Alcohol enhances its toxicity.

1. Assessment

   a. Subjective

     1) History of present illness

       a) Agent ingested; short or long acting

       b) Route: PO, IM, IV

       c) Other drugs ingested: narcotics, hallucinogens, alcohol

       d) Symptoms

         (1) Mild: drowsiness, euphoria, impaired memory and judgment

         (2) Excessive use: CNS depression, shock/hypotension, arrhythmias

(3) Withdrawal symptoms
 (a) Within 24 hours: insomnia, nausea and vomiting, nightmares, depression, diaphoresis, tremors
 (b) After 48 hours: jerking of extremities leading to seizure activity, hallucinations, delirium, agitation
 (c) Abatement of symptoms: 7 to 14 days later
  2) Medical history
 a) Psychiatric: e.g., suicidal intent
 b) Seizures
  b. *Objective*
   1) Physical exam
 a) Cardiac: dysrhythmias, hypotension
 b) Skin: hypothermia, "barb blisters" (hemorrhagic blisters over areas of pressure that develop at about 4 hours after ingestion)
 c) Neurological: ataxia, slurred speech, flaccid muscle tone
   2) Diagnostic procedures
 a) Laboratory: urine/serum toxicology screen, glucose level
 b) Cardiac: monitor, 12- to 15-lead ECG
 c) Radiography: CXR to rule out pulmonary edema and pneumonia
 d) Other: temperature monitoring, pulse oximetry, ABGs to assess for acidosis

2. Analysis: differential nursing diagnosis/collaborative problems
  a. *Ineffective airway clearance related to altered LOC*
  b. *Cardiac output, decreased related to dysrhythmias*
  c. *Potential for poisoning: barbiturates related to ingestion*

3. Planning/interventions
  a. *Maintain airway, breathing, circulation: do not induce emesis because of respiratory depression*
   1) Consider multidose charcoal, especially with phenobarbital; it shortens half-life of drug
   2) Consider hemodialysis or peritoneal dialysis
   3) Maintain patent airway: consider intubation if needed
   4) Initiate IV access
   5) Provide urine alkalinization with sodium bicarbonate to promote ion binding of phenobarbital and increase drug excretion
  b. *Monitor cardiac function and maintain cardiac output*
   1) Monitor for dysrhythmias and treat per protocol
   2) Stabilize blood pressure: fluid challenge, vasopressors (dopamine); consider pulmonary artery catheter and/or arterial catheter placement
  c. *Decrease toxicity*
   1) Monitor temperature and rewarm as needed
   2) Treat barb blisters as second-degree burns
   3) Psychiatric consult when alert
   4) Treat withdrawal syndrome aggressively

4. Expected outcomes (see Appendix B)

5. Age-related considerations
  a. *Pediatrics*
   1) Infants born to addicted mothers will also be physically dependent on drug; they will show signs of withdrawal within 72 hours of birth such as a high-pitch cry, vomiting, diarrhea, tremors, seizures; infants are treated with tapered doses of phenobarbital

N. Iron poisoning

Iron toxicity is an important cause of morbidity and mortality, especially in children. Most cases of poisoning involve the accidental ingestion of prenatal vitamins or children's vitamins by toddlers. Adults absorb about 15 mg of iron daily from food and vitamins; however, the body can only lose 1 mg per day. Therefore, the serum iron level may be greater than the iron-binding capacity level, causing toxicity. Toxicity depends on the amount of elemental iron found in the preparation. An iron overdose can produce GI hemorrhage and result in cardiovascular collapse.

1. **Assessment**
   a. *Subjective*
      1) History of present illness
         a) Number and kind of tablets ingested (e.g., prenatal vitamins, children's tablets)
         b) Type of iron in compound: 60 mg/kg elemental iron can lead to severe symptoms
         c) Time of exposure and reason
         d) Postingestion emesis and amount
         e) Concurrent ingestion
         f) Symptoms
            (1) Lethargy
            (2) Diarrhea
            (3) Hematemesis
      2) Medical history
         a) Pregnancy
         b) Anemia or other chronic disease
         c) Medications used
   b. *Subjective*
      1) Physical exam
         a) LOC
         b) Vital signs: hypotension, tachycardia, tachypnea
         c) Occult blood: stool, emesis
         d) Phases of toxicity
            (1) Phase I ($<$ 6 hours after ingestion): corrosive effects of iron on GI tract (bloody diarrhea/emesis, abdominal pain, lethargy)
            (2) Phase II (6–48 hours): "recovery phase"; patient will seem to improve
            (3) Phase III (12–48 hours after ingestion): cardiovascular collapse, shock, metabolic acidosis, coma, GI bleeding
            (4) Phase IV (2–5 days later): onset of liver failure (jaundice, hepatic coma, coagulation defects); this stage is rare
            (5) Phase V (2–6 weeks after ingestion): very rare stage causing small bowel obstruction from corrosive effects of iron
      2) Diagnostic procedures
         a) Laboratory: serum iron peak is 3 to 5 hours after ingestion
            (1) Serum: total iron-binding capacity (TIBC)
            (2) Occult blood studies: stool, emesis, urine
            (3) LFTs, PT/PTT
         b) Radiographs
            (1) Abdominal films: tablets are radiopaque
         c) Other
            (1) ABG: assess acidosis
            (2) Type and cross-match to replace blood loss if needed

(3) Cardiac monitor

2. **Analysis: differential nursing diagnosis/collaborative problems**

   a. *Fluid volume deficit related to blood loss*

   b. *Anxiety/fear related to prognosis*

   c. *Potential for poisoning: iron overdose related to ingestion*

3. **Planning/interventions**

   a. *Maintain airway and provide GI decontamination*

   1) Prevent absorption: syrup of ipecac; initiate within 30 minutes of ingestion (rule out GI bleed before administration)

      a) Lavage: difficult to remove iron tablets because of their size

      b) Do not use activated charcoal because it does not bind iron

   2) Enhance elimination

      a) Antidote therapy: administer deferoxamine IV/IM; this chelation therapy binds iron and increases its renal excretion; observe "vin rosé" colored urine (pink-red) with a positive chelating response to deferoxamine

      b) Consider hemodialysis or peritoneal dialysis

   b. *Correct fluid volume losses*

   1) IV access initiated for fluid challenges to maintain blood pressure and to administer chelation therapy

   2) Order type and cross-match and administer blood as ordered

   3) I&O to maintain urine output to prevent anuria

   4) Monitor for cardiac dysrhythmias, hypotension, and seizures

   5) Monitor stool samples for blood

   c. *Decrease poisoning potential*

   1) Maintain nonjudgmental attitude and explain all procedures to parent/guardian and patient

   2) Allow significant adults to be with patient to decrease anxiety and fear

   3) Instruct caregivers on the following:

      a) Toxicity of iron

      b) Keeping ipecac at home and general poison prevention strategies

      c) Keeping poison control center's number handy

   4) Contact poison control center for treatment information

   5) Consider psychiatric consult if appropriate

4. **Expected outcomes** (see Appendix B)

O. Heavy metal poisoning

Poisoning from heavy metals (e.g., zinc, lead, mercury, and arsenic) may affect every body system, including the CNS, heart, lungs, liver, and kidney. These metals deposit themselves in the body and are excreted slowly. Children often eat chipped paint, exposing themselves to lead.

1. **Assessment**

   a. *Subjective*

   1) History of present illness

      a) Reason for exposure: accidental, intentional, occupational (plumber, steel welders, glass workers [metal fume fever])

      b) Route of exposure: inhalation, oral (lead), dermal

      c) Type of product

      d) Symptoms

         (1) Neurological: irritability, lethargy, insomnia, headaches, confusion, ataxia, paresthesias around lips and mouth

         (2) GI: anorexia, nausea and vomiting, metallic taste, thirst

(3) Cardiac: palpitations, substernal pain
2) Medical history
    a) Chronic exposure from occupation or pre-1960 residence with lead-painted surfaces
    b) Neurological history: seizures
  b. *Objective*
    1) Physical exam
      a) Neurological: seizures, myalgia, ataxia, diminished deep tendon reflexes (DTRs); LOC (e.g., malaise, confusion, coma)
      b) Cardiac: T-wave changes, VT, ventricular fibrillation (VF)
      c) GI: emesis, constipation, diarrhea (watery rice-like with arsenic)
      d) Renal: anuria, proteinuria, glycosuria
      e) Pulmonary: shortness of breath, hemoptysis
      f) Dermal (with zinc): burns, corneal changes
      g) Metal fume fever: inhaling metal oxides causes fever, chills, vomiting
      h) Lead poisoning: fatigue, lethargy, headaches, anorexia, abdominal pain, seizure, coma; long-term exposure may cause hyperactivity and retarded mental development
    2) Diagnostic procedures
      a) Laboratory: CBC, electrolytes, UA
      b) Other: arsenic—serum arsenic, 24-hour urine, LFTs, renal panel; mercury—serum mercury, 24-hour urine; zinc, no specific labs; lead—serum lead (Pb), 24-hour urine, erythrocyte protoporphyrin level, abdominal radiographs (lead particles are radiopaque)

2. Analysis: differential nursing diagnosis/collaborative problems
  a. *Risk for poisoning: heavy metals related to exposure*
  b. *Knowledge deficit of occupational protective devices/gear*

3. Planning/interventions
  a. *Maintain airway, breathing, circulation and use antidote therapy*
    1) Arsenic: chelation therapy—BAL, d-penicillamine (do not give BAL to patients allergic to peanuts; drug solution contains peanut oil)
      a) Alkalinize urine
      b) Hemodialysis
    2) Mercury: chelation therapy—BAL, d-penicillamine
      a) Treat seizures
    3) Zinc: chelation therapy—EDTA, BAL
      a) Treat metal fume fever with antipyretics and analgesics
      b) Observe for pulmonary edema
    4) Lead: chelation therapy—oral succimer, parenteral BAL, EDTA
      a) Treat seizure activity
      b) Correct iron deficiency anemia if present
  b. *Prevent occupational exposure*
    1) Wear correctly fitting respirators, protective clothing and gloves
    2) Properly handle, store and label heavy metals
    3) Follow agency/state regulations regarding workplace practices
  c. *Education regarding lead poisoning*
    1) Report exposure to health department to determine source of lead poisoning in children
    2) Avoid residences with pre-1960 lead-base paint; avoid crayons made in China
    3) Observe child for pica (consuming nonedible starchlike products) and frequent hand-to-mouth activity

4) Screening of all asymptomatic children younger than 6 years is recommended (serum lead)
4. **Expected outcomes** (see Appendix B)

P. Acids and alkali burns

Corrosives such as acids and alkalis cause severe burns. *Acids* include sulfuric, hydrochloric, and nitric acid. They are found in batteries, drain cleaners, and toilet bowl cleaners. Acids produce coagulation-type necrosis when in contact with the body tissue, especially in the stomach. The oral cavity and esophagus tend not to be significantly inflamed as a result of the short duration of contact with the agent. Acids cause severe emesis, which may continue for up to 90 minutes. *Alkalis* include sodium, potassium, and ammonium hydroxide, which may be found in drain cleaners, alkaline batteries, and fertilizers. Alkalis cause severe tissue necrosis, particularly to the esophagus, immediately on contact. Even small quantities can produce serious injury such as perforation and infection. Liquid alkalis produce rapid and deeply penetrating injuries. Alkali injuries to the eye cause corneal erosion and damage to the anterior chamber.

1. **Assessment**
   a. *Subjective*
      1) History of present illness
         a) Circumstances of exposure: occupational, accidental, intentional
         b) Nature of agent (acid, alkali) and concentration
         c) Amount and route of exposure: dermal, oral, inhalation
         d) Prehospital treatment: milk given to neutralize; never use ipecac
         e) Symptoms
            (1) Pain
            (2) Burns, blisters
            (3) Emesis, retching
            (4) Shortness of breath, stridor
            (5) Visual disturbances: decreased vision
      2) Medical history
         a) Chronic illness
         b) Psychiatric history: depression, suicidal
   b. *Objective*
      1) Physical exam
         a) Dermal findings: burns, blisters
         b) Oral cavity: drooling, burns, dysphagia (occurs soon after ingestion), blisters
         c) GI distress: nausea/vomiting, hematemesis
         d) Pulmonary: stridor, dyspnea, pulmonary edema (especially with acid ingestion, occurs after several hours)
         e) Ocular: decreased vision, corneal erosion, blindness, pale conjunctiva
      2) Diagnostic procedures
         a) Laboratory: CBC, type, and cross-match if hemodynamically unstable
         b) Radiographs: CXR, abdominal films; rule out pulmonary edema and perforation
         c) Other: esophagoscopy within 24 hours after alkali ingestion
2. **Analysis: differential nursing diagnosis/collaborative problems**
   a. *Pain related to burns*
   b. *Risk for poisoning: acids/alkali burns related to exposure*
   c. *Impaired skin integrity related to burns/ blisters*
3. **Planning/interventions**

    a. Emetics, charcoal, and cathartics are never indicated; never insert nasogastric or orogastric tube with alkali ingestion because of risk of perforation

      1) Alkali

        a) Dilute and neutralize with milk/water if ingested orally

        b) Consider steroid administration to reduce esophageal stricture formation (controversial)

        c) Administer analgesia to decrease pain

        d) Debride sloughed tissue to decrease infection

        e) Apply supplemental oxygen if inhalation injury

        f) Ocular injury: irrigate with normal saline for 1 hour or until pH has returned to 7.2 to 7.4 (normal range); ophthalmic exam; consider topical antibiotic to decrease infection

      2) Acid

        a) Oral: do not neutralize with water; this produces heat and steam, causing further tissue necrosis; do not induce emesis

        b) Ocular: irrigate with normal saline for a minimum of 15 minutes

        c) Dermal: wash exposed area with soap and water

        d) Administer analgesics to decrease pain

  4. Expected outcomes (see Appendix B)

Q. Cyanide poisoning

    Cyanide is a very lethal poison that causes death within 2 minutes when inhaled as a gas, thus its effectiveness as a form of capital punishment. Cyanide interferes with cellular respiration, causing decreased utilization of oxygen by the tissues. This effect causes bright-colored venous blood with unusual oxyhemoglobin saturation. Cyanide may be ingested orally or inhaled and is found in industrial fumigants, insecticides, and silver polish. It is also present in the pits of stone fruits such as cherries, peaches, and apricots (laetrile). Medically, cyanide may be generated from the long-term use of nitroprusside.

  1. Assessment

    a. Subjective

      1) History of present illness

        a) Circumstances of exposure: occupational, intentional, accidental, medical, corporal punishment

        b) Route: oral, inhaled

        c) Time of exposure

        d) Symptoms

          (1) Headache, dizziness

          (2) Nausea, confusion

          (3) Burning sensation in mouth and throat

      2) Medical history

        a) Medication use contributing to cause: laetrile, nitroprusside

        b) Psychiatric history: suicidal ideation

        c) Occupational hazard

    b. Objective

      1) Physical exam

        a) Breath odor: characteristic odor of bitter almonds

        b) Cardiac: hypertension, bradycardia followed by hypotension and tachycardia

        c) Respiratory: rapid initially, then slow and labored followed by respiratory arrest

        d) Neurological: seizure activity

2) Diagnostic procedures
a) Serum cyanide
b) Serum lactate
c) Electrolytes and hemoglobin
d) Other: venous blood gases and ABGs
e) Cardiac: monitoring, 12- to 15-lead ECG, pulse oximetry

2. **Analysis: differential nursing diagnosis/collaborative problems**
   a. *Impaired gas exchange related to cyanide toxicity*
   b. *Risk for poisoning: cyanide toxicity*

3. **Planning/interventions**
   a. *Improve gas exchange by maintaining airway, breathing, circulation*
      1) Do not do mouth-to-mouth resuscitation; protect yourself from the cyanide
      2) Administer 100% oxygen by mask
      3) Establish IV access for antidote therapy
      4) Administer cyanide antidote kit: induces methemoglobinemia to bind the cyanide
         a) Amyl nitrite: apply nasally or inside mask
         b) Sodium nitrite: IV
         c) Sodium thiosulfate: IV
   b. *Improve tissue perfusion*
      1) Monitor cardiac rhythm and pulse oximetry
      2) Monitor ABG results to assess acid-base status
      3) Consider vasopressor initiation to increase blood pressure
      4) Control seizure activity with diazepam/lorazepam
   c. *Decrease poisoning potential*
      1) Prevent absorption: do not delay antidote for these measures
         a) Remove contaminated clothing
         b) Decontaminate eyes
         c) Do not induce emesis because of rapid onset of seizure activity
      2) Instruct patient on the following:
         a) Proper storage, handling, labeling, and disposal of cyanide in occupational setting
         b) Prevention measures: rubber gloves, respirator use, protective clothing
         c) Encourage work site evaluations by county/state agencies if unsafe practices exist

4. **Expected outcomes** (see Appendix B)

R. Petroleum distillates poisoning

Also known as hydrocarbons, petroleum distillates include gasoline, kerosene, paint thinner, motor oil, and mineral sea oil (found in furniture polish). Some insecticides have a petroleum base. Toxicity depends on viscosity. Highly viscous products such as motor oil and heavy greases have a low toxicity, whereas low-viscosity products such as mineral sea oil are highly toxic because of the potential for aspiration. These products spread over lung surfaces, causing chemical pneumonitis.

1. **Assessment**
   a. *Subjective*
      1) History of present illness
         a) Route: oral, inhalation, dermal
         b) Circumstances: accidental, intentional, occupational
         c) Type of product: pure petroleum distillates or products mixed with heavy metal or insecticides
         d) Symptoms

             (1) Cough, choking, shortness of breath

             (2) Nausea and vomiting, abdominal pain, belching

             (3) Tremors, seizures

             (4) Burns on skin

        2) Medical history

           a) Chronic illness: neurological, cardiac, GI

           b) Respiratory problems

     b. *Objective*

        1) Physical exam

           a) Neurological: euphoria, ataxia, hallucinations, vertigo, seizures, fever

           b) Pulmonary: coughing, choking, tachypnea, pulmonary edema

             (1) Pulmonary edema with hemoptysis is common

             (2) Check for aspiration pneumonia on radiograph

           c) GI: nausea, vomiting, bloody diarrhea, belching

           d) Breath odor: check for characteristic odor

           e) Cardiac: arrhythmia

        2) Diagnostic procedures

           a) Laboratory: CBC, electrolytes, glucose, LFTs

           b) Radiographs: CXR

           c) Cardiac: 12- to 15-lead ECG, monitoring, pulse oximetry

           d) Other: ABGs

2. Analysis: differential nursing diagnosis/collaborative problems

     a. *Impaired gas exchange related to ventilation-perfusion imbalance*

     b. *Ineffective breathing pattern related to impaired gas exchange*

     c. *Impaired skin/ocular tissue integrity related to chemical exposure*

     d. *Risk for poisoning: petroleum distillate toxicity related to exposure*

3. Planning/interventions

     a. *Maintain airway, breathing, circulation and gas exchange*

        1) Initiate cardiac monitoring to assess for dysrhythmias

        2) Monitor pulse oximetry, and assist with airway maintenance if pulmonary edema or aspiration pneumonia develops

        3) Initiate IV access

     b. *Maintain effective respiratory pattern*

        1) Monitor patient for signs of aspiration, especially with emesis

        2) Monitor ABGs and treat metabolic acidosis

        3) Provide supplemental oxygen

     c. *Maintain skin integrity from chemical burns*

        1) Remove contaminated clothing

        2) Copiously wash skin with soapy water to remove residue

     d. *Prevent poisoning and further absorption*

        1) Do not administer ipecac or lavage unless a large ingestion (> 30 mL) has occurred as hydrocarbons are intestinal irritants and pass quickly

        2) If ipecac/lavage techniques are used, be cautious for risk of aspiration

        3) Observe patient closely for onset of delayed symptoms: respiratory distress, dysrhythmias

        4) Consider psychiatric consult before disposition

        5) Discuss proper handling, storage, and labeling of petroleum products

   4. Expected outcomes (see Appendix B)

S. Organophosphate poisoning

    Toxicity from organophosphates causes a cholinergic crisis whereby the substance binds to acetylcholinesterase, resulting in accumulation of acetylcholine at the receptor sites. This accumulation causes excess stimulation and hypersecretion of bodily fluids, resulting in excess diaphoresis, urination, lacrimation, salivation, and diarrhea. Organophosphates are found in insecticides and range in toxicity from highly toxic (e.g., parathion) to low toxicity (e.g., malathion, diazinon).

1. **Assessment**
   a. *Subjective*
      1) History of present illness
         a) Route of exposure: dermal, ocular, ingestion, inhalation
         b) Circumstances of exposure: accidental, intentional, occupational
         c) Symptoms: MUDDLES
            (1) *M*iosis
            (2) Increased *u*rination
            (3) *D*efecation
            (4) *D*iaphoresis
            (5) *L*acrimation
            (6) *E*xcitation
            (7) *S*alivation
      2) Medical history
         a) Chronic exposure
         b) Chronic illness
   b. *Objective*
      1) Physical exam
         a) Neurological: fasciculations, flaccid paralysis, seizures
         b) LOC: confusion to coma
         c) Hypersecretion: lacrimation, salivation, urination, defecation, vomiting and diarrhea
         d) Cardiac: bradycardia, hypotension
      2) Diagnostic procedures
         a) Serum/urine drug screen
2. **Analysis: differential nursing diagnosis/collaborative problems**
   a. *Ineffective airway clearance related to altered LOC*
   b. *Altered pattern of elimination related to hypersecretion*
   c. *Ineffective breathing pattern related to altered LOC*
   d. *Risk for poisoning: organophosphate toxicity related to exposure*
3. **Planning/interventions**
   a. *Maintain airway, breathing, circulation*
      1) Suction oropharynx of excess secretions as needed
      2) Assist with intubation if needed
      3) Apply supplemental oxygen
      4) Monitor cardiac status for dysrhythmias
   b. *Prevent further poisoning*
      1) Administer antidote therapy
         a) Atropine: it may take several milligrams to ease symptoms
         b) Pralidoxime (2-PAM): releases binding of insecticide
   c. *Promote effective breathing*
      1) Monitor pulse oximetry
      2) Keep head of bed elevated to drain secretions
      3) Monitor lung sounds for pulmonary edema
   d. *Promote adequate elimination patterns*
      1) Monitor I&O
      2) Consider urinary catheter if patient is unable to void
   e. *Instruct patient on proper use, handling, and storage of insecticides*

     f. Instruct patient to wear protective clothing and respirator when in contact with organophosphates

  4. Expected outcomes (see Appendix B)

T. Digoxin toxicity

     Digitalis and digoxin are commonly prescribed drugs in the middle-aged and elderly population used to increase myocardial contractility. Digoxin enhances cardiac output and reduces cardiac rate. It is useful in the treatment of atrial fibrillation and paroxysmal atrial tachycardia. Digoxin toxicity may result from an overdose, hypokalemia, advanced heart disease with conduction disturbances, or a combination of these. It may also result from decreased renal elimination of the drug. Digoxin toxicity is very common because the toxic level is slightly higher than the therapeutic serum level. Digoxin is absorbed from the GI tract.

  1. Assessment
    a. Subjective
      1) History of present illness
        a) Circumstances of exposure: intentional, accidental, recent surgery
        b) Acute versus chronic ingestion
        c) Diuretic therapy causing hypokalemia
        d) Recent myocardial infarction or cardiac event
        e) Symptoms
          (1) Mild: anorexia, PVCs or bradycardia, nausea and vomiting, malaise and depression
          (2) Acute: blurred vision, color changes in vision (yellow/green), halos around lights, confusion, delirium, disorientation, personality changes
      2) Medical history
        a) Renal failure
        b) Psychiatric history
        c) Electrolyte imbalance
        d) Cardiac disease: congestive heart failure, coronary artery disease
        e) Age of patient: elderly predisposed to ventricular dysrhythmias
    b. Objective
      1) Physical exam
        a) Vision changes: photophobia, decreased visual acuity, mydriasis
        b) GI: abdominal pain, nausea, vomiting
        c) Neurological: weakness, disorientation
        d) Cardiac: hypotension, dysrhythmias, bradycardia (children)
      2) Diagnostic procedures
        a) Laboratory
          (1) Serum digoxin level
          (2) Electrolytes, especially potassium, calcium, and magnesium
          (3) Renal panel, LFTs
        b) ECG: any change in rhythm may be result of toxicity, cardiac monitor
  2. Analysis: differential nursing diagnosis/collaborative problems
    a. Decreased cardiac output related to dysrhythmias
    b. Risk for poisoning: digoxin toxicity related to ingestion
    c. Knowledge deficit regarding health maintenance: digoxin use
  3. Planning/interventions
    a. Improve cardiac output
      1) Apply supplemental oxygen therapy as indicated
      2) Assess serum electrolyte levels and replace deficient potassium, magnesium

3) Closely monitor cardiac rhythm and ECGs
    a) Treat dysrhythmias with lidocaine or phenytoin
    b) Discontinue digoxin until serum levels are within normal range
    c) Consider pacemaker insertion for continuing heart block, external pacing at bedside
4) Discontinue diuretic therapy and monitor serum potassium
5) Avoid beta blockers and quinidine administration: effects will be additive with digoxin

b. *Decrease risk for poisoning*
1) Prevent absorption
    a) Consider gastric lavage with documented recent overexposure: lavage may stimulate bradycardia, requiring pretreatment with atropine
    b) Administer charcoal or cholestyramine to bind drug in intestines
    c) Consult poison control center or toxicologist if patient remains symptomatic
2) Consider antidote therapy
    a) Administer digoxin immune Fab (Digibind): for treatment of life-threatening dysrhythmias caused by digoxin overdose
    b) Administer 10 vials in 50-mL NS IV over 30 minutes for acute ingestion (may be repeated)

c. *Educate patient regarding effects of digoxin on body*
1) Instruct patient on safe storage and use of digoxin
2) Instruct patient to take digoxin daily as scheduled and not to discontinue medicine without notifying care provider

d. *Contact care provider with symptoms of toxicity (see prior discussion)*

4. Expected outcomes (see Appendix B)

5. Age-related considerations
a. *Pediatrics*
1) Toxicity manifested as atrial arrhythmias
2) Digibind may be administered to symptomatic pediatric overdose patients

U. Calcium channel blocker toxicity

Calcium channel blockers, also known as slow channel blockers or calcium antagonists, inhibit the movement of calcium across the cell membrane. Because calcium is needed for generating an action potential and for contractility, inhibition of this process causes a decrease in contractility, automaticity (impulse formation), and conduction velocity. Calcium channel blockers dilate the coronary arteries and reduce arterial resting blood pressure but are known to cause reflex tachycardia. They also decrease coronary artery spasm and increase oxygen delivery. Common medications include verapamil, nifedipine, and diltiazem. The toxic-therapeutic margin is small; thus, toxicity results in severely decreased cardiac output and junctional rhythms or heart block.

1. Assessment
a. *Subjective*
1) History of present illness
    a) Circumstances of exposure: accidental, intentional
    b) Route: dermal, oral, parenteral
    c) Type of preparation: sustained release
    d) Symptoms
        (1) Irregular heart rate
        (2) Dizziness
        (3) Nausea, diarrhea (nifedipine)

(4) Constipation (verapamil)
  2) Medical history
    a) Chronic renal or liver abnormalities
    b) Use of beta-adrenergic blocking agents: may slow heart rate
    c) Psychiatric history
    d) Cardiac history
  b. *Objective*
    1) Physical exam
      a) Cardiac: junctional rhythms, bradycardia, heart blocks
      b) Respiratory: shortness of breath
      c) Vital signs: marked hypotension
      d) Metabolic: hyperglycemia (secondary to the blockage of insulin release), metabolic acidosis
    2) Diagnostic procedures
      a) Laboratory
        (1) CBC, electrolytes, glucose
      b) Cardiac: monitor, 12- to 15-lead ECG
      c) Other: ABG, pulse oximetry
2. **Analysis: differential nursing diagnosis/collaborative problems**
  a. *Decreased cardiac output related to dysrhythmias*
  b. *Tissue perfusion, altered cardiac related to decreased cardiac output*
  c. *Risk for poisoning: calcium channel blocker toxicity related to ingestion*
3. **Planning/interventions**
  a. *Improve cardiac output*
    1) Maintain airway, breathing, circulation
    2) Apply supplemental oxygen
    3) Continuous cardiac monitoring for bradycardia or dysrhythmias
    4) Administer antidote therapy
      a) Calcium chloride or calcium gluconate IV to reverse effects of depressed contractility
      b) Vasopressors to maintain blood pressure: dopamine, epinephrine, amrinone
      c) Atropine: for acute treatment of bradycardia
    5) Keep external pacing equipment at bedside
  b. *Improve cardiac tissue perfusion*
    1) IV access and fluid challenges to maintain blood pressure
    2) Consider use of cardioversion, lidocaine, or procainamide if patient has rapid ventricular rate
    3) Monitor cardiac rhythm, respiratory function, and pulse oximetry
  c. *Decrease risk for poisoning*
    1) Prevent absorption
      a) Gastric lavage/syrup of ipecac
      b) Activated charcoal with or without cathartics
      c) Consider whole bowel irrigation or multidose charcoal if sustained-release preparations
    2) Psychiatric evaluation if intentional overdose
    3) Instruct patient regarding effects of calcium channel blockers on body
4. **Expected outcomes** (see Appendix B)

V. Beta-blocker toxicity

Beta-adrenergic receptor blocking agents inhibit both the beta$_1$ (cardiac muscle) and beta$_2$ (bronchial and vascular musculature) receptors, causing a decreased heart rate, decreased cardiac output at rest and with exercise, and hypotension. These effects make the drugs useful in the treatment of angina and hypertension. Recent literature promotes the use of beta blockers to enhance survival after a myocardial infarction. The cardioprotective effects are thought to prevent reinfarction. Beta blockers have also been used in the treatment of migraines. An overdose of beta blockers causes severe hypotension and bradycardia. Abrupt withdrawal causes a rebound hyperactivity, leading to unstable angina and a myocardial infarction. The drugs must be tapered. Death results from asystole. Common agents include propranolol, metoprolol, and atenolol.

1. **Assessment**
   a. *Subjective*
      1) History of present illness
         a) Circumstances of exposure: accidental, intentional
         b) Concurrent therapy: calcium channel blockers
         c) Symptoms
            (1) Irregular heart rate
            (2) Chest pain, shortness of breath, palpitations
            (3) Dizziness, fatigue, vertigo
            (4) Nausea and vomiting, abdominal pain
      2) Medical history
         a) Cardiac: myocardial infarction, angina, hypertension
         b) Migraine history
         c) Asthma
   b. *Objective*
      1) Physical exam
         a) Cardiac: bradycardia, AV block, asystole, hypotension, and cardiogenic shock
         b) Respiratory: dyspnea, pulmonary edema, respiratory depression, bronchospasm
         c) Neurological: decreased LOC from delirium to coma, seizures (especially with propranolol)
         d) Metabolic: hypoglycemia
      2) Diagnostic procedures
         a) Laboratory: electrolytes (especially potassium), serum glucose
         b) Radiograph: CXR to rule out pulmonary edema
         c) Cardiac: monitor, 12- to 15-lead ECG
         d) Other: pulse oximetry, ABG
2. **Analysis: differential nursing diagnosis/collaborative problems**
   a. *Decreased cardiac output related to dysrhythmias*
   b. *Altered tissue perfusion, cardiac related to decreased cardiac output*
   c. *Ineffective breathing pattern related to altered LOC*
   d. *Risk for poisoning: beta-blocker toxicity related to ingestion*
3. **Planning/interventions**
   a. *Improve cardiac output*
      1) Correct bradycardia with atropine or glucagon IV (increases heart rate)
      2) Continuously monitor for dysrhythmias and wide QRS
      3) External cardiac pacing equipment at bedside
      4) Treat dysrhythmias with phenytoin-lidocaine: avoid quinidine or procainamide, which may further depress cardiac function
      5) Treat torsades de pointes with isoproterenol (Isuprel), magnesium sulfate, and external pacing if present
   b. *Improve tissue perfusion*
      1) Intravenous access and fluid boluses to increase blood pressure

2) Consider vasopressor therapy: dopamine, dobutamine
3) Continually monitor blood pressure, and consider arterial catheter or pulmonary artery catheter placement
4) Treat seizures with phenytoin/diazepam
5) Monitor serum glucose for hypoglycemia and treat with D50W if needed
c. *Decrease ineffective breathing pattern*
1) Monitor ABGs for acidosis
2) Monitor lung sounds and CXR for evidence of pulmonary edema
3) Correct bronchospasms with a beta$_2$-stimulating agent if needed: albuterol
d. *Decrease poisoning risk*
1) Prevent absorption
a) Emesis/lavage
b) Charcoal with or without cathartic
2) Monitor vital signs for changes in condition
3) Consider psychiatric consult
4) Discuss effects of beta blockers on body
4. **Expected outcomes** (see Appendix B)

W. Plant poisonings

There are many kinds of plant poisonings of which one should be aware. Cardiac glycoside plants such as the oleander, foxglove, and lily of the valley cause a loss of cardiac excitability and hyperkalemia. Plants with anticholinergic properties antagonize acetylcholine at the neuroreceptor site. This causes a typical anticholinergic presentation of tachycardia, mydriasis, and fever. Plants in this category include jimsonweed, deadly night shade, and potato leaves. Plants that contain oxalic acids produce severe pain when ingested from the crystal needles of the calcium oxalate. These plants include *Dieffenbachia,* philodendron, and rhubarb.

1. **Assessment**
a. *Subjective*
1) History of present illness
a) Type of plant ingested, part of plant (bulb, blossoms, leaves)
b) Acute versus chronic exposure
c) Symptoms
(1) Cardiac glycosides: vomiting
(2) Anticholinergic: agitation, delirium, disorientation, visual hallucinations
(3) Oxalic acid: bloody emesis and diarrhea, pain, and burning sensation orally
2) Medical history
a) Cardiac or GI history
b) Psychiatric history
c) Age of patient
b. *Objective*
1) Physical exam
a) Cardiac glycosides: bradycardia with heart block
b) Anticholinergics
(1) Neurological: seizures, mydriasis, blurred vision
(2) Cardiac: tachycardia, hypertension
(3) Metabolic: hyperpyrexia
(4) GI: dry mouth, decreased gastric motility
(5) Genitourinary: urinary retention
(6) Skin: hot, dry and flushed

        c) Oxalic acids
           (1) Head, eyes, ears, nose, and throat: swelling of the mouth, tongue, throat; increased salivation
           (2) Respiratory: shortness of breath if edema develops
           (3) Neurological: hypocalcemia, tetany
      2) Diagnostic procedures
        a) Cardiac glycosides: serum potassium, 12- to 15-lead ECG
        b) Anticholinergics: LFTs, 12- to 15-lead ECG
        c) Oxalic acid: UA for calcium oxalate crystals, serum calcium

2. Analysis: differential nursing diagnosis/collaborative problems

    a. Decreased cardiac output related to dysrhythmias
    b. Risk for poisoning: plants related to exposure

3. Planning/interventions

    a. Maintain airway, breathing, circulation and cardiac output
      1) Monitor ECG and airway patency
      2) Initiate IV access
      3) Treat electrolyte imbalances (hyperkalemia)
      4) Consider atropine, cardiac pacing for bradycardia
      5) Treat dysrhythmias with phenytoin
    b. Maintain mucous membrane and skin integrity
      1) Apply ice to lips and oral area to decrease swelling
      2) Administer milk or water to flush out oxalic acid crystals from oral cavity
    c. Prevent risk of further poisoning
      1) Consider ipecac or lavage for anticholinergic overdose
      2) Administer charcoal with or without catharsis
      3) Consider physostigmine for anticholinergic overdose as antidotal therapy
      4) Instruct all patients/caregivers regarding poison prevention measures in the home: keep plants out of reach

    4. Expected outcomes (see Appendix B)

BIBLIOGRAPHY

Barker, L. R., Burton, J., & Zieve, P. (Eds.). (1995). *Principles of ambulatory medicine.* Baltimore: Williams & Wilkins.

Bozzuto, T. (1993). Poisonings and overdoses. In G. Hamilton (Ed.), *Presenting signs and symptoms in the emergency department: Evaluation and treatment* (pp. 238–247). Baltimore: Williams & Wilkins.

Brown-Beasly, M. (1998). After fen-phen/Redux: Cardiac and pulmonary sequelae implications for patient assessment. *Journal of Emergency Nursing, 24*(1), 62–65.

Brueske, P. (1997). ED management of cyanide poisoning. *Journal of Emergency Nursing, 23*(6), 569–573.

Dambro, M. (1997). *Griffith's 5 minute clinical consult.* Baltimore: Williams & Wilkins.

Ellenhorn, M. (1997). *Ellenhorn's medical toxicology* (2nd ed.). Baltimore: Williams & Wilkins.

Erickson, T., Goldfrank, L., & Kulig, K. (1997). How to treat the poisoned patient. *Patient Care,* 90–113.

Espeland, K. (1995). Identifying the manifestations of inhalant abuse. *Nurse Practitioner, 20*(5), 49–53.

Huston, C. (1996). Carbon monoxide poisoning. *American Journal of Nursing, 96*(1), 48.

Litovitz, T. L., Felberg, L., White, S., et al. (1995). 1995 Annual report of the American Association of Poison Control Centers toxic exposure surveillance system. *American Journal of Emergency Medicine, 14,* 487–537.

Olson, K. (1994). *Poisoning and drug overdoses* (2nd ed.). East Norwalk, CT: Appleton & Lange.

Tintinalli, J., Ruiz, E., & Krome, R. (Eds.). (1996). *Emergency medicine, comprehensive study guide* (4th ed.). San Francisco: McGraw-Hill.

Weintraub, B. (1997). A fatal case of acid ingestion. *Journal of Emergency Nursing, 23*(5), 413–416.

Zimmerman, P. (1997). Tricylic antidepressant overdose. *American Journal of Nursing, 97*(10), 39.

Barbara M. Mitchell, RN, MSN

CHAPTER **21**

Wound Management Emergencies

MAJOR TOPICS

General Strategy

Specific Wound Management Emergencies

Lacerations

Abrasions

Avulsions

Puncture Wounds

Foreign Bodies

Missile Injuries

Human Bites

Wound-Related Infections

I. GENERAL STRATEGY

A. Assessment

1. **Primary survey/resuscitation (see Chapter 1)**
2. **Secondary survey (see Chapter 1)**
3. **Psychological, social, and environmental factors**
   a. *Exposure- or injury-prone activities*
   b. *Socioeconomic factors that may result in*
      1) Exposure to certain types of injuries (e.g., stab wounds)
      2) Inadequate follow-up care
   c. *Pathophysiological disorders that prolong bleeding*
   d. *Pathophysiological disorders that affect healing*
      1) Diabetes
      2) Chronic steroid use
      3) Host immunocompromise
      4) Poor tissue perfusion
      5) Predisposition to frequent infections (axiom: wounds resulting from compressive forces are 100 times more susceptible to infection than those from sharp instruments)
      6) Extended time between injury and treatment
   e. *Poor nutritional status*
   f. *Medications that prolong bleeding*

    g. *Anxiety or panic related to*
       1) Extent of injury
       2) Extent of bleeding
       3) Potential threat to life or limb
       4) Pain and other symptoms
       5) Cause of injury
       6) Treatment and hospitalization procedures
       7) Concern expressed by significant others
    h. *Fear of disfigurement or scarring*
    i. *Denial of severity of symptoms*
    j. *Concern regarding*
       1) Body image
       2) Alterations in function
       3) Impact on work and lifestyle
    k. *Anger or fear related to*
       1) Being victim of assault or violence
       2) Authorities (e.g., police, legal system)

4. Focused survey
    a. *Subjective data*
       1) History of present condition
          a) Chief complaint
            (1) Description of injury
            (2) Cause of injury
            (3) Mechanism of injury (e.g., angle of blow; direction of fall; deceleration of vehicle)
            (4) Time elapsed since injury
          b) Region of body affected
          c) Anatomical structures involved
          d) Bleeding
            (1) Estimated amount at time of assessment and since injury
            (2) Venous and/or arterial
            (3) Systemic responses
          e) Pain
            (1) Provocation related to activity/movement
            (2) Quality and type
            (3) Radiation/region of body
            (4) Severity, including changes since onset
            (5) Time of onset
          f) Numbness/tingling in immediate area or in other parts of body
       2) Medical history
          a) Age
          b) Calluses in area of injury
          c) Stains on skin, both old and new
          d) Scars: location and type
          e) Needle marks: number and location
          f) Circulatory status: general and in extremities
          g) Nutritional status
            (1) General appearance and grooming
            (2) Hypovitaminosis, particularly vitamin C
               (a) Hemorrhages
               (b) Loose teeth
               (c) Gingivitis
            (3) Obesity

h) Medication history
  (1) Immunization status
  (2) Aspirin
  (3) Steroids
  (4) Immunosuppressive drugs
  (5) Anticoagulants
  (6) Other drugs
  (7) Allergies

b. *Objective data*
  1) Physical examination
    a) General survey of patient
      (1) Level of consciousness
      (2) Vital signs
      (3) Body size
      (4) Stage of growth, development
      (5) Concurrent and associated injuries, problems
    b) Inspection
      (1) Color: pallor, cyanosis, discoloration
      (2) Edema of surrounding tissues
      (3) Characteristics of wound
      (4) Location of wound or injury
      (5) Underlying structures
      (6) Thinness of skin
      (7) Type of exposure of body part
      (8) Effect on function of involved part
        (a) Blood vessel involvement
        (b) Arterial and venous flow
        (c) Lymphatic drainage
        (d) Nerve involvement
        (e) Tendon involvement
        (f) Bone injury
      (9) Extent of wound contamination
      (10) Presence of necrotic tissue
      (11) Presence of foreign bodies
    c) Palpation
      (1) Areas of tenderness
      (2) Bony deformity
      (3) Circulation: test distal pulses and, if indicated, capillary refill
      (4) Sensation: identify absence or deficiencies in sensation
      (5) Tendon function: identify whether patient can move involved joints through full range of motion
      (6) Temperature of affected area
  2) Diagnostic procedures
    a) Laboratory studies: in general, diagnostic studies are not obtained for surface trauma; in select instances, the following diagnostic studies may be considered
      (1) Grossly infected wounds: consider wound culture and sensitivity (C&S) and complete blood count (CBC) with differential
      (2) In setting of either coagulopathy or profuse bleeding consider platelet count, prothrombin time (PT), type, cross-match
    b) Radiographic studies are used in specific cases to identify foreign bodies, fractures, soft tissue gas

B. Analysis: differential nursing diagnosis/collaborative problems

1. Anxiety/fear
2. Body image disturbance
3. Impaired skin integrity
4. Knowledge deficit
5. Risk for fluid volume deficit
6. Risk for infection
7. Risk for injury

C. Planning/interventions

1. **Determine priorities**
   a. *Maintain airway, breathing, circulation*
   b. *Control local bleeding*
   c. *Control pain*
   d. *Relieve anxiety or apprehension*
   e. *Educate patient and significant others*
2. **Develop nursing care plan specific to patient's presenting emergency**
3. **Obtain and set up necessary equipment and supplies**
4. **Institute appropriate interventions based on nursing care plan**

D. Expected outcomes/evaluation

1. **Monitor patient's responses and outcomes, adjusting nursing care plans as indicated**
   a. *Specific interventions*
   b. *Disposition and discharge planning*
2. **Record data as appropriate**
3. **If positive outcomes are not demonstrated, assessment and/or plan of care needs re-evaluation**

E. Age-related considerations

1. **Pediatric**
   a. *Growth- and development-related factors*
      1) Pediatric healing responses are more rapid than those of adults
      2) Close fluid monitoring is essential
      3) Major heat loss can occur in young child if unclothed for period of time as a result of large body surface area
      4) High metabolic rate and low glycogen stores in infants can lead to hypoglycemia during stress
   b. *"Pearls"*
      1) It is important to develop and maintain relationship with family, along with child, because security for most children comes from parents
      2) It is essential to communicate at child's level of understanding whenever possible
      3) Child's need to remain covered should be respected
      4) Possible child abuse should always be considered because surface trauma often is associated with or is most evident sign of nonaccidental injuries in children
2. **Geriatric**
   a. *Aging-related factors*

1) Reduced elasticity of skin, decreased subcutaneous fat layer, and reduced perfusion
2) Limited mobility and joint flexion as a result of osteoarthritis
3) Capillary fragility, leading to large ecchymoses
4) Adaptive responses take longer to occur
5) Poor tolerance for cold as result of peripheral vascular changes and diminished thermoregulatory ability
6) Loss of visual acuity
7) Hearing impairments
8) Diminished temperature sensation
9) Frequent chronic dysrhythmias
10) Reduced lung mass and elasticity, decreased vital capacity, and reduced ability to cough

II. SPECIFIC WOUND MANAGEMENT EMERGENCIES

A. Lacerations

Lacerations are open wounds that result from tearing or sharp cutting. They usually extend into the deep epithelial tissue, may involve some of the underlying structures, and vary in length and depth. Within 6 hours of wound injury, platelet deposition and vasospasm mitigate local bleeding. Epithelialization (i.e., growth of epithelial cells across the surface of a laceration) occurs within 48 hours of wound injury and makes most lacerations watertight by that time. Fibroblasts deposit procollagen into wounds, which is transformed into collagen. However, fibroblast activity does not maximize until about 1 week after wound injury. Consequently, laceration tensile strength is not adequate at the time of suture removal. For this reason, the use of tapes is generally recommended after suture removal.

1. **Assessment**
   a. *Subjective data*
      1) History of present condition
         a) Description of injuring instrument
         b) Extent of contamination of instrument
         c) Time lapse since injury
         d) Location of injury
         e) Extent of bleeding
         f) Pain
            (1) Location
            (2) Radiation
            (3) Relation to activity
         g) Care measures before arrival
      2) Medical history
         a) Immunization status
         b) Allergies
         c) Medications
   b. *Objective data*
      1) Physical examination
         a) Continued bleeding: check for arterial injury
         b) Depth, length of laceration
         c) Structures involved
         d) Extent of necrotic tissue
         e) Apparent wound contamination

   f) Function of involved part

   g) Associated injuries

  2) Diagnostic procedures

   a) Culture and white blood cell (WBC) count if

    (1) Wound contaminated

    (2) Wound more than 8 to 12 hours old

   b) Radiological examination if

    (1) Possible associated bony injury

    (2) Nonobservable foreign body in wound

2. Analysis: differential nursing diagnosis/collaborative problems

 a. Risk for fluid volume deficit related to blood loss

 b. Impaired skin integrity related to wound

 c. Risk for infection related to open wound and contamination

 d. Pain related to laceration of skin and underlying tissues/structures

 e. Anxiety/fear related to injury, treatment, and effects on activities of daily living

 f. Knowledge deficit related to therapeutic regimen and self-care

3. Planning/interventions

 a. Maintain airway, breathing, circulation

 b. Control local bleeding

  1) Direct pressure

  2) Elevation of part

 c. Continue monitoring vital signs

 d. Establish intravenous (IV) catheter with crystalloid solution if blood loss is great or patient is hypotensive

 e. Place affected part in position of comfort

 f. Shave area, removing as little hair as necessary (never shave eyebrows because regrowth may be distorted)

 g. Cleanse/irrigate skin around wound with antiseptic solution

 h. Assist with administration of local anesthetic

 i. Administer sedation as adjunct to local anesthesia as ordered

 j. Cleanse wound thoroughly with mild antiseptic soap

 k. Irrigate skin and wound per order

 l. Assist with debridement

 m. Ensure appropriate dressing

 n. Apply splint if partial immobilization of part is indicated

 o. Administer appropriate immunizations and/or antibiotics per standard guidelines

 p. Provide verbal/written instructions to patient or significant others, including directions to

  1) Elevate affected part

  2) Apply ice or heat, as directed

  3) Provide wound care instructions, which include keeping wound and dressing clean and dry: keep covered for the first 48 hours

  4) Change dressing if wet and/or soiled

  5) Observe for redness, swelling, heat (fever), discharge

  6) Take medications according to directions, if ordered

  7) Return or make appointment for follow-up care as indicated

  8) Have sutures removed as directed

  9) Use sunblock over wound for at least 6 months (sun protection factor [SPF] of 15 or stronger)

4. Expected outcomes/evaluation (see Appendix B)

B. Abrasions

Abrasions are partial-thickness denudations of an area of skin. These common injuries result from falls, scrapes, and particularly cycle accidents, and are quite painful.

1. Assessment
  a. *Subjective data*
    1) History of present condition
      a) Description of accident
      b) Time lapse since injury; dirt and debris must be removed within 4 to 6 hours from extremity and within 8 hours from face
      c) Location of injury
      d) Amount of pain or discomfort
    2) Medical history
      a) Immunization status
      b) Allergies
      c) Medications
  b. *Objective data*
    1) Physical examination
      a) Extent of denuded tissue
      b) Depth of injury
      c) Presence of embedded dirt and debris
      d) Associated injuries
    2) Diagnostic procedures, as indicated if related injuries
2. Analysis: differential nursing diagnosis/collaborative problems
  a. *Impaired skin integrity related to wound*
  b. *Risk for infection related to open wound and contamination*
  c. *Pain related to wound and exposed nerve endings*
  d. *Anxiety/fear related to injury, treatment, and effects of activities of daily living*
  e. *Knowledge deficit related to therapeutic regimen and self-care*
3. Planning/interventions
  a. *Administer appropriate immunizations*
  b. *Place affected part in position of comfort*
  c. *Cleanse skin around abraded area*
  d. *Provide verbal/written instructions to patient and significant others, including directions to*
    1) Change dressing and apply ointment as indicated and recommended
    2) Wash facial area four times a day and reapply ointment
    3) Avoid direct sunlight to area for 6 months, because of risk of pigmentary changes
    4) Take or use medication according to directions
    5) Return or make appointment for follow-up care, as indicated
4. Expected outcomes/evaluation (see Appendix B)

C. Avulsions

Avulsions are characterized by full-thickness tissue loss that prevents wound edge approximation. This injury is commonly seen in finger tip and nose tip injuries. Hemostasis is the immediate problem. Small avulsions will usually heal by secondary intention. Larger avulsed areas may require split-thickness grafting. One type of severe avulsion is a "degloving" injury, in which the full thickness of skin is peeled away from a finger, hand, or foot or an area of a limb, resulting in devascularization of the skin and potential damage to underlying tissues. Flap replacement and grafting are frequently required.

1. **Assessment**
   a. *Subjective data*
      1) History of present condition
         a) Description of accident
         b) Time lapse since injury
         c) Location of injury
         d) Efforts made to preserve avulsed tissue
         e) Amount of pain or discomfort
         f) Care measures of wound and amputated tissue before arrival
      2) Medical history
         a) Immunization status
         b) Allergies
         c) Medications
   b. *Objective data*
      1) Physical examination
         a) Amount of bleeding
         b) Extent of injury: structures involved
         c) Associated injuries
      2) Diagnostic procedures: radiological examination if degloving injury with possible associated fracture

2. **Analysis: differential nursing diagnosis/collaborative problems**
   a. *Impaired skin integrity related to avulsion injury*
   b. *Risk for infection related to open wound and possible contamination*
   c. *Pain related to exposed nerve endings and tissue trauma*
   d. *Anxiety/fear related to injury, pain, possible disfigurement*
   e. *Knowledge deficit related to therapeutic regimen and self-care*

3. **Planning/interventions**
   a. *Elevate part*
   b. *Apply sterile, saline-soaked gauze*
   c. *Apply steady pressure*
   d. *Care for amputated tissue*
      1) Home care
         a) Do not allow tissue to come in contact with ice or iced water
         b) Keep tissue as clean and moist as possible
         c) Wrap in gauze soaked in tap water or saline, if available
         d) Transport to emergency facility as soon as possible
      2) Emergency setting care
         a) Wrap in gauze moistened with sterile normal saline
         b) Seal in either sterile container or plastic bag
         c) Place container in bath of iced saline or water (ensure that iced saline does not come in contact with tissue)
   e. *Cleanse wound with antiseptic soap and irrigate thoroughly*
   f. *If small avulsion*
      1) Apply petrolatum (Vaseline) gauze or other nonadhering material
      2) Apply pressure dressing
   g. *If large avulsion*
      1) Apply petrolatum (Vaseline) gauze or other nonadhering material to avulsed area and donor site
      2) Apply layered dressing
      3) Apply metal protector, if indicated
   h. *If degloving injury*

       1) Realign soft tissue to prevent further damage
       2) Cover with sterile dressing
       3) Prepare to transfer to operating room for debridement and grafting
    i. Administer appropriate immunizations and antibiotics, as indicated
    j. Provide verbal/written instruction to patient and significant others, including directions to
       1) Elevate part to reduce bleeding
       2) Apply ice as indicated
       3) Care for wound and dressing
       4) Observe for signs of infection
       5) Take medications, as ordered
       6) Return or make appointment for follow-up care
  4. Expected outcomes/evaluation (see Appendix B)

D. Puncture wounds

    Puncture wounds occur when tissue is penetrated by sharp or blunt objects. Such wounds most commonly result from stepping on nails, tacks, needles, or broken glass. Running into or being assaulted with sharp objects also causes these injuries. Characteristically, puncture wounds bleed minimally and tend to seal off, creating a high infection potential.

    Puncture wounds near joints place those joints at risk for bacterial inoculation and sepsis. A puncture wound on the plantar aspect of the foot places the host at risk for cellulitis, chondritis, and osteomyelitis (0.4–0.6% of cases). Plantar puncture wounds through shoes increase the risk of *Pseudomonas* infection and osteomyelitis, a particularly virulent infection.

  1. Assessment
    a. Subjective data
       1) History of present condition
         a) Description of accident
         b) Location of injury
         c) Type of injuring object
         d) Length or depth of penetration
         e) Degree of contamination
         f) Time elapsed since injury
         g) Amount of pain/discomfort
       2) Medical history
         a) Immunization status
         b) Allergies
         c) Medications
    b. Objective data
       1) Physical examination
         a) Estimation of wound depth
         b) Possible presence of foreign body or material
         c) Extent of injury: structures involved
       2) Diagnostic procedures
         a) Radiological examination if embedded foreign body is suspected and cannot be easily located: involves use of soft tissue films with special composition that give clear images with marker placed near suspected entry site

  2. Analysis: differential nursing diagnosis/collaborative problems
    a. Impaired skin integrity related to puncture wound
    b. Risk for infection related to open wound and possible contamination

     c. *Pain related to wound*

     d. *Anxiety/fear related to injury, pain, and possible sequelae*

     e. *Knowledge deficit related to therapeutic regimen and self-care*

  3. Planning/interventions

     a. *Assist in administration of local anesthetic if puncture wound is to be explored*

     b. *Administer mild analgesia as ordered*

     c. *Remove or assist with removal of foreign body if present (see section II.E.3. for specific interventions)*

     d. *Assist with opening, debriding, irrigating, and packing severely contaminated wound*

     e. *Apply appropriate dressing*

     f. *Administer appropriate immunizations*

     g. *Administer antibiotic, if ordered*

     h. *Provide verbal and written instructions to patient and significant others, including directions to*

       1) Soak wound in warm, soapy water two or three times a day for 2 to 4 days (unless packing in place)

       2) Observe for signs of infection

       3) Return or make appointment for follow-up care, if indicated

  4. Expected outcomes/evaluation (see Appendix B)

E. Foreign bodies

    Foreign bodies include wood and metal splinters, glass, clothing, fragments from gunshot wounds, pins and needles, rubber from tennis shoes, fishhooks, and many other items that become embedded in various parts of the body. Occasionally, objects that are difficult to find but not likely to cause a tissue reaction are left in place (e.g., glass, metal). Vegetative foreign bodies (e.g., thorns, wood) are highly reactive, lead to infection, and should be removed as quickly as possible. Unfortunately, vegetative foreign bodies are also more difficult to visualize on plane radiographs and may require computed tomographic (CT) scans, ultrasonograms, and local wound exploration.

  1. Assessment

     a. *Subjective data*

       1) History of present condition

         a) Description of injury

         b) Characteristics of suspected foreign body

         c) Location of injury

         d) Direction of entry

         e) Time elapsed since injury

         f) Extent of contamination by foreign body

         g) Amount of pain and discomfort

       2) Medical history

         a) Immunization status

         b) Allergies

         c) Medications

     b. *Objective data*

       1) Physical examination

         a) Extent of injuries: structures involved

       2) Diagnostic procedures: radiology

         a) Not useful for pieces of clothing, natural wood splinters

         b) Fluoroscopy may be required for needle removal

  2. Analysis: differential nursing diagnosis/collaborative problems

a. *Impaired skin integrity related to penetration of foreign body*

b. *Risk for infection related to open wound and presence of contaminated foreign body*

c. *Pain related to injury and presence of foreign body*

d. *Anxiety/fear related to injury, pain, and procedure to remove foreign body*

e. *Knowledge deficit related to therapeutic regimen*

3. **Planning/interventions**

a. *Cleanse area around entry site thoroughly with mild antiseptic solution; do not soak part of body containing a wooden splinter because wood absorbs liquid and may disintegrate during removal*

b. *Apply gentle, careful traction with small forceps to remove objects that lie close to or protrude through skin (anesthesia may not be needed)*

c. *Assist in administration of local anesthetic if puncture wound is to be explored*

d. *Assist with administration of regional anesthesia and removal of foreign bodies that are embedded in deeper tissues or are difficult to find*

e. *Administer mild analgesia, if required*

f. *Apply appropriate dressing*

g. *Administer appropriate immunizations*

h. *Administer antibiotics if ordered*

i. *Provide verbal/written instructions to patient and significant others, including directions to*

   1) Soak wound in warm, soapy water two or three times a day for 2 to 4 days

   2) Watch for signs of infection

   3) Return or make appointment for follow-up care, if indicated

4. **Expected outcomes/evaluation** (see Appendix B)

F. Missile injuries

Missile injuries include stab wounds, gunshot wounds, and other high-pressure, penetrating wounds. Bullet wounds, especially those of high velocity, may cause bony, neurovascular, and soft tissue injuries remote from the projectile's path. Remain alert to the potential for occult neurovascular injury, especially in high-velocity injuries of the arm and leg.

Forensic considerations include appropriate reporting to law enforcement agencies, careful documentation of patient's condition with accurate description of injury, careful removal of clothing (including not cutting through areas of "evidence"), and appropriate handling and disposition of bullets and weapons.

Patients experiencing high-pressure injection injuries generally are taken immediately to surgery for debridement and extensive irrigation because serious problems result from the injected material spreading along fascial planes, neurovascular bundles, and tendon sheaths.

1. **Assessment**

a. *Subjective data*

   1) History of present condition

      a) Stab wounds

         (1) Type of instrument (e.g., knife, ice pick)

         (2) Location of wound

         (3) Estimate of length of instrument

         (4) Estimate of depth inserted

         (5) Angle of entrance

         (6) Direction of force

      b) Gunshot wounds

         (1) Location of wound

          (2) Characteristics
            (a) Movement of the bullet
            (b) Tissue characteristics (e.g., resistance, ricochet potential)
            (c) Type of weapon used
            (d) Distance of victim from weapon
            (e) Characteristics of bullet
          (3) Similar injuries
            (a) Bolt from high-powered machine
            (b) Rock thrown by lawn mower
        c) High-pressure injection wounds (paint and grease guns, staple or nail guns)
          (1) Location of wound (most commonly index finger of nondominant hand)
          (2) Amount of pressure
          (3) Type of material in gun
        d) General information
          (1) Extent of bleeding
          (2) Amount of discomfort
          (3) Time elapsed since injury
     2) Medical history
        a) Immunization status
        b) Allergies
        c) Medications
   b. *Objective data*
     1) Physical examination
        a) Stab wounds
          (1) Amount of bleeding (assess for arterial injury)
          (2) Depth, length of wound
          (3) Structures involved
          (4) Extent of necrotic tissue
          (5) Apparent wound contamination
          (6) Function of involved part
        b) Gunshot wounds
          (1) Observe lacerations (entry and exit sites)
          (2) Consider degree and extent of injury resulting from cavity formation from energy shock waves
          (3) Consider tissue and bone destruction caused by burning and expanding gases
          (4) Estimate wound depth
        c) High-pressure injection wounds
          (1) Estimate wound depth
          (2) Estimate amount of substance injected
     2) Diagnostic procedures
        a) Radiological examination for location of bullet or other objects
        b) Routine laboratory tests if patient is to be admitted to hospital
        c) If injury is associated with crime, photographs before cleaning or destroying of evidence may be indicated

2. Analysis: differential nursing diagnosis/collaborative problems
   a. *Risk for fluid volume deficit related to possible blood loss*
   b. *Impaired skin integrity related to penetration of object through skin*
   c. *Risk for infection related to open wound, contamination, and tissue damage*
   d. *Pain related to tissue damage from penetrating injury*
   e. *Anxiety/fear related to pain, treatment, outcome of injury*

  f. Knowledge deficit related to therapeutic regimen
3. **Planning/interventions**
  a. Control local bleeding
   1) Direct pressure
   2) Elevation of part
   3) Ligation of major bleeding points if other methods fail (avoid masses of ligatures)
  b. Cleanse and irrigate skin around wound with mild antiseptic solution
  c. Assist in administration of local anesthetic if wound is to be explored
  d. Assist with administration of regional anesthesia and removal of missiles that are embedded in deeper tissues or are difficult to find
  e. Assist with debriding, irrigating, removal of missile, packing, and closing procedures as needed
  f. Administer analgesia, if required
  g. Apply appropriate dressing
  h. Administer appropriate immunizations
  i. Administer antibiotic if ordered
  j. Maintain calm, efficient manner
  k. Explain all procedures in simple terms
   1) Transport patient to operating room if required
  l. Permit calm significant others to accompany patient in treatment area if appropriate
  m. Provide verbal and written instructions to patient and significant others, including directions to
   1) Elevate affected part
   2) Keep wound and dressing clean and dry
   3) Change dressing if wet or soiled
   4) Observe for redness, swelling, heat (fever), discharge
   5) Take medications, if ordered, according to directions
   6) Return or make appointment for follow-up care as indicated
4. **Expected outcomes/evaluation** (see Appendix B)

G. Human bites

  These lacerations or puncture wounds are at increased risk of infection because of the multiple organisms found in the human mouth. These injuries may be self-inflicted or may result from person-to-person contacts. Puncture wounds or deep lacerations that cannot be cleaned adequately are at particular risk of wound sepsis. Clenched-fist injuries (i.e., human bites over the metacarpophalangeal joint) typically occur during a fight and are at increased risk of joint penetration and infection.

1. **Assessment**
  a. Subjective data
   1) History of present condition
    a) Description of incident
    b) Time elapsed since injury
    c) Location of bite
    d) Extent of bleeding
    e) Amount of discomfort
   2) Medical history
    a) Immunization status
    b) Allergies
    c) Medications
  b. Objective data

1) Physical examination
   a) Size of wound
   b) Estimated depth of wound
   c) Structures involved
   d) Extent of necrotic tissue
   e) Function of involved part
2) Diagnostic procedures
   a) Saliva residue samples (swabs)
   b) Culture of wound
   c) WBC if wound infected
   d) Radiological examination if bone involvement

2. **Analysis: differential nursing diagnosis/collaborative problems**
   a. *Impaired skin integrity related to break in skin secondary to bite*
   b. *Risk for infection related to grossly contaminated open wound*
   c. *Pain related to tissue destruction and inflammatory response*
   d. *Anxiety/fear related to pain, cause of injury, treatment, and outcome*
   e. *Knowledge deficit related to therapeutic regimen and self-care*

3. **Planning/interventions**
   a. *Place affected part in position of comfort*
   b. *Consider taking photographs before cleaning if injury associated with crime*
   c. *Cleanse wound thoroughly with mild antiseptic soap*
   d. *Irrigate extensively with normal saline*
   e. *Apply topical anesthetic*
   f. *Administer injectable local anesthetic if topical anesthetic is not effective*
   g. *Assist with wound debridement, as needed*
   h. *Assist with suture placement, if required; delayed closure is preferred*
   i. *Apply appropriate dressing*
   j. *Administer appropriate immunizations*
   k. *Administer antibiotics, as ordered*
   l. *Assist in admitting patient to hospital for treatment with systemic antibiotics if wound is infected*
   m. *Maintain calm, efficient manner*
   n. *Explain all procedures in simple terms*
   o. *Permit calm significant others to accompany patient in treatment area*
   p. *Provide verbal and written instructions to patient and significant others, including directions to*
      1) Carry out specific wound care instructions based on situation
      2) Change dressings, as indicated
      3) Watch for signs of infection and other complications
      4) Take antibiotic medication, as ordered
      5) Return or schedule appointment for follow-up care

4. **Expected outcomes/evaluation** (see Appendix B)

H. Wound-related infections

Infections related to wounds of the integumentary system may be the initial problem or may occur after an injury. The common localized infections are treated in the emergency setting. Patients experiencing major systemic infections are admitted to the hospital for general support and definitive treatment. The emergency nurse's role includes intervention to assist in resolution of the infection. Prophylaxis, however, constitutes the overriding challenge.

1. **Characteristics of common wound-related infections**
   a. *Staphylococcus* infections

    1) *Staphylococcus aureus* gram-positive bacteria

    2) Associated with most skin infections

    3) Usually localized abscesses in superficial subcutaneous tissues

    4) Infection may become systemic

 b. *Pasteurellosis*

    1) *Pasteurella multocida*

    2) Necrotizing infection associated with animal bites

    3) Progresses to cellulitis, osteomyelitis, sinusitis, pleuritis

 c. *Cat-scratch fever*

    1) Unknown etiological organism

    2) Associated with cat or dog scratches

    3) Regional or local lymphadenitis, self-limiting

 d. *Wound botulism*

    1) Anaerobic *Clostridium botulinum*

    2) Associated with crush injuries or major trauma

    3) Incubation period 4 to 14 days

    4) Symptoms

      a) Weakness

      b) Blurred vision

      c) Difficulty speaking/swallowing

      d) Dry mucous membranes

      e) Dilated fixed pupils

      f) Progressive muscular paralysis

 e. *Gas gangrene*

    1) Anaerobic *Clostridium perfringens*

    2) History of intestinal or gallbladder surgery or minor trauma to old scar containing spores

    3) Incubation period 1 day to 6 weeks

    4) Symptoms

      a) Rapidly developing woody, hard edema, leading to hypoxia

      b) Thrombosis of local vessels

      c) Soft tissue crepitus (hydrogen sulfide and carbon dioxide in tissues)

      d) Severe pain

      e) Thin, watery, brown or brown-gray drainage

      f) Low-grade fever

      g) Increased pulse rate

      h) Anorexia

      i) Vomiting

      j) Diarrhea

      k) Coma

 f. *Tetanus*

    1) Anaerobic *Clostridium tetani*

    2) Organism found in soil and in human and animal intestines

    3) Entry to body through break in skin

    4) Incubation period 2 days to several months (mean, 6–14 days)

    5) Prodromal symptoms

      a) Restlessness

      b) Headache

      c) Muscle spasms

      d) Pain (initially in back, neck, or face)

      e) Low back pain

    6) Progression of disease

      a) Extreme stiffness

        b) Tonic spasms of voluntary muscles

        c) Exaggerated reflex activity

        d) Generalized convulsions

        e) Respiratory depression

   g. *Rabies*

      1) Neurotoxic virus acquired from saliva of rabid animal

      2) Major source of virus: skunks, raccoons, bats, squirrels, opossums

      3) Incubation period 10 days to several months

      4) Children younger than 12 years most susceptible

      5) Symptoms

        a) General malaise

        b) Fever

        c) Headache

        d) Lymphadenitis

        e) Photophobia

        f) Muscle spasm

        g) Coma

        h) Osteomyelitis

        i) Abscess

        j) Necrotizing fasciitis

2. Assessment

   a. *Subjective data*

      1) History of present condition

        a) Description of recent injury or wound

        b) Time elapsed since injury

        c) Reported signs and symptoms

      2) Medical history

        a) Immunization and antibiotic history related to injury

        b) Allergies

        c) Medications

        d) Chronic medical disease

   b. *Objective data*

      1) Physical examination

        a) Appearance of wound

        b) Temperature, pulse, respirations

        c) Blood pressure

        d) Presence of cardinal signs of infection

          (1) Pain

          (2) Heat

          (3) Redness

          (4) Swelling

        e) Signs and symptoms of infection related to specific organism (see section II.H.1.a–g of this chapter)

      2) Diagnostic procedures

        a) Laboratory tests including WBC

        b) C&S: aerobic and/or anaerobic

3. Analysis: differential nursing diagnosis/collaborative problems

   a. *Impaired skin integrity related to initial injury and infectious process*

   b. *Pain related to infection/inflammatory response*

   c. *Anxiety/fear related to symptoms, treatment, prognosis, outcome*

   d. *Knowledge deficit related to therapeutic regimen and self-care*

4. Planning/interventions

   a. *Provide meticulous wound care*

b. *Apply topical anesthetic, if needed*

c. *Assist with incision and drainage to relieve pressure and provide for drainage*

d. *Administer antibiotics, as ordered, if wound is severely contaminated and has potential for anaerobic infection*

e. *Administer mild analgesic, if needed*

f. *Encourage all individuals to maintain current diphtheria, pertussis, and tetanus (DPT) immunization status according to current Recommendations of the Immunization Practices Advisory Committee, Centers for Disease Control and Prevention (CDC)*

g. *Avoid overimmunization because of hypersensitivity reactions to tetanus when antibody titers are high; signs include*
   1) Rash
   2) Serum sickness
   3) Anaphylaxis

h. *Administer (at time of injury according to current Recommendations of the Immunization Practices Advisory Committee, CDC)*
   1) Tetanus-diphtheria toxoid booster for active immunity
   2) Human tetanus immune globulin (TIG), if patient not adequately immunized, to provide passive immunity for 1 month (may be repeated at end of month if needed)

i. *Institute prophylactic rabies therapy if it appears that animal causing bite may have been rabid, following CDC guidelines*
   1) Human diploid cell vaccine (HDCV) initially and on days 3, 7, 14, and 28 after exposure to provide active immunity
   2) Human rabies immune globulin (RIG) as soon as possible, one half of vaccine into and around wound site and one half intramuscularly in buttocks to achieve passive immunity
   3) If HDCV not obtainable, duck embryo vaccine (DEV) may be substituted; antirabies serum equine (ARS) may be given if RIG unavailable; skin testing must be done before administration

j. *Maintain calm, efficient manner*

k. *Explain all procedures in simple terms*

l. *Permit calm significant others to accompany patient in treatment area*

m. *Provide verbal and written instructions to patient and significant others, including directions to*
   1) Maintain adequate drainage through use of warm saline soaks
   2) Continue specific wound care measures as indicated
   3) Take mild analgesic, if needed
   4) Observe for signs of continuing infection
   5) Observe for side effects of administered vaccine
   6) Return or make an appointment for follow-up care; completion of immunization series

   5. Expected outcomes/evaluation (see Appendix B)

BIBLIOGRAPHY

Berk, W., Welch, R., & Bock, B. (1992). Controversial issues in clinical management of the simple wound. *Annals of Emergency Medicine, 21*, 72–80.

Cummings, P., & Del Beccaro, M. (1995). Antibiotics to prevent infection of simple wounds: A meta-analysis of randomized studies. *American Journal of Emergency Medicine, 13*, 396–400.

Fishbein, D., & Robinson, L. (1993). Rabies. *The New England Journal of Medicine, 329*, 1632–1638.

Newman, J. (1998). Bites and stings. In J. Howell, M. Altieri, A. Jagoda, J. Prescott, J. Scott, & T. Stair (Eds.), *Emergency medicine* (pp. 1585–1597). Philadelphia: W. B. Saunders.

Pigman, E. (1998). Wound management. In J. Howell, M. Altieri, A. Jagoda, J. Prescott, J. Scott, & T. Stair (Eds.), *Emergency medicine* (pp. 1117–1124). Philadelphia: W. B. Saunders.

Susan Engman Lazear, RN, MN, CEN, CFRN

CHAPTER **22**

Emergency Patient Transfer and Transport

MAJOR TOPICS

System Components

Components of the Emergency Medical Services (EMS) System

Medical Control

Prehospital Triage Decision Scheme

Interhospital Triage Criteria

Policies and Procedures for All Phases of Transfer

Consolidated Omnibus Budget Reconciliation Act (COBRA)

Transfer Agreements

Protocols for Treatment and Transport

Responsibility for Decision to Transfer

Mode of Transport

Transport Team Personnel

Communication

Family Members and Friends

Patient Care Components

Transport Physiology

Stabilization and Preparation for Transport

Nursing Care During Transport

Arrival at Receiving Facility

Intrafacility Transports

Sample Transfer Form

I. SYSTEM COMPONENTS

A. Components of emergency medical services (EMS) system

1. **Provision of human resources: number of health professionals with adequate training and experience to provide EMS 24 hours a day, 7 days a week**
2. **Training of personnel: training programs must be coordinated within system to provide initial certification/licensure and continuing education**
3. **Communications: system provides connections with all personnel within system and with surrounding EMS systems**
4. **Transportation: distribution of appropriate number of equipped emergency vehicles to meet needs of area**

5. **Emergency facilities:** necessary number and types of emergency department facilities with specialized inpatient services (levels I, II, and III trauma centers, burn centers, neonatal intensive care units, poison center)

6. **Critical care units:** necessary number and types of specialized units within system (trauma, newborn, cardiac, behavioral, burn, pediatric)

7. **Public safety agencies:** these provide for effective usage and sharing of public resources and personnel and disaster operating procedures

8. **Consumer participation:** goal is to involve lay persons in system components as much as possible

9. **Accessibility of care:** system must provide emergency medical care to all patients regardless of ability to pay

10. **Transfer of patients:** provisions must be made for efficient transfer of patients between emergency medical care facilities and critical care units through standing agreements and transfer protocols within particular area

11. **Standardized record keeping:** helps track patient's care from scene through final discharge; assists with evaluation of entire system

12. **Public information and education:** includes programs to educate public about goals and objectives and proper mechanisms of access and utilization of system

13. **System review and evaluation:** must provide for periodic, comprehensive review and evaluation of quality of emergency health care services provided by system

14. **Disaster planning:** coordinated approach for handling episodes where demand for EMS exceeds available resources (see Chapter 23)

15. **Mutual aid arrangements:** EMS providers and public safety agencies coordinate response of resources necessary to handle natural disaster situations and other mass casualty incidents

B. Medical control

1. **EMS medical director**

   The medical director supervises and monitors all medical aspects of the EMS system.

   a. *Ensures that protocols are medically sound*

   b. *Evaluates triage decisions and management for appropriateness*

   c. *Ensures that medication and treatments are rendered according to protocols*

2. **Off-line medical control**

   Off-line medical control includes the administrative components of medical control. It provides the framework, standards, and protocols for the system operations.

   a. *Protocols: set of policies and procedures that provide standardized approach for management of various medical conditions*

   b. *Standing orders: emergency interventions that may be performed by prehospital personnel before contacting direct medical control physician*

3. **On-line medical control**

   Supervision of patient care and treatment orders via direct voice contact to prehospital personnel from a medical control or base station hospital

   a. *Medical control communications may be delegated to mobile intensive care nurse (MICN), who has completed advanced training in system components, treatment protocols, and communication policies and procedures*

b. *A base station hospital is a fixed location that contains a transmitter and receiver with single or multiple radio channels used for communications between prehospital personnel and medical control, or it may be an associate hospital with landline connections to the base station. Resource hospital communications may also be completed using cellular phone connections*

C. Prehospital triage decision scheme

This scheme is used to assess the severity of the patient's condition and determine the available regional resources to treat the patient.

1. **Trauma categories**

    The following parameters indicate that a patient should be transported to a trauma center.

    a. *American College of Surgeons Committee on Trauma (1993)*

    1) Physiological parameters

        a) Glasgow Coma Scale (GCS) score (see Appendix C) less than 14 or
        b) Systolic blood pressure less than 90 mm Hg or
        c) Respiratory rate less than 10 or greater than 29 breaths/min or
        d) Revised trauma score less than 11 or
        e) Pediatric trauma score less than 9

    2) Anatomical parameters

        a) Penetrating injuries to head, neck, torso, and extremities proximal to elbow and knee
        b) Flail chest
        c) Combination of trauma with burns over 10% of body or inhalation injuries
        d) Two or more proximal long bone fractures
        e) Pelvic fractures
        f) Limb paralysis
        g) Amputation proximal to wrist and ankle

    3) Mechanism of injury

        a) Ejection from automobile
        b) Death in same passenger compartment: associated fatality
        c) Extrication time more than 20 minutes
        d) Falls from heights of more than 20 feet
        e) Vehicle rollover
        f) High-speed automobile crash
        g) Automobile-pedestrian injury with significant (> 5 mph) impact
        h) Pedestrian thrown or run over
        i) Motorcycle crash occurring at speed greater than 20 mph or with separation of rider and bike

    4) Historical information

        a) Age less than 5 or more than 55 years
        b) Known cardiac or respiratory disease
        c) Diabetic patient taking insulin; patient with cirrhosis, malignancy, obesity, or coagulopathy
        d) Pregnancy

2. **Nontrauma categories**

    These categories are based on a match between the patient's care requirements and the facility's ability to provide care. These may include psychiatric, pediatric, neurological, cardiac, neonatal, spinal cord, or burn cases in which the patients require specialized care centers.

D. Interhospital triage criteria

1. **American College of Surgeons Committee on Trauma (1993) recommends using the following guidelines for transferring trauma patients to higher level of optimal care**
   a. *Central nervous system injury*
      1) Head injury
         a) Penetrating injury or depressed skull fracture
         b) Open injury with or without cerebrospinal fluid leak
         c) GCS score less than 13 or GCS deterioration
         d) Lateralizing signs
      2) Spinal cord injury
   b. *Chest injury*
      1) Widened mediastinum
      2) Major chest wall injury
      3) Cardiac injury
      4) Patients requiring protracted ventilation
   c. *Pelvic injury*
      1) Unstable pelvic ring disruption
      2) Pelvic ring disruption with shock and evidence of hemorrhage
      3) Open pelvic injury
   d. *Multiple system injury*
      1) Severe facial injury with head injury
      2) Chest injury with head injury
      3) Abdominal or pelvic injury with head injury
      4) Burns with associated injuries
      5) Multiple fractures
   e. *Evidence of high-energy impact*
      1) Automobile crash or pedestrian injury: velocity greater than 25 mph
      2) Rearward displacement of front axle or front of car (20 inches)
      3) Ejection of patient or vehicle rollover
      4) Death of occupant in same car: associated fatality
   f. *Comorbid factors*
      1) Age less than 5 years or more than 55 years
      2) Known cardiorespiratory or metabolic diseases
   g. *Secondary deterioration*
      1) Mechanical ventilation required
      2) Sepsis
      3) Single- or multiple-organ system failure (deterioration in central nervous, cardiac, pulmonary, hepatic, renal, or coagulation system)
      4) Major tissue necrosis

E. Policies and procedures for all phases of transfer

1. **Patients to be transferred**
2. **Medical authority regarding transfer (i.e., who decides)**
3. **Most appropriate facility for specific needs: not closest facility**
4. **Appropriate mode of transport**
5. **Personnel and equipment to accompany patient**
6. **Protocols or standing orders for transport personnel**
7. **How to arrange transfer and transportation**
8. **How family and friends are to be included in transfer**
9. **Forms used before, during, and after transfer**

10. Records to be sent with patient
11. Documentation during transport
12. Special circumstances: vehicle breakdown, long detours, patient deterioration, death
13. Financial responsibility

F. Emergency Medical Treatment and Active Labor Act (EMTALA) (see Chapter 24, Legal Issues)

G. Transfer agreements

1. Formalized between referring and receiving facilities
2. Developed cooperatively
3. Include transport service

H. Protocols for treatment and transport

1. Established in cooperation with receiving facility
2. Based on facility category, capabilities and limitations of staff, and patient's needs
3. Special situations
   a. Burns
   b. Head injury
   c. Spinal injury
   d. Multiple system trauma
   e. Limb avulsion
   f. Infants and children
   g. Psychiatric emergencies
   h. Cardiovascular emergencies
   i. Obstetric-gynecological emergencies
   j. Respiratory emergencies
   k. Snake bites
   l. Transport of prisoners
   m. Combative or violent patients
   n. Administration of blood products

I. Responsibility for decision to transfer

1. Emergency department physician
2. Private attending physician
3. Surgeon
4. Referring physician has responsibility for patient during transfer and transport; however, transfer/transport may be collaborative effort between referring/receiving physicians regarding preparation of patient and care en route to tertiary facility

J. Mode of transport

1. Options
   a. Ground ambulance
      1) Basic life support (BLS): level of care involving noninvasive life support measures

        a) Cardiopulmonary resuscitation (CPR)

        b) Use of pneumatic antishock garment (PASG)

        c) Basic airway management and hemorrhage control

        d) Childbirth

        e) Extrication skills

    2) Advanced life support (ALS): level of care involving techniques, invasive skills, and medications to support life to the critically ill or injured adult, child, or infant

        a) Advanced airway maneuvers: use of bag-valve-mask devices and intubation

        b) Intravenous (IV) catheter placement

        c) Cardiac dysrhythmia recognition

        d) Cardiac defibrillation and cardioversion

        e) Drug therapy

  b. Air ambulance

    1) Rotary wing (helicopter): usually less than 150 miles; ability to provide field response, including scene management and extrication skills; unpressurized cabin generally not compromising to patient because altitude gains are not significant

    2) Fixed wing (propeller or jet): usually more than 150 miles; may provide state-to-state or international patient transfer; most airplanes used in air transport are pressurized, thus limiting effects of altitude on patient; if unpressurized aircraft is used, risk of patient compromise increases greatly

2. Major considerations for choosing type of transport

  a. Patient care requirements

    1) Urgent need for rapid access to definitive care

  b. Patient's potential response or contraindications

    1) Air transport

        a) Patient may be fearful of flying

        b) Combative or violent patients are hazardous, and flight crew may opt to abort mission or transport

        c) Stresses in flight: see section II.A. Transport Physiology

  c. "Out-of-hospital" transit time: air transport time is approximately half that of ground transport for same distance; ground transport time may be increased by heavy traffic or poor road conditions

  d. Work space required versus work space available: the more complex the patient's condition and medical care required, the more personnel and equipment are needed

    1) Air transport: may be limited to two care providers; restricted access to patient; some equipment may not fit in vehicle treatment space (e.g., traction, splints)

    2) Ground transport: room for additional care providers, access to all parts of patient, space for extra and/or large equipment

  e. Personnel qualifications

    1) BLS versus ALS skills

    2) Crew configuration: registered nurse (RN)-physician, RN/respiratory therapist, RN/paramedic, etc.

  f. Necessary equipment available

  g. Weather conditions

  h. Terrain and/or road conditions

  i. Need to transport family member

K. Transport team personnel

1. **Must be qualified to continue advanced level of assessment and intervention initiated at referring facility**
2. **Must be qualified to perform additional advanced interventions as needed during transport**
3. **Team member options**
   a. *Physician*
   b. *Emergency nurse*
   c. *Flight nurse*
   d. *Adult/pediatric/neonatal intensive care nurse*
   e. *Respiratory therapist*
   f. *Paramedic*
   g. *Emergency medical technician (EMT)*
   h. *First responder*
   i. *Others to assist, as needed*

L. Communication

1. **Before transport**
   a. *Referring physician to receiving physician*
      1) Patient identification
      2) History of incident
      3) Initial findings, procedures, treatments
      4) Estimated time of departure and arrival
   b. *Primary nurse to receiving charge nurse*
   c. *Referring facility administrator to receiving facility administrator, as needed*
   d. *Referring and/or receiving physician to transferring personnel*
      1) Airway and ventilatory maintenance
      2) Volume replacement and management
      3) Special procedures
      4) Transfer orders
2. **During transport**
   a. *Contact from vehicle or aircraft to sending and/or receiving facility*
   b. *Third-party relay contact if direct contact is not possible*
3. **After transport**
   a. *Follow-up report from transport team to referring physician*
   b. *Follow-up report from receiving physician, nurse, facility to referring facility*
   c. *Combined medical audits to identify deficits in care*
   d. *Educational resources to remove deficits in care*
   e. *Interfacility-interdisciplinary conference to redesign system or problem solve*
   f. *Ongoing monitoring process to evaluate effectiveness of system*

M. Family members and friends

1. **Crisis intervention: involve chaplain, social worker, and psychiatric personnel in care when possible**
2. **Need explanation of condition and reason for transfer**
3. **Obtain consent for transfer as necessary**
4. **Not responsible for arranging emergency transfer**
5. **Remain at initial facility until patient leaves**
6. **Need opportunity for brief interaction with patient before departure**

7. Maps and written directions to receiving facility and parking area are helpful
8. Family members who accompany patient in transport must be oriented to transport vehicle, safety procedures, and so forth; family members must be instructed as to what they can and cannot do during transport in regard to patient management

II. PATIENT CARE COMPONENTS

A. Transport physiology

1. **Complications that occur in transport are dependent on**
   a. *Motion of transport vehicle*
   b. *Changes in atmospheric conditions (generally problematic in air transport)*
   c. *Vehicle design and configuration*
   d. *Patient condition before transport*
   e. *Combination of one or more of these problems*

2. **Hypoxia**
   a. *Four types: hypoxic hypoxia, histotoxic hypoxia, anemic hypoxia, and stagnant hypoxia (note: patient may have one or more types)*
   b. *Hypoxic hypoxia: occurs with ascent of air transport vehicle; as altitude increases, available oxygen decreases secondary to decreased partial pressure of oxygen (greatest concern in unpressurized airplanes)*
   c. *Histotoxic hypoxia: occurs when available hemoglobin is bound by chemicals other than oxygen (e.g., carbon monoxide poisoning and cyanide poisoning)*
   d. *Anemic hypoxia: occurs when there is inadequate amount of circulating hemoglobin (e.g., hemorrhagic shock, anemia) (note: oxygen saturation does not accurately reflect level of hypoxia)*
   e. *Stagnant hypoxia: occurs secondary to inadequate circulation of oxygen-saturated hemoglobin (e.g., low-flow states, low cardiac output states, hypovolemic shock states)*

3. **Gas expansion**
   a. *Occurs with ascent of the air transport vehicle, based on Boyle's law, which states that volume of gas increases as pressure decreases*
   b. *Example: 100 mL of gas at sea level will expand to*
       130 mL at 6000 feet
       200 mL at 18,000 feet
       400 mL at 34,000 feet
   c. *Free air will expand, potentially compromising patient's condition (Table 22–1)*

4. **Dehydration**
   a. *Occurs with increase in altitude as well as in pressurized airplane cabin*
   b. *Causes drying of respiratory secretions and enhances evaporative losses in diaphoretic patient*

5. **Temperature changes**
   a. *Temperature drops are caused by increases in altitude*
   b. *Additionally, patient is exposed to multiple changes in environmental conditions throughout duration of transport*
   c. *Temperature changes also impact gas expansion: with temperature increases, gas expands; for example, air inside air splints will expand when the patient is transported from cold outside air into warm emergency department, leading to enhanced risk of compromised circulatory response*

6. **Acceleration and deceleration forces**

Table 22–1   EFFECTS OF GAS EXPANSION AT ALTITUDE*

Location of Gas	Effects	Consequence	Intervention
Pneumothorax	Size ↑	Worsening respiratory effort	Decompress before transport
GI tract	Peristalsis ↑	GI motility ↑	Monitor patient
	Pressure on diaphragm ↑	Worsening respiratory effort	NG tube to suction
Open head injury	Risk of herniation ↑	Worsening neurological status	Position to decrease ICP
Air splints, PASG	Pressure on limbs ↑	Circulation to affected area ↓	Decrease pressure at altitude
ETT cuff	Cuff pressure ↑	Tracheal damage	Decrease pressure at altitude
Gas gangrene	Rupture of gas bubbles	Exacerbation of disease process	Incise and drain before transport

GI, gastrointestinal; ET, endotracheal; PASG, pneumatic antishock garment; NG, nasogastric; ICP, intracranial pressure; ↑, increased; ↓, decreased.

*Any intervention undertaken during transport must be reversed when altitude is decreasing (i.e., pressure in ETT cuff must be increased on descent).

     a. Acceleration forces occur during aircraft take-off and climb-out as well in ground ambulance, which is increasing in speed

     b. Deceleration forces occur during slowing, stopping, descent, and landing

     c. Acceleration and deceleration forces produce momentary changes in hemodynamic status of patient

     d. Effects of acceleration and deceleration forces on patient are dependent on speed and angle of force, duration, and patient's individual tolerance

  7. Prolonged immobilization

     a. Transported patients need to be safely secured to transport stretcher, requiring multiple belts and securing devices to prevent free movement of extremities, etc; immobilization is established early during patient's course and may continue until all potential injuries are ruled out; thus, duration of immobilization is much greater than that of transport itself

  8. Motion sickness

     a. Occurs secondary to changes in inner ear equilibrium

     b. Enhanced by hypoxia, foul odors, turbulence, stress and fear, heat, excessive visual stimuli, poor diet as well as gastric gas expansion

  9. Noise and vibration

     a. Inherent in transport vehicle secondary to design

     b. Produce irritability, changes in vital signs that are difficult to distinguish as being changes secondary to worsening patient condition or secondary to excessive input

  10. Stabilization measures before transport can reduce and/or eliminate many of these consequences

B. Stabilization and preparation before interfacility transport within capabilities of staff and facilities

  1. Patent airway support with simultaneous cervical spine (C-spine) precautions

     a. Positioning

     b. Artificial airway

       1) Oropharyngeal-nasopharyngeal

       2) Endotracheal tube (ETT)

     c. Suction

    d. Stomach decompression with nasogastric or orogastric tube, unless contraindicated

  2. Breathing support
    a. Positioning
    b. Bag-valve-mask device, as needed
    c. Supplemental oxygen
    d. Mechanical ventilation, as needed
    e. Decompression of pneumothorax or hemothorax
      1) Needle thoracostomy
      2) Chest tube insertion (Heimlich valve may be used to prevent re-expansion of pneumothorax with inadvertent disconnection of water-seal drainage set)

  3. Circulatory support
    a. Control external bleeding
    b. Two IV catheters with large-bore catheters
    c. Fluid replacement with crystalloid and/or blood products
      1) Pack blood products in ice for transport, and monitor time outside of blood bank (recommend use of blood within 1 hour)
    d. Monitor cardiac rhythm
    e. Indwelling catheter to monitor urinary output: drain urinary collection bag before transport

  4. Spine precautions
    a. Long backboard
    b. Special immobilization of head and neck
      1) Cervical immobilization device
      2) Towel rolls and tape or lateral immobilization device
      3) Cervical traction devices
        a) Use with caution: acceleration and deceleration forces during transport tend to swing free-hanging weights, altering tension of traction and possibly injuring occupants in vehicle; locking pulley systems are preferred
        b) Rotational stability of neck should be controlled even if long traction is applied; may be done by placing towel rolls or stabilization devices along each side of head and neck and securing to stretcher with tape

  5. Splinting of injured extremities
    a. Posterior gutter
    b. Plaster: casts should not be circumferential unless bivalved before fixed-wing transport
    c. Traction: devices may be large and bulky; anticipate problems in transport vehicles with limited working space
    d. Pneumatic antishock garment (PASG)
    e. Preserve access to distal pulse for monitoring
    f. Use air splints with caution; contraindicated for air transport secondary to gas expansion

  6. Wound care
    a. Critical life-threatening problems have priority for care
    b. Control bleeding
    c. Limited initial cleansing
    d. Sterile dressing
    e. Tetanus prophylaxis and antibiotics, when indicated
    f. Burn wounds
      1) No topical ointment or ice applied before transfer
      2) Follow local burn center protocols

3) Prevent hypothermia: cover patient with warm blankets, apply heat packs and warming lights as needed

7. **Psychosocial responses of patient**
   a. *Fear, anxiety, anger, grief*
   b. *Continuously provide patient (and family) with information*
      1) What happened: details of accident or illness
      2) What is currently happening: step-by-step description of events
      3) What to expect next: plans for treatment and procedures
   c. *Interpret sounds, voices, procedures for patient as needed*
   d. *Allow patient to see family and significant others*

8. **Baseline diagnostic studies**
   a. *Radiographs*
      1) Chest: repeat chest radiograph for ETT placement, if indicated
      2) C-spine: Ensure visualization of seven cervical vertebrae before transport
      3) Pelvis
      4) Suspicious extremities
      5) Other, as indicated
   b. *Laboratory studies*
      1) Hemoglobin (Hgb)
      2) Hematocrit (Hct)
      3) Electrolytes
      4) Arterial blood gases (ABGs)
      5) Urinalysis (UA)
      6) Urinary chorionic gonadotropin (UCG), as indicated
      7) Ethanol (ETOH) and drug of abuse urine screen
   c. *Electrocardiogram (ECG)*

9. **Documentation to accompany patient**
   a. *Patient identification: arm band*
   b. *Prehospital care record*
   c. *Initial facility record*
   d. *Radiographs and other studies*
   e. *Valuables: location and list of items*
   f. *Transfer record (Fig. 22–1)*
      1) Patient demographic data, including next of kin
      2) History of illness/mechanism of injury
      3) Patient condition on admission
      4) Diagnostic impressions
      5) Results of diagnostic studies
      6) Treatments rendered
      7) Status of patient at time of transfer
      8) Management during transport
      9) Name and telephone number of referring physician
      10) Receiving physician and facility
      11) Transfer orders
   g. *Emphasis on initial assessment, treatment rendered, and responses to treatment*
   h. *Consent for transfer and/or surgery (see Chapter 24)*

C. Nursing care required during transport

1. **Age and developmental differences may require varying assessment and intervention skills**
   a. *Pediatric population*

(Addressograph stamp)

All Sections Must Be Completed Prior To Transfer

1. **Physicial Certification.** The undersigned physician has examined and evaluated.

_____
Patient's Name

(Check One)

( ) *Nonmedical Nonrequested Transfer*
On the basis of this examination and the information available to me at this time, I have concluded as of the time of the transfer, within reasonable medical probability, that the transfer or delay caused by the transfer will not create a material deterioration in or jeopardize the patient's medical condition or expected chances for recovery of the patient or, if pregnant, the patient's unborn child.

( ) *Requested Transfer*
Patient or (when unable or incompetent) the patient's legal representative requests the transfer.

( ) *Medical Transfer*
On the basis of this examination and the information available to me at this time, I have concluded that the medical benefits reasonably expected from the provision of appropriate medical treatment at the other medical facility outweigh the increased risk, if any, to the patient and, if pregnant, to the patient's unborn child from effecting the transfer. A summary of the risks and benefits of transfer is as follows:

_____

_____

The reasons for my conclusion are *(check all appropriate)*:

( ) The patient's vital signs are stable.
( ) The patient's condition is not immediately life threatening.
( ) The patient is safe for transport with appropriate intratransport monitoring.
( ) For a pregnant woman who presented in contractions, delivery of the infant has occurred, including the placenta.

( ) Other: _____

I also certify that I have been informed by the receiving facility that it has available space and qualified personnel for the treatment of the patient, that the receiving facility has agreed to accept transfer and to provide appropriate medical treatment, and that the patient will be transferred by qualified personnel and transportation as required, including the use of necessary and medically appropriate life support.

Transferring physician name: _____

Transferring physician office address: _____

Receiving facility: _____

Receiving facility physician consenting to transfer: _____

Date and time of consent (of receiving physician): _____

Name of any on-call physician who failed to appear within a reasonable time and therefore necessitated the transfer: _____

Mode of transport and attendant: _____
(e.g., paramedic unit, EMT unit, Lifeflight)

Updated Status of Patient's Condition *(to be completed 15 minutes prior to transfer)*

Transfer date: _____   Transfer time: _____

Copy of applicable medical records included: Yes No   If not, why: _____

Vital signs: BP: _____   P: _____   RR: _____   T: _____

Patient condition: ( ) Stable   ( ) Satisfactory to transfer now

_____   _____
Attending physician   Date   Other treating physician   Date

FIGURE 22–1. Emergency department transfer form.

EMERGENCY DEPARTMENT
TRANSFER SUMMARY
(Page 2)

(Addressograph stamp)

1. **Patient Acknowledgment.** I understand that I have a right to receive medical screening, examination, and evaluation by a physician, or other appropriate personnel, without regard to my ability to pay, prior to any transfer from this hospital and that I have a right to be informed of the reasons for any transfer from this hospital. I acknowledge that I have received medical screening, examination, and evaluation by a physician, or by the appropriate personnel, and that I am being transferred for the following reasons:

(   )   A special care unit is required that is not available at this hospital (e.g., burn unit). Specify: _____

(   )   The HMO/prepaid health plan in which I am enrolled contracts for health care services at the receiving institution.

(   )   I am a medically indigent adult. I understand that my primary provider of medical care is the county hospital of _____ County, where I reside.

(   )   I (or my representative) have requested the transfer. I acknowledge that I have been informed of the risks and consequences of the transfer, this hospital's obligations to provide emergency services and care, the possible benefits of continuing treatment at this hospital, and the alternatives (if any) to the transfer I am requesting. I hereby release the attending physicians involved in my (the patient's) care, this hospital and its physicians, agents, and employees from all responsibility for any ill effects that may result from the transfer or delay involved in the transfer.

(   )   Other reason: _____

_____
Date

_____
Time

_____
Witness

_____
Patient or legal representative

_____
Relationship if other than patient

(   )   Patient not available because of mental or physical condition, and no patient representative available.

Should you have any complaints concerning the services you have received from the hospital, you may contact:

Department of Health Services
Licensing and Certification

FIGURE 22–1. *Continued*

1) Security comes from parents: allow parents to stay with patient when possible
2) If parents not allowed to ride in transport vehicle, allow them to explain their travel arrangements and plans to patient
3) Allow child to carry a toy during transport
4) Speak clearly and slowly: children may become anxious and fearful from loud and excited movements and voices
5) Be honest in providing explanations of care; explain every procedure step by step
6) Reassure child that you are there to help, not hurt
7) Respect feelings of modesty, especially with school-aged children and adolescents

   b. Geriatric population

     1) Consider deterioration of senses: vision, hearing, touch, and thermoregulation

       a) Provide direct eye contact in clear line of vision

b) Speak loudly, clearly, and slowly; phrase questions simply, avoid medical jargon

c) Touch patient gently but firmly to reinforce verbal communication

d) Elderly people experience poor tolerance to cold; prevent hypothermia

2) Information and sensory overload, short-term memory losses, and delay in information processing may contribute to acute confusion

3) Underlying medical problems may affect responses to treatment

2. **Assessment**

a. *Noise and vibration levels require extensive use of sight and touch*

b. *Airway and breathing: observe and feel quality and symmetry of chest wall expansion, use portable pulse oximeter to monitor oxygen saturation*

c. *Circulation: palpate pulses, determine blood pressure, observe skin moisture, observe color, use Doppler to assess pulse quality and blood pressure*

d. *Portable electronic monitoring of heart rate and rhythm*

e. *Direct observation of urine output: volume and color*

f. *Stimulation of patient and observation of response in relation to level of consciousness*

3. **Interventions**

a. *Maintain airway and ventilatory support with supplemental oxygen, bag-valve-mask device, or mechanical ventilation*

b. *Maintain cardiac output with volume replacement*

c. *Administer medications or procedures as indicated by established protocols or as ordered by physician*

d. *Prevent hypothermia with warm environment, blankets, fluids*

e. *Maintain control in coordinating movement of patient into and out of facilities and transport vehicle*

f. *Provide for safety of transport crew members*

g. *Provide safety precautions for patient by applying safety straps and securing transport equipment*

h. *Institute measures to prevent problems in transport (see section II.A. Transport Physiology)*

4. **Evaluation: monitor patient responses for signs of improvement or deterioration**

5. **Documentation: maintain accurate records of transport events; document responses to transport stressors**

D. Arrival at receiving facility

1. **Accompany patient into facility, providing interventions as needed**
2. **Provide receiving team with verbal report and documentation listed previously**
3. **Close interactions with patient**
4. **Speak to family or friends if they have arrived**
5. **Notify referring facility and patient family (as appropriate) of safe arrival of patient at receiving facility**
6. **Collect equipment used for transport**
7. **Close interactions with receiving facility staff**

E. Intrafacility transports

Intrafacility transport of patients requires the same preplanning and organization as interfacility transports. The stresses of transport are greatly reduced; many previously discussed stressors occur only in out-of-hospital situations. Much of the same battery-operated, lightweight portable equipment can be used to ease transition of the patient from one location to another. Additional equipment, medications, and so on should be readily available if time in transport exceeds expectations.

1. **Airway support**
   a. *Airway management equipment should accompany patient at all times*
   b. *Suction equipment should be present and functional*
2. **Ventilatory support**
   a. *Supplemental oxygen should be continued or readily available for patient not currently on supplemental oxygen therapy*
   b. *Pulse oximetry can be used to monitor trends in oxygen saturation*
3. **Circulatory support**
   a. *Adequate volume should accompany patient to replace all completed IV fluids*
   b. *Cardiac monitoring should be considered using portable monitor*
4. **Support equipment and personnel**
   a. *Other equipment that may accompany patient includes medications and infusion devices*
   b. *Critically ill or injured patients must not be left unattended with personnel not trained in ALS measures; nurses caring for patient should remain with patient until appropriately trained personnel can accept patient transfer of care*

F. Sample transfer form: see Figure 22–1

REFERENCES

American College of Surgeons Committee on Trauma. (1993). *Resources for optimal care of the injured patient.* Chicago: American College of Surgeons.

American College of Surgeons Committee on Trauma. (1998). *Advanced trauma life support for doctors.* Chicago: American College of Surgeons.

Cardona, V. D., Hurn, P. D., Bastnagel Mason, P. J., Scanlon, A. M., & Veise-Berry, S. W. (1994). *Trauma nursing: From resuscitation through rehabilitation* (2nd ed.). Philadelphia: W. B. Saunders.

Emergency Nurses Association. (1996). *Standards of emergency nursing practice* (4th ed.). St. Louis, MO: C. V. Mosby-Year Book.

Emergency Nurses Association. (1998). *Sheehy's emergency nursing principles and practice* (4th ed.). St. Louis, MO: C. V. Mosby.

Jaimovich, D. G., & Vidyasagar, D. (1996). *Handbook of pediatric and neonatal transport medicine.* Philadelphia: Hanley & Belfus.

McCloskey, K. A., & Orr, R. A. (1995). *Pediatric transport medicine.* St. Louis, MO: C. V. Mosby.

National Flight Nurses Association. (1995). *Standards of practice for flight nurses* (2nd ed.). St. Louis, MO: C. V. Mosby.

National Flight Nurses Association. (1996). *Flight nursing: Principles and practice* (2nd ed.). St. Louis, MO: C. V. Mosby.

National Flight Nurses Association. (1997). *Core curriculum for flight nurses.*

Jorie Klein, RN

CHAPTER **23**

Disaster Preparedness/Disaster Management

MAJOR TOPICS

Emergency Preparedness:
Assessment

Emergency Preparedness: Disaster
Plan

Emergency Disaster Response

Weapons of Mass Destruction:
Nuclear, Biological, Chemical

Testing or Exercising Disaster
Preparedness

Emergency nurses have a responsibility to take an active role in disaster preparedness and disaster management. A disaster is defined as a situation or event, natural or manmade, that overwhelms a community's or institution's ability to respond with existing resources. Disasters produce human death, suffering, and changes in the community environment affected. Understanding the emergency medical system (EMS) response at the local, state, and federal levels and the potential for military interfacing is part of disaster preparedness. The following outline provides a framework that the emergency nurse can use to evaluate the disaster preparedness plan as well as the training required to address injuries or the human impact of such events, allocate needed resources existing in their facility, and provide an organized approach in a chaotic disaster environment.

I. EMERGENCY PREPAREDNESS: ASSESSMENT

A. Definition of disaster: community

1. **Any situation, natural or manmade, that overwhelms community's ability to respond with existing resources**
2. **Three-tier classification**
   a. *Multiple-patient incident*
      1) Event resulting in fewer than 10 casualties (usually single-hospital response)
      2) Common
   b. *Multiple-casualty incident*
      1) Results in 100 or fewer casualties (single- or multiple-hospital response)

      2) Strains but does not overwhelm existing health care facilities

      3) Occurs less commonly

      4) Occurs in mass transportation and natural events such as floods, tornadoes, hurricanes, snowstorms, fires

      5) Occurs in manmade environmental events such as radiation or biological contamination, hostage, or terrorist events

   c. *Mass casualty incident*

      1) Results in more than 100 casualties (multiple-hospital response)

      2) Significantly overwhelms existing health care facility/facilities

      3) Occurs with major earthquakes, volcanic eruptions, structural failures, fires in densely populated areas, certain hazardous materials, radiation, chemical, or biological contamination

      4) Occurs least commonly

      5) Causes greatest amount of deaths, injuries, and property damage

B. Definition of disaster: institutional

1. **Any situation that results in health care facility becoming partially or totally inoperable**

   a. *Partial or total evacuation required*

   b. *Physical plant sustains damage so severe that occupancy is unsafe*

C. Disaster response assessment

1. **Loss of life**

   a. *Probable number of victims in surrounding communities that may be affected*

   b. *Expectations for morgue facilities*

2. **Physical injuries**

   a. *Index of injury severity*

   b. *Determines volume and types of supplies to have on hand*

   c. *Defines triage resource needs*

3. **Psychological trauma**

   a. *Plan for staff critical incident stress management*

   b. *Care for "walking wounded"*

   c. *Care for families and bystanders*

4. **Property damage**

   a. *Health care facility itself*

   b. *Structural, nonstructural, and vital equipment*

   c. *Communication capabilities*

5. **Environmental destruction**

   a. *Contamination from hazardous substances*

   b. *Impact on health care resources*

   c. *Impact on community's water, electrical power, waste processing, or other utility service*

   d. *Transportation*

6. **Economic/business loss**

   a. *Loss of income during response and recovery phase of incident*

   b. *Cost of recovery of information and data systems*

   c. *Cost of supplies/equipment used to respond*

   d. *Cost of staff overtime, special resources*

D. Internal disaster situation

1. **Hospital/clinic facility's structure and routine operations impaired**

2. May be caused by fire, earthquake, storm, explosion, terrorist activity, radiation, chemical spill, flood, and so forth
3. Loss of electrical power or loss of oxygen source may require evacuation of existing inpatients because of structural damage or resource interruption (e.g., power, oxygen, water)
4. May require outside providers to respond to facility

E. External disaster situation

1. Takes place external to facility but may impair routine operations
2. Requires activation of facility's disaster plan to either receive casualties or to evacuate patients
3. May require evacuation of existing inpatients to provide resources for incoming disaster casualties
4. May be caused by earthquake, flood, hurricane, tornado, explosion, transportation catastrophes, hostage or terrorist action, chemical spill, and so forth

II. EMERGENCY PREPAREDNESS DISASTER PLAN

A. Essential elements

1. Organized disaster/safety management committee
2. Elements
   a. *Authority, system for activation of disaster response*
   b. *Pre-established hospital operation centers per policy*
   c. *Communication*
   d. *Coordination of patient care*
   e. *Security*
   f. *Aftermath*
      1) Deactivation of disaster response
      2) Return to normal patient flow
      3) Critique of disaster response
      4) Critical incident stress management/intervention

B. Disaster command center (DCC) (Fig. 23–1)

1. Responsible for disaster decision making, organization, and communication flow
2. Location
   a. *Consider physical setup needs when choosing location, such as space for defined staff, adequate communication (television monitor, radios, telephones, data lines), wall space communication boards, rest rooms, adequate electrical outlets, back-up generator power*
   b. *Alternative or secondary location for the DCC should be identified if primary site is not accessible*
   c. *Choose location convenient to emergency department (ED)*
3. DCC staffing
   a. *Disaster medical director*
   b. *Chief executive officer (CEO)/designee*
   c. *Community/public relations representative*
   d. *Representatives for each defined operations centers (emergency, operating room [OR], nursing, administration, personnel, security)*

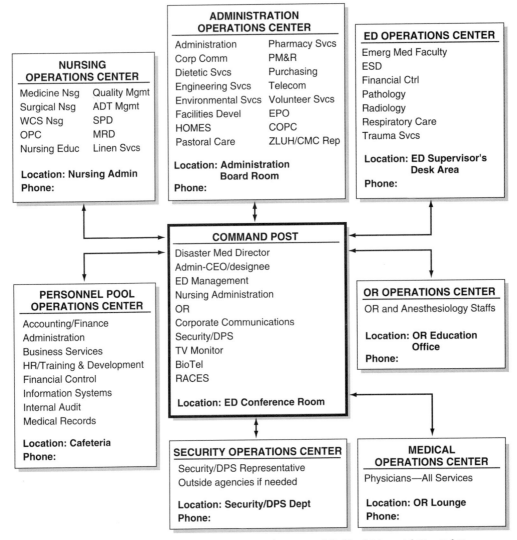

FIGURE 23–1. Possible disaster command center structure. (Courtesy of Parkland Memorial Hospital Emergency Services Department, Dallas, TX.)

  e. Safety management representative
  f. Liaisons or runners for operations centers
  g. Secretarial or clerical assistants
 4. Responsibilities for each DCC member include decision making for respective operations center and will be variable, depending on nature of disaster
 5. Communications
  a. Voice and data lines
  b. Color-tagged telephone lines (direct to operations centers)
  c. Two-way radios (DCC to triage, ED, OR)
  d. Amateur radio capability
  e. Television monitor
  f. Computer lines

    g. Fax machines

6. **Authority**

    a. Notification and deactivation of disaster plan

    b. Initiation of evacuation

    c. Limiting or expanding disaster response

    d. Media response and interview scheduling

    e. Implementing specialty plans or resources

    f. Overall coordination of care provided, interaction and integration with other facilities

7. **DCC supplies**

    a. DCC resource guide for staff member

    b. Flashlights with batteries

    c. Emergency telephone lists (home, car, beepers, cellular telephones, vendors, community resources)

    d. Telephone books, facility and community

    e. Hand-held radios with chargers

    f. Map of region

    g. Floor plan of hospital

    h. Erasable write-on board, bulletin board

    i. Marking pens for board

    j. Pens

    k. Fax machine, computer or CRT terminals, printer access, paper

    l. Public radio, television, or amateur radio capability suggested

    m. Internal departmental disaster response plans

    n. Disaster plan synopsis for quick reference

C. Administrative operations center (AOC)

1. **Location in administrative suite (hospital may combine with DCC)**
2. **Coordination by CEO**
3. **Coordinates facility or resource needs such as water, food, waste, medications**
4. **Coordinates media release and interviews**
5. **Coordinates release of information to families**
6. **Coordinates telephone response for casualties' families and responding agencies**
7. **Coordinates response with affiliated facilities and agencies**
8. **Coordinates with clinic and community response**
9. **Coordinates inspection of facility for structural damage, utility interruption**
10. **Communicates all findings to DCC for updates related to**

    a. Administrative staff

    b. Dietary

    c. Engineering

    d. Patient services (translators, social workers, case managers)

    e. Pharmacy

    f. Materiel management and purchasing

    g. Telecommunications

    h. Volunteer services

    i. Pastoral care

    j. Community relations

    k. Rehabilitation

D. Medical operations center

1. Located in designated area
2. Coordinated by the chief of medical staff/designee
3. Coordinates physician response and allocation of physician resources in ED, OR, intensive care unit (ICU), and patient care units for patient follow-through and discharge planning
4. Coordinates specialty services response and needs
5. Number of physicians notified and requested to respond is dependent on type of event

E. Nursing operations center

1. Located in nursing administration suite (may be combined with DCC)
2. Coordinated by nursing administration
3. Coordinates the housewide nursing response
4. Ensures appropriate nursing and staff mix ratios for inpatient units
5. Ensures competency of nurses assigned to specialty areas
6. Coordinates patient discharges, bed availability, and patient needs
7. Participating or communicating staff
   a. *Medicine services*
   b. *Surgical services*
   c. *Women and children services*
   d. *Outpatient clinic*
   e. *Nursing education*
   f. *Quality management*

F. OR operations center

1. Located in designated OR such as a conference room
2. Coordinated by chief of anesthesiology and nursing director/manager
3. Coordinates OR utilization, room assignments, and room turnover
4. Coordinates staff resource needs
5. Coordinates diagnostic resource needs
6. Participating staff
   a. *OR management*
   b. *Anesthesiology*
   c. *OR nurse educator*
   d. *Environmental services*
   e. *OR triage officer (re-evaluates and defines priority of surgical intervention)*

G. Personnel operations center

1. Located in specified area of the hospital such as cafeteria
2. Coordinated by assigned manager
3. Coordinates assignments and staffing for loggers, runners, non-nursing and unassigned staff

H. Security operations center

1. Located in security office
2. Coordinated by chief of security
3. Centralizes all security activities

   4. Secures transportation access to hospital to prevent street jams
   5. Secures defined areas for access and entry (e.g., medical control, helipad, ED, OR)
   6. Coordinates outside police agency activities
   7. Ensures overall safety in facility
   8. Limits media access to patient treatment areas

I. ED operations center

   1. Located in or near ED
   2. Coordinated by nursing manager/director and medical director or designee
   3. Coordinates ED patient triage, communication, resource utilization, acquisition of specialty resources, and patient management
   4. Coordinates initial data management and patient tracking
   5. Participating staff
      a. *Chaplain*
      b. *Radiology*
      c. *Pathology*
      d. *Respiratory services*

III. EMERGENCY DISASTER RESPONSE

A. Confirm disaster activation response

   1. Notification from administration or EMS medical control
   2. Nature of disaster, location
   3. Potential number of casualties, potential injury, human impact
   4. Lead responding agency
   5. Estimated time of patient arrival
   6. Disaster equipment supplies
   7. Disaster packets

B. ED operations center

   1. Assignments of on-duty supervisor
      a. *Notify ED management staff*
      b. *Initiate staff notification*
      c. *Ensure prompt notification of support services*
      d. *Establish ED disaster operations center*
   2. Staff assignments
      a. *ED ambulance dock or alternate site for triage of patients*
      b. *Disaster casualty registration/loggers*
      c. *Helipad for triage of patients arriving by helicopter*
      d. *Charge nurse for treatment areas*
      e. *Physicians in charge of treatment areas*
      f. *Staff pool coordinator*
      g. *Security screening of arriving personnel*
      h. *Temporary morgue*
   3. Evacuation of patients from ED
      a. *Assess less acute current ED patients for retriage to designated area*
         1) Treatment areas

        2) Waiting room

        3) Record patients retriaged

        4) Coordinate movement with appropriate papers, medical record

    b. Admitted patients

        1) Notify receiving floor

        2) Notify family

        3) Coordinate patient transfer

    c. Discharge patients

    d. Organize remaining patients

        1) Cluster patients to facilitate assignment of staff and physicians

        2) Allocate needed resources

        3) Facilitate dispositions

        4) Evacuate family

4. Secure environment

    a. Screen responding staff

    b. ED badge required for ED access

    c. Media to designated area

    d. Casualty families to defined area

    e. Responding hospital staff to designated area

5. ED staffing considerations

    a. Responding staff to ED staff pool area

    b. Staffing needs for incoming shift

    c. Payroll documentation

    d. Assignments

6. Communication

    a. Communication with EMS/medical control

    b. Charge nurse assesses area and assignments for staffing, equipment, supply, and resource needs by radio

    c. All requests for additional resources are routed to ED operations center

    d. ED operations center notifies DCC by radio, phone, computer, or runner, if not together

C. Disaster casualty patient coordination

1. Triage through ED ambulance dock or helipad

2. Acuity assessment

    a. Immediate (emergent)

    b. Delayed (urgent or nonurgent)

3. Alternate assessment triage categories

    a. Red: critical

    b. Yellow: urgent

    c. Green: walking wounded

    d. Black: dead, imminent death

4. Assignment of disaster number and packet

    a. Patient identification (ID) tagged on entry with area assignment and acuity assessment

    b. Prenumbered packet used for ID, charting in patient care areas

        1) Disaster patient care chart

        2) Prenumbered laboratory, radiology requisitions

5. Registration log (Fig. 23–2)

6. Treatment area assigned for evaluation

7. All documentation on disaster packet

PARKLAND MEMORIAL HOSPITAL

Dallas County Hospital District
Emergency Services Department

DISASTER REGISTRATION LOG

(To be Completed by Registration Clerk at Patient's Point of Entry)

TIME	DISASTER #	HOW ARRIVED	RACE	SEX M	SEX F	CHILD	ADULT	AREA TRIAGED	CARE IMMEDIATE	CARE DELAYED	REMARKS	FINAL DISPOSITION
		DFD-Dallas Fire Dept. OA-Other Ambulance H-Helicopter P-Private	B-Black H-Hispanic W-White O-Other					M-Medicine S-Surgery				*NOTE Secretary #2 will enter final disposition utilizing disaster log information.

This form will be banded with five disaster packets and coinciding disaster numbers and case numbers. When complete, the registrar will give to the runner and it will be sent to the triage desk nurse, then the Emergency Department Operations Center.

- **DELIVER TO TRIAGE DESK NURSE (ORIGINAL)**
- **DELIVER TO ESD OPERATIONS CENTER (COPY)**

(DISASTER REGISTER - pg. 26)
ESD STAFF

FIGURE 23–2. Disaster registration log. (Courtesy of Parkland Memorial Hospital Emergency Services Department, Dallas, TX.)

8. Tracking by disaster number, registration loggers in defined areas (e.g., radiology, morgue)
9. Family interventions by chaplain or designated staff
10. Admission or discharge by disaster number
11. Tracking by ED operations center
12. ED operations center notifies DCC, if not together

D. Data management

1. Registration logs
2. Disaster number and disaster packet
3. Treatment area room assignment
4. Area registration loggers
5. Computer program
6. ED operations center forwards information to DCC

E. Stress management

1. Stress reducers
   a. *Five-minute breaks every hour*
   b. *Rotate front-line, critical care personnel with arriving staff, if possible*
2. Assess staff during breaks or rounds
   a. *Shaking, trembling*
   b. *Loss of coordination*
   c. *Visual difficulties*
   d. *Respiratory difficulties*
   e. *Confusion, disorientation*
3. Signs of excessive stress
   a. *Relieve immediately*
   b. *Provide immediate supportive counseling*
   c. *Refer for critical incident stress management, post-traumatic stress evaluation*
4. Educate staff regarding delayed stress reaction
   a. *Provide handout with referral numbers*
   b. *Signs and symptoms*
      1) Feelings of loss, grief, guilt
      2) Wanting to fix blame
      3) Withdrawal from social/coworker contact
      4) Irritability
      5) Denial of feelings
      6) Difficulty in concentrating, mild confusion, difficulty in remembering
      7) Visual flashbacks
      8) Cannot stop talking about it
      9) Sleep disturbances, nightmares
      10) Mild nausea
      11) Decreased sexual interest
      12) Decreased appetite
      13) Constant fatigue
      14) Concern over coworkers who change negatively
      15) Use of alcohol/drugs

Table 23–1   PHASES OF CRITICAL INCIDENT STRESS DEBRIEFING

Phase	Description
Initial	Introduction of confidentiality; debriefing the team
Fact	Helps individuals find out the facts; everyone is encouraged to talk
Thought	Expression of personal feelings related to the incident; speaking is voluntary
Reaction	Discussion of the worst part of the incident
Symptom	Discuss possible unresolved emotional issues from past incidents; participants are observed for possible follow-up needs with mental health providers
Teaching	Stress reduction and communication techniques
Re-entry	Final questions are answered; debriefing is complete

    5. **Schedule debriefing sessions for all staff** (Table 23–1)

F. Ongoing needs

    1. **Refer all media inquiries to designated area**
    2. **Coordination of supplies and equipment**
    3. **Secured access to ED**
    4. **Access for ED nondisaster patients**
    5. **Tracking of patients**
    6. **Communication**

G. Deactivation

    1. **All casualties evacuated from scene; be advised that even though "scene" may be clear, hospital may still be in midst of disaster response and still receive patients**
    2. **Activities returning to normal operations**
    3. **Support resources meeting demand**
    4. **Staff-patient ratio exceeds need**
    5. **Institutional needs assessment**
    6. **Communicate findings to DCC**
    7. **DCC initiates internal deactivation**
    8. **Staff pool dismisses staff**

H. Critique

    1. **ED operations center review: what worked, what needs improvement?**
    2. **ED staff: what worked, what needs improvement?**
    3. **Communication: what worked, what needs improvement?**
    4. **Security: what worked, what needs improvement?**
    5. **Patient management: what worked, what needs improvement?**
    6. **Patient tracking**
    7. **Deactivation**
    8. **Coordination with DCC**
    9. **Schedule department critique to gain staff input**
    10. **Participation in institutional critique**
    11. **Participation in EMS/System–wide critique**

I. Revisions of disaster plan

IV. WEAPONS OF MASS DESTRUCTION AND EFFECT: NUCLEAR, BIOLOGICAL, CHEMICAL

A. Overview

1. **Activation of disaster notification and response**
2. **Identification of route, exposure, specific agent, dose, or concentration, population at risk**
3. **Phases of management**
   a. *Decontamination*
   b. *Assessment*
   c. *Treatment*
4. **Specific ED entrance with decontamination capabilities**
5. **Personal protective equipment**
   a. *Disposable gown (may not be adequate)*
   b. *Mask*
   c. *Head covering*
   d. *Eye protection*
   e. *Butyl rubber or fluorelastomer (Viton) gloves*
   f. *Shoe coverings*
   g. *Respiratory protection*
6. **Assessment after field decontamination**
7. **Special precautions for patient's bodily secretions/airborne spread for certain pathogens (plague)**
8. **Admission to decontamination room**
9. **Life-threatening situation assessment**
   a. *Primary survey/resuscitation*
      1) Airway patency
      2) Breathing
         a) Rate
         b) Effort, symmetry
         c) Lung sounds
      3) Circulation
         a) Cardiac rate, rhythm
         b) Signs of shock
         c) Life-threatening injuries
   b. *Secondary survey: complete secondary survey necessary for all exposed patients to identify signs of injury occurring during exposure*
10. **Psychological, social, and environmental factors**
11. **Focused survey**
    a. *History of exposure*
       1) Specific nature of exposure
       2) Route of exposure
          a) Estimated amount of exposure
          b) Duration of exposure
          c) Prehospital decontamination and care
    b. *Presence of distinct symptoms related to specific exposure*
    c. *Medical history*
       1) Illness and injury
       2) Medication
       3) Allergies
       4) Pre-exposure health status
    d. *Ongoing evaluation*
       1) Vital signs (in most instances, contamination does not cause change; if change occurs, assess for other injuries or illnesses)

    2) Respiratory status

        a) Increase or change in respiratory effort

        b) Peak flow

    3) Cardiovascular changes: organic solvents may cause cardiac arrest

    4) Neurological changes

        a) Altered mental status

        b) If organic solvent exposure: depression, euphoria, disorientation, and confusion

    5) Dermatological factors

        a) Open or closed wounds

        b) Skin absorption factors: state of hydration of skin; skin temperature; pH; presence of surfactants; degree to which substance directly disturbs skin integrity; and evidence of frostbite (potential exists with exposure to liquid and compressed gases)

    6) Diagnostic procedures

        a) Laboratory

            (1) Complete blood count (CBC) with differential leukocyte count

            (2) Arterial blood gas (ABG) (initial and repeated with inhalation exposure)

            (3) Urine toxin screen

            (4) Blood toxin screen

            (5) Liver function tests (for exposure to organic solvents)

            (6) Oxyhemoglobin level (for carbon monoxide exposure)

            (7) Pulse oximetry

        b) Chest radiograph (primarily for inhalation injury)

        c) Electrocardiogram (ECG)

e. *Provide further decontamination as needed*

    1) Remove all jewelry as well as clothing

    2) Save all effects in appropriate receptacle

    3) Save all irrigation run-off and bodily fluids in appropriate self-contained receptacles

f. *For contact exposure, clean skin with soap and water*

    1) Start with cool water, proceed to warm (to prevent further skin absorption)

    2) Pay special attention to nail beds, hair, and skinfolds

    3) Avoid further contamination of open wounds

    4) Avoid vigorous scrubbing to prevent further breakdown of skin integrity

    5) Irrigate open wounds with copious amounts of water

g. *Treat ocular exposure*

    1) Irrigate with copious amounts (1 L minimum) of water or saline solution

    2) Note that any pulmonary irritant is also likely to be eye irritant

h. *Treat ingestion*

    1) Emesis as appropriate; contraindications include

        a) Petroleum distillates

        b) Organic solvents

        c) Pulmonary irritants

    2) Nasogastric lavage with or without activated charcoal and cathartics

i. *Keep patient quiet*

j. *Maintain normal body temperature*

k. *Assess continuously for delayed effects to specific toxin*

l. *Encourage patient to verbalize fears*

    1) Address anxiety-provoking concern

2) Inform and educate patient/significant others regarding immediate plan of care (emergent phase)
   m. *Medicate for pain as appropriate*
   n. *Treat specific sources of pain*
   o. *Coordinate room cleanup and decontamination with environmental services and engineering*

B. Radiation exposure

1. **Activation of disaster notification and response**
2. **Incidents commonly industrial**
3. **Varies in nature and severity**
   a. *Depends on dose*
   b. *Measure of rad (radiation absorbed dose)*
   c. *Dose rate*
   d. *Dose distribution*
   e. *Individual susceptibility*
4. **Symptoms of nausea, vomiting, or bloody diarrhea within 3 hours are indications of a significant dose**
5. **The higher the dose, the earlier the onset**
6. **Clinical phases of radioactive contamination**
   a. *Prodome*
   b. *Latent phase*
   c. *Manifest illness*
   d. *Recovery*
7. **ED responses**
   a. *Type of radiation incident*
   b. *Number and condition of causalities*
   c. *Name of isotopes involved*
   d. *Expected time of arrival*
   e. *Radiation incident team responsibilities*
      1) Emergency physician responsible for medical evaluation
      2) Radiation safety officer coordinates decontamination
      3) Decontamination responsibilities
         a) Floor of route to decontamination room protected with paper floor covering
         b) Secure with 2-inch masking tape, rope off area, place radioactive marking
         c) Nonessential equipment removal or protection with plastic covering
         d) Light switches and handles on cabinet and doors protected by masking tape
         e) Establish buffer zone around decontamination area
         f) Preparation of stretcher, decontamination tub
         g) Preparation of containers with plastic bags for receiving contaminated disposable supplies
         h) Disaster supply cart
         i) Geiger counter monitor in buffer zone for monitoring all personnel, equipment, samples, crossing at clean line
         j) Evaluate Geiger counter's battery and background radiation before patient's arrival
         k) Geiger counter protection with plastic bag
         l) Evaluation of ventilation system by radiation officer
8. **Control point**

     a. Second portable cart for backup supplies

     b. Larger plastic lined barrel for contaminated supplies/waste

  9. Security monitors restricted areas

     a. Referral of family members to identified waiting area

     b. Referral of media to designated area

10. Decontamination team preparation

     a. Film badge with name

     b. Full surgical dress

       1) Surgical trousers and top

       2) Surgical hood

       3) Waterproof shoe covers

       4) Surgical gown

       5) Surgical gloves (secure with tape to sleeves and cuffs to show covers)

       6) Second pair of surgical gloves (not taped to facilitate washing or changing if contaminated)

       7) Surgical mask, eye protection

       8) Penlight

11. Circulating nurse assists evaluating physician

12. Control nurse monitors buffer zone

13. Monitoring nurse

     a. Vital signs

     b. Collecting specimens

       1) Laboratory: blood work, urinalysis, etc

       2) Swabbing of contaminated area

14. Radiation safety officer

     a. Assigns person for control point monitoring

     b. Monitors prehospital providers, pathway from ambulance, patient, and ED personnel

     c. Decontaminates with nursing staff

     d. Analyzes all specimens taken of potentially contaminated area

     e. Disposes of any contaminated item or water

     f. Examines all film badges/dosimeters and coordinates follow-up

15. Patient arrival

     a. Decontamination stretcher at entrance

     b. Evaluation by ED physician and radiation officer in ambulance

     c. Removal of all clothing

     d. Decontamination stretcher receives contaminated patient from ambulance

     e. Assessment of ambulance, supplies, prehospital providers for contamination by radiation officer

16. Planning/interventions

     a. Priorities of care

       1) Treatment of life-threatening emergencies according to specific exposure

       2) Decontamination

       3) Fluid management

       4) Pain management

     b. Primary intervention: ensure airway, breathing, and circulation

     c. Decontamination

       1) Remove any remaining patient clothing and jewelry

       2) Place in sealed container marked "radioactive waste"

       3) Clean skin with soap and water

       4) Repeat until dosimeter readings are acceptable

     d. Clean open wounds first: irrigate with copious amounts of water, remembering to prevent contamination of surrounding body surface area e. Irrigate contaminated eyes with water from medial aspect outward

    f. Irrigate contaminated ear canals gently with small amounts of water to prevent vertigo

    g. Rinse contaminated nares or mouth gently with small amounts of water, turning patient's head to side and suctioning frequently; do not allow patient to swallow water

    h. Suction stomach contents with nasogastric tube and monitor ingestion of contaminant

    i. Administer analgesia for pain

    j. Encourage patient to verbalize fears

    k. Inform and educate patient or significant others regarding immediate plan of care (emergency phase)

    l. Continuation of care/specific to illness or injury

C. Chemical exposure (Table 23–2)

    1. Industrial incident

    2. Terrorist incident

    3. Preparedness

        a. Recognition of agent

        b. Patient decontamination

        c. Patient management and transport

    4. Routine industrial chemicals

        a. Phosgene

        b. Cyanide

        c. Anhydrous ammonia

        d. Chlorine

    5. Vesicants

        a. Mustard

        b. Lewisite

        c. Phosgene oxime

    6. Riot control agents

        a. Tear gas

        b. Mace

        c. Pepper spray

    7. Personal protective equipment

        a. Atmospheric contamination

            1) Air-purifying respirator for removal of contaminants

            2) Clothing protection for liquid and vapor

        b. Chemicals or substance with potential inhalation hazard

            1) Full liquid and vapor protective clothing, hood

            2) Supplied air respirator (SAR)

            3) Necessary for hospital personnel for decontamination of chemical exposure

        c. Hot zone chemical release, air concentrations that are immediately dangerous to life and health

            1) Self-contained breathing apparatus

            2) Clothing fully encapsulated

            3) Resistant to liquid and vapor

            4) Risk

                a) Claustrophobia

                b) Heat stress

Table 23-2   EXAMPLES OF INHALED CHEMICALS KNOWN TO CAUSE PULMONARY INJURY

Chemical	Sources of Exposure	Injury Produced
Acetaldehyde	Plastics, synthetic rubber industry	Primarily upper airway Rarely causes delayed pulmonary edema Also a central nervous system depressant
Acrolein	Plastics, textiles, and pharmaceuticals manufacturing	Diffuse airway and parenchyma
Ammonia	Fertilizer, chemical, and pharmaceutical manufacturing, refrigeration, and oil refining	Primarily upper airway burn; occasionally causes bronchiectasis
Anhydrides	Chemical, paint, and plastics industries; components of epoxy resins	Rhinitis, airway injury, asthma, pulmonary hemorrhage after high-dose exposure
Antimony trichloride, antimony pentachloride	Steel industry, organic catalysts	Pulmonary edema
Boranes	Aircraft fuel, welding, fungicide	Airway injury, pulmonary edema after high-concentration exposure
Bromine (hydrogen bromide)	Petroleum refining, chemical industry (as a catalyst)	Upper airway injury, rare pulmonary edema
Cadmium	Electroplating, paint and pesticide manufacturing, cutting plated metals	Diffuse airway and lung injury, renal injury, lung carcinogen
Chlorine	Chemical industry, transportation accidents, gas evolved from mixing chlorine bleach with acid cleaners, swimming pools	Diffuse airway and lung injury
Chromium	Alloy production, chrome plating, welding chromium-containing metals	Asthma, diffuse airway injury, lung carcinogen
Cobalt	Metal alloy manufacture, especially tungsten carbide, catalyst	Acute inhalation can cause pulmonary edema, chronic exposure may cause interstitial fibrosis
Copper sulfate	Vineyard sprayers	Patchy pneumonitis
Hydrochloric acid	Fires, welding, rubber manufacturing, and metal refining	Upper airway injury
Hydrogen fluoride	Etching, welding, metal refining	Primarily upper airway, rarely causes pulmonary edema
Isocyanates	Polyurethane production, paints, varnishes, roofing, bathtub refinishing	Asthma, diffuse airway injury, hypersensitivity pneumonitis
Lithium hydride	Rocket fuel, chemical industry, nuclear power plants	Pulmonary edema
Manganese dioxide	Chemical battery manufacturing	Parenchyma injury
Methyl bromide	Refrigeration, produce fumigation	Diffuse airway and lung injury Also causes central nervous system depression and seizures
Nickel carbonyl	Metal alloys, electroplating, welding	Pulmonary edema; also causes headache, nausea, and vomiting
Nitrogen dioxide	Grain silos, mining fires, missile fuels	Airway injury, bronchiolitis obliterans, pulmonary edema
Osmium	Metal, chemical industries	Upper airway injury
Ozone	Welding, high-altitude aircraft cabins, paper bleaching	Airway injury, pulmonary edema at high concentrations

Table continued on following page

Table 23–2   EXAMPLES OF INHALED CHEMICALS KNOWN TO CAUSE PULMONARY INJURY Continued

Chemical	Sources of Exposure	Injury Produced
Polyvinyl chloride	Plastics, meat wrapping	Asthma, pulmonary fibrosis
Phosgene	Welding, chemical industry, paint removal	Pulmonary edema
Phosphine	Welding, chemical industry	Pulmonary edema
Selenium hydrochloride	Metal industry, paint, glass production	Airway injury
Sulfur dioxide	Smelters, pulp mills, wineries, oil refineries, power plants	Bronchoconstriction, mucus secretion; airway injury at high concentration
Titanium tetrachloride	Dyes, pigments, sky writing	Upper airway injury
Trichloroethane	Waterproofing sprays	Probable airway injury
Zinc chloride	Taxidermy, oil refining, galvanizing iron	Pulmonary edema

Adapted from Murray, J. F., & Nadel, J. A. (1988). *Textbook of respiratory medicine.* Philadelphia: W. B. Saunders (pp. 1636–1637). Used with permission.

8. **Decontamination**
   a. *Mechanical removal*
   b. *Absorption*
   c. *Degradation*
   d. *Dilution*
      1) Most applicable to hospital environment
      2) Showering with large quantities of water dilutes agent
      3) Reduces patient's skin contamination load
      4) Need collection system for irrigating water for prevention of further decontamination
      5) Portable showers outside facility
9. **Response team**
   a. *Emergency physician*
   b. *Toxicologist*
   c. *ED nurses*
   d. *Respiratory therapist*
   e. *Pulmonologist*
   f. *Disaster medical director*
   g. *Safety officer*
10. **Formal training**
    a. *Agent recognition*
    b. *Patient decontamination*
    c. *Antidote therapy*
    d. *Personal protective equipment*
11. **Specific agents**
    a. *Nerve agents*
       1) Tabun
       2) Sarin
       3) Soman
       4) VX
       5) Initial diagnosis by clinical signs and symptoms, confirmation by laboratory findings
       6) Symptoms
          a) Increased saliva

       b) Tearing

       c) Runny nose

       d) Secretions in airway

       e) Secretions in gastrointestinal tract

       f) Sweating

       g) Fasciculation

       h) Twitching

       i) Weakness

       j) Flaccid paralysis

       k) Tachycardia or bradycardia

       l) Hypertension or hypotension

       m) Loss of consciousness

       n) Seizures

       o) Apnea

       p) Psychological effects

  7) Treatment

       a) Self-protection

       b) Decontamination

       c) Atropine (intravenous [IV], intramuscular, endotracheal tube)

       d) Airway/ventilation

          (1) Endotracheal intubation with positive-pressure ventilation

          (2) Frequent suctioning

          (3) Repetitive atropine dosages until shortness of breath (SOB) resolves, and secretions and airway resistance are reduced to tolerable levels.

       e) Pralidoxime chloride (2-PAMCl)

          (1) Administration must be within 4 to 6 hours for sarin exposure and within 60 hours after VX exposure

          (2) Mark 1 kit (atropine and pralidoxime chloride autoinjector kit, military usage)

       f) Diazepam or other benzodiazepines for seizure activity and control

b. *Cyanide*

  1) Types

       a) Hydrogen cyanide

       b) Cyanogen chloride

       c) Cyanide salts

  2) Acute cyanide poisoning symptoms (nonlethal)

       a) Anxiety, hyperventilation, headache, dizziness, vomiting, loss of consciousness

       b) Flushed or cherry-red skin

  3) Clinical improvements with agent removal

c. *Cyanide toxicity*

  1) Symptoms

       a) Respiratory distress

       b) Metabolic acidosis

       c) Concentrated serum cyanide levels

  2) High concentration

       a) 15 seconds: hyperpnea

       b) 30 seconds: seizures

       c) 3 to 5 minutes: breathing ceases

       d) 5 to 10 minutes—asystole, death

  3) Treatment

       a) Amyl nitrite

  b) Sodium nitrite
  c) Sodium thiosulfate (cofactor for enzyme rhodanese for detoxification)
   (1) Oxygen, hyperventilate, IV sodium bicarbonate, IV fluids
   (2) Monitor for arrhythmias
 d. *Phosgene*
  1) Characteristic odor of freshly mowed lawn or hay
  2) Hazard by inhalation, carbonyl group
  3) Signs and symptoms
   a) Irritation of eyes, nose, throat, upper airway, and bronchi
   b) Dry cough
   c) Shortness of breath as result of alveolocapillary damage
   d) Hypoxia and apnea
  4) Treatment
   a) Intubation and positive end-expiratory pressure (PEEP), oxygen
   b) Gentle hydration
   c) Bronchodilators
 e. *Chlorine*
  1) Significant irritant to eyes and respiratory tract
  2) Characteristic pungent odor
  3) Signs and symptoms
   a) Eye irritation, cough, SOB, wheezing
   b) Within 12 to 24 hours, noncardiogenic pulmonary edema
   c) Sudden death resulting from hypoxia
  4) Treatment
   a) Remove from source
   b) Initiate management for airway, breathing, and circulation
   c) Decontaminate
   d) Flush skin and eyes with copious water
   e) Oxygen, cool mist, bronchodilators
   f) Intubate, PEEP
   g) Hydration
 f. *Ammonia*
  1) Colorless, highly water-soluble, alkaline gas with pungent odor
  2) Rapidly absorbed by mucosal surfaces
  3) pH less than 12 (household ammonia): limited damage
  4) pH greater than 12 (anhydrous ammonia): severe damage
  5) Corrosive when combined with water: liquefactive necrosis
  6) Signs and symptoms
   a) Burning, tearing, severe eye pain with potential injury to cornea and lens
   b) Cough, SOB, chest pain, wheezing, laryngitis with mild exposure
   c) Blister formation, pain, deep burns to skin
   d) Nausea, vomiting, abdominal pain
   e) Edema to lips and mouth with potential airway obstruction
   f) Esophageal strictures and perforations
  7) Treatment
   a) Removal from exposure
   b) Decontaminate
   c) Irrigate eyes, slit-lamp examination with fluorescein
 g. *Vesicants*
  1) Sulfur mustard (vapor inhalation or liquid contact)
   a) Causes signs and symptoms of cellular damage

(1) Injury to eyes, skin, airway, and internal organs

(2) Delayed reaction

(3) Death resulting from airway injury, sepsis caused by impaired immune system

b) Onset time of 1 to 2 minutes; clinical effects do not begin for hours

c) Decontamination

(1) Physical removal of all clothing, jewelry

(2) Soap, water, or 1/10 solution of household bleach

(3) Flush with copious water

(4) Cellular damage begins within 2 minutes of exposure

(5) Decontamination produces no change in clinical course but prevents cross-contamination of providers

d) Treatment

(1) Silver sulfadiazine (Silvadene) for blisters

(2) Oral or intravenous pain medication

(3) Fluid management

(4) Irrigation of eyes

(5) Severe upper airway involvement

(a) Intubation and positive-pressure and expiratory pressure or continuous positive airway pressure

(b) Bronchodilators

(6) No antidote

2) Lewisite

a) Symptoms of vesicant similar to those associated with sulfur mustard

(1) Significant irritation with initial exposure

(2) Quickly produces visible lesions

b) Treatment

(1) Decontamination with hypochlorite (bleach) or soap and water

(2) Antidote: British anti-Lewisite

h. *Riot control agents (tear gas)*

1) Eye, nose mouth, skin, and respiratory tract irritant

2) Transient effect (usually 30 minutes)

3) Treatment

a) Irrigation of eyes, removal of contact lenses

b) Bronchodilators for wheezing

c) Oxygen therapy

D. Biological agents

1. **Occur naturally in environment**
2. **Some toxins or bacteria may be employed as biological weapons**
3. **Agents may be more deadly on a per weight basis than chemical agents (botulinum toxins)**
4. **Types of biological agents**
   a. *Bacteria: anthrax, plague, tularemia*
   b. *Viruses: smallpox, Venezuelan equine encephalitis (VEE), viral hemorrhagic fever (VHF), Ebola, and so forth*
   c. *Toxins: botulinum toxin, ricin, staphylococcal enterotoxin B (SEB), and so forth*
5. **Primary route of infection or "portal of entry" by inhalation, high disease-infection ratio**
6. **Modes of dissemination**

a. *Industrial sprayers*
b. *Aerosol generator*
c. *Airplane or boat traveling upwind*

7. **Meteorological constraints**
   a. *Sunlight*
   b. *Wind*
   c. *Temperature*
   d. *Desiccation*

8. **Potential impact of biological contamination**
   a. *Widespread illness and death*
   b. *Extensive and prolonged need for medical services*
   c. *Possibility of quarantine*

9. **Bacterial exposure**
   a. *Bacteria*
      1) *Bacillus anthracis*
      2) Plague
      3) Tularemia
   b. *Anthrax: Bacillus anthracis, gram-positive, rod-shaped organism*
      1) Symptoms begin within 1 to 6 days of exposure; toxins produce edema and tissue necrosis
      2) Early symptoms: fever, muscle aches, cough, malaise, chest discomfort
      3) Symptoms may seem to improve, then severe respiratory distress, shock, and death follow
      4) Treatment
         a) Universal precautions
         b) Ciprofloxacin and/or
         c) Doxycycline
         d) Oral prophylaxis
         e) Treatment usually fails once severe symptoms develop
   c. *Plague:* Yersinia pestis, *gram-negative, rod-shaped organism*
      1) Common infection in rodents
      2) Symptoms: fever, chills, headache, cough, bloody sputum
      3) Plague treatment
         a) Respiratory isolation, universal precautions
         b) Prophylaxis administration of tetracycline or doxycycline in exposed persons with close contact
         c) Antibiotics must be administered within 24 hours of symptoms
         d) Plague pneumonia treated with streptomycin, doxycycline, ciprofloxicin
         e) Plague meningitis treated with chloramphenicol
      4) Supportive care
      5) Vaccine for preventing bubonic plague; not effective against aerosol exposure
   d. *Tularemia:* Francisella tularensis, *gram-negative coccobacillus*
      1) Signs and symptoms
         a) Abrupt onset of fever, chills, headache, myalgias, swollen lymph nodes, nonproductive cough, and pneumonia within 2 to 10 days of exposure
         b) Ingestion produces painful, tender regional lymphadenopathy with or without skin ulcers
      2) Tularemia treatment
         a) Universal precautions
         b) Antibiotic therapy for 10 days with streptomycin
         c) Prophylaxis with tetracycline or doxycycline

E. Viral agents

1. **Examples of viruses**
   a. Smallpox
   b. Venezuelan equine encephalomyelitis (VEE)
   c. Viral hemorrhagic fever (VHF)
2. **General characteristics**
   a. Ribonucleic acid (RNA) or deoxyribonucleic acid (DNA) within protein coat
   b. Require a host
   c. May attack specific cell types
3. **Signs and symptoms**
   a. Onset 7–17 days
   b. Muscle pain
   c. Fever
   d. Vomiting
   e. Headache
   f. Backache
   g. Rash
4. **Treatment**
   a. Quarantine
   b. Supportive
   c. Vaccine
   d. Immune globulin
   e. No approved antiviral medication
5. **Venezuelan equine encephalomyelitis**
   a. Alphavirus spread by mosquitoes (may be aerosolized as a weapon)
   b. Endemic to Central and South America, Mexico, and Florida
   c. Signs and symptoms
      1) Onset, 1–5 days
      2) Fever, severe headache, fatigue, "encephalitis" symptoms
      3) Mortality may be higher with aerosol
      4) VEE treatment
         a) Supportive
         b) No antiviral available
6. **Viral hemorrhagic fever**
   a. Acute febrile illness with increased vascular permeability
   b. Viruses
      1) Ebola
      2) Marburg
      3) Dengue
      4) Yellow fever
      5) Crimean-Congo hemorrhagic fever
      6) Hantavirus
      7) Lassa and others
   c. Signs and symptoms
      1) Early: fever, myalgias, prostration
      2) Exacerbation: shock; generalized mucous membrane hemorrhage; involvement of respiratory, hematopoietic, and central nervous systems; conjunctival infection, petechial hemorrhage
      3) Abnormal renal and liver function test; multiple organ system involvement and failure
      4) Poor prognosis
      5) Treatment
         a) Universal precautions or isolation; respiratory protection if copious bleeding/coughing
         b) Supportive ICU monitoring

   c) Comfort measures
   d) Blood replacement
   e) Ribavirin (not effective against Ebola or Marburg)

F. Toxin agents

1. Toxins
   a. Botulinum
   b. Ricin
   c. Staphylococcal enterotoxins

2. Botulinum
   a. Neurotoxin (7 similar toxins)
   b. Blocks release of acetylcholine (ACh) at three places in presynaptic terminal of neuromuscular junction and receptors in the autonomic nervous system
   c. Similar effects whether inhaled or ingested
   d. Signs and symptoms
      1) Dry mouth, difficulty swallowing
      2) Blurred vision, diplopia
      3) Skeletal muscle weakness, starting on upper body and moving downward, cranial nerve palsy
      4) Progression to acute respiratory failure in 24 hours to 2 days
   e. Treatment
      1) Supportive: long-term ventilation
      2) Antitoxin administration as early as possible
      3) Vaccine: investigational (prevents disease)

3. Ricin
   a. Potent toxin: byproduct of castor bean processing blocks protein synthesis within the cell
   b. Signs and symptoms
      1) Onset 8 to 24 hours, cough, dyspnea in aerosol exposure
      2) Airway necrosis and edema leading to death in aerosol exposure
      3) Nausea, vomiting, severe diarrhea, gastric hemorrhage, necrosis of the liver, spleen, kidney in gastrointestinal exposure
      4) Injection produces marked muscular necrosis and multiple-organ failure
   c. Treatment
      1) Supportive: oxygenation and hydration
      2) No antitoxin or vaccine currently available
      3) Activated charcoal lavage after ingestion

4. Staphylococcal enterotoxins
   a. Signs and symptoms
      1) Sudden onset of high fever, headache, and chills in aerosol exposure
      2) Severe SOB, chest pain with larger doses
      3) Nausea, vomiting, diarrhea, mild to severe in gastrointestinal exposure
   b. Treatment
      1) Supportive: oxygenation and hydration
      2) Ventilatory support

V. TESTING OR EXERCISING DISASTER PREPAREDNESS

A. Philosophy of disaster preparedness and training must be developed and adopted

B. Realistic acceptance of potential for natural or manmade events

C. Disaster preparedness philosophy and training for

1. Administration
2. Nursing staff
3. Medical staff
4. ED staff
5. Support departments
6. Security
7. Facilities management

D. Types of exercise

1. Major exercise
   a. *Entire facility/staff*
   b. *Community resources*
   c. *Victims/volunteers*
   d. *EMS and other public agencies*
   e. *News media*
   f. *Multiple hospitals*

E. Disaster drill event

1. Defined goals of practice
2. Two drills or actual events per year/Joint Commission on Accreditation of Healthcare Organizations (JCAHO) requirement (one with patients)
3. All participants involved in critique
4. Realistic

F. Disaster drill planning principles

1. Purpose of drill
2. Defined goals and objectives
3. Assignments, responsibilities, timelines
4. Structure: staged or free flowing
5. Critique

BIBLIOGRAPHY

Boffard, K. K., & MacFarlane, C. (1993). Urban bomb blast injuries: Patterns of injury and treatment. *Annals of Surgery, 25*(1), 29–47.

Borowitz, J. L., Kanthasamy, A. K., & Isom, G. E. (1992). Toxicodynamics of cyanide. In S. Somani (Ed.), *Chemical warfare agents* (pp. 209–236). San Diego: Academic Press.

Bourg, P., Sherer, C., & Rosen, P. (1986). Surface trauma: Radioactive contamination. In P. Bourg, C. Sherer, & P. Rosen (Eds.), *Standardized nursing care plans for emergency departments* (pp. 277–281). St. Louis, MO: C. V. Mosby.

Brackett, D. (1996). *Holy terror, Armageddon in Tokyo.* New York: Weatherhill.

Cole, L. (1996). The specter of biological weapons. *Scientific American, 275,* 60–65.

Cooper, C. J., et al. (1983). Casualties of terrorist bombings. *Journal of Trauma, 23,* 955–967.

Defense Protective Service, Pentagon. (1996). *10–90*

gold NBC response plan: Procedures and support activities developed by the Defense Protective Service for response to a nuclear, biological, or chemical incident within DPS jurisdiction. Washington, DC: Pentagon.

Dinerman, N. (1990). Disaster preparedness: Observations and perspectives. *Journal of Emergency Nursing, 16,* 4.

Federal Emergency Management Agency. (1989). *Nonstructural earthquake hazard mitigation for hospitals and other health care facilities.* Washington, DC: FEMA.

Gans, L., & Kennedy, T. (1996). Management of unique clinical entities in disaster medicine. *Emergency Medical Clinics of North America, 14,* 301–326.

Gross, P. L., Weber-Bornstein, N., Castronovo, F. P., & Baker, A. S. (1989). Environmental hazards. In E. W. Wilkins, J. J. Dineen, P. L. Gross, C. J. McCabe, A. C. Moncure, & P. J. O'Malley (Eds.), *Emergency medicine scientific foundations and current practice* (3rd ed., pp. 186–196). Baltimore: Williams & Wilkins.

Hafen, B. Q., & Karren, J. J. (1989). Hazardous materials emergencies. In B. Hafen & J. Karren (Eds.), *Prehospital emergency care and crisis intervention* (pp. 503–517). Englewood, CO: Morton.

Institute of Medicine and Board on Environmental Studies and Toxicology; National Research Council (1999). Chemical and biological terrorism: Research and development to improve civilian medical response (pp. 125–154, 261–264). Washington, D.C.: National Academy Press.

Jarrett, D. G. (1996). Nuclear nightmares. *Emergency Medical Services*, 65–91.

Jimmerson, CL. (1992). Environmental emergencies. In S. B. Budassi (Ed.), *Emergency nursing* (3rd ed., pp. 383–411). St. Louis, MO: Mosby-Year Book.

Klein, J., & Wigelt, J. (1991). Disaster management: Lesson learned. *Surgical Clinics of North America, 71*(2), 257–266.

Lee, R. J., et al. (1996). Personal defense sprays: Effects and management of exposure. *Journal of the American Optometric Association, 67,* 548–560.

Mallonee, S., et al. (1996). Physical injuries and fatalities resulting from the Oklahoma City bombing. *Journal of the American Medical Association, 276,* 382–387.

Mathur, B. B., & Krishna, G. (1992). Toxicodynamics of phosgene. In S. Somani (Ed.), *Chemical warfare agents* (pp. 237–254). San Diego: Academic Press.

Mettler, F. A., Jr., et al. (1990). *Medical management of radiation accidents.* Boca Raton, FL: CRC Press.

National Council on Radiation Protection and Measurements. (1980). *NCRP report no. 65: Management of persons accidentally contaminated with radionuclides.* Washington, DC: National Council on Radiation Protection and Measurements.

Nozaki, H. (1995). A case of VX poisoning and the difference from sarin [Letter to the editor]. *Lancet, 346,* 698–699.

Ruhl, C. M., et al. (1994). A serious skin sulfur mustard burn from an artillery shell. *Journal of Emergency Medicine, 12,* 159–166.

Sidell, F. R. (1992). Clinical considerations in nerve agent intoxication. In S. Somani (Ed.), *Chemical warfare agents* (pp. 155–194). San Diego: Academic Press.

Sidell, F. R., Hurst, C. G. (1992). Clinical considerations in mustard poisoning. In S. Somani (Ed.), *Chemical warfare agents* (pp. 51–66). San Diego: Academic Press.

U. S. Army MRICD. (1995). *Medical management of chemical casualties handbook.* Aberdeen, MD: Chemical Casualty Care Office, MRICD.

Waeckerie, J. (1991). Disaster planning and response. *New England Journal of Medicine, 432,* 815–821.

Yokoyama, K., Yamade, A., et al. (1996). Clinical profiles of patients with sarin poisoning after the Tokyo subway attack. *American Journal of Medicine, 100,* 586.

Genell Lee, JD, MSN, RN

CHAPTER **24**

Legal Issues

MAJOR TOPICS

This chapter contains a discussion of general principles of law. To determine whether these principles have been modified for a particular state, it is necessary to refer to the applicable state law or case law for the state in question. Federal law should be consulted for federal facilities.

For specific emergency department (ED) situations, such as telephone advice, it is wise to obtain the position papers of the Emergency Nurses Association to assist in the formulation of institutional policy. Additionally, ED managers should have access to the hospital legal counsel to obtain advice on the development of policies and procedures to address medical or legal ED issues.

I. GENERAL OVERVIEW

A. Sources of law

Legal issues relevant to emergency nursing are predicated on a variety of sources of law. The sources of law that have an impact on nursing include constitutional law (federal and state), common (case) law, statutory law (federal and state), ordinances, and administrative law.

1. Constitutional law

The U.S. Constitution is the supreme law of the land. No activity or other law may conflict with the Constitution. The Supreme Court is the judicial body that decides the constitutionality of particular activities (e.g., abortion).

Each state also has a constitution that describes the protections available to citizens of that state. A state constitution may provide greater protection for its citizens, but it cannot provide less protection than the federal Constitution.

2. Common (case) law

Common law is the body of law formed by judicial decisions in the various courts. When a court hears a case and the judge issues a decision, that decision joins the body of common, or case, law. That decision becomes a precedent that may be relied on to support or oppose a point of law in a pending case with similar facts. For example, if a school district went to court to request segregation of its schools, the opposing side would use the case of Brown v. Board of Education (1954) to argue that integration is the law as settled by this precedent-setting case. A precedent is not absolute, and a later court may overrule a case previously established as a precedent.

3. Statutory law

Statutory law is the law made by the U.S. Congress (legislative branch) and the state legislatures. The laws passed by these bodies are called statutes. The Medicare law is an example of a federal statute. Nurse Practice Acts and some safety belt laws are examples of state statutes.

As is true in constitutional law, federal statutes will pre-empt or override state statutes in authority; therefore, state statutes may not conflict with federal statutes.

4. Ordinances

Ordinances are laws passed by cities or other local jurisdictions. These laws regulate such things as parking, sanitation services, and other issues of local concern. Both federal and state statutes pre-empt a conflicting ordinance.

5. Administrative law

Administrative laws are created by administrative agencies through power delegated to them by the federal or state legislature. An administrative agency is empowered to enact only laws specific to the functions of the agency. For example, regulatory boards for nursing are created with the state Nurse Practice Acts. These regulatory boards are then given the power to promulgate rules and regulations specific to the practice of nursing.

To ensure that these administrative agencies are held accountable for their actions, they have specific rules and regulations that detail their responsibilities and limitations. A common requirement is that administrative agencies must publish notice of proposed rules and allow for public comment.

B. Types of law

The law is divided into two types: civil and criminal.

1. Civil law

Civil law addresses injury to individuals and/or their property. The remedy sought for civil wrongs is generally monetary compensation. Another remedy sought may be the order to stop the activity causing injury (i.e., an injunction).

2. **Criminal law**

Criminal law addresses injury to society. For a society to flourish, its citizens must be able to live free from the fear of harm. Therefore, a criminal act against an individual threatens the societal orderliness essential to ensuring stability and advancement. The remedy sought for a criminal act is incarceration or payment of a fine by the guilty individual(s).

Remedies for civil and criminal wrongs are not mutually exclusive. For example, if a patient draws a gun and shoots an ED employee, that patient could be charged with violation of the criminal law and a civil suit could be filed by the employee's family for money damages in the loss of life.

C. Specific laws

1. **Torts**

Torts (Prosser, 1991) are civil wrongs committed against an individual or the property of an individual. Torts are divided into intentional and nonintentional categories.

a. *Intentional torts: these torts require that the person committing the tort have the intent to commit the act (e.g., assault, battery, and false imprisonment).*

   1) Assault is the intention to cause harm to an individual with the ability to carry through the threat immediately (e.g., a nurse raises her hand to a patient and states, "If you do that again, I will slap you").

   2) Battery is the nonconsensual, offensive touching of another individual. For example, when a competent adult refuses a pain injection but has it administered against his or her will, the nurse administering the injection might have committed a battery.

   3) False imprisonment is the placement of restraints on an individual's freedom of movement. For example, a competent adult is brought to the ED after an automobile collision. She is found to have a laceration on her palm that requires sutures but has no other physical problems. The patient declines to have the laceration sutured. The ED staff then proceed to restrain her and perform the procedure. This would be a case of false imprisonment and battery.

b. *A nonintentional tort is a civil injury caused without intent by the defendant. Professional negligence (commonly referred to as medical malpractice) is a nonintentional tort. State law governs what the plaintiff-patient must prove and the type of evidence allowed. In federal facilities, the Federal Tort Claims statute is followed. A negligence lawsuit will fail in the absence of any of the following four elements, which must be pleaded and proved by the individual bringing the lawsuit (plaintiff-patient):*

   1) Duty, or the presence of a relationship between the plaintiff-patient and the defendant-health care professional

   2) Breach of duty: the plaintiff-patient complains that the care rendered was below accepted standards of care (i.e., the expected duty was breached)

   3) Proximate cause: proof that breach of duty was the probable cause of the injury; if the patient is going to die regardless of interventions and a negligent intervention occurs, there is no proximate cause because the death (injury) would have occurred irrespective of the negligent intervention

   4) Injury: the plaintiff-patient must be able to demonstrate an injury (dam-

ages) that occurred because of the negligence of the defendant; damages may include compensation for pain and suffering, medical expenses, and lost wages; if state law allows, the plaintiff-patient may seek punitive damages, meant to punish or deter wrongful conduct

c. *Application of negligence elements*

   1) Duty

      a) Wilmington General Hospital v. Manlove (1961): this court decision held that if a hospital has an ED, it has the duty to provide emergency care. Internal hospital policies cannot be used to negate the duty owed to the community at large.

      b) Hill-Burton Act (1946): this federal law required hospitals that received federal funds under this act to provide care to patients regardless of ability to pay.

      c) Lunsford v. Board of Nurse Examiners (1983): in this Texas case, the court held that nurses have a duty to patients just as physicians owe a duty; that duty stems from the privilege granted by the state in nurse licensure

      d) Nurse Practice Acts: this is a statutory law in each state that defines the legal parameters for the practice of nursing. A copy of the statute and the administrative rules and regulations can generally be obtained for a small fee from the State Board of Nursing.

   2) Breach of duty

      a) Nursing care provided to the plaintiff-patient is alleged to have been below the standard of care.

      b) The standard of care is that degree of care that a reasonable, prudent professional would exercise in the same or similar circumstances.

      c) The standard of care is presented in court through the use of expert witnesses and documents, such as the state Nurse Practice Act, institutional policies and procedures, and learned treatises. For ED nursing negligence, the ENA Standards of Nursing Practice may be used. State law may specify requirements for expert witnesses. In a case against an ED nurse, for example, an expert nurse witness without ED experience might be disqualified as an expert.

   3) Proximate cause: the defendant's conduct was responsible for the injury sustained by the patient. A direct causal relationship must exist between the defendant's negligence and the injury that occurred. For example, a 21-year-old woman is admitted to the ED after a 20-foot fall. She is diagnosed with a ruptured spleen and must undergo surgery. During the preoperative preparation, the ED nurse shears off an intravenous catheter in the patient's vein. Several days later, the patient requires reoperation for removal of the catheter. The injury, prolonged hospitalization, and a second injury was proximately caused by the nurse's negligence.

   4) Injury

      a) The plaintiff-patient must have sustained some type of injury (damage) as a result of the negligent action.

      b) The injury can be either physical or psychological.

      c) In the example for proximate cause, the injury was the extended hospitalization and the need for a second operation.

D. Other relevant legal concepts

1. Respondeat superior

This legal term describes the vicarious liability that employers have for the negligent acts of their employees who act within the scope of their employment.

   a. The hospital employer is held legally liable for the acts of its staff while they are performing work duties

   b. For example, an improperly administered injection that results in nerve damage would be a situation in which the hospital would maintain liability for the nurse's negligent act. However, if an ED nurse leaves work and stops to render care at a crash site, any legal action for negligence would be the responsibility of the nurse only. The care given was outside the scope of employment.

2. **Good Samaritan laws**

   Good Samaritan laws were passed to encourage rendering of assistance in emergency situations outside the hospital without fear of liability. Some states have laws that mandate that nurses and physicians stop and provide emergency care. (Check with local law school libraries to obtain copies of the state Good Samaritan statute. There may be a charge for this service.) Good Samaritan laws vary greatly among states and may not apply if the health care professional was grossly negligent or received compensation for the service provided.

3. **Indemnification**

   If an employee is found liable for professional negligence and the employer, through vicarious liability, is required to pay the settlement, the employer has the ability to require indemnification from the employee for the loss. Essentially, the employer could require the employee to repay the employer the money that was lost in a professional negligence action. Although this is not a frequent occurrence for nurses, it is an option that employers have available.

4. **Malpractice insurance**

   Malpractice insurance is available to cover the costs associated with litigation of professional negligence cases and the expenses of the settlement or verdict. Malpractice insurance is generally carried by the hospital for its employees, but it is also available to nurses on a personal basis. Each nurse should be clearly informed of the pros and cons of obtaining personal malpractice insurance. A pamphlet is available for a small charge from The American Association of Nurse Attorneys (TAANA) at 720 Light Street, Baltimore, Maryland 21230-3826. This pamphlet provides comprehensive information that will assist in the decision about obtaining personal malpractice insurance coverage.

5. **Captain of the ship**

   This legal rule holds that the physician was the "captain of the ship," and that any negligence that occurred would be attributed to the physician because of his or her role. For example, if an ED nurse gave the wrong dosage of medication, the physician would be liable for the negligent act under this rule. This rule has generally lost favor in the legal system. It is not possible to impute to one person the legal responsibility for the negligent acts of other licensed personnel. If, however, the nurse is practicing as a physician extender under the physician's supervision, the physician will generally be held liable for negligent acts.

II. CONSENT

A. Types of consent

1. **Express consent**

   This is the voluntary consent of an individual seeking medical treatment. The ability of the individual to provide express consent is predicated on the patient's competency. Patient competency is often a judgment made by ED personnel.

Issues related to patient competency must be well documented. For example, a competent individual presents to the ED with a forearm laceration and requests medical care. The admitting personnel give the patient a standardized consent form to sign. The patient's signature constitutes express consent for treatment. Express consent does not waive the patient's ability to sue for presumed negligence that may have occurred during the treatment.

2. **Implied consent**

   Consent is implied when an individual is in a life- or limb-threatening situation and is unable, because of unconsciousness or incompetency, to provide express consent. For example, a critically injured patient is transported to the ED unconscious, unresponsive, and hemodynamically unstable. The patient requires immediate operative intervention to save her life. No family members are available, and the patient is unable to give consent. The law will assume implied consent is present for the life-saving surgery. As soon as possible, every attempt should be made to obtain express consent from the family or the patient.

3. **Involuntary consent**

   Consent is involuntary when the individual refuses to consent to needed medical treatment, and yet another individual (physician or police) can ensure that the individual receives treatment. For example, a patient brought to the ED after a suicide attempt refuses medical care. An ED physician, often in consultation with a psychiatrist, can sign papers that will hold the patient for treatment for a specified period of time (usually not more than 48 hours). If medical care is needed in excess of the original 48 hours, most states require that a hearing be held in front of a judge, who can make the determination that the patient will continue to be hospitalized regardless of the patient's refusal to consent to the extended hospitalization.

4. **Informed consent**

   Informed consent has three essential components that must be presented to the patient by the physician before a procedure. For the patient to make an informed decision, the physician must (1) describe the procedure to be performed, (2) explain the alternatives available to the procedure, and (3) detail the risks of the procedure. Most states mandate by statute that physicians have the responsibility to provide the information required to obtain informed consent. A surgical procedure performed without consent is battery. A surgical procedure performed without informed consent is negligence.

B. Consent dilemmas

1. **Minors**

   The age of consent varies, depending on state statutes. Each ED should have a policy available to all personnel that details the state law on age of consent. If a minor is emancipated (e.g., economically independent, married), the minor may be allowed to consent to medical treatment regardless of his or her age. Most states have laws that allow minors of any age to consent to such things as birth control counseling and treatment of sexually transmitted diseases. ED policy manuals should contain this information from the applicable state laws.

2. **Refusal to consent based on religious conviction**

   Individuals who may be in need of medical treatment may refuse the treatment based on religious convictions. A common occurrence of this situation is the Jehovah's Witness who has the medical indications to require a blood transfusion. Most states will allow competent adults to refuse even life-saving care if they make that decision based on complete knowledge of the risks of the refusal. If the death of the adult would leave minor children without a parent, the social policy considerations may override the patient's wishes. If the patient is a minor and the parents are refusing medical care, it is necessary to involve hospital administration and/or legal counsel to consider obtaining a court order to treat. There must be a policy available in the General Policy and Procedure Manual that provides information on how to proceed should this issue arise on the evening or night shift or when hospital administrative staff are not in-house.

3. **Managed care**

   a. *In a managed-care participating hospital, an on-call physician or the patient's primary physician may be called on to approve or authorize payment for admission. The interaction between ED personnel, the patient, and the managed care physician should be documented.*

   b. *In a nonparticipating hospital, the managed-care plan provider is frequently contacted by ED personnel before treatment. The managed-care plan provider can authorize (or refuse) payment, but the consent for treatment and refusal of treatment remains the sole responsibility of the patient. Conflict can occur and the ED/institutional policies should provide guidance should the conflict occur between the managed-care plan's payment decision and the patient's need for treatment. (See section III.A. for a discussion of restrictions in delaying treatment to obtain financial information.)*

4. **Refusal of treatment/leaving against medical advice**

   a. *If a patient refuses treatment that is medically indicated, it is essential that a determination be made regarding the patient's competency to make such a decision.*

   b. *If the patient is found to be competent, the ED physician must provide a comprehensive explanation of the risks involved in refusing treatment. The details of the patient conference must be thoroughly documented in the medical record.*

   c. *The patient should be requested to sign a "release of responsibility" form. If the patient refuses to sign the form, document the refusal in the medical record.*

   d. *If the patient's refusal of treatment puts the patient at risk and there is a question of the patient's competency, contact the hospital administrator or designee to consider court-ordered treatment.*

5. **Patients in custody of law enforcement**

   a. *Consent for treatment generally remains with the individual, not law enforcement personnel.*

   b. *Conflict may occur if the patient is in custody for suspected alcohol or drug intoxication or ingestion. State law governs whether the individual in custody can refuse consent for withdrawal of blood and other body fluid specimens for police or forensic purposes.*

   c. *Invasive surgical procedures to remove suspected ingested balloons or bags of illegal drugs generally require a court order if the patient refuses removal. The court may not order the removal because of the risk associated with the surgery. The court weighs the interests of the state and the individual in custody.*

   d. *Legal counsel should be consulted for specific direction for policy development.*

C. Consent regarding withholding or withdrawal of life support

1. **Patient Self-Determination Act**

   The Patient Self-Determination Act is a federal law that became effective in December 1991. The basis of the law is to provide hospitalized patients with information about advance directives. Under provisions of the law, the patient must be asked during the admission phase whether he or she has an advance directive. If the patient does not have an advance directive, information about advance directives must be provided. The interaction must then be documented in the medical record. For ED admissions, the responsibility for compliance with this law may fall to ED personnel. If this is the case, in-services must be provided to existing personnel along with inclusion of the material into orientation for new employees. Patient information booklets on this topic are also helpful.

2. **Durable power of attorney for health care decisions/living wills**

The most current form of advance directives is the "durable power of attorney for health care decisions" ("durable power"). Durable power has replaced "living wills" in many states as the advance directive of choice. Durable power allows individuals to select someone (attorney-in-fact) to act for them in the area of health care decisions should they become unable to make their own decisions. The attorney-in-fact (who does not have to be an attorney-at-law) assumes the responsibility to speak for the individual regarding all treatment decisions unless his or her power is specifically limited in the durable power. Durable power is preferred over a living will because it allows an individual to discuss the options with the medical team. If the living will was signed several years before, the question arises whether the patient would choose differently given the changes in technology. Because durable power provides an individual who is speaking with the written authorization of the patient, the courts allow great deference to the decisions. Each state has different requirements for durable powers of attorney for health care decisions or living wills, and an ED must have information on its particular state requirements.

III. PATIENT TRANSFER ISSUES

A. Emergency Medical Treatment and Active Labor Act (EMTALA)

1. **EMTALA**

This is a portion of the Medicare law designed to prevent inappropriate transfers ("dumping") of individuals who seek ED care or who are in active labor.

2. **ED requirements**

a. *Hospitals with EDs must provide an "appropriate" medical screening examination for every individual who comes to the ED and requests care.*
   1) This requirement is not limited to the ED: any area on hospital property is included.
   2) Hospital-owned ambulance services are hospital property for purposes of this requirement.
b. *The examination cannot be delayed to inquire about insurance status or method of payment.*
c. *The screening examination must include the ancillary services routinely available to the ED.*
d. *If the individual is diagnosed with an emergency medical condition or is in active labor, the hospital must either provide stabilizing treatment or transfer the individual to another medical facility ensuring compliance with transfer guidelines. Once an individual meets the described conditions for EMTALA protection, the law will apply unless the patient refuses treatment or transfer.*
e. *If an individual refuses treatment or transfer, the hospital must make every effort to obtain a written informed consent of the refusal by the individual.*
f. *All Medicare-participating EDs must have a sign posted prominently in the waiting/admission/triage area that specifies the patient's rights with respect to examination and treatment for emergency medical conditions. If an ED serves*

> *a bilingual or multilingual population, there should be signs in the languages of the most frequent visitors.*

> g. *EDs must maintain a list of on-call physicians who are available in a reasonable time period to provide care to these patients. If an on-call physician fails to respond or to respond in a reasonable time, his or her name and contact information must be sent with the individual transferred to the receiving hospital.*

3. **Transfer requirements**
   a. *An individual who has an unstabilized emergency condition should not be transferred unless*
      1) A physician certifies in writing that, based on information available at the time of the contemplated transfer, the medical benefits of the transfer outweigh the risks of the transfer to the individual or unborn child. Certification must contain a summary of risks and benefits of transfer.
      2) The transferring hospital has provided medical treatment within its capability to ensure that the risks of the transfer are minimized.
      3) The receiving medical facility has agreed to accept the individual and provide appropriate medical treatment.
      4) The receiving medical facility has available space and qualified personnel for the treatment of the individual.
      5) All medical records (or copies) related to the emergency medical condition, available at the time of transfer, are sent to the receiving hospital.
      6) The transfer is effected using qualified personnel and appropriate vehicle and equipment as required to provide care during the transfer.
      7) There is compliance with other requirements that may be imposed by the Secretary of the Department of Health and Human Services to ensure the health and safety of the transferred individuals (see Fig. 21–1, Patient Transfer Form)

4. **Penalties**
   a. *$50,000.00 fine against the responsible hospital and/or physician; $25,000.00 fine against qualified rural hospital*
   b. *Potential loss of Medicare provider status*
   c. *Potential for liability in civil litigation by the injured individual or hospital that inappropriately received the transfer*

5. **Special requirements**
   a. *Medicare-participating hospitals that have specialized capabilities or facilities (e.g., burn units, trauma centers, neonatal ICUs, and, with respect to rural areas, regional referral centers) cannot refuse to accept an appropriate transfer of an individual who requires such specialized facilities or capabilities as long as the hospital has the capacity to treat the individual.*

IV. REPORTABLE SITUATIONS

A. Requirements

1. **Each state has defined by law certain situations that require health care professionals to breach patient confidentiality and report the situation to a specified agency or individual.**
2. **Because of the variance by state, each ED needs to obtain copies of its particular state laws related to mandatory reporting requirements.**
3. **Examples: some common examples of mandatory reporting include homicide or suicide attempts, child or elder abuse, rape, communicable diseases, and deaths within 48 hours of hospital admission.**

B. Nursing responsibility

1. If the situation requires either a physician or a nurse to report the incident, nurses should not assume that the physician will be the person responsible. The nurse shares equally in this legal responsibility.
2. If the nurse believes in good faith that the incident meets the statutory reporting requirements but the physician disagrees, it remains the nurse's responsibility to report to the designated authority.

V. DOCUMENTATION

A. Medical record requirements

1. A medical record should be initiated and maintained on every individual who seeks emergency care.
2. The medical record serves a variety of functions, including a communication system for health care professionals providing patient care, a chronicle of the patient's progress, and the medical-legal record of all care provided.
3. The requirements for what must be included in medical record documentation vary on an institutional basis. Hospitals accredited by the Joint Commission on the Accreditation of Healthcare Organizations (JCAHO) are required to have certain information on the medical record. Trauma centers are often required to track specific information on the medical records of injured patients.
4. State law may dictate the minimum requirements for what is included in medical records.

B. Documentation variances

1. Many hospitals have implemented or are exploring the possibility of implementing alternative methods of charting (e.g., documentation by exception).
2. No laws mandate that all charting must be done using the SOAP method (*s*ubjective, *o*bjective, *a*ssessment, *p*lan).
3. In a court of law, if the medical record documentation is at issue, it is necessary to be able to present a cogent discussion on the documentation used. The discussion should be based on the presence of an institutional policy (in the hospital manual) that confirms the methodology used in the documentation.
4. As long as the defendant-health care professional can demonstrate that the documentation method used is adequate to answer the complaint, there should not be a problem with documentation alternatives.

C. Confidentiality

The contents of the medical record are confidential and cannot be discussed outside the medical care setting without breaching patient confidentiality. State law should be reviewed to determine specific requirements. Special federal laws serve to protect the confidentiality of medical records for patients undergoing alcohol or drug abuse treatment in federally funded programs. Technological advances in documentation and communication via computers, networks, fax transmission, and electronic mail require enhanced attention to confidentiality. Inattention to or disregard of confidentiality principles could lead to liability for invasion of the right to privacy, defamation (slander or libel), and, in some states, infliction of emotional distress.

D. Discharge instructions

1. The standard of care for every ED discharge is that the patient should receive written and oral discharge instructions. A copy of the discharge instructions must be a permanent part of the medical record. There should also be documented evidence that the written instructions were discussed with the patient and that the patient indicated that he or she understood them.
2. The language of the discharge instructions should not be more complex than sixth-grade reading level.
3. If an ED sees a large number of non–English-speaking patients, discharge instructions should be available in the predominant languages.

E. Special concerns in ED documentation

1. Documentation should reflect that past medical records were ordered and received.
2. When rapid interventions are occurring, it is optimal to have someone making contemporaneous and chronological documentation.
3. Critically ill or injured ED patients should have documented evidence that intensive nursing care via the frequent recording of vital signs or interventions were being performed.
4. Unusual occurrences or problems should be documented on incident reports, not in the patient's medical record.
5. If a problem is found (e.g., esophageal intubation), the resolution should also be documented (e.g., endotracheal tube [ET] replaced into trachea, with equal breath sounds).
6. All communication with or attempted communication with physicians, supervisors, or administrators regarding the patient's status should be documented. Proper use of chain of command to benefit the patient is the focus in many lawsuits.
7. Documentation must be present to reflect compliance with state laws (e.g., evidence of organ request in the case of death and documentation of the patient's decision regarding life support for the patient admitted from the ED).
8. All appropriate forms and consents must be included in the ED medical record.

VI. TRAUMA CENTER ISSUES

A. Application to emergency departments

1. If an ED is in a hospital that is a designated or verified trauma center, it will be held legally accountable to provide the resources described nationally as applicable to its designation level. For example, a Level 1 trauma center is required to have an attending surgeon meet the injured patient on arrival in the ED (American College of Surgeons, 1990).
2. Nondesignated hospitals are not required to have all the resources available that designated centers have. However, with the availability of

trauma-related continuing education, a nondesignated hospital is expected to provide rapid intervention or transfer of the patient to a hospital that can provide the care. (The transfer would have to meet EMTALA guidelines.)

3. Under federal law, trauma centers are required to accept appropriate transfers of injured patients if the capacity is present to provide care.
4. If a hospital claims to be a trauma center, it will be held legally accountable to the standards of a trauma center.

BIBLIOGRAPHY

American College of Surgeons. (1990). *Optimal resources for injured patients.* Chicago: American College of Surgeons.

Brown v. Board of Education, 347 U.S. 483 (1954), Suppl. 349 U.S. 294.

Emergency Medical Treatment and Active Labor Act (EMTALA) (Suppl. 1995). 42 U.S.C.A. section 1395dd.

Emergency Nurses Association. (1995). *Standards of emergency nursing practice* (3rd ed.). St. Louis, MO: C. V. Mosby.

Fischbach, F. T. (1991). *Documenting care: Communication, the nursing process, and documentation standards.* Philadelphia: F. A. Davis.

Krebs-Markrich, J., Coffey, J. E., & Korjus, J. L. W. (1995). *EMTALA: The next generation. Health Lawyer,* 8, 1.

Lunsford v. Board of Nurse Examiners, 648 SW 2d 391 (Tex. App. 3 Dist., 1983).

Meisel, A. (1992). *The right to die.* New York: Wiley.

Patient Self-Determination Act (PSDA). (Suppl. 1995). 42 U.S.C.A. section 1395.

Prosser, W. L. (1991). *Handbook on the law of torts* (4th ed.). St. Paul, MN: West.

Roach, W. H., Jr., & Aspen Health Law Center. (1994). *Medical records and the law* (2nd ed.). Gaithersburg, MD: Aspen.

Rothenberg, M. A. (1994). *Emergency medicine malpractice* (2nd ed.). New York: Wiley. (Supplement published 1997)

Rozovsky, F. A. (1990). *Consent to treatment: A practical guide* (2nd ed.). Boston: Little, Brown.

Rozovsky, F. A. (1995). *Consent to treatment: A practical guide* (2nd ed., suppl.). Boston: Little, Brown.

Wilmington General Hospital v. Manlove, 194 A.2d 135 (State Court, Delaware, 1961).

Frank L. Cole, PhD, RN, CEN, CS, FNP

CHAPTER **25**

Research

MAJOR TOPICS

Purpose of Research

Research Function of Nurses

Research Projects

Research Methodologies

How to Get Started

Steps in Qualitative Research
Process

Steps in Quantitative Research
Process

Research Ethics

Application of Research to Clinical
Practice

Critiquing Quantitative Research
Studies

Critiquing Qualitative Research
Studies

The scientific basis of nursing practice is established through research. Research in the emergency department (ED) identifies nursing interventions that are effective and produce the desired outcome in patient care. Therefore, research provides a means for the emergency nurse to demonstrate that high-quality patient care is delivered by nursing staff. Research also helps to develop nursing knowledge about situations, people, and circumstances unique to the practice of emergency nursing. The scientific basis of emergency nursing practice is constantly changing and requires that new knowledge be developed and that existing knowledge be validated and revalidated through research.

I. PURPOSE OF RESEARCH

A. Improves nursing care by establishing scientific bases for practice

B. Validates scope of emergency nursing practice

C. Facilitates evaluation of emergency care concepts and practice

D. Provides basis for accountability

E. Documents contribution of emergency nursing to health care

F. Assesses outcomes of emergency nursing care

G. Validates and refines existing emergency nursing knowledge

H. Generates new knowledge related to nursing care of emergency patients

I. Describes and promotes understanding human experiences

II. RESEARCH FUNCTION OF NURSES

A. Educational institutions incorporate various research activities into their programs to familiarize nurses with research process and related responsibilities

B. The American Nurses Association Commission on Nursing Research (1981) delineated the following research roles for nurses

1. **Associate degree in nursing**
   a. *Demonstrates awareness of value or relevance of research in nursing*
   b. *Assists in identifying problem areas in nursing practice*
   c. *Assists in collection of data within established structure format*

2. **Diploma in nursing**
      Although the diploma in nursing was not mentioned in the ANA (1981) report, the following investigative functions of diploma nurses are identified:
   a. *Identifies nursing problems that need investigation*
   b. *Assists in collection of data within well-defined structured format*
   c. *Explains relevance of research in practice*

3. **Baccalaureate degree in nursing (BSN)**
   a. *Reads, interprets, and evaluates research for applicability to nursing practice*
   b. *Identifies nursing problems that need to be investigated and participates in implementation of scientific studies*
   c. *Uses nursing practice as means of gathering data for refining and extending practice*
   d. *Applies established findings of nursing and other health-related research to nursing practice*
   e. *Shares research findings with colleagues*

4. **Master's degree in nursing**
   a. *Analyzes and reformulates nursing practice problems so that scientific knowledge and scientific methods can be used to find solutions*
   b. *Enhances quality and clinical relevance of nursing research by providing expertise in clinical problems and by providing knowledge about the way in which these clinical services are delivered*
   c. *Facilitates investigation of problems in clinical settings through such activities as contributing to climate supportive of investigative activities, collaborating with others in investigations, and enhancing nurses' access to clients and data*
   d. *Conducts investigations for practice of nursing in clinical setting*
   e. *Assists others to apply scientific knowledge in nursing practice*

5. **Doctorate degree in nursing or related discipline**
   a. *Graduate of a practice-oriented doctoral program*

1) Provides leadership for integration of scientific knowledge with other sources of knowledge for advancement of practice

2) Conducts investigations to evaluate contribution of nursing activities to well-being of clients

3) Develops methods to monitor quality of practice of nursing in clinical setting and to evaluate contributions of nursing activities to well-being of clients

b. *Graduate of a research-oriented doctoral program*

1) Develops theoretical explanations of phenomena relevant to nursing by empirical research and analytical processes

2) Uses analytical and empirical methods to discover ways to modify or extend existing scientific knowledge so that it is relevant to nursing

3) Develops methods for scientific inquiry of phenomena relevant to nursing

III. RESEARCH PROJECTS

A. Clinical problem solving

1. Uses trial and error method
2. Generally involves one problem or a set of problems
3. Is not theory based
4. Generally does not use high-level statistical analysis
5. Is not concerned with issues of validity or reliability
6. Provides possible solutions to specific problems

B. Research study

1. Uses formal plan to study problem
2. Looks for several solutions simultaneously
3. Is based on theory or generates a theory
4. Uses statistical analysis for quantitative research and uses words as basis for analysis with qualitative research
5. Is concerned with issues of reliability and validity in quantitative research and auditability, creditability, and fittingness in qualitative research
6. May suggest solutions with wide applications with quantitative research or describe and give meaning to life experiences with qualitative research

IV. RESEARCH METHODOLOGIES

A. Qualitative

1. Described as a systematic, interactive, and subjective approach
2. Uses words, not numbers, to give meaning to data
3. Used to describe life experiences and give them meaning
4. Is less frequently used as a research method but has been gaining popularity since the late 1970s
5. Types (see Section VI)
   a. *Phenomenological*
   b. *Grounded theory*
   c. *Ethnographic*
   d. *Historical*

B. Quantitative

1. Described as a formal, objective, and systemic process
2. Uses numerical data to understand world
3. Used to describe variables, examine relationships among variables, and determine cause-and-effect interactions between variables
4. Is most frequently used method of research studies
5. Types (see Section VII)
   a. *Descriptive*
   b. *Correlational*
   c. *Quasiexperimental*
   d. *Experimental*

V. HOW TO GET STARTED

A. The steps involved in getting started on a research project vary depending on whether research method to be used is qualitative or quantitative

1. Identify problem to be investigated in quantitative studies or phenomenon, culture, idea, or topic for qualitative studies
2. Identify the significance and importance of the problem, phenomenon, culture, idea, or topic to be studied
3. For quantitative research studies, review literature to determine whether an answer exists and/or to find possible theoretical frameworks or instruments. A review may also resolve the study's problem by providing possible solutions. In general, the literature is not reviewed in qualitative studies until the researcher is giving meaning to the data
4. Put the problem in question form: e.g., "What is the effect of discharge plans on patient awareness about his or her condition?" The way a research question is worded depends on whether a qualitative or quantitative study is being conducted. Moreover, the type of qualitative study also influences how the question is asked
5. Once a question has been formulated, seek out someone with research experience to act as a preceptor, mentor, or chairperson for the research proposed. This person can carefully analyze the research and prevent undue work and anxiety
6. If the project involves a health care agency, communicate research intent to appropriate people
7. Plan a budget (time and money) for the project
8. Identify how to use findings generated by the research study (e.g., impact on practice)
9. Examine legal and ethical implications involved (e.g., privacy act, malpractice)

VI. STEPS IN QUALITATIVE RESEARCH PROCESS

A. Phenomenology

1. Identify the phenomenon to be explored (e.g., chest pain in persons experiencing MI in ED)
2. Develop research question (e.g., What is the meaning of chest pain to persons experiencing a myocardial infarction [MI] in the ED?)
3. Obtain a sample: identify sources of the phenomenon and individuals willing to describe the experience

4. Collect data through observation, interactive interviews, videotapes, and/or written descriptions
5. Analyze data: initiated with first data gathered and influences decisions related to further data collection
   a. *Read all information to gain sense of the whole*
   b. *Re-read all information, looking for changes in meaning and note themes or "meaning units"*
   c. *Examine meaning units for redundancy, clarification, and relationships between other meaning units*
   d. *Meaning of units is assessed*
   e. *Develop description of phenomenon*
6. Develop theoretical statement related to research question

B. Grounded theory

1. Steps occur simultaneously and involve observing, collecting data, organizing data and forming theory
2. Data collected by interview, observations, and/or written descriptions
3. Data coded from the beginning
   a. *Development of categories*
   b. *Saturation of categories*
   c. *Development of concept*
   d. *Search for additional categories*
   e. *Reduce categories*
   f. *Link categories*
   g. *Examine literature to assess fit of categories with theories and other studies*
   h. *Determine core concept of theory to be developed*
4. Develop theory that explains phenomenon under study

C. Ethnography

1. Select culture to be examined
2. Identify significant variables to be studied
3. Review literature
4. Gain entrance into culture
5. Immerse oneself into culture
6. Acquire informants
   a. *Seek out people willing to interpret culture*
7. Gather data through observation and interviews; data are written in field notes
8. Analyze data through intuition, introspection, and reasoning to determine meaning of activities, events, rituals, etc. in culture
9. Describe culture
10. Results may be applied to existing theory, or new theory of culture may be developed

D. Historical

1. Formulate idea or topic for study and limit time period
2. Develop research questions
3. Develop inventory of sources of data
4. Obtain data sources
5. Clarify validity and reliability of data sources

6. **Develop research outline**
   a. *Includes broad topics to be examined*
   b. *Serves as filing system for data collected*
7. **Collect data**
8. **Analyze data**
   a. *Synthesis of collected data*

VII. STEPS IN QUANTITATIVE RESEARCH PROCESS

A. Formulation of research questions or problem

1. **Definition of problem or question**
   a. *Can be declarative or interrogative*
   b. *Yields facts, not opinions*
   c. *Will add to body of nursing knowledge*
   d. *Will improve nursing practice*
   e. *Will solve existing nursing problem*
   f. *Will provide solutions that will explain, describe, identify, or predict behaviors*
   g. *Is current and pertains to present and future of nursing*
   h. *Is relevant to issues facing nursing today*
   i. *Is clear, concise, and cogent*
   j. *Provides direction for rest of research project*
   k. *Demands activity from researcher (e.g., observations or experiments)*
2. **Research question**
   a. *Directs research*
   b. *Includes one topic per question*
   c. *Provides basis for study and narrows focus*
   d. *Example: "What effect does the teaching of nonpharmacological pain interventions have on the number of emergency visits by patients with migraine headaches?"*
3. **Types of questions**
   a. *Type I research question*
      1) No prior knowledge exists about topic
      2) Stem question begins with "what is" or "what are"
      3) The topic is the expression of a single entity or concept
      4) Exploratory research concerning what exists on the topic
      5) Example: "What are emergency nurses' attitudes toward overdose patients?"
   b. *Type II research question*
      1) Looks at relationships between concepts or variables
      2) Usually includes "What is the relationship...?" as part of question
      3) Examines two or more concepts or variables
      4) Generally uses descriptive research methods
      5) Builds on type I research
      6) Example: "What is the relationship between basic educational preparation of emergency nurses and their job satisfaction level when caring for patients with psychiatric problems?"
   c. *Type III research question*
      1) Builds on type I and type II research and elicits a cause-and-effect relationship
      2) Uses an experimental design

3) Asks "why"
4) Example: "Why does an increase in the number of patients with emergency psychiatric complaints decrease the self-reported level of emergency nurses' job satisfaction and overall job performance?"

B. Problem statement

1. **Definition**
   a. *Introduction of research topic*
   b. *Explanation of importance of problem*
   c. *What the study hopes to investigate*
   d. *Full exposure of idea that needs to be studied*
   e. *Logical ordering of thoughts about problem*
2. **Elements of problem statement**
   a. *Initial literature search*
      1) Substantiates rationale for development and narrowing of problem
      2) Provides references that support researcher's justification for studying problem
   b. *Rationale for developing research question includes*
      1) Why is there a need for this particular research topic?
      2) Why is an answer for this question so imperative?
      3) How will the findings be applied to practice?
   c. *Theoretical or conceptual framework*
      1) Both describe framework for study
      2) Theoretical frameworks are composed of a set of concepts in which the relationships among concepts are described
      3) Conceptual frameworks are the building blocks of theoretical frameworks; they may include multiple concepts related to a common theme (e.g., child abuse, anger) and tend to be more global and less testable than theoretical frameworks
      4) Not all research studies have a fully developed conceptual or theoretical framework (e.g., descriptive or exploratory research studies)
      5) Findings from type I questions can generate conceptual frameworks
      6) Type II questions have conceptual frameworks to explain relationships between concepts or ideas
      7) Type III questions require a theoretical framework that answers the question "why": explains cause and effect of behavior

C. Identification of dependent and independent variables

1. **Dependent variables: what the researcher is interested in exploring, understanding, and measuring; it is the answer or outcome response**
2. **Independent variables: what the researcher believes to be cause of or influence on dependent variables; variable manipulated by the researcher; it is the treatment or intervention**
3. **Example: "what effect is there on turnover among emergency nurses who work in Level I trauma centers versus those who work in freestanding centers?"**
   a. *Dependent variable: turnover rates of emergency nurses*
   b. *Independent variable: type of emergency setting (Level I trauma or freestanding centers)*

D. Review of literature

1. **A critique or analysis of existing research that should help researcher assemble or evaluate data from previous research studies; can provide or examine three types of information**
   a. *Findings from previous studies*
   b. *Theoretical or conceptual basis*
   c. *Sources of methodology: instruments to be used to measure variables*
2. **Steps to use when critiquing a research study for review of literature**
   a. *Usefulness of study*
      1) Can literature reviewed be used in research study?
         a) Appropriate topic?
         b) Currency (less than 5 years old)?
         c) Credible investigator?
         d) Ethical or feasible?
         e) Applicable to practice?
      2) Is the research being reviewed clear, and is it related to proposed study?
      3) Was the literature being reviewed written logically, and is it understandable?
      4) Did this research literature further increase nursing's knowledge base?
   b. *Completeness*
      1) Does study being reviewed follow sequence expected of a research study?
      2) Do steps in research process flow in logical order, and are they described in appropriate depth and scope in reviewed study?
      3) Are all questions in review answered?
      4) Are subjects' rights protected?
      5) Is method consistent with and supportive of what was described in problem statement and hypothesis?

E. Formulation of hypothesis, if appropriate

1. **Requires theoretical basis**
2. **Is appropriate when researcher is able to predict outcomes of research study**
3. **Is used as a method to test a "scientific hunch" or idea**
4. **Is method of showing a relationship among two or more variables**
5. **Example: "an emergency nursing–sponsored community health program on bicycle safety and helmet use will result in a decreased number of head injuries in those who attend all six sessions"**

F. Definition of terms

1. **Terms used in research study are clearly defined, so that there is no question as to how the researcher has used these terms**
2. **Operational definitions: specify what the researcher wants to study and how he or she wants to study it (e.g., an emergency nurse can be operationally defined as a registered nurse with a BSN who works in an emergency care facility)**
3. **Theoretical definitions: abstract definitions that arise from theory or conceptual framework used (e.g., an emergency nurse can be theoretically defined as a person who provides nursing care to patients in an emergency care facility)**

G. Methodology

1. **Research approaches**
    The selection of a specific approach depends on research purposes. Approaches can be categorized as follows:
    a. *Descriptive*
    b. *Correlational*
        1) Prospective
        2) Retrospective
    c. *Quasiexperimental*
    d. *Experimental*
2. **Research instruments**
    a. *Methods used to collect, measure, and record data*
    b. *Types of research instruments include*
        1) Interviews: involve interview with each participant in the study; interviews are recorded for further analysis
        2) Questionnaires: involve written responses of participants to open or closed questions
        3) Observational tools: entail recording observations of patients, families, or staff by the researcher for later analysis
        4) Physiological tools: involve both in vitro methods, such as an electrocardiogram (ECG), or in vivo measurements, such as serum blood values
        5) Record analysis: involves careful auditing of charts and records to obtain data for analysis
    c. *Reliability and validity of instrument or tool*
        1) Researcher needs to show reliability and validity of instrument that is being used
        2) Reliability of instrument or tool is support for how consistently tool measures what it is supposed to measure; various forms of reliability are as follows:
            a) Test–retest
            b) Parallel form
            c) Internal consistency
            d) Inter-rater
            e) Intra-rater
        3) Validity of instrument or tool refers to extent to which tool or instrument measures what it is supposed to measure; there are several ways to measure an instrument's validity
            a) Content
            b) Criterion related
            c) Construct
                (1) Contrasted group
                (2) Experimental manipulation
                (3) Multitrait or multimethod
3. **Sample and population**
    a. *The population includes all persons who fit specific characteristics the researcher wants to study; it serves as basis for sample selections*
    b. *Not every member of a population can be studied, so the researcher takes a sample of the population (e.g., it might be difficult to study the diet habits of every MI patient who is admitted from ED; therefore, a sample of this population is used)*
    c. *Population needs to be carefully defined with regard to critical variables to delineate clearly objects of research study (e.g., does researcher want to*

> *study dietary habits of every MI patient who is admitted from ED or only a certain age group, ethnic background, or sex?)*

   d. *Sample and population must be of adequate size and depend on the research design and problem to be investigated*
   e. *Sample methodology depends on financial resources, available time, and availability of subjects; various methods of sample selection are as follows:*
      1) Probability
         a) Random
         b) Stratified random
         c) Cluster
         d) Systematic
      2) Nonprobability
         a) Convenience
         b) Quota
         c) Purpose

4. **Informed consent** (Box 25–1)
   a. *Protection of human subjects, particularly when outcomes are unknown*
   b. *ANA Commission on Nursing Research Guidelines (1985) proposes*
      1) Discussion of all instruments or tools, proposals, and techniques with prospective subjects and research assistants and workers
      2) Safeguards to be established to ensure that no unanticipated physical, psychological, or social disadvantage occurs to subjects during research or as a result of dissemination of findings
      3) Anonymity to be ensured
      4) Confidentiality to be ensured
      5) Consent to participate in research be obtained from each subject; each consent is expected to cover an explanation of study, procedures used,

---

Box 25–1   ESSENTIAL ELEMENTS OF AN INFORMED CONSENT

- A statement that the study involves research with explanations of the purpose, expected duration of the subject's participation, procedures to be followed, and identification of any procedures that are experimental

- A description of any reasonably foreseeable risks or discomforts

- A description of any benefits to the subject or to others that may reasonably be expected from the research

- A disclosure of appropriate alternative procedures or courses of treatment, if any, that might be advantageous to the subject

- A statement describing the extent, if any, to which confidentiality of records identifying the subject will be maintained

- For research involving no more than minimal risk, an explanation as to whether any compensation is available and an explanation as to whether any medical treatments are available if injury occurs and, if so, what they consist of or where further information may be obtained.

- An explanation of whom to contact for answers to pertinent questions about the research and research subject's rights, and whom to contact in the event of a research-related injury to the subject

- A statement that participation is voluntary, that refusal to participate will involve no penalty or loss of benefits to which the subject is otherwise entitled, and that the subject may discontinue participation at any time without penalty or loss of benefits to which the subject is otherwise entitled.

Adapted from *The Federal Register, 46*(16), 8390, 1981.

        description of any discomfort or risk, any invasion of privacy and threat to dignity, methods used to ensure anonymity and confidentiality

  c. Bilingual forms are available when appropriate

  d. Approval for research is obtained from appropriate institutional review board, as required:

    1) Examines researcher's efforts to determine whether proposed study protects subjects' rights

    2) Returns comments and decision of support or nonsupport to researcher

  e. Safeguards subjects' personal privacy

  f. Weighs benefits and risks to patients and clients participating in study

  g. Provides confidentiality and anonymity

  h. Free choice is offered, no coercion; subjects may withdraw without prejudice (see sample consent form, Box 25–2)

H. Analysis of data

1. **Summarizes all data collected from research study**
2. **Analysis of numerical data**
   a) Descriptive analysis
     1) Provides description of data collected from sample
     2) Usually used with descriptive or exploratory research designs
     3) Describes what was seen or found in sample
     4) Example: median, mode, range, standard deviation, correlation coefficients
   b) Inferential analysis
     1) Based on analysis and derives inferences about population from sample
     2) Tests hypothesis to determine whether scientific hunch was correct
     3) Depending on sample, can use either parametric or nonparametric statistics
3. **Analysis of non-numerical data**
   a) Used to provide a description of people, places, situations, happenings, opinions, attitudes, or behavior
   b) Can be used to generate theory or hypothesis for future testing
   c) Data usually come from written documents or notes related to unstructured interviews, observations, medical records, open-ended responses to questions on questionnaire, and other written accounts
   d) Involves reviewing written material for categories, themes, or patterns in data
   e) For example, analysis of interviews with patients about care received in the ED may reveal the following themes: patients were satisfied with nursing care received, patients were dissatisfied with their waiting time to be seen, and nurses were viewed as being concerned about patient's condition or illness

I. Results, conclusions, recommendations

1. **Results are merely stated as clear-cut data in tables, graphs, and so forth**
2. **Answers to research questions are provided in support/nonsupport of hypothesis**
3. **Based on results of data analysis, certain conclusions are made**
4. **Based on study's results and conclusions, recommendations are made for future research**
5. **Limitations are acknowledged**

Box 25–2   HUMAN RESEARCH REVIEW BOARD GUIDELINES FOR DRAFTING CONSENT FORM FOR PARTICIPATION IN RESEARCH

The following components must be included in a consent form for subject participation in research:

1. I, _____, agree to participate in the investigation

_____

2. *Purpose* of the study.
3. *Procedures* to be followed. Identify the *experimental aspects* of the study.
4. *Participation:* Identify the subject's extent of participation in the study.
5. *Risks:* Identify any discomforts or risks that may be reasonably expected.
6. *Benefits:* Identify possible benefits of participation in the study.
7. *Alternative Procedures:* If the research involves treatment protocols, identify alternative treatments available to the subject.
8. *Answer Inquiries:* Identify, by name, the person who has explained the research to the subject and who will be available to answer questions during the course of the study.
9. *Confidentiality:* Identify procedures to be used that will ensure the maintenance of confidentiality and conditions under which information from the study will be disclosed.
10. *Financial Benefits:* Identify, if appropriate.
11. *No Prejudice:* Indicate that subjects may withdraw from the study at any time and this will not jeopardize present or future relationships with MCMC.
12. *Compensation for Injuries:* Identify, if appropriate.
13. *Further Information:* Identify by name persons available to answer questions regarding study.

The Human Research Review Board of Milwaukee County Medical Complex has reviewed and approved this study.

_____

(Signature of Subject or Legal Guardian) (Date)

_____

(Signature of Witness) (Date)
I have defined and fully explained the study as described herein to the subject.
Type or Print:

_____

(Name of Principal Investigator or Authorized Representative)

_____

(Position Title)

_____

(Signature) (Date)
ASSENT OF MINOR: (Add only if appropriate)
In my opinion the child has not reached the age of assent.

_____

(Signature of Principal Investigator) (Date)
The above has been explained to me and I agree to participate.

_____

(Signature of Minor) (Date)

_____

From Luske, A. M. (1986). *Clinical nursing research: A guide to understanding and using research in nursing practice* (pp. 89–90). Rockville, MD: Aspen Systems Corp. Used with permission.

J. Communication of research findings

This is the final step of the research process, which is necessary if research findings are to be integrated into practice.

1. Professional journals (e.g., *Journal of Emergency Nursing; Nursing Research*)
2. Professional meetings (e.g., Annual Scientific Assembly Research Presentation)

VIII. RESEARCH ETHICS

A. Human subjects and ethical guidelines

1. Resulted from unethical treatment and harm of subjects in earlier research studies, such as withholding treatment to persons with syphilis to study effects of the disease
2. Institutional review boards (IRBs) were developed to review all research studies to ensure that patients' or research subjects' rights and safety are maintained
3. Department of Health and Human Services instituted the following regulations in 1983:
   a) *Requirements for and documentation of informed consent*
   b) *IRB review of research proposals*
   c) *Procedures for expedited and exempt reviews*
   d) *Criteria for IRB approval of research proposals*
4. Human rights to be maintained while participating in a research project:
   a) *Right to self-determination*
   b) *Right to privacy and dignity*
   c) *Right to anonymity and confidentiality*
   d) *Right to fair treatment*
   e) *Right to protection from discomfort and harm*
5. Protection of human rights is actualized through informed consent (see section VII.G.4.)

B. Animal subjects and ethical guidelines

1. Rights of animals used in research are controlled by legislation in the United States
2. Animal care and use committees (ACUCs) are the equivalent of the IRB for protecting animal rights
3. Research involving animals must be approved by the ACUC

C. Scientific fraud and misconduct

1. Includes the following circumstances:
   a) *Inventing data for a project*
   b) *Falsifying or altering data*
   c) *Reporting another researcher's results as one's own*
   d) *Plagiarism*
   e) *Violating animal or human rights*
2. Agencies exist to investigate allegations of scientific misconduct or fraud

IX. APPLICATION OF RESEARCH TO CLINICAL PRACTICE

Before the findings of a research study can be used in clinical practice, several questions need to be answered.

A. Do study findings address current clinical problems?

B. Does study include a reliable and valid subject population?

C. Were subjects' rights protected?

D. Was study ethical, legal, and feasible?

E. Was a critical review of the literature done?

F. Is study's setting similar to or different from intended practice setting?

G. Is sample similar to intended population to which you hope to apply findings?

H. Is the tool used reliable and valid?

I. Are findings consistent with practice?

J. Do other studies report similar or different findings?

X. CRITIQUING QUANTITATIVE RESEARCH STUDIES

A. Title

1. Readily understood
2. Intent of study is clear to reader
3. Related to content of study (variables, population)

B. Abstract

1. General impressions of study
2. Problem or purpose, hypothesis, or questions are outlined clearly and concisely
3. Methodology is identified and described briefly
4. Analysis of data is summarized
5. Conclusions are clear
6. Description is clear versus vague
7. Describes important findings

C. Problem statement/purposes

1. Precise information about variables studied
2. General problem statement is narrowed to a specific statement
3. Information is clear and concise
4. Definitions of terms are complete
5. Background information clearly and concisely describes importance of study
6. Definite statement of problem and purposes of study
7. Limitations of study are listed
8. Assumptions of study are listed

D. Review of literature

1. Information specific to problem and purpose of study
2. Primary sources were used more often than secondary sources
3. Recent and past literature was reviewed
4. Empirical work was emphasized
5. Literature reviewed was adequate in number (20–30)
6. Literature reviewed was taken from professional journals, books, and general scientific sources
7. Review of literature is clear, concise, and logically organized
8. Review of literature concludes with synopsis of literature and its implications for this research study; authors of study are authorities in their fields
9. Research used in literature review is critically analyzed

E. Framework: theoretical-conceptual

1. Linkage of problem to theory or concept
2. Selected framework makes sense and is relevant to research focus
3. Deductions from theory or conceptual framework are clear, correct, and well defined
4. Framework is understandable

F. Hypothesis and questions of research study

1. Does the study list and identify hypothesis or questions for the research proposed?
2. Does each question or hypothesis show a relationship between two or more variables?
3. Are hypothesis and questions testable?
4. Are hypothesis and questions worthy of study?

G. Methodology

1. Research design
   a. *Experimental*
      1) Subjects are randomly assigned
      2) Design is adequately described
      3) There is a rationale for the selection of the design
      4) Design is the best approach for addressing hypothesis or questions
      5) There is adequate control for threats to internal validity of the study
   b. *Quasiexperimental*
      1) Comparison groups are described clearly
      2) Steps are taken to ensure equal group participation
      3) If there is no comparison group, why not?
      4) How are the results interpreted?
      5) Internal validity is ensured
      6) Is design appropriate for this study?
   c. *Nonexperimental*
      1) Are there comparison groups in this study?
      2) Are the groups equally compared?
      3) Are groups equivalent?
      4) Are all variables controlled?

5) Has best design been used?
2. **Research procedure**
   a. *Researcher describes method used to execute design selected*
   b. *Researcher ensures internal consistency in data collection process*
   c. *Contamination of groups is adequately prevented*
   d. *Research is conducted in proper setting*
   e. *Subjects are protected*
3. **Subjects**
   a. *Appropriate sample size*
   b. *Sample was representative of population studied*
   c. *Population was defined and described*
   d. *Description provided of how population was selected*
4. **Data selection**
   a. *Instruments or tools used are clearly defined and described*
   b. *Instruments or tools are reliable and valid*
   c. *Instrument or tools ask questions that are in line with hypothesis or questions of study*
   d. *Methods used to collect the data are appropriate*
   e. *Intervening variables are controlled*
   f. *If instruments or tools were newly developed, there is evidence that they were properly tested and described*
   g. *Statistical methods for data analysis are described and are appropriate for the study*
   h. *Confidentiality was provided for and ensured*
5. **Data analysis**
   a. *Detailed description of how the data were analyzed*
   b. *Were statistics used appropriate for this instrument or tool?*
   c. *Were results reported and interpreted correctly?*
   d. *Was hypothesis or question(s) answered?*
   e. *Were tables and graphs set up clearly, correctly, and concisely?*
   f. *Can readers look at tables and graphs and determine results or make an analysis?*
   g. *Was there consistency in data interpretation and table construction?*

H. Conclusions

1. **Clearly stated**
2. **Substantiated by data analysis**
3. **Methodological problems are discussed**
4. **Conclusions are specifically related to hypothesis or research questions**
5. **Results are generalizable to population identified in study**

I. Implications for further research

1. **Clear and applicable**
2. **Based on data analysis**
3. **Meaningful and realistic**

XI. CRITIQUING QUALITATIVE RESEARCH REPORTS

A. Context of study

1. Are research questions and purpose of study well written and easily understood?
2. Is phenomenon, idea, culture, or topic clearly defined?
3. Is there adequate description of people, places, events, and/or site of study?
4. Is the philosophical basis for study described?

B. Research method

1. Is qualitative method used to collect data identified and described in detail?
2. Is method consistent with research questions and purpose?
3. Does researcher follow method consistently?
4. Are sampling procedures explained?
5. Are sampling procedures appropriate for type of qualitative method used?
6. Will subjects selected be able to provide data required for this project (i.e., have they experienced the phenomenon or been a member of the culture under study)?
7. Was sample size adequate to ensure redundancy in data or to provide a complete picture of the culture, behavior, or events?
8. Are steps used to collect data described?
9. Are data collection strategies consistent with research method selected?
10. Will data collection strategies provide the type of data required for this study?
11. Are human subjects protected?
12. Did researcher identify the decision trail used in the study?

C. Data analysis

1. Did researcher follow the data analysis strategy required for selected method used?
2. Are steps in data analysis comprehensively detailed?

D. Results

1. Do results flow from the data collected and the analysis?
2. Do results fit within the data analysis codes, categories, or patterns identified by researcher?
3. Did subjects who participated provide evidence that results represent their experience?
4. Are people who were not in the study able to recognize the experience from the results provided?
5. Are results presented as description of the phenomenon or culture and/or a conceptual/theoretical framework (i.e., do the results answer the research question)?
6. Are results consistent with the data analysis method used and data collected?
7. Is there a visual representation of the results in the form of a diagram or table?
8. Are results linked to existing knowledge?

E. Conclusions

1. Are results applicable to nursing and clinical practice?
2. Does researcher describe usefulness of the results?
3. Does researcher identify areas in need of further research?
4. Are limitations to the study discussed?

BIBLIOGRAPHY

American Nurses Association Commission on Nursing Research. (1985). *Guidelines for the investigative function of nurses.* Kansas City, MO: ANA.

American Nurses Association. (1985). *Human rights guidelines for nurses in clinical and other research* (Publication No. D-465M). Kansas City, MO: Author.

Brink, P., & Wood, M. (1988). *Basic steps in planning nursing research: From question to proposal* (3rd ed.). Belmont, CA: Jones and Bartlett.

Burns, N., & Grove, S. K. (1997). *The practice of nursing research* (3rd ed.). Philadelphia: W. B. Saunders.

Hawley, D. J., & Jeffers, J. M. (1992). Scientific misconduct as a dilemma for nursing. *Image: The Journal of Nursing Scholarship, 24,* 51–55.

Isaac, S., & Michael, W. (1982). *Handbook in research and evaluation* (2nd ed.). San Diego, CA: Edits.

Lincoln, Y., & Guba, E. (1985). *Naturalistic inquiry.* Beverly Hills, CA: Sage.

LoBiondo-Wood, G., & Haber, J. (1998). *Nursing research: Methods, critical appraisal, and utilization* (4th ed.). St. Louis, MO: C. V. Mosby.

Polit, D. F., & Hungler, B. P. (1995). *Nursing research: Principles and methods* (5th ed.). Philadelphia: J. B. Lippincott.

Waltz, C. F., & Bausell, R. B. (1983). *Nursing research: Design, statistics, and computer analysis.* Philadelphia: F. A. Davis.

Linda Jacobson Bracken, RN, BS, MEd, MPA, CEN
Robin Rosser Martinez, RN, MS

CHAPTER **26**

Education

MAJOR TOPICS

Emergency nurses have the opportunity to interface with and educate large numbers of patients on a daily basis. Emergency nursing expertise encompasses knowledge specific to all age groups and specialties of medicine. The attainment of this information and knowledge is a nursing responsibility that enhances practice, patient care, and the community.

I. EDUCATION OF THE EMERGENCY DEPARTMENT (ED) NURSE

A. Distinctions of the educational needs of the emergency nurse

1. **Knowledgeable in every discipline**
   a. *Pediatrics*
   b. *Obstetrics*
   c. *Medicine*
   d. *Cardiology*
   e. *Trauma*
   f. *Orthopedics*
   g. *Oncology*
   h. *Infectious disease*
   i. *Psychiatry*
   j. *Others*
2. **Knowledgeable in caring for all age groups**
   a. *Newborns*
   b. *Infants, toddlers*
   c. *Childhood*
   d. *Adolescence*
   e. *Adult*
   f. *Geriatric*
3. **Functions efficiently and safely in high-stress situations**
4. **Adapts to unexpected increase in workload**
5. **Works effectively as a team player**
6. **Skillfully practices triage of patients**
7. **Provides crisis intervention for patients and families**
8. **Delivers pediatric and adult trauma care**
9. **Mastery of technology and equipment used in ED**
10. **Proficient in public relations and customer service techniques**
11. **Assists public in appropriately accessing health care system**
12. **Participates as a resource for medical instruction**
13. **Interfaces effectively with prehospital care providers (i.e., emergency medical technicians [EMTs], paramedics, firefighters, and law enforcement officers)**
14. **Facilitates social service for the indigent and homeless**
15. **Knowledgeable in providing treatment for exposure to hazardous materials**
16. **Skilled in activation and implementation of hospital and community disaster management**
17. **Knowledgeable in ways to control violence in ED**
18. **Cognizant of legal implications as they relate to patient care (i.e., psychiatric "holds," EMTALA)**

19. Keeps up to date on reimbursement issues
20. Skilled in radio/phone communication

B. Facilitators of learning in ED

1. **Clinical nurse specialist**
   a. *Educator: serves as resource to staff, nursing students, and other health care personnel in the acquisition of knowledge and skills related to nursing practice*
   b. *Consultant: collaborates with clinical nurses and other members of the health care team to resolve complex clinical situations for specialty needs of emergency patients*
   c. *Researcher: critically analyzes current nursing research and disseminates relevant findings to staff to improve patient care and patient outcomes; facilitates and/or conducts nursing research*
   d. *Clinical expert: models excellence in emergency nursing practice through use of assessment, planning, implementation, and evaluation; assists and provides direction to nursing staff with clinical decision making, priority setting, stabilization, and resuscitation*

2. **Nurse educator**
   a. *Organizes and implements orientation program*
   b. *Develops and executes educational programs for ED personnel*
   c. *Serves as resource to staff*

3. **Nurse manager**
   a. *Supports and encourages staff's involvement in education process within ED*
   b. *Organizes committees and projects that support education*
   c. *Holds staff accountable for complying with educational requirements of ED*

C. Concepts of adult learning (Malcolm Knowles)

1. **Basic assumptions about adults as learners**
   a. *Adult learner is independent and self-directed and appreciates rationale for the existence of learning experience (e.g., knowledge of basic thrombolytic pharmacokinetics enables nurse to administer a new thrombolytic therapy protocol competently)*
   b. *Adult learner has past experiences in life that enable adaptation to new information (e.g., past experience with invasive forms of temporary cardiac pacing enables nurse to adapt to new technology of external pacing)*
   c. *Adult learner expects and appreciates learning that is immediately applicable to present work situation (e.g., including special blood product delivery techniques in an ED educational program for factor administration for hemophiliacs)*
   d. *Adult learns best from education that is problem centered (e.g., an increase in drug errors in ED may prompt a program on drug calculations)*
   e. *Adults have extrinsic and intrinsic motivators for learning (e.g., salary incentives, promotion, self-fulfillment, achievement)*

2. **Ideal conditions for adult learning**
   a. *Climate conducive to learning is helpful, comfortable, and respectful*
   b. *Learner has innate desire to learn*
   c. *Course objectives help learner recognize the experience as one that is applicable to practice*
   d. *Learner should help plan and implement the content*
   e. *Learning program should appeal creatively to different learning styles*

f. *Learner's past experiences are taken into account*
g. *Learner has sense of personal progress toward objectives*

D. Approaches to nurse orientation in ED

1. **Review of specific institutional policies and procedures**
2. **Review of ED's standards of care**
3. **Checks skills with return demonstration**
4. **Preceptor-sponsored orientation: a preceptor is a specially trained nurse who serves as a role model and resource person for new employee**
5. **Modularized education: self-instructional orientation program**
6. **Competency-based orientation (CBO)** (Fig. 26–1)
   a. *An organized system of assessing a new nurse's ability to perform proficiencies, tasks, skills (competency) required for baseline job performance*
   b. *Essential competencies are given to nurse on arrival to ED; at end of orientation, nurse must understand, complete, and demonstrate successful achievement of these competencies*
   c. *Essential components of CBO*
      1) Skill and knowledge assessment
      2) Competence standards: behavioral objectives based on performance outcomes
      3) Critical behaviors: criterion-referenced behaviors that denote ability to safely perform skills
      4) Learning options: a guide to resources available for utilization
      5) Time frames, completion dates
   d. *Management of CBO completion, determination of clinical competence*
      1) Clinical nurse specialist
      2) Nurse educator
      3) Preceptor
      4) Peer review (based on seniority)
   e. *Determination of department specific competencies*
      1) High-volume procedures performed in ED
      2) High-risk procedures performed in ED
      3) Unusual or rare procedures should be considered
   f. *Copies of all competencies should be available within ED for staff to use for reference and review*
   g. *Competencies should complement and correlate with ED's ongoing quality improvement program*

E. Certification/verification: validation of essential knowledge base for practice

1. **Certification**
   a. *Certified emergency nurse (CEN)*
   b. *Certified flight registered nurse (CFRN)*
2. **Verification**
   a. *Advanced cardiac life support (ACLS)*
   b. *Trauma nursing core course (TNCC)*
   c. *Emergency nurse pediatric course (ENPC)*
   d. *Pediatric advanced life support (PALS)*
   e. *Institution specific (e.g., trauma, triage)*

COMPETENCY: Safely and efficiently assists with insertion and management of chest tube.

Critical Behaviors:

Critical Behavior	Date Completed	Validated By
1. Assembles appropriate equipment: Chest tube tray Povidone-iodine solution Chest tube Sterile gloves for MD Chest drainage unit 2″ pink tape Wall suction Local anesthetic as requested		
2. Sets up chest drainage unit according to manufacturer's instructions.		
3. Preps skin insertion site with povidone-iodine.		
4. Aseptically hands off chest tube to physician when ready.		
5. Connects collection chamber tubing to the thoracic catheter after it is placed by the physician.		
6. Initiates suction by slight increments until continuous bubbling appears in the suction chamber. Confirms desired amount of suction with physician (15–20 cc of water for adult).		
7. Marks the collection chamber to indicate date/time of insertion. Marks/times drainage levels at intervals.		
8. Tapes connections securely with pink waterproof tape.		
9. Obtains x-ray post chest tube placement.		
10. Applies occlusive dressing around chest tube insertion site after physician has sutured chest tube. Applies benzoin to skin and allows to dry. Secures a gauze dressing with 2″ pink tape.		
11. Assesses functioning of chest drainage system: A. Auscultates breath sounds before and after insertion. B. Identifies fluctuation in water seal chamber with inspiration/expiration. (Checks this with suction disconnected). C. Monitors bubbling in the water seal chamber: *Appropriate:* Small amount of bubbles expected with pneumothorax as device evacuates excess air from pleural cavity. *Inappropriate:* Large amounts of bubbles or continuous bubbling. D. If inappropriate bubbling occurs, attempts to isolate the air leak: 1. Checks/tightens all connections. 2. Clamps tubing momentarily at various points beginning at the chest and working toward drainage unit. Notes that bubbling stops when clamp is placed between water seal and air leak.		
12. Maintains normal function of unit: A. Keeps drainage below patient's chest. B. Avoids dependent loops in tubing. C. Transports the patient without suction unless continuous suction is ordered. D. States would AVOID CLAMPING the chest tube at any time unless specifically ordered. E. Ensures constant slow bubbling in suction chamber if suction is ordered.		
13. If chest tube becomes dislodged: A. Immediately applies pressure over site with petrolatum gauze and stack of 4×4s. B. Notifies physician immediately.		

Name: _____

Classification: RN   LVN
(circle one)

FIGURE 26–1. Assist with chest tube insertion. (Reprinted with permission from Stanford University Hospital.)

F. Teaching strategies for emergency nurse education

1. In-services, classes, lectures
2. Seminars, conferences, workshops, symposia
3. Panel discussions, debates
4. Bedside teaching, dialogue, nursing rounds
5. Role modeling
6. Questioning
   a. *Lecture*
   b. *Clinical practice*
   c. *Discussion*
7. Autotutorial learning module/instructional package (e.g., review of assessment skills for pediatric patients)
8. Equipment update, drug update
9. Demonstration/skill review (e.g., new chest tube set-up)
10. Case studies (e.g., snakebite care)
11. Mock scenarios (e.g., pediatric code)
12. Games, simulations (e.g., equipment "scavenger hunt" for new nurse)
13. Posters (e.g., special equipment assembly, such as pediatric arterial catheter)
14. Staff meeting (e.g., education updates)
15. Committee work (e.g., education committee, customer service committee)
16. Fact sheets, newsletter
17. Brainstorming (e.g., tackling staffing problems)
18. Learning resource center (e.g., books, journals, tapes, videos)
19. Portable education cart
20. Video or closed-circuit television
21. Computer literacy (e.g., teaching basic skills needed for computer use in ED)
22. Computer-assisted instruction (e.g., learning modules)
23. Interactive video: screen-displayed accounts of clinical situations in which interactive process enables validation or correction of nurse's treatment plan

G. Potential obstacles to education process

1. Staffing patterns not conducive to education programs
2. Institutional funding for education and educators
3. Staff's attitudes toward learning
4. Nurses with multiple commitments
   a. *Family constraints*
   b. *Additional employment*
5. Fatigue of nurse
6. Nursing burnout
7. Philosophical differences
8. ED patient overload
9. Inappropriate needs assessment
10. Morale

H. Continuing education for emergency nurse

1. Purpose

a. *Promotes competence in nursing (e.g., electrocardiogram [ECG] course improves rhythm interpretation skills)*
b. *Enhances nurse's working knowledge (e.g., trauma nurse core curriculum)*
c. *Advances skills in education, research, administration, and theory development*
d. *Improves health care to the client (e.g., emergency nurse pediatric course increases proficiency in pediatric care)*
e. *Fosters personal and professional development as well as career goals (e.g., management course for new managers)*

2. **Beneficiaries of education**
   a. *Nurse*
   b. *Employer*
      1) Increased competence
      2) Decreased liability
      3) Advanced expertise to benefit patient care
   c. *Profession*
      1) Increased adherence to standards of practice
      2) Strengthened image of nurse
   d. *Public*
      1) Improved patient care
3. **Means of obtaining continuing education**
   a. *Self-learning/self-study*
   b. *Home study/correspondence courses*
   c. *Institution-sponsored continuing education*
   d. *Workshops, seminars*
   e. *Organizational meetings (e.g., ENA)*
   f. *Degree advancement*
   g. *Computer-assisted instruction*

I. Nursing research and application to practice

1. **Incorporates research findings into clinical practice**
2. **Encourages unit-based research**
3. **Implements unit-based research**

II. EDUCATION OF THE PATIENT IN ED

A. Distinctiveness of patient teaching in ED

1. **Patient education defined: patient education is an ongoing process during the visit in ED; information imparted in ED should effect changes in patient's knowledge, attitudes, and skills in relation to his or her health or illness**
2. **Patient teaching encompasses all disciplines of medicine**
3. **Patient teaching information has to be customized to patient's age and developmental level**
4. **Families and significant others are included in teaching**
5. **Teaching should be adapted to patient's culture and ethnicity**
6. **Effective teaching may depend on conquering language barriers**
7. **Teaching is a "one-moment, one-visit" opportunity**
   a. *Must be short and concise*
   b. *Must be immediately understandable*
   c. *Nurse must have teaching information committed to memory*

8. **All opportunities for teaching must be used during ED visit**
   a. *Teaching begins at triage*
   b. *Teaching is required before treatment and during treatment*
   c. *Teaching is required before and after medication is administered*
   d. *Teaching opportunities generally end at time of discharge*
9. **Time and energy are at a premium in ED; patient will benefit from a focus on key items, as opposed to information overload**

B. Education: a patient's right and a nurse's legal obligation

1. **Nurse Practice Acts include health guidance and health education as a part of nurse's role and responsibility**
2. **Patients have right to be educated about their disease process or injury**
3. **Nurse must ensure that teaching has taken place before any procedure or medication**
4. **Nurse is legally responsible for teaching content and is, therefore, open to potential litigation**

C. Assessment of need for patient teaching

1. **Data gathering**
   a. *Observations of patient during entire visit*
   b. *Old medical records (previous hospital visits)*
   c. *Patient's support systems (family and friends)*
   d. *Interview, discussions with patient throughout visit*
2. **Sort data informally**
3. **Determine what patient wants to know**
4. **Ascertain what will enhance patient's ability and motivation to learn**
5. **Devise and tailor teaching plan, keeping in mind that approach to learning is determined by past experiences, lifestyle, and personality**

D. Adaptations of adult learning principles to ED teaching

1. **Adult patients bring life experiences that will contribute to understanding of new material: consider patient's experience before teaching**
2. **Patient will more readily learn material that is meaningful to him or her as an individual**
3. **Patient who is physically comfortable will more readily focus on educational material (pain relief, warm blanket, position of comfort)**
4. **Acknowledge each patient's need for support and anxiety about learning new behaviors**
   a. *Patient may be afraid to disclose lack of knowledge*
   b. *Patient may be afraid to make mistakes (e.g., during return demonstration)*
   c. *During crisis or period of stress, patients may test nurse's willingness to aid them, yet may want additional information*
5. **Adult learning is problem centered**
   a. *Help patient to recognize problem (patient may not be able to do this independently)*
   b. *Work with patient to assist him or her in knowing what to do about problem*
   c. *Assist patient in feeling competent to deal with problem*
6. **Use methods that increase recall of learning**
   a. *Shorter words and sentences*

  b. *Repetition*

  c. *Concrete, specific statements (e.g., instead of "No weight-bearing on the affected limb," use "Do not walk on your sprained foot")*

  d. *Goal-related suggestions*

7. **Impaired patients (physical state, drug or alcohol use, medications)**

  a. *Family and friends should be included in teaching process*

  b. *Teaching may be delayed until patient is clear-minded*

8. **Teaching is reinforced with written discharge instructions as mandated by regulatory agencies**

  a. *Patient may be too nervous, stressed, or distracted to absorb information in ED*

  b. *Allows for later reference*

  c. *Legal record*

E. Potential obstacles to teaching in ED

1. **Lack of privacy**
2. **Time constraints**
3. **Effective nurse–patient rapport**
4. **Nurse's knowledge deficit or teaching finesse**
5. **Deficiency in involvement of family of impaired patient**
6. **Opportunity to establish continuity and to follow up for reinforcement and evaluation**

F. Barriers to learning in ED

1. **Physiological barriers: pain, restlessness, age, prognosis, critical illness**
2. **Psychological barriers: intelligence, anxiety, denial, depression, psychosis**
3. **Environmental barriers: lack of privacy, separation from family, noise level, lack of sleep**
4. **Sociocultural barriers: language barrier, ethnic background, lack of education**
5. **Sight or hearing deficits**
6. **Illiteracy**
7. **Patient's desire to take responsibility for health care**
8. **Cognizance of patient's needs and desire to learn**

G. Learning activities in ED

1. **Patient teaching methods**

  a. *Demonstration and return demonstration (e.g., crutch training)*

  b. *One-on-one discussion between nurse and patient*

  c. *Use of preprinted information sheets for patient (Fig. 26–2)*

  d. *Reiteration of physician's instructions*

  e. *Questioning*

  f. *Final written instructions*

2. **Educational information located in lobby or hallways**

  a. *Display on bulletin boards: drawings, photographs*

  b. *Signs, posters, cartoons*

  c. *Educational coloring books for children*

  d. *Video or educational television in lobby*

  e. *Pamphlets in lobby and examination rooms on various medical topics*

The patient involved has sustained a head injury that is not of sufficient degree to warrant hospitalization at this time.

However, in a small percentage of cases, subsequent symptoms may appear that make further close observation necessary.

The following is a list of symptoms for which the person who has sustained the injury should be observed:

1. **Severe or persistent** headache.
2. **Repeated** nausea and vomiting.
3. Excessive sleepiness or difficulty in arousing from sleep. (It is suggested that the person involved not be allowed to sleep for periods longer than 2 hours following the injury.)
4. Unequal pupils, double vision, or change in ability to see or hear.
5. Dizziness.
6. Weakness or paralysis of arms or legs.
7. Confusion, irritabilty, or personality change.
8. Drainage of fluid or blood from ears or nose.

Avoid all sedatives, narcotics, and alcohol. Aspirin or Tylenol may be used for pain.

If any or all of these symptoms appear, return patient to the Emergency Department immediately.

FIGURE 26–2. Instructions for patients with minor head injuries. (Reprinted with permission from Stanford University Hospital.)

H. Evaluation of patient teaching

Patient education should result in positive behavior and attitude changes in relation to health and well-being.

1. **Ask learner to restate (in own words) what has been taught**
2. **Ask patient a question about what has been taught to test understanding of learning**
3. **Learning will be increased if teaching is related to something with which the patient is familiar**
4. **Return demonstration by patient will indicate need for correction and feedback**
5. **Follow-up telephone call can help nurse determine effectiveness of patient teaching**
6. **Follow-up questionnaire with specific questions helps nurse assess teaching effectiveness**

I. Guidelines for relating information and providing feedback to patient

1. **Be specific rather than general (e.g., instead of saying "Watch for signs of infection," state specific signs of infection)**
2. **Focus on behavior, not on the person (e.g., maintain respect for patient as a person and give corrective advice in a positive manner)**
3. **Avoid use of absolute words such as "always" and "never"**
4. **Direct feedback toward behavior or situation that learner has the ability to change (e.g., encourage condom use for "safe sex" as opposed to advising abstinence)**
5. **Do not overload patient or learner with information**
6. **Do not argue with patient**
7. **First give positive feedback and then discuss weaknesses**

J. Patient compliance

1. **Patient has right to choose whether or not to follow nurse's advice**
2. **Compliance with teaching depends on**
   a. *Recall ability*
   b. *Comprehension*

c. Desire to comply
d. Ability to perform

K. Reinforcement of discharge instructions

1. Give written discharge instructions
2. Read over discharge instructions with patient
3. Answer questions
4. Clarify unclear items
5. Explain medical terms and directions
6. Request that physician return to clarify patient needs
7. Involve family and significant others in interaction
8. Explain rationale for prescribed medication (e.g., include drug actions, side effects, and so forth)
9. Offer specific instruction with medication (e.g., "Do not drive while taking this medication")

L. Arrangements for follow-up after discharge

1. Private physician appointment
2. Clinic appointment
3. Return visit to ED
4. Home health care
5. Social service referral
6. County/charity hospital
7. Psychiatric facility
8. Drug/alcohol detoxification centers

III. EMERGENCY NURSE'S ROLE IN COMMUNITY EDUCATION

A. General health education for the visiting public within ED

1. Educational pamphlets, reading material, health-related magazines and posters in ED
   a. Lobby
   b. Hallways
   c. Examination rooms
2. Ongoing instructional video in ED lobby
3. Health information resource center, library
   a. On hospital grounds
   b. Outside of hospital
4. Telephone line advice or directions given by knowledgeable personnel (dependent on hospital, state policy, protocol)
   a. First aid advice
   b. Public health guidance (e.g., flu vaccine)
   c. Counsel, recommendation during an epidemic (e.g., measles outbreak)
   d. Direction during disaster

B. Injury prevention programs: school, workplace, community-based education programs

1. Traffic injuries
   a. Motor vehicle occupants

        b. Pedestrians
        c. Motorcyclists
        d. Bicyclists

2. **Residential injuries**
     a. Falls
     b. Fire and burns
     c. Poisoning
     d. Suffocation

3. **Recreational injuries**
     a. Drowning
     b. Aquatic spinal cord injuries
     c. Boating
     d. Playground
     e. Fireworks
     f. Amateur competitive sports
     g. All-terrain vehicles

4. **Occupational injuries**
5. **Violence, assault**
6. **Domestic assault: battery**
7. **Rape and sexual assault**
8. **Firearm injuries**
9. **Child abuse, neglect**
10. **Elder abuse**
11. **Suicide**
12. **Alcohol, drug use**
     a. Correlation with all modes of injury

C. Persuasion programs: designed to change human behavior using real-life scenarios

1. **ED nurse giving slide presentation and lecture to junior high school, high school**
     a. Injury prevention
     b. Drug use
     c. Alcohol use
2. **Focus on what transpires during emergency treatment and rehabilitation**

D. Marketing nursing as career

1. **Provision of ED, hospital tours, and information for students**
2. **Junior high, high school classroom visits (e.g., Career Day participation)**

E. Health fair to instruct, demonstrate, and distribute literature regarding helpful topics

1. **Access and appropriate use of emergency health care system**
2. **Injury prevention**
3. **Education and awareness about acquired immunodeficiency syndrome (AIDS)**
4. **Warning signs of illness (e.g., cancer, heart disease)**
5. **Vital signs and laboratory testing**

F. Paramedic/EMT training

1. Serves as instructor for medics in classroom settings
2. Serves as preceptor in clinical setting

G. Legislative advocate for health care issues

H. Cardiopulmonary resuscitation (CPR) instructor

1. Schools
2. Workplace
3. Civic groups
4. Community organizations

I. Red Cross volunteer

1. Staffing local events
2. Disaster work

J. Disaster management

1. ED nurse as member of regional disaster team
   a. *Active involvement in planning medical components of disaster management before event*
      1) Schools, workplace, and community
2. Stimulates, organizes, or acts as resource for teaching programs for hospital disaster team
   a. *Clinical and management skills during disaster*
3. Organizes or participates in critical incident stress debriefing after incident

BIBLIOGRAPHY

Abruzzese, R. S. (1996). *Nursing staff development: Strategies for success*. St. Louis, MO: Mosby-Year Book.

Bastable, S. B. (1997). *Nurse as educator*. Boston: Jones and Bartlett.

Benware, S. N. (1995). A self-paced case study approach to continuing education. *Journal of Emergency Nursing, 21*(3), 258–261.

Burns, C., & Harm, N. J. (1993). Emergency nurses' perceptions of critical incident stress debriefing. *Journal of Emergency Nursing, 19*(5), 431–436.

Emergency Nurses Association. (1994). *Standards of emergency nursing practice* (3rd ed.). St. Louis, MO: Mosby-Year Book.

Emergency Nurses Association. (1997a). *Position statement: CEN credentialing and review courses*. Park Ridge, IL: Author.

Emergency Nurses Association. (1997b). *Position statement: Telephone advice*. Park Ridge, IL: Author.

Flaherty, L., & McLean, S. (Eds.). (1996). *Crash course in motor vehicle prevention*. Park Ridge, IL: Emergency Nurses Association.

Flynn, J. P. (Ed.). (1997). *The role of the preceptor: A guide for nurse educators and clinicians*. New York: Springer Verlag.

Hamric, A. B., Spross, J. A., & Hansen, C. M. (1996). *Advanced nursing practice: An integrative approach*. Philadelphia: W. B. Saunders.

Knowles, M. S. (1970). *The modern practice of adult education*. New York: Association Press.

Lewis, C. P., & Aghababian, R. V. (1996). Disaster planning, part I: Overview of hospital and emergency department planning for internal and external disasters. *Emergency Medicine Clinics of North America, 14*(2), 439–451.

Martinez, R. (1996). Creating the future: The emergency nurse's role in injury prevention. *Journal of Emergency Nursing, 22*(4), 265–266.

McBee, M. J. (1996). Pocket guide to emergency department orientation. *Journal of Emergency Nursing, 22*(5), 446–450.

Melnykovich, P. (1994). Developing self-teaching packages for the emergency department staff. *Journal of Emergency Nursing, 20*(3), 239–240.

Newberry, L. (1998). *Sheehy's emergency nursing: Principles and practice* (4th ed.). St. Louis, MO: C. V. Mosby.

Rankin, S. H., & Stallings, K. D. (1996). *Patient education: Issues, principles, practices* (3rd ed.). Philadelphia: J. B. Lippincott.

Ready, R. W. (1994). Clinical competency testing for emergency nurses. *Journal of Emergency Nursing, 20*(1), 24–32.

Redman, B. K. (1997). *The practice of patient education* (8th ed.). St. Louis, MO: C. V. Mosby.

Robinson, S. M., & Barberis-Ryan, C. (1995). Competency assessment: A systematic approach. *Nursing Management, 26*(2), 40–44.

Schure, B. L., Dunn, S. C., Clark, H. M., Soled, S. W., & Gilman, B. R. (1991). The effects of inter-active video on cognitive achievement and attitude toward learning. *Journal of Nursing Education, 30*(3), 109–113.

Stanford University Hospital Emergency Department. (1997). *Competency-based orientation manual.* Stanford, CA: Author.

Trautman, D., & Watson, J. E. (1995). Implementing continued clinical competency evaluation in the emergency department. *Journal of Nursing Staff Development, 11*(1), 41–47.

Polly Gerber Zimmermann, RN, MS, MBA, CEN
Laura Skidmore Rhodes, BSN, MSN

CHAPTER **27**

Professionalism and Leadership

MAJOR TOPICS

Concepts

Standards

Emergency Nursing Practice

Professional Performance

Professional Behaviors

Specialized Professional Nursing Roles

Professionalism is a foundation in the development of the standard of practice for emergency nursing. Professional standards, characteristics, and behaviors are expected in every emergency nurse.

I. CONCEPTS (ENA, 1999)

A. Definition (ENA 1996, 1999)

1. A registered nurse who has specialized education and experience in caring for emergency patients
2. A specialist in rapid assessment and treatment, particularly during the initial phase of acute illness and trauma
3. Role-specific rather than site-specific

B. Scope of Practice

1. Occurs and exists whenever and wherever an emergency patient and an emergency nurse interact
2. Covers the entire span of age, acuity, and interaction from a single individual to communities
3. Core: The scope of emergency nursing practice involves the assessment, diagnosis, outcome identification, planning, and implementation of interventions and evaluations of human responses to perceived, actual or

potential, sudden or urgent, physical or psychosocial problems that are primarily episodic or acute and that occur in a variety of settings

4. **Dimensions: Multidimensional characteristics unique to emergency nursing practice include the aforementioned core, triage and prioritization, emergency operations preparedness, stabilization and resuscitation, crisis intervention for unique patient populations, provision of care in uncontrolled or unpredictable environments, and consistency (as much as possible) across the continuum of care**

5. **Boundaries**
   a. *External*
      1) Legislation/regulations
      2) Social demands
      3) Economic climate
      4) Health care delivery trends
      5) States' Nurse Practice Acts
   b. *Internal*
      1) Professional forces
   c. *Dynamic*

6. **Intersections: Emergency nurses participate for the common purpose of improving health care through education, administration, consultation, and collaboration in practice, research, and policy decisions with professional and governmental groups outside the domain of nursing**

C. Emergency Nurses Association (ENA, 1998b)

1. **Role**
   a. *The specialty organization for professional nurses committed to the advancement of emergency nursing*
   b. *The authority, advocate, lobbyist, and voice for emergency nursing*

2. **Purpose and mission: To provide visionary leadership for emergency nursing and emergency care**

3. **Vision: To define the future of emergency nursing and emergency care through advocacy, expertise, innovation, and leadership**

4. **Value statements of the ENA mission**
   a. *All individuals have a right to high quality emergency care delivered with compassion*
   b. *Respect for diversity of patients and colleagues is inherent to emergency nursing practice and emergency care*
   c. *Prevention of illness and injury and promotion of wellness are essential components of emergency nursing practice and emergency care*
   d. *Discipline of emergency nursing includes a defined and an evolving body of knowledge based on research*
   e. *Continuing education and professional development are fundamental to emergency nursing practice and emergency care*
   f. *Emergency nursing practice is both independent and collaborative*

5. **Objectives**
   a. *To promote the specialty of emergency nursing*
   b. *To work collaboratively with other health-related organizations toward the improvement of emergency care*
   c. *To serve as a resource for emergency nursing education and research*
   d. *To define and disseminate education and research resources toward the stated standards*

e. To provide a networking structure to address professional emergency nursing issues

f. To serve as a patient advocate for the consumer through public education and other mechanisms

g. To affirm the philosophy of the American Nurses' Association's Ethical Principles

h. To promote the common interests of the Emergency Nurses Association's members and to improve the business conditions for emergency nurses within the health care industry

II. STANDARDS (ENA, 1998b)

A. Definition: Recommended goals and general guidelines of care, education, and experience levels for emergency nurses, representing the philosophy, mission, values, and vision of the ENA

B. Development

1. The ENA supports Nursing's Social Policy Statement (ANA, 1995) that charges specialty nursing organizations with defining their individual scope of practice
2. ENA endorsed and adapted the 1998 ANA Standards of Clinical Nursing Practice as generic nursing standards and used them as the basis for further development of emergency nursing specialty standards

C. Application Criteria

1. Competency level: The level of performance an emergency nurse or an institution should consider in establishing goals for the nurse's professional practice
2. Excellent level: The practice that surpasses the competent level and contributes to the growth of emergency nursing practice

III. EMERGENCY NURSING PRACTICE (ENA, 1998)

A. Assessment

B. Diagnosis

C. Outcome Identification

D. Planning

E. Implementation

F. Evaluation

G. Triage

IV. PROFESSIONAL PERFORMANCE (ENA, 1998)

A. Comprehensive Standard VIII: Quality of Care

1. Emergency nurse evaluates the quality and effectiveness of emergency nursing practice

    a. Develops and implements a comprehensive plan for assessing and improving the quality of care for emergency patients

    b. Continually assesses and evaluates the care delivery system using quality improvement principles and practices

       1) Assesses customer needs to maximize customer satisfaction

B. Comprehensive Standards IX: Performance Appraisal

  1. The emergency nurse adheres to established standards of practice, including activities and behaviors that characterize professional status

    a. Accountable for own actions

    b. Participates in clinical and peer review to evaluate practice

C. Comprehensive Standards X: Education

  1. The emergency nurse recognizes self-learning needs and opportunities and is accountable for maximizing professional development and optimal emergency nursing practice

    a. Responsible for acquiring and demonstrating attainment of a defined body of nursing knowledge

       1) Attains provider status in

          a) Basic Life Support (BLS)

          b) Advanced Cardiac Life Support (ACLS) and/or Pediatric Advanced Life Support (PALS)

          c) Certification in Emergency Nursing (CEN)

          d) Trauma Nurse Core Curriculum (TNCC) as the minimum for caring for trauma patients

          e) Emergency Nurse Pediatric Curriculum (ENPC) as the minimum for caring for pediatric patients

       2) Becomes an instructor

       3) Attends programs in Concepts in Advanced Trauma Nursing (CATN)

       4) Develops, implements, monitors, and evaluates competency-based staff education

    b. Obtains ongoing education consistent with the role and area of practice

       1) Competency is demonstrated by sound clinical judgment in autonomous practice (ENA, 1998b)

D. Comprehensive Standards XI: Collegiality

  1. The emergency nurse engages in activities and behaviors that characterize a professional

    a. Supports the professional development of nursing by promoting understanding of nursing roles and responsibilities

       1) Participating member of ENA

       2) Assumes leadership role in ENA

       3) Acts as liaison to groups

    b. Possesses an understanding of current and proposed legislation and regulations related to emergency care and the practice of emergency nursing

    c. Fosters a professional image of nursing

    d. Responsible for public education regarding emergency nursing and the emergency care system

    e. Facilitates learning experiences for peers, other health care providers, students, and volunteers

    1) Participates in orientation and mentoring

    2) Develops, implements, and evaluates orientation, mentoring, and educational programs

    3) Aware of Emergency Nurses Care (EN CARE): ENA–affiliate that uses trained volunteers to present injury prevention

   f. Promotes wellness in the workplace

E. Comprehensive Standards XII: Ethics

1. **Emergency nurse provides care based on philosophical and ethical concepts. These concepts include reverence for life; respect for the inherent dignity, worth, autonomy, and individuality of each human being; and acknowledges the diversity of all people**

   a. Provides care that demonstrates ethical beliefs and respect for patient rights

    1) Advocates for patients and their significant others

    2) Develops and implements policies, procedures, and programs related to ethics and advanced directives

   b. Functions autonomously to the extent that knowledge, skills, and role permit

   c. Exercises authority congruent with the state's Nurse Practice Act and is knowledgeable about local, state, and federal laws that govern the delivery of care

    1) Understands and implements proper informed consent, use of restraints, advanced directives, and interfacility transfers

    2) Defines standards of emergency practice

2. **Code of Ethics for Emergency Nurses (ENA, 1996)**

   a. Provides care with compassion and respect for human dignity and individual uniqueness

   b. Maintains competence within and accountability for emergency nursing practice

   c. Acts to protect the individual when health care and safety are threatened by the incompetent, unethical, or illegal practice of any person

   d. Exercises sound judgment in accepting responsibility, delegating, and seeking consultation

   e. Respects the individual's right to privacy and confidentiality

   f. Continues to study, implement, and promote scientific knowledge

   g. Collaborates with other health care professionals and the public in meeting community and national health needs

F. Comprehensive Standard XIII: Collaboration

1. **Emergency nurse ensures open and timely communication with emergency patients and their significant others and with other health care providers through professional collaboration**

   a. Ensures open communication with patients and their significant others

   b. Participates in community education related to emergency care

   c. Utilizes education of the patients and their significant others to clarify learning needs and optimize outcomes

   d. Functions as a facilitator and liaison among health care providers and health care agencies, respecting their limits, abilities, and responsibilities

2. **Collaborates with other professional groups in educational activities, disaster planning, domestic violence, organ and tissue procurement, injury prevention campaigns, and pre-hospital care**

G. Comprehensive Standards XIV: Research

1. **Emergency nurse recognizes, supports, and utilizes research to enhance emergency nursing practice**
   a. *Uses information from research literature to improve practice*
   b. *Participates in research to expand the body of validated knowledge related to emergency nursing*
   c. *Collaborates with colleagues in other disciplines engaged in research in the practice setting*
2. **Principles for ethical conduct in research (Polit and Hungler, 1995)**
   a. *Principles of beneficence*
      1) Freedom from harm
      2) Freedom from exploitation
   b. *Principles of respect for human dignity*
      1) Right to self-determination
      2) Right to full disclosure
   c. *Principles of justice*
      1) Right to fair treatment
      2) Right to privacy

H. Comprehensive Standard XV: Resource Utilization

1. **The emergency nurse collaborates with other health care providers to deliver patient-centered care in a manner consistent with safe, efficient, and cost-effective resource utilization**
   a. *Ensures that necessary supplies and equipment are readily available and appropriate charges are generated for their use*
   b. *Takes appropriate measures to optimize the safety of peers, patients, their significant others, other health care providers, and self in the emergency care setting*
   c. *Assigns and delegates care that reflects the needs of patients and is in the scope of practice of other health care providers*

V. PROFESSIONAL BEHAVIORS

A. Autonomy (ENA, 1997b)

1. **Nursing is an autonomous profession with an independent scope of practice of which emergency nursing is a recognized specialty**
2. **Registered nurses are independently licensed by and accountable to state boards of nursing to make clinical and management decisions regarding nursing care irrespective of the practice setting**
   a. *Only registered nurses should supervise and evaluate emergency nurses*
   b. *Nursing's autonomy is carried out with collaboration and interdependent practice of shared values, mutual acknowledgment, and respect for each other's contributions to health care*

B. Critical Thinking (Luckman, 1997)

1. **Uses the information from a wide variety of sources in a manner that raises questions, identifies assumptions, and develops new connections so that the scope of possible solutions is broadened**
2. **Traits**

    a. *Uses elements of reasoning*
    b. *Thinks in nonlinear steps*
    c. *Has an attitude of openness and inquisitiveness*
    d. *Uses cognitive skills*
    e. *Examines environmental context*
    f. *Understands how one is thinking*

C. Leadership

1. **A set of qualities attributed to those who are perceived as successfully achieving, with and through others, the outcome of goals and new shared reality (Malone, 1997)**
   a. *Can occur within a specialized job title or any nursing position*
   b. *Components (Smeltzer and Bare, 1996)*
      1) Decision-making
      2) Relating
      3) Influencing
      4) Facilitating
   c. *Differentiate from a pure management role that keeps an organization's complex systems running optimally in line with established criteria (Hughes, Ginnett, and Curphy, 1993)*
2. **Characteristics (Malone, 1997)**
   a. *Vision*
   b. *Boundary management*
   c. *Risk taking*
   d. *Empowerment of followers*
   e. *Mentoring: Intense career building, mutually beneficial relationship between two individuals of unequal power in an organization*
3. **Beneficial skills**
   a. *Team building*
   b. *Communication*
   c. *Negotiation*
   d. *Conflict management*
   e. *Knowledge of corporate language*
   f. *Knowledge of financial and budgetary concepts*
   g. *Knowledge of computers and technology*
   h. *Change manager with flexibility*
4. **Personality traits**
   a. *Effectiveness*
   b. *Dominance*
   c. *Self-confidence*
   d. *Achievement orientation*
   e. *Dependability*
   f. *High energy and activity level*
   g. *Self-monitoring*
   h. *Locus of control*
   i. *Tolerance for ambiguity*
   j. *Adjustment*
   k. *Sociability*
   l. *Agreeableness*
   m. *Creativity*
5. **ENA Foundation: Leadership is developed, not discovered**

a. *Mission: To enhance emergency care services by identifying and supporting funding priorities in education, research, and program development*

b. *Encourage nurses to become active in emergency nursing, serve as role models, and expand professional knowledge*

D. Delegating (ANA, 1992; ANA, 1994; ENA, 1997a; Zimmermann, 1996)

1. **Retaining the ultimate responsibility, accountability, and legal liability for proper delegation, potential problems, and completion of interventions in an act of nursing**

   a. *Tasks that can always be delegated are technical—repetitive, supportive, and non-nursing (Hansten and Washburn, 1995)*

   b. *Tasks that can never be delegated are professional activities involving the specialized knowledge, judgment, or skill of the nursing process (ANA, 1994; ENA, 1994)*

   1) Patient assessment
   2) Triage
   3) Formulating a nursing diagnosis or care goal
   4) Establishing a nursing plan of care
   5) Extensive teaching or counseling
   6) Telephone advice
   7) Evaluating outcome
   8) Discharging patients

2. **Factors to consider when delegating (Zimmermann, 1996)**

   a. *Patient's condition*
   b. *Complexity of the task*
   c. *Capabilities of the non-RN*
   d. *Amount of problem solving necessary*
   e. *Infection control precautions*
   f. *Safety precautions*
   g. *Potential for harm*
   h. *Extent of patient interaction*
   i. *Environment*

3. **Differentiation (ANA, 1992; ANA, 1994)**

   a. *Supervision: Directing, guiding, and influencing the outcome of an individual's performance*

   1) Either on-site or off-site
   2) Verbal or written

   b. *Assignment: Shift of an activity from one person to another person of similar skill, knowledge, and judgment*

   1) Includes responsibility and accountability
   2) Activity must be within receiving person's legal authority or regulatory scope of practice

4. **Steps in delegation**

   a. *Identify purpose*
   b. *Know the non-RN's job qualifications, description, and qualifications*
   c. *Spell out the what, whom, how, and when, possibly including reportable parameters and rationales*
   d. *Establish priorities*
   e. *Verify comprehension*

5. **Principles of delegation and coordination of care (ENA, 1997a)**

   a. *Registered nurse ultimately decides the appropriateness of delegation, although the non-RN, employers, or administrators may make suggestions b. The non-RN caregiver cannot re-delegate a delegated act*

    c. The laws that establish prehospital practice standards for non-RN caregivers do not authorize comparable practice in the emergency department

6. **Standards of care for use of non-RN caregivers (ENA, 1997)**

    a. The nursing profession defines and supervises the education, training, and utilization of any non-RN caregiver providing delegated nursing care

    b. Nursing management/administration is accountable for ensuring that utilization complies with established standards of care

    c. Written job description for non-RN caregivers clearly delineates appropriate duties, responsibilities, qualifications, skills, and requirements for registered nurse supervision

    d. Performance expectation and mechanism for ongoing appraisal are established and maintained

    e. Orientation and training are appropriate for performance expectation and role responsibility

    f. One registered nurse is always available in the emergency department and a ratio of non-RN caregivers to registered nurses ensures high quality care

    g. Impact of non-RN caregivers on patient outcome and adherence to standards of care is monitored and evaluated by registered nurses on a regularly scheduled basis

VI. Specialized Professional Nursing Roles

A. Advanced Practice Nurse (APN) (ENA, 1996)

1. **ENA supports APN role as it improves access to quality, cost-effective, primary health care and specialized nursing care requirements of patients with increasingly complex needs**

2. **ENA considers masters' prepared Clinical Nurse Specialists (CNS) and Nurse Practitioners (NP) as APNs, although masters' prepared case managers and trauma coordinators could also be in this category**

B. Clinical Nurse Specialist (CNS)

1. **Purpose: Primarily provides improved quality nursing care delivered at the bedside**

2. **Focus: Education, system analysis, research, and search utilization, and provision of direct and indirect nursing care**

C. Nurse Practitioner (NP)

1. **Purpose: Primarily direct patient care**

2. **Focus: Diagnosis and treatment, increasing access to primary care, and decreasing physician shortages**

D. Flight Nurses

1. **Discipline of emergency nursing that renders nursing practice to all clients who are transported in all environments**

2. **Standards of Flight Nursing Practice**

3. **Certified Flight Registered Nurse (CFRN) administered by the Board of Certification in Emergency Nursing (BCEN)**

E. Telephone Triage/Advice (ENA, 1998a)

1. **Essentials of an established telephone triage program**

   a. *Uses experienced, professional registered nurses with specialized education*

   b. *Has mandatory continuing education for staff*

   c. *Establishes clearly defined protocols*

   d. *Develops policies and procedures*

   e. *Maintains continuous quality improvement program*

2. **ENA maintains that wherever an established telephone triage program is not in place, no advice is to be given over the telephone**

   a. *Life-threatening urgency may be assessed to assist in life-saving measures (e.g., CPR) and to access the Emergency Medical Services (EMS)*

   b. *Document each conversation and recommendation*

BIBLIOGRAPHY

American Nurses Association (1994). *Registered professional nurses and unlicensed assistive personnel.* Washington, DC: American Nurses Publishing.

American Nurses Association (1995). *Nursing: a social policy statement.* Washington, DC: Author.

American Nurses Association (1998). *Standards of clinical nursing practice*, 2nd ed. Washington, DC: American Nurses Publishing.

Emergency Nurses Association (1996). *Code of ethics for emergency nurses.* Park Ridge, IL: Author.

Emergency Nurses Association (1994). *Delegation: what every emergency nurse needs to know.* Park Ridge IL: Author.

Emergency Nurses Association (1996a). *Emergency Nurses Association on advanced practice nursing.* Park Ridge, IL: Author.

Emergency Nurses Association (1996b). *Scope of emergency nursing practice.* Park Ridge, IL: Author.

Emergency Nurses Association (1997a). *Position statement: The use of non-registered nurse (non-RN) caregivers in emergency care.* Park Ridge, IL: Author.

Emergency Nurses Association (1997b). *Position statement: autonomous emergency nursing practice.* Park Ridge, IL: Author.

Emergency Nurses Association (1998). *Policy statement: Customer satisfaction.* Park Ridge, IL Author.

Emergency Nurses Association (1998a). *Position statement: Telephone advice.* Park Ridge, IL: Author.

Emergency Nurses Association (1998b). *Standards of emergency nursing practice*, 4th ed. Park Ridge, IL: Author.

Emergency Nurses Association (1998c). *Emergency Nurses Association bylaws.* Park Ridge, IL: Author.

Emergency Nurses Association (1999). *Emergency nursing* (The brochure.) Park Ridge, IL: Author.

Hansten, R., & Washburn, M. (1995). Knowing how to delegate. *American Journal of Nursing* 95:16H–16I.

Hughes, R.L., Ginnett, R.C., & Curphy G.J. (1993). *Leadership: Enhancing the lessons of experience.* Homewood, IL: Irwin.

Luckmann, J. (1997). *Saunders manual of nursing care* (pp. 3 and 4). Philadelphia: W.B. Saunders.

Malone, B.L. (1997). Nurses in non-nursing leadership positions. In McCloskey, J.C., & Grace, H.K. *Current issues in nursing*, 5th ed, pp. 355–363. St. Louis: Mosby.

Polit, D.F., & Hungler, B.P. (1995). *Nursing research principles and methods*, 5th ed (pp. 117–125). Philadelphia: J.B. Linppincott.

Smeltzer, S.C., & Bare B.G. (1996). *Brunner and Suddarth's textbook of medical-surgical nursing*, 8th ed, (p. 12). Philadelphia: J.B. Lippincott.

Zimmermann, P.G. (1996). Delegating to assistive personnel. *Journal of Emergency Nursing* 22(3), 206–212.

NANDA-Approved Nursing Diagnoses

This list represents the NANDA-approved nursing diagnoses for clinical use and testing.

PATTERN 1: EXCHANGING

	1.1.2.1	Altered Nutrition: More Than Body Requirements
	1.1.2.2	Altered Nutrition: Less Than Body Requirements
	1.1.2.3	Altered Nutrition: Risk for More Than Body Requirements
	1.2.1.1	Risk for Infection
	1.2.2.1	Risk for Altered Body Temperature
	1.2.2.2	Hypothermia
	1.2.2.3	Hyperthermia
	1.2.2.4	Ineffective Thermoregulation
	1.2.3.1	Dysreflexia
°	1.2.3.2	Risk for Autonomic Dysreflexia
†	1.3.1.1	Constipation
	1.3.1.1.1	Perceived Constipation
	1.3.1.1.2	Colonic Constipation (deleted in 1998)
†	1.3.1.2	Diarrhea
†	1.3.1.3	Bowel Incontinence
°	1.3.1.4	Risk for Constipation
	1.3.2	Altered Urinary Elimination
	1.3.2.1.1	Stress Incontinence
†	1.3.2.1.2	Reflex Urinary Incontinence
	1.3.2.1.3	Urge Incontinence
†	1.3.2.1.4	Functional Urinary Incontinence
	1.3.2.1.5	Total Incontinence
°	1.3.2.1.6	Risk for Urinary Urge Incontinence
	1.3.2.2	Urinary Retention
‡	1.4.1.1	Altered Tissue Perfusion (Specify type: Renal, Cerebral, Cardiopulmonary, Gastrointestinal, Peripheral)
°	1.4.1.2	Risk for Fluid Volume Imbalance
	1.4.1.2.1	Fluid Volume Excess
	1.4.1.2.2.1	Fluid Volume Deficit
	1.4.1.2.2.2	Risk for Fluid Volume Deficit
	1.4.2.1	Decreased Cardiac Output
†	1.5.1.1	Impaired Gas Exchange
†	1.5.1.2	Ineffective Airway Clearance
†	1.5.1.3	Ineffective Breathing Pattern
	1.5.1.3.1	Inability to Sustain Spontaneous Ventilation

	1.5.1.3.2	Dysfunctional Ventilatory Weaning Response
	1.6.1	Risk for Injury
	1.6.1.1	Risk for Suffocation
	1.6.1.2	Risk for Poisoning
	1.6.1.3	Risk for Trauma
	1.6.1.4	Risk for Aspiration
	1.6.1.5	Risk for Disuse Syndrome
†	1.6.1.6	Latex Allergy Response
†	1.6.1.7	Risk for Latex Allergy Response
	1.6.2	Altered Protection
‡	1.6.2.1	Impaired Tissue Integrity
†	1.6.2.1.1	Altered Oral Mucous Membrane
‡	1.6.2.1.2.1	Impaired Skin Integrity
‡	1.6.2.1.2.2	Risk for Impaired Skin Integrity
°	1.6.2.1.3	Altered Dentition
	1.7.1	Decreased Adaptive Capacity: Intracranial
	1.8	Energy Field Disturbance

PATTERN 2: COMMUNICATING

‡	2.1.1.1	Impaired Verbal Communication

PATTERN 3: RELATING

	3.1.1	Impaired Social Interaction
	3.1.2	Social Isolation
	3.1.3	Risk for Loneliness
†	3.2.1	Altered Role Performance
†	3.2.1.1.1	Altered Parenting
†	3.2.1.1.2	Risk for Altered Parenting
	3.2.1.1.2.1	Risk for Altered Parent/Infant/Child Attachment
	3.2.1.2.1	Sexual Dysfunction
†	3.2.2	Altered Family Processes
†	3.2.2.1	Caregiver Role Strain
	3.2.2.2	Risk for Caregiver Role Strain
	3.2.2.3.1	Altered Family Processes: Alcoholism
	3.2.3.1	Parental Role Conflict
	3.3	Altered Sexuality Patterns

PATTERN 4: VALUING

	4.1.1	Spiritual Distress (Distress of the Human Spirit)
°	4.1.2	Risk for Spiritual Distress
	4.2	Potential for Enhanced Spiritual Well-Being

PATTERN 5: CHOOSING

†	5.1.1.1	Ineffective Individual Coping
†	5.1.1.1.1	Impaired Adjustment
	5.1.1.1.2	Defensive Coping
	5.1.1.1.3	Ineffective Denial
	5.1.2.1.1	Ineffective Family Coping: Disabling
	5.1.2.1.2	Ineffective Family Coping: Compromised
	5.1.2.2	Family Coping: Potential for Growth

	5.1.3.1	Potential for Enhanced Community Coping
†	5.1.3.2	Ineffective Community Coping
	5.2.1	Ineffective Management of Therapeutic Regimen: Individuals
	5.2.1.1	Noncompliance (specify)
	5.2.2	Ineffective Management of Therapeutic Regimen: Families
	5.2.3	Ineffective Management of Therapeutic Regimen: Community
	5.2.4	Effective Management of Therapeutic Regimen: Individual
	5.3.1.1	Decisional Conflict (specify)
	5.4	Health-Seeking Behaviors (specify)

PATTERN 6: MOVING

†	6.1.1.1	Impaired Physical Mobility
	6.1.1.1.1	Risk for Peripheral Neurovascular Dysfunction
	6.1.1.1.2	Risk for Perioperative Positioning Injury
	6.1.1.1.3	Impaired Walking
	6.1.1.1.4	Impaired Wheelchair Mobility
°	6.1.1.1.5	Impaired Transfer Ability
	6.1.1.1.6	Impaired Bed Mobility
	6.1.1.2	Activity Intolerance
†	6.1.1.2.1	Fatigue
	6.1.1.3	Risk for Activity Intolerance
†	6.2.1	Sleep Pattern Disturbance
	6.2.1.1	Sleep Deprivation
	6.3.1.1	Diversional Activity Deficit
	6.4.1.1	Impaired Home Maintenance Management
	6.4.2	Altered Health Maintenance
	6.4.2.1	Delayed Surgical Recovery
	6.4.2.2	Adult Failure to Thrive
†	6.5.1	Feeding Self-Care Deficit
†	6.5.1.1	Impaired Swallowing
	6.5.1.2	Ineffective Breastfeeding
	6.5.1.2.1	Interrupted Breastfeeding
	6.5.1.3	Effective Breastfeeding
	6.5.1.4	Ineffective Infant Feeding Pattern
†	6.5.2	Bathing/Hygiene Self-Care Deficit
†	6.5.3	Dressing/Grooming Self-Care Deficit
†	6.5.4	Toileting Self-Care Deficit
	6.6	Altered Growth and Development
	6.6.1	Risk for Altered Development
	6.6.2	Risk for Altered Growth
	6.7	Relocation Stress Syndrome
	6.8.1	Risk for Disorganized Infant Behavior
†	6.8.2	Disorganized Infant Behavior
	6.8.3	Potential for Enhanced Organized Infant Behavior

PATTERN 7: PERCEIVING

‡	7.1.1	Body Image Disturbance
	7.1.2	Self-Esteem Disturbance
	7.1.2.1	Chronic Low Self-Esteem
	7.1.2.2	Situational Low Self-Esteem
	7.1.3	Personal Identity Disturbance

‡	7.2	Sensory/Perceptual Alterations (Specify: Visual, Auditory, Kinesthetic, Gustatory, Tactile, Olfactory)
	7.2.1.1	Unilateral Neglect
	7.3.1	Hopelessness
	7.3.2	Powerlessness

PATTERN 8: KNOWING

	8.1.1	Knowledge Deficit (Specify)
	8.2.1	Impaired Environmental Interpretation Syndrome
	8.2.2	Acute Confusion
	8.2.3	Chronic Confusion
	8.3	Altered Thought Processes
	8.3.1	Impaired Memory

PATTERN 9: FEELING

	9.1.1	Pain
	9.1.1.1	Chronic Pain
°	9.1.2	Nausea
	9.2.1.1	Dysfunctional Grieving
	9.2.1.2	Anticipatory Grieving
°	9.2.1.3	Chronic Sorrow
	9.2.2	Risk for Violence: Directed at Others
	9.2.2.1	Risk for Self-Mutilation
	9.2.2.2	Risk for Violence: Self-Directed
†	9.2.3	Post-Trauma Syndrome
†	9.2.3.1	Rape-Trauma Syndrome
	9.2.3.1.1	Rape-Trauma Syndrome: Compound Reaction
	9.2.3.1.2	Rape-Trauma Syndrome: Silent Reaction
°	9.2.4	Risk for Post-Trauma Syndrome
‡	9.3.1	Anxiety
°	9.3.1.1	Death Anxiety
‡	9.3.2	Fear

°New diagnoses accepted in 1998.

†Revised diagnoses submitted and approved in 1998.

‡Diagnoses revised by small work groups at the 1996 Biennial Conference on the Classification of Nursing Diagnoses; changes approved and added in 1998.

Nursing Diagnoses and Desired Expected Outcomes

The following nursing diagnoses and desired patient outcomes represent the most frequently used in the emergency department setting. For a comprehensive list of the NANDA-approved nursing diagnoses and desired patient outcomes, the reader is referred to a nursing diagnosis textbook.

Nursing Diagnosis	Desired Expected Outcome
Airway clearance, ineffective related to: Decreased energy, fatigue Effects of anesthesia, medication, perceptual-cognitive impairment, presence of an artificial airway, trauma Inability to cough effectively Tracheobronchial secretions or obstruction Aspiration of foreign matter Environmental pollutants Inhalation of toxic fumes or substances	***The patient will maintain a patent airway as evidenced by:*** Regular rate, depth, and pattern of breathing Bilateral chest expansion Effective cough-gag reflex Absence of signs, symptoms of airway obstruction: stridor, dyspnea, hoarse voice Clear sputum without abnormal color or odor Absence of signs and symptoms of retained secretions (e.g., fever, tachypnea)
Anxiety/fear related to: Effects of actual or perceived loss of significant others Threat to or change in health status, role functioning, support systems, environment, self-concept, or interaction patterns Situational and maturation crises Unmet needs Threat of death, actual or perceived Lack of knowledge Loss of control Feelings of failure Disruptive family life Threat to self-concept Pain	***The patient, significant others will experience decreasing anxiety/fear as evidenced by:*** Absence of fear related behaviors (e.g., crying, agitation) Verbalizes decreased anxiety/fear Utilizes effective coping skills Vital signs within normal limits Communicates fears to others

Nursing Diagnosis	Desired Expected Outcome

Aspiration, risk for related to:
Decreased level of consciousness
Depressed cough and gag reflexes
Presence of tracheostomy or endotracheal tube
Medication administration
Situations hindering elevation of upper body
Increased intragastric pressure
Impaired swallowing
Facial, oral, or neck trauma
Wired jaw

The patient will not experience aspiration as evidenced by:
A patent airway
Clear and equal bilateral breath sounds
Regular rate, depth, and pattern of breathing
Arterial blood gas (ABGs) within normal limits
Clear chest x-ray film without evidence of infiltrates
Ability to handle secretions independently

Breathing pattern, ineffective related to:
Decreased energy, lung expansion
Effects of anesthesia, cognitive-perceptual impairment, medications (e.g., sedatives, narcotics), neuromuscular-musculoskeletal impairment
Obesity
Immobility, inactivity
Inflammatory processes
Pain, discomfort
Tracheobronchial obstruction
Anxiety

The patient will have an effective breathing pattern as evidenced by:
Normal rate, depth, and pattern of breathing
Absence of dyspnea, cyanosis, orthopnea, shortness of breath
Clear and equal bilateral breath sounds
Arterial blood gases (ABGs) within normal limits
Absence of use of accessory muscles or nasal flaring

Cardiac output, decreased related to:
Reduction in stroke volume as a result of electrical factors: alteration in conduction, rate, and/or rhythm
Reduction in stroke volume as a result of mechanical factors: alteration in afterload, preload, and/or inotropic changes in heart
Structural problems secondary to congenital abnormalities or trauma

The patient will maintain adequate cardiac output as evidenced by:
Appropriate heart rate for age
Adequate blood pressure for age
Strong, palpable peripheral pulses
Level of consciousness: awake and alert
Skin color normal, skin warm and dry
Urinary output appropriate for age and weight
Electrocardiogram (ECG) with normal sinus rhythm, absence of dysrhythmias

Communication, impaired verbal related to:
Altered thought processes
Auditory impairment
Effects of trauma
Inflammation
Physical barriers: intubation
Language barrier
Anxiety/fear

The patient will demonstrate an effective communication method as evidenced by:
Use of an alternate method of communication
Use of slower speech
Use of short phrases
Use of appropriate responses to questions

Constipation related to:
Less than adequate dietary, fiber, and/or fluid intake
Gastrointestinal lesions
Pain, discomfort on defecation
Effects of aging, diagnostic procedures, medications, neuromuscular-musculoskeletal impairment, presence of anatomical obstruction
Immobility or less than adequate physical activity
Chronic use of laxatives and enemas
Personal habits
Anxiety, stress

The patient will demonstrate improved bowel elimination as evidenced by:
Expressed knowledge of appropriate dietary interventions
Expressed knowledge of appropriate and prescribed pharmacological interventions
Reported feelings of increased comfort or decreased fullness

Nursing Diagnosis	Desired Expected Outcome
Coping, ineffective individual related to: Effects of acute or chronic illness Loss of control over body part or body function Lack of support systems Separation from or loss of significant other Low self-esteem Major changes in lifestyle Unrealistic perceptions Situational or maturation crisis Knowledge deficit regarding therapeutic regimen, disease process, prognosis Sensory overload	**The patient will demonstrate effective coping as evidenced by:** Verbalizing feelings to others Engaging in open communication Seeking methods of to improve coping skills Seeking external support
Diarrhea related to: Allergies Effects of medications, radiation, surgical intervention Infectious process Inflammatory process Malabsorption syndrome Nutritional disorders Anxiety and stress Excessive use of laxatives	**The patient will demonstrate improved bowel elimination as evidenced by:** Expressed knowledge of various potential sources of infectious causes of diarrhea Expressed knowledge of routes of contamination Decreased report of stool frequency
Dysreflexia related to: Bladder distention Bowel distention Constipation Skin irritation Knowledge deficit	**The patient will not demonstrate signs of dysreflexia as evidenced by:** Appropriate blood pressure for age Appropriate heart rate for age Skin warm and dry
Fluid volume deficit related to: Active fluid volume loss (e.g., vomiting/diarrhea, blood loss) Failure of regulatory mechanisms	**The patient will have an adequate fluid volume as evidenced by:** Balanced intake and output Appropriate blood pressure for age Appropriate heart rate for age Appropriate urinary output for age and weight Strong, palpable peripheral pulses Level of consciousness: awake and alert Skin color normal, skin warm and dry Moist mucous membranes Hematocrit and hemoglobin at baseline Central venous pressure reading 5–10 cm H_2O No evidence of external bleeding

Nursing Diagnosis	Desired Expected Outcome

Fluid volume excess related to:
Compromised regulatory mechanisms: antidiuretic hormone, renin-angiotensin-aldosterone
Effects of age extremes, medications, pregnancy
Excessive fluid or sodium intake
Low protein intake

The patient will have an adequate fluid volume as evidenced by:
Balanced intake and output
Appropriate blood pressure for age
Appropriate heart rate for age
Appropriate urinary output for age and weight
Normal rate, depth, and pattern of breathing
Absence of dyspnea, cyanosis, orthopnea, shortness of breath
Clear and equal bilateral breath sounds
Arterial blood gases (ABGs) within normal limits

Gas exchange, impaired related to:
Ventilation-perfusion imbalance
Altered blood flow, oxygen-carrying capacity of the blood, oxygen supply
Alveolar capillary membrane changes
Aspiration of foreign matter
Decreased surfactant production
Effects of anesthesia, medications
Hypo- or hyperventilation
Inhalation of toxic fumes or substances

The patient will maintain adequate gas exchange as evidenced by:
Arterial blood gases (ABGs) within normal limits
Level of consciousness: awake and alert
Regular rate, depth, and pattern of breathing
Skin color normal, skin warm and dry

Grieving, related to:
Actual or anticipated losses associated with recent injury or illness

The patient/significant other(s) will begin the grieving process as evidenced by:
Expressing signs of the grieving process
Participating in decision making
Recognizing reasons for feelings
Verbalizing feelings to others
Seeking external support

Hyperthermia related to:
Exposure to hot environment
Increased metabolic rate
Effects of medications, illness, or trauma involving temperature regulation, aging, obesity
Dehydration
Inability or decreased ability to perspire
Vigorous activity
Inappropriate clothing

The patient will maintain a normal core body temperature as evidenced by:
Core temperature measurement of 36°–37.5°C (98°–99.5°F)
Skin color normal, skin warm and dry
Vital signs within normal limits
Level of consciousness: awake and alert

Hypothermia related to:
Exposure to cold environment
Decreased metabolic rate
Effects of medications, illness, or trauma involving temperature regulation, aging
Malnutrition
Inactivity
Consumption of alcohol
Inappropriate clothing

The patient will maintain a normal core body temperature as evidenced by:
Core temperature measurement of 36°–37.5°C (98°–99.5°F)
Skin color normal, skin warm and dry
Vital signs within normal limits
Level of consciousness: awake and alert

Nursing Diagnosis	**Desired Expected Outcome**

Infection, high risk for related to:

Inadequate primary defenses
    Broken skin
    Traumatized tissue
    Decreased ciliary action
    Stasis of body fluids
    Change in pH of secretions
    Altered peristalsis
Inadequate secondary defenses
    Decreased hemoglobin
    Leukopenia
    Suppressed inflammatory response
Tissue destruction and increased environmental exposure
Effects of
    Chronic disease
    Immunosuppression
    Inadequate acquired immunity
    Invasive treatment, procedures
    Malnutrition
    Pharmaceutical agents
    Trauma
Insufficient knowledge to avoid exposure to pathogens

The patient will remain free from infection as evidenced by:

Core temperature measurement of 36°–37.5°C (98°–99.5°F)
Absence of systemic signs of infection
Wounds free from erythema, edema, pain, and purulent drainage
Leukocyte count and differential within normal limits

Injury, high risk for related to:

Internal
    Biochemical factors
    Regulatory dysfunction (sensory, integrative, effector dysfunction; tissue hypoxia)
    Malnutrition
    Immune, autoimmune dysfunction
    Abnormal blood profile (leukocytosis, leukopenia, altered clotting factors, thrombocytopenia, sickle cell anemia)
    Physical impairment (broken skin, altered mobility)
    Developmental age
    Psychological factors
External factors
    Biological (immunization level of community, microorganism)
    Chemical factors (pollutants, poisons, drugs, pharmaceutical agents, alcohol, caffeine, nicotine, preservatives)
    Nutrients (vitamins, food types)
    Physical factors (design, structure, and arrangement of community, building, and/or equipment)
    Mode of transport, transportation

The patient will remain free from injury as evidenced by:

Absence of physical signs of injury
Awareness of limitations
Knowledge of injury prevention
Requesting assistance as needed

Nursing Diagnosis	Desired Expected Outcome

Knowledge deficit related to:
Effects of aging, sensory deficits, language barrier, cognitive limitations
Information misinterpretation
Unfamiliarity with information resources
Lack of interest in learning, exposure recall
Denial
Substance abuse
Self-destructive patterns
Inadequate economic resources

The patient will demonstrate an adequate knowledge level as evidenced by:
Accurate perception of the problem
Accurate follow-through of instruction
Accurate explanation of therapeutic regimen
Request for information
Accurate repeat demonstration
Accurate verbalization of discharge instructions
Identification of risk factors and behaviors to prevent further episodes

Mobility, impaired physical related to:
Neuromuscular impairment
Sensory-perceptual impairment
Fatigue, decreased strength and endurance
Intolerance to activity
Effects of trauma
Inflammation
Pain
Obesity
Side effects of medications
Depression, anxiety
Fear of movement
Lack of assistive devices

The patient will maintain adequate mobility as evidenced by:
Willingness to attempt movement as prescribed
Use of safety, assistive devices as instructed
Ability to describe measures to increase mobility
Active participation in measures designed to increase mobility

Noncompliance related to:
Acceleration of illness symptoms
Nonadherence to therapeutic regimen
Making of inappropriate choices
Failure to seek care when disease state warrants
Failure to keep appointments
Economic difficulties
Lack of support system
Knowledge deficit
Powerlessness
Impaired ability to perform tasks
Denial
Depression

The patient will demonstrate compliant behavior as evidenced by:
Absence of symptom exacerbation and/or complications
Progression toward wellness
Resolution of health problems
Adherence to therapeutic regimen and follow-up instructions
Seeking out appropriate health care
Seeking out appropriate community resources

Oral mucous membrane, altered related to:
Dehydration
Effects of medications
Immunosuppression
Inadequate oral hygiene
Infection
Malnutrition
Trauma

The patient will maintain an intact oral mucous membrane as evidenced by:
Absence of signs of inflammation, infection: redness, ulceration, pain
Signs of progressive healing
Ability to maintain oral intake

Pain related to:
Inflammation
Muscle spasm
Effects of trauma
Immobility
Obstructive process
Infectious process
Experience during diagnostic tests
Injury agents: biological, chemical, physical, psychological

The patient will experience absence of pain as evidenced by:
Communication of pain descriptors (verbal or coded)
Absence of physiological indicators of pain: pallor, tachycardia, tachypnea, diaphoresis, increased blood pressure, restlessness
Absence of nonverbal cues of pain: crying, grimacing, inability to assume position of comfort
Ability to cooperate and participate in care

Nursing Diagnosis	Desired Expected Outcome

Rape-trauma syndrome related to:
Assault

The patient will demonstrate appropriate coping as evidenced by:
Decreased anxiety and fear
Ability to focus on tasks and procedures
Cooperation and participation with care
Accepts referral for follow-up care

Sensory-perceptual alterations (visual, auditory, kinesthetic, gustatory, tactile, olfactory) related to:
Sleep deprivation
Pain
Effects of aging, stress and/or neurological impairment
Visual
   Restriction of head, neck motion
   Failure to use eye protection
   Inflammation
   Infection
Auditory
   Effects of certain antibiotics
   Excessive earwax, fluid, or foreign body
   Failure to use ear protection
Kinesthetic
   Inner ear inflammation
   Side effects of medications
   Sleep deprivation
Gustatory
   Inflammation of nasal mucosa
   Side effects of medications
   Trauma to the tongue
Tactile
   Circulatory impairment
   Inflammation
   Effects of burns
Olfactory
   Inflammation of the nasal mucosa
   Foreign body in the nose

The patient will maintain adequate sensation, perception as evidenced by:
Ability to verbalize limitations in sensation/perception
Verbalizes methods used to safely perform activities of daily living (ADLs)
Verbalizes appropriate follow-up care
Verbalizes discharge instructions accurately

Skin integrity impaired related to:
External
   Chemical substance
   Hyper- or hypothermia
   Mechanical factors
   Immobilization
   Trauma
Internal
   Altered circulation, metabolism, nutritional state, sensation
   Developmental factors
   Effects of medications
   Immunological deficit

The patient will maintain intact skin integrity as evidenced by:
Absence of signs of irritation: erythema, blanching, itching
Absence of signs of infection: erythema, edema, purulent drainage, odor, and pain

Swallowing, impaired related to:
Effects of neuromuscular impairment
Mechanical obstruction
Excessive or inadequate salivation
Fatigue
Inflamed oropharyngeal cavity

The patient will maintain adequate swallowing as evidenced by:
Absence of coughing, choking
Adequate oral intake and hydration
Absence of evidence of aspiration
Reported absence of pain

Nursing Diagnosis	Desired Expected Outcome
Tissue perfusion, altered renal, cardiopulmonary, cerebral, gastrointestinal, peripheral (specify type), related to: Exchange problems Hypervolemia Hypovolemia Interruption of flow: arterial or venous	*The patient will maintain adequate tissue perfusion as evidenced by:* Absence of ischemic pain Normal sinus rhythm or return to baseline cardiac rhythm Level of consciousness: alert and oriented or baseline Vital signs within normal limits Strong and equal peripheral pulses Adequate urinary output Skin color normal, warm and dry

Trauma, high risk for related to:
Internal (individual)
  Balancing difficulties
  Confusion
  Fatigue
  Hypotension
  Pain
  Sensory-perceptual alterations
  Reduced mobility
  Weakness
  Substance abuse
  Lack of safety education and precautions
  Language barrier
  Developmental age
External (environmental)
  Electrical hazards
  Fire hazards
  Safety hazards
	The patient will remain free from trauma as evidenced by:
	Knowledge of injury prevention
	Behaviors designed to promote an injury-free environment
	Active participation in medical care to reduce risk factors

Urinary elimination, altered patterns related to: Anatomical obstruction Constipation, fecal impaction Dehydration Fatigue Obesity Mechanical trauma Pain, spasm in bladder, abdomen Urinary tract infection Effects of medication Fear Inability to express needs Change in environment Effects of aging, immobility, indwelling catheter, medications, sensorimotor impairment	*The patient will maintain adequate urinary output as evidenced by:* Ability to communicate the need to urinate Absence of urinary tract infection Absence of urinary incontinence Decreased complaints of urinary symptoms Absence of a distended bladder

Data from Taptich, B., Iyer, P., & Bernocchi-Losey, D. (1994). *Nursing diagnosis and care planning.* Philadelphia: W. B. Saunders.

Glasgow Coma Scale and Modified Infant Coma Scale

GLASGOW COMA SCALE*

Response Finding	Score
Best eye opening	
Spontaneous	4
To voice	3
To pain	2
None	1
Best verbal	
Oriented	5
Confused	4
Inappropriate words	3
Incomprehensible words	2
None	1
Best Motor	
Obeys commands	6
Localizes to pain	5
Withdraws from pain	4
Flexion to pain	3
Extension to pain	2
None	1
Total score	**3–15**

*Obtain best score in each category, then determine total score. Highest total score obtainable is 15, lowest is 3. (Selfridge-Thomas, J. [1997]. *Emergency Nursing: An essential guide for patient care.* [pp. 202–203]. Philadelphia: W.B. Saunders.)

MODIFIED INFANT COMA SCALE*

Response Finding	Score
Best eye opening	
Spontaneous	4
To speech	3
To pain	2
None	1
Best verbal	
Coos, babbles	5
Irritable cry	4
Cries to pain	3
Moans to pain	2
None	1
Best motor	
Normal spontaneous movements	6
Withdraws to touch	5
Withdraws to pain	4
Abnormal flexion	3
Abnormal extension	2
None	1
Total score	**3–15**

*Obtain best score in each category, then determine total score. Highest total score obtainable is 15, lowest is 3. (Selfridge-Thomas, J. [1997]. *Emergency Nursing: An essential guide for patient care.* [pp. 202–203]. Philadelphia: W.B. Saunders.)

Glossary

AB	Abortion
ABCs	Airway, breathing, circulation
ABE	Acute bacterial endocarditis
ABGs	Arterial blood gases
ACE	Angiotensin-converting enzyme
ACLS	Advanced cardiac life support
ACP	Ambulatory casualty post
ACS	American College of Surgeons
ACSCOT	American College of Surgeons, Committee on Trauma
ADH	Antidiuretic hormone
ADLs	Activities of daily living
AF	Atrial fibrillation
AIDS	Acquired immunodeficiency syndrome
ALS	Advanced life support
AP	Anteroposterior
ARDS	Adult respiratory distress syndrome
ASA	Aspirin
AV	Atrioventricular
BCLS	Basic cardiac life support
BCPs	Birth control pills
BLS	Basic life support
BP	Blood pressure
BPM	Beats per minute
BVM	Bag-valve-mask (for ventilation)
C	Centigrade (Celsius)
CEN	Certified emergency nurse
CHF	Congestive heart failure
CID	Cervical immobilization device
CISD	Critical incident stress debriefing
CNS	Central nervous system
CO$_2$	Carbon dioxide
COBRA/ OBRA	Consolidated Omnibus Budget Reconciliation Act (also known as Emergency Medical Treatment and Active Labor Act [EMTALA])
COPD	Chronic obstructive pulmonary disease
CPAP	Continuous positive airway pressure
CPR	Cardiopulmonary resuscitation
CSF	Cerebrospinal fluid
C-spine	Cervical spine
CT	Computed tomography
CVA	Cerebrovascular accident
CVP	Central venous pressure
CXR	Chest x-ray
D&C	Dilation and curettage
DCC	Disaster control center
DIC	Disseminated intravascular coagulation
DOA	Dead on arrival
DOE	Dyspnea on exertion
DTR	Deep tendon reflexes
Dts	Delirium tremens
ECG	Electrocardiogram
ED	Emergency department
EDC	Estimated date of confinement

EDT	Emergency department technician (also known as Emergency Care Technician [ECT])
EEG	Electroencephalogram
EGTA	Esophageal gastric tube airway
EMD	Electromechanical dissociation
EMS	Emergency medical system
EMTLA	Emergency Medical Treatment and Active Labor Act
ENT	Ear, nose, throat
EOA	Esophageal obturator airway
EOM	Extraocular movement
ETT	Endotracheal tube
F	Fahrenheit
FEMA	Federal Emergency Management Agency
FEV$_1$	Forced expiratory volume in 1 second
FHT	Fetal heart tones
FTE	Full-time equivalent
FVC	Forced vital capacity
GCS	Glasgow Coma Scale
GI	Gastrointestinal
HCO$_3$	Bicarbonate
Hg	Mercury
HIV	Human immunodeficiency virus
H$_2$O	Water
H$_2$O$_2$	Hydrogen peroxide
HOB	Head of bed
HTN	Hypertension
ICP	Intracranial pressure
ICS	Intercostal space
IICP	Increased intracranial pressure
IM	Intramuscular
I&O	Intake and output
IU	International unit
IUD	Intrauterine device
IV	Intravenous

IVP	Intravenous pyelogram
J	Joules
JCAHO	Joint Commission on Accreditation of Healthcare Organizations
JVD	Jugular venous distention
KUB	Kidney-ureter-bladder
LMP	Last menstrual period
LNMP	Last normal menstrual period
LOC	Level of consciousness
LSB	Left sternal border
LSD	Lysergic acid diethylamide
LV	Left ventricle
LPN	Licensed practical nurse
LVN	Licensed vocational nurse
MCL	Midclavicular line
MI	Myocardial infarction
MICN	Mobile intensive care nurse
mm Hg	Millimeters of mercury
MVC	Motor vehicle crash
NP	Nurse practitioner
NPO	Nothing per os (orally)
O$_2$	Oxygen
OCP	Oral contraceptive pills
OES	Office of Emergency Services
OR	Operating room
OTC	Over the counter (medications)
PA	Posteroanterior
PA	Public address
PA	Pulmonary artery
PAC	Premature atrial contraction
PAPs	Pulmonary artery pressures
PASG	Pneumatic antishock garment
PAWP	Pulmonary artery wedge pressure
PCP	Phencyclidine poisoning
PEEP	Positive end-expiratory pressure
PFT	Pulmonary function test

PMI	Point of maximal impulse
PND	Paroxysmal nocturnal dyspnea
PO	Per os, orally
PQRST	*P*rovocation, *q*uality, *r*adiation, *r*egion, *s*everity, *t*ime of onset
PR	Pulse rate
PSVT	Paroxysmal supraventricular tachycardia
PTS	Pediatric trauma score
PVB	Premature ventricular beat
PVC	Premature ventricular contraction
QA	Quality assurance
QI	Quality improvement
RAS	Reticular activating system
Rh	Rhesus factor
RL	Ringer's lactate
RN	Registered nurse
ROM	Range of motion
RPP	Reserve personnel pool
RR	Respiratory rate
RSI	Rapid-sequence intubation (also known as rapid-sequence induction)
RTS	Revised trauma score
SA	Sinoatrial
SBE	Subacute bacterial endocarditis
SCI	Spinal cord injury
SIDS	Sudden infant death syndrome
SOB	Shortness of breath
STD	Sexually transmitted disease
TIA	Transient ischemic attack
TMJ	Temporomandibular joint
TSS	Toxic shock syndrome
UHF	Ultrahigh frequency
URI	Upper respiratory tract infection
VD	Venereal disease
VF	Ventricular fibrillation

VHF	Very high frequency
VPB	Ventricular premature beat
VQ scan	Ventilation-perfusion scan
VT	Ventricular tachycardia
WNL	Within normal limits

Laboratory Studies

ABGs	Arterial blood gases
BUN	Blood urea nitrogen
Ca^{++}	Calcium
CBC	Complete blood count
CBC with differential	Complete blood count with smear analysis
CK	Creatine kinase
CK-MB	Creatine kinase isoenzymes
Cl	Chloride
CO$_2$	Carbon dioxide
CPK	Creatine phosphokinase
C&S	Culture and sensitivity
ESR	Erythrocyte sedimentation rate
ETOH	Alcohol (ethanol)
Hb	Hemoglobin
Hct	Hematocrit
K$^+$	Potassium
KOH	Potassium hydroxide
LDH	Lactate dehydrogenase
LFT	Liver function test
Mg	Magnesium
Na	Sodium
Paco$_2$	Partial pressure of carbon dioxide, arterial
Pao$_2$	Partial pressure of oxygen, arterial
Pco$_2$	Partial pressure of carbon dioxide
Po$_2$	Partial pressure of oxygen
PT	Prothrombin time
PTT	Partial thromboplastin time
RBC	Red blood cell count

SGOT	Serum glutamic-oxaloacetic transaminase	**VDRL**	Venereal Disease Research Laboratory (test for venereal disease)
SGPT	Serum glutamate pyruvate transaminase	**WBC**	White blood cell count
UA	Urinalysis		

Advisory Committee on Immunization Practices (ACIP) Recommended Schedule of Vaccinations for Children and Recommended Schedule of Vaccinations for Adults

RECOMMENDED CHILDHOOD IMMUNIZATION SCHEDULE

Vaccines are listed under the routinely recommended ages. Bars indicate range of acceptable ages for vaccination. Shaded Bars indicate *catch-up vaccination:* at 11–12 years of age, hepatitis B vaccine should be administered to children not previously vaccinated, and Varicella vaccine should be administered to children not previously vaccinated who lack a reliable history of chickenpox.

Age ► Vaccine ▼	Birth	1 mo	2 mos	4 mos	6 mos	12 mos	15 mos	18 mos	4–6 yrs	11–12 yrs	14–16 yrs
Hepatitis B	Hep B-1	Hep B-2			Hep B-3					Hep B	
Diphtheria, Tetanus, Pertussis			DTaP	DTaP	DTaP		DTaP		DTaP	Td	
H. influenzae type b			Hib	Hib	Hib	Hib					
Polio			IPV	IPV		Polio			Polio		
Measles, Mumps, Rubella						MMR			MMR or MMR		
Varicella Zoster Virus Vaccine						Var				Var	
Rotavirus			RV	RV	RV						

Approved by the Advisory Committee on Immunization Practices (ACIP), the American Academy of Pediatrics (AAP), and the American Academy of Family Physicians (AAFP). (Modified.)

ACIP RECOMMENDED SCHEDULE OF VACCINATIONS FOR ADULTS*

Vaccine	Who?	When?	Why? Because the Disease Can Cause:
Measles, mumps, rubella (MMR)†	*Everyone* born after 1956 should have one dose of MMR Some adults should have two doses of measles vaccine‡	Any time after the first birthday Second dose at least 1 month after the first, if needed	*Measles:* diarrhea, ear infections, pneumonia, and infections of the brain (encephalitis) *Mumps:* deafness, inflammation of the testes, and infections of the brain and covering of the brain (meningitis) *Rubella (in pregnancy):* loss of sight and hearing, retardation, and heart defects in the infant
Hepatitis B†	High-risk groups are health care workers, certain travelers, sexually active adults with multiple partners, intravenous drug users	Three-shot vaccine series at any age for people at risk	Inflammation of the liver, tiredness, nausea, vomiting, scarring (cirrhosis) of the liver, liver cancer, liver failure
Tetanus, diphtheria toxoid†	*Everyone*	Booster at 14–16 years of age, then boosters every 10 years for life	*Tetanus:* severe muscle spasms leading to inability to open the jaw ("lockjaw"), difficulty in breathing, and death *Diphtheria:* severe sore throat leading to a gray coating across the windpipe and death
Influenza (flu)	All people aged 65 years or older; people of any age with chronic disease of the heart, lungs, or kidneys, anemia, or diseases that interfere with the body's immune system; people living in nursing homes; people who have contact with those who are at high risk	Each year before flu season	Fever, chills, headache, sore throat, dry cough, runny nose, and body aches; pneumonia, the most common complication of flu
Pneumococcal disease	All people aged 65 years or older; people of any age who have a chronic illness (similar to those listed for influenza)	One dose for most people at risk; a second dose every 6 years for people at highest risk and those with certain kidney diseases	Serious infections of the lungs (pneumonia), the blood stream (bacteremia), and the covering of the brain (meningitis)
Polio†	Boosters for certain travelers§	Boosters when necessary	Paralysis, weakness, inability to swallow or talk

*Refer to ACIP recommendations for more details.
†Primary series of these vaccines is given in childhood.
‡College students, health care workers, and susceptible travelers need two doses of measles vaccine unless immunity is confirmed by physician diagnosis or a blood test.
§Certain susceptible travelers to high-risk areas may need these vaccines.

Mini-Mental Status Exam

MINI-MENTAL STATE EXAMINATION

Patient _____

Examiner _____

Date _____

Maximum Score	Score	
		Orientation
5	_____	What is the (year) (season) (date) (day) (month)?
5	_____	Where are we: (state) (country) (town) (hospital) (floor)?
		Registration
3	_____	Name 3 objects: 1 second to say each. Then ask the patient all 3 after you have said them. Give 1 point for each correct answer. Then repeat them until he learns all 3. Count trials and record.
		Trials _____
		Attention and Calculation
5	_____	Serial 7's. 1 point for each correct. Stop after 5 answers. Alternatively spell "world" backwards.
		Recall
3	_____	Ask for the 3 objects repeated above. Give 1 point for each correct.
		Language
9	_____	Name a pencil and watch (2 points).

Repeat the following "No ifs, ands, or buts." (1 point).
Follow a 3-stage command: "Take a paper in your right hand, fold it in half, and put it on the floor." (3 points).
Read and obey the following:
 Close your eyes (1 point).
 Write a sentence (1 point).
 Copy a design (1 point).

Total Score _____

Assess level of consciousness along a continuum

Alter	Drowsy	Stupor	Coma

Instructions for Administration of Mini-Mental State Examination Orientation

1. Ask for the date. Then ask specifically for part omitted (e.g., "Can you also tell me what season it is?"). One point for each correct.
2. Ask in turn "Can you tell me the name of this hospital?" (town, county, etc.). One point for each correct.

Registration

1. Ask the patient if you may test his memory. Then say the name of 3 unrelated objects, clearly and slowly, about 1 second for each. After having said all 3, ask him to repeat them. This first repetition determines his score (0–3), but keep saying them until he can repeat all 3, up to 6 trials. If he does not eventually learn all 3, recall cannot be meaningfully tested.

Attention and Calculation

1. Ask the patient to begin with 100 and count backwards by 7. Stop after 5 subtractions (93, 86, 79, 72, 65). Score the total number of correct answers.
2. If the patient cannot or will not perform this task, ask him to spell the word "world" backwards. The score is the number of letters in correct order (e.g., DLROW = 5; DLORW = 3).

Recall

1. Ask the patient if he can recall the 3 words you previously asked him to remember. Score 0–3.

Language

1. Naming: Show the patient a wrist watch and ask him what it is. Repeat for pencil. Score 0–2.
2. Repetition: Ask the patient to repeat the sentence after you. Allow only one trial. Score 0 or 1.
3. 3-Stage command: Give the patient a piece of plain blank paper and repeat the command. Score 1 point for each part correctly executed.
4. Reading: On a blank piece of paper print the sentence "Close your eyes," in letters large enough for the patient to see clearly. Ask him to read it and do what it says. Score 1 point only if he actually closes his eyes.
5. Writing: Give the patient a blank piece of paper and ask him to write a sentence for you. Do not dictate a sentence; it is to be written spontaneously. It must contain a subject and a verb and be sensible. Correct grammar and punctuation are not necessary.
6. Copying: On a clean piece of paper, draw intersecting pentagons, each side about 1 inch, and ask him to copy it exactly as it is. All 10 angles must be present, and 2 must intersect to score 1 point. Tremor and rotation are ignored.

Scoring:

APPENDIX **G**

Drug Calculations for Vasoactive Medications

When administering vasoactive medications (e.g., Intropin [dopamine HCL], Dobutrex [dobutamine HCL]), the nurse must determine rate of infusion based on kilograms of body weight. The following formulas can be used to determine rate of infusion and microgram per kilogram of drug infusing.

Calculating cc's per hour based on μg/kg/min

$$\text{Rate} = \frac{\mu g \times kg \times 60 \text{ (minutes)}}{\mu g/cc}$$

CLINICAL EXAMPLE: To determine how many cubic centimeters per hour to infuse a Brevibloc (esmolol) IV infusion, which is to be maintained at 100 μg/kg/min for a 90-kg patient.

Determine how many μg/cc:

1. Find out how many milligrams (mg) in 1 cc (i.e., total mg ÷ total volume of solution)
2. Convert mg/cc to μg/cc × 1000)

In the example above, Brevibloc is mixed, resulting in 2.5 g of Brevibloc in 285 cc of solution.

$$2500 \text{ mg} \div 285 = 8.77 \text{ mg/cc}$$

$$8.77 \text{ mg/cc} \times 1000 = 8770 \text{ μg/mL}$$

$$\text{Therefore: } \frac{100 \times 90 \times 60}{8770 \text{ μg/cc}} = \frac{540,000}{8770} = 61.5, \text{ or } 62 \text{ cc/hr}$$

Determining μg/kg/min when rate known

$$\mu g/kg/min = \frac{(\mu g/cc \times cc/hr) \div 60}{kg}$$

CLINICAL EXAMPLE: To determine how many micrograms per kilogram per minute are infusing for a 70-kg patient with a single-strength dopamine HCL IV infusion running at 32 cc/hr.

1. Find out how many milligrams (mg) in 1 cc (i.e., total mg ÷ total volume of solution)
2. Determine number of milligrams delivered per hour (mg/cc × rate = mg/hr)
3. Convert milligrams per hour to micrograms per hour (mg/hr × 1000 = μg per hour)
4. Determine micrograms per minute (μg/hr ÷ 60 = μg/min)
5. Calculate micrograms per minute per kilogram (μg/min ÷ kg = μg/min/kg)

Dopamine HCL (single strength) is mixed at 200 mg in 250 cc of solution:

1. 200 ÷ 250 = 0.8 mg/cc
2. 0.8 × 32 = 25.6 mg/hr
3. 25.6 × 1000 = 25,600 μg/hr
4. 25,600 ÷ 60 = 426 μg/min
5. 426 μg/min ÷ 70 = 6.09 μg/kg/min

APPENDIX H

Rapid-Sequence Intubation

Rapid-sequence intubation (RSI) is defined as the procedure used to induce rapid paralysis and/or anesthesia for the purpose of initiating an advanced definitive airway.

Indications for RSI are as follows:

- Uncooperative patient
- Head injury
- Suspicion of an injury to a major vessel but without active bleeding
- Asthma exacerbation
- Reactive airway disease

Contraindications to RSI are as follows:

- Distorted anatomy
- Obstruction
- Major facial, laryngeal trauma
- Angioedema

RSI EQUIPMENT AND PERSONNEL REQUIREMENTS

At least two individuals must be available to safely initiate RSI, one being a skilled intubationist. Other personnel will be responsible for preparing the patient and equipment.

Overview:

Brief history and assessment
↓
Preparation: medications, oxygenation, patient, team
↓
Preoxygenation
↓
Premedication: atropine, lidocaine, defasciculating dose of paralyzing agent, sedative
↓
Administer neuromuscular blocking agent
↓
Cricoid pressure
↓
Intubate
↓
Provide post-intubation assessment and care
Confirm tube placement
Maintain sedation and paralysis

Step 1: prepare equipment and team.

A. **Equipment**

Oxygen source
Suction equipment
Endotracheal tubes
Bag-valve-mask device
Laryngoscope and blades
Stylet
Cardiac monitor
Pulse oximeter

End-tidal carbon dioxide monitor
Temperature probe
Alternative airway equipment (available in case of failed intubation)
Laryngeal mask airway, transtracheal jet ventilation set-up, cricothyroidotomy equipment

B. Team

Assign roles and responsibilities; leader, intubation, cricoid pressure, monitoring, medications.

Step 2: perform a brief history and assessment.

A. Use the mnemonic AMPLE:

Allergies, Medications, Past medical history, Last meal, Existing circumstances.

B. Primary and secondary assessments should be conducted.

Step 3: make final preparations.

A. Assemble all equipment and ensure personnel are available.
B. Draw up all necessary medications in labeled syringes.
C. Record preinduction vital signs:

- Cardiac monitor
- Pulse oximeter
- Core body temperature probe
- End-tidal carbon dioxide detector

Step 4: preoxygenate the patient.

A. Preoxygenate a patient with spontaneous respirations with 100% oxygen via a well-fitting mask for 3 to 5 minutes if possible.
B. The goal of preoxygenation is to create an oxygen reservoir in the functional residual capacity of the lungs. This reservoir permits continued oxygenation of blood circulating through the pulmonary vascular bed during apnea induced by neuromuscular blocking agents.
C. If a patient is unable to breath adequately on his or her own or presents with apnea, use a bag-valve-mask device to preoxygenate. Use the Sellick maneuver when ventilating the patient to avoid gastric distention.

Step 5: premedicate the patient.

A. Intubation stimulates the body in a number of ways causing:

- In the brain increased intracranial pressure (ICP)
- In the eyes increased intraocular pressure (IOP)
- In the heart bradycardia in pediatric patients, hypertension and tachycardia in adults

B. Premedication may be given depending on the amount of time available and the particular patient situation.
C. Lidocaine may be given to counteract a potential increase in ICP, especially in head trauma cases.
D. Atropine may be administered to decrease the occurrence of vagal stimulation during laryngoscopy and from the administration of succinylcholine.
E. A sedative-hypnotic is administered at this time to a conscious patient to provide analgesia and sedation and to induce amnesia. Sedation is required to eliminate awareness of pending paralysis.
F. Limit stimulation as much as possible because the patient may exhibit a period of excitement

- Keep voices quiet
- Limit unnecessary conversation
- Limit tactile stimulation while offering emotional support

Step 6: administer neuromuscular blocking agent.

A. Neuromuscular blocking agents cause muscle paralysis; they ideally have a rapid onset and a short duration and are reversible.
B. If succinylcholine is to be used, muscle twitching (fasciculations) of the major muscle groups are to be expected; this can cause muscle pain, hyperkalemia, rhabdomyolysis, myoglobinuria, increased intragastric pressure, and ICP.
C. Fasciculations can be blocked by administering a minidose of a nondepolarizing muscle

relaxant such as pancuronium or vecuronium; this should be administered 2 to 3 minutes before paralyzing the patient.

Step 7: intubate the patient.

A. Bag-valve-mask ventilation should be available if hypoxia occurs with intubation attempts.
B. The Sellick maneuver should be used. This maneuver consists of gentle downward pressure on the cricoid cartilage to make visualization of the vocal cords and tube placement easier. It also prevents passive regurgitation of stomach contents.
C. Intubation should be performed by a skilled intubationist when the muscles are fully relaxed. This usually occurs 45 to 120 seconds after the neuromuscular blocking agent is administered.

Step 8: provide post-intubation care.

A. Confirm tube placement clinically via auscultation of bilateral breath sounds and end-tidal carbon dioxide detector.
B. Inflate endotracheal tube cuff. Secure tube and obtain chest film.
C. Assist ventilations via bag-valve-mask device or ventilator.
D. Monitor oxygenation via pulse oximetry.
E. Check vital signs and monitor.
F. Many anesthetic agents depress the hypothalamus and the patient's temperature control center, thus allowing hypothermia to develop. External warming measures should be applied to maintain the patient's body temperature.
G. The anesthetized patient cannot assist in positioning and loses protective mechanisms such as blinking. After the airway is secured, scan the patient to ensure there is no undue pressure on any body part, and that extremities are not in danger of injury from moving parts of the stretcher or other equipment.
H. Consider adding eye lubrication and taping the lids shut to prevent corneal abrasions.

From Twedell, D. M. (Ed.). (1997). *Slide script series: RSI.* Park Ridge, IL: Emergency Nurses Association. Used with permission.

RAPID SEQUENCE INTUBATION MEDICATIONS

Medication	Dosage	Caution/Contraindications
Atropine	0.01–0.02 mg/kg IV	
Etomidate	0.2–0.4 mg/kg IV	Pain on injection, myotonic or myoclonic activity
Fentanyl	3–8 μg/kg IV	
Ketamine	1.0–2.0 mg/kg IV	Head injury patients
Lidocaine	1.5–3 mg/kg IV	
Midazolam	0.1–0.2 mg/kg IV	
Pancuronium	0.01 mg/kg IV (defasciculating dose) 0.1 mg/kg IV (standard paralyzing dose)	Normotensive patients with eye or head injuries or patients with a history of cardiovascular disease
Propofol	0.5–2 mg/kg IV	Allergy to eggs
Rocuronium	0.5–0.8 mg/kg IV	
Succinylcholine	1–2 mg/kg IV	Neuromuscular disease, ocular injury, burns, hyperkalemia
Thiopental	2 mg/kg IV	Hypotension, laryngospasm in nonparalyzed patient, asthma
Vecuronium	0.1–0.2 mg/kg IV (defasciculating dose) 0.1 mg/kg IV (paralyzing dose)	Normotensive patients with eye or head injuries or patients with a history of cardiovascular disease

From Twedell, D. M. (Ed.). (1999). *Slide script series: RSI.* Park Ridge, IL: Emergency Nurses Association. Used with permission; Howell, J. M., Altieri M., Jagoda A., Prescott, J. (1998). *Emergency medicine.* Philadelphia: W.B. Saunders, 1998.

Advanced Practice

The health care environment changes continuously. Changes in this environment have provided new opportunities for emergency nurses to diversify their role. One role that has taken on a more active role in the emergency care setting is that of the advanced practice registered nurse (APRN).

The Emergency Nurses Association (ENA) defines an APRN as "a nurse who has completed a master's degree in a specialty area of nursing and is clinically active in the area of specialty" (ENA, 1996). Specific advanced practice roles in emergency care, identified by the Emergency Nurses Association Advanced Nursing Practice Committee, include nurse practitioner and clinical nurse specialist. The fifth edition of the *Core Curriculum* has incorporated this appendix to assist in addressing the needs of the APRN.

The purpose of this appendix is to give nurses working in emergency advanced practice roles or those seeking such a role a guide to the clinical, educational, leadership, administrative, research, and professional competencies important to the role. It should be stressed that the content of this section is intended as a foundation for APRNs and is not comprehensive. It should be used to guide those seeking further education to look at specific content areas they may want to study to assist in their role. For current practitioners, this guide can be used to assist in evaluating their practice, and possibly seeking new educational opportunities to increase their current role. Scope of practice issues are state specific, and mastery of competencies does not constitute a legal right to practice as an APRN. Additionally, skills listed are those that some or most APRNs use on a daily basis; they should not be constituted as an absolute.

The following outline contains major areas of emphasis. The outline should be considered an extension to the content of the previous chapters. There is an assumption that APRNs will have the basic content of the core as a foundation to the following pages.

SECTION 1: CLINICAL

The advanced technical skills listed are the major skills identified by APRNs. A clinical nurse specialist may be called on to educate the nursing staff regarding these procedures including the potential complications and patient management surrounding the procedure.

I. CRITICAL THINKING SKILLS

APRNs will need to use expert reasoning based on their acquired knowledge. On the basis of their educational focus, APRNs will apply advanced reasoning to look beyond the immediate situation and focus on future outcomes.

A. Synthesis of assessment and diagnostic findings
B. Prediction of patient outcomes considering complex variables
C. Differential diagnosis
D. Innovative problem solving

II. APRN PROTOCOLS

A. Clinical guidelines

      1. Creation
      2. Evaluation

B. Process protocols

III. PHARMACOLOGY

A. Drug selection
B. Drug interaction
C. Adverse reaction

      1. Recognition
      2. Management

D. Prescriptive authority

      1. State legislation
      2. Regulations
      3. Responsibilities

IV. ADVANCED TECHNICAL SKILLS

For each skill the APRN will understand the following: a knowledge of diagnostic conditions, when to apply, how to do procedure, complications to look for, patient management during procedure, and discharge instructions when applicable.

A. Advanced airway management

      1. Intubation
      2. Cricothyroidotomy

B. Anoscopy
C. Arterial catheter insertion
D. Chest tube insertion, needle decompression
E. Diagnostic peritoneal lavage
F. Epistaxis control

      1. Packing
      2. Cautery
      3. Balloons

G. Gastric tube replacement
H. Intraosseous catheter insertion
I. Lumbar puncture
J. Pacemakers

      1. External
      2. Internal

K. Pelvic exam

      1. Sexually transmitted diseases
      2. Sexual assault evidence collection

L. Pericardiocentesis

M. Slit-lamp exam

1. Fluorescein stain
2. Foreign body removal
3. Intraocular pressure measurement

N. Venipuncture

1. Peripheral intravenous catheter insertion
2. Central catheter insertion/peripherally inserted central catheter

O. Wound repair/management

1. Debridement
2. Incision and drainage
3. Nail avulsion
4. Suture techniques
   a. Simple interrupted suture
   b. Horizontal mattress suture
   c. Vertical mattress suture
   d. Continuous suture
5. Skin staples
6. Wound adhesives
7. Local anesthesia
8. Digital nerve blocks

P. Orthopedic procedures

1. Dislocations, fracture management
2. Splints

SECTION 2: EDUCATION

I. ADULT LEARNING PRINCIPLES

APRNs are in a unique position to educate both patients and staff. They are usually responsible for education of the staff and, therefore, must have a working knowledge of how to create educational materials.

II. METHODS

The following is a list of the various types of educational offerings APRNs should be familiar with and able to apply based on the learning needs of their audience.

A. Lecture
B. Group discussion
C. Role-playing
D. Self-study modules
E. Computer-based learning
F. Grand rounds

   G. Demonstration, return demonstration
   H. One-to-one bedside teaching

III. CURRICULUM DEVELOPMENT
A. Needs assessment tools

   1. **Psychomotor skills**
   2. **Cognitive skills**
   3. **Interpersonal skills**

B. Program planning

   1. **Objectives**
   2. **Identifying audience**
      a. Identifying type of presentation to meet the needs of the audience
      b. Formal versus informal
   3. **Course length**
   4. **Identifying speakers**
      a. Speaker selection
         1) Initial arrangements
         2) Letter of confirmation
         3) Copy of conference agenda
         4) Level of audience
      b. Honorarium
   5. **Course budget**
   6. **Course agenda**
   7. **Locating classroom space**
      a. Room set-up
      b. Audiovisual needs
   8. **Course evaluation**

C. Instructional media

   1. **Type of materials that should be used for presentation**
      a. Slides
      b. Overheads
      c. Other media
   2. **Trouble-shooting equipment**
   3. **Handouts**

IV. CONTINUING EDUCATION
A. Application process

   1. **State nurses association**
   2. **Professional association**
   3. **Understanding the requirements**
      a. Time constraints
      b. Financial needs
      c. Record keeping

V. PRESENTATION SKILLS

A. Comfort level

1. Experience
2. Practice

B. Public speaking courses
C. Knowledge of subject

1. Level of audience dictates level of information
2. Research

VI. BARRIERS TO EDUCATION

A. Institutional funding
B. Staff schedules
C. Staff attitudes

1. Internal need versus external issue
2. Relevance of material

D. Inconsistency between information provided and that desired by audience

SECTION 3: LEADERSHIP/ADMINISTRATIVE

Many times APRNs are in a position to assist the leadership of the department to advance the delivery of care for the emergency department patients. APRNs affect quality by influencing others, developing policies and procedures, as well as working with staff. Therefore, it is important for the APRN to appreciate and understand the management issues involved in ensuring that the emergency department runs effectively.

I. JOINT COMMISSION ON THE ACCREDITATION OF HEALTHCARE ORGANIZATIONS (JCAHO) REQUIREMENTS

A. Policy and procedure development
B. Record keeping
C. Continuous process improvement (CPI) activities

1. Creating indicators
2. Interpreting data gathered
3. Reporting data results

II. CASE MANAGEMENT, OUTCOME MANAGEMENT

A. Development of critical pathways
B. Implementation of pathways
C. Evaluation of pathways
D. Coordination of patient care

III. ELEMENTS OF LEADERSHIP

A. Visionary
B. Risk taker

    1. Change agent

C. Mentor

    1. Empowerment
    2. Coach

D. Communication skills

    1. Articulation of ideas
    2. Delivery of message
    3. Feedback
    4. Written reports

IV. FINANCIAL MANAGEMENT

A. Budget

    1. Operational budget
    2. Staffing budget
    3. Productivity

B. Reimbursement

    1. Health Care Financing Administration (HCFA) guidelines
       a. Medicare
       b. Urban and rural practices
       c. Documentation guidelines
    2. Public aid
    3. Managed-care plans
       a. Health Maintenance Organization (HMO)
       b. Preferred provider organization (PPO)
       c. Capitated contracts
    4. Private insurance
    5. Reimbursement rates

C. Diagnostic coding

    1. ICD-9-CM
    2. Physician's current procedural terminology (CPT) codes
       a. Documentation requirements for levels of care
          1) History
          2) Physical examination
          3) Medical decision making
          4) Counseling
          5) Coordination of care
       b. Modifiers for APRNs

V. DEVELOPMENT OF A BUSINESS PLAN

A. Objectives
B. Fit of work setting with objectives

      1. Community and institutional needs

C. Assessment of institutional strengths

      1. Resources available
      2. Support services needed
      3. Institutional trends

D. Operational readiness

      1. Capital requirements
      2. Education, training requirements

E. Market analysis and plan

      1. Estimate demands for service
      2. Market assessment, opportunity, and plan

F. Financial analysis and projections

      1. Revenues
      2. Reimbursement
      3. Expenses

G. Conclusions and recommendations

      1. Opportunities
      2. Assessment of risk

VI. STRATEGIC PLANNING
A. Evaluate institutional needs
B. Develop plan to address needs with measurable outcomes

      1. Long- and short-term goals
      2. Define outcomes
      3. Key players and staff input

C. Submit proposal

      1. Identify key players
      2. Seek support

D. Negotiate proposal
E. Evaluate effectiveness of performance by monitoring predetermined outcomes

SECTION 4: RESEARCH

The role of researcher has been intimately linked with advanced practice. The role of researcher needs to be incorporated into all APRN job descriptions as a defining difference to their practice.

I. RESEARCH ROLES

A. Use of research as the foundation of practice

1. **Identifies nursing practice problems and forms a research question**
   a. *Literature review*
   b. *Development of policies, procedures, standards of care*
2. **Helps others apply research in daily practice**

B. Evaluating practice using simple research designs and replication activities

1. **Conducts research studies**
2. **Replicates studies**
3. **Tests research findings in daily practice**

C. Generation of new knowledge

1. **Participates in research by designing studies**
2. **Participates in others' research by gathering and interpreting data**

SECTION 5: PROFESSIONAL DEVELOPMENT

One of the most important aspects of the APRN role is professional development. It is essential that the APRN has an understanding of how to market the role, negotiate for a contract, form a network, and finally evaluate the role. These activities help strengthen the role in the health care system by positioning the APRN as a viable health care provider.

I. MARKETING ONESELF

A. Resume

1. **Work history**
2. **Key components**
   a. *Objective*
   b. *Qualification summary*
   c. *Employment history: brief description of roles and responsibilities with major accomplishments*
   d. *Education*
   e. *Memberships and associations*
   f. *Personal data*

B. Curriculum vitae

1. **Academic history**
2. **Key components**
   a. *Position sought*
      1) Accent professional experiences
      2) Qualification and career objectives
      3) Strengths and areas of growth
      4) Short- and long-term goals
      5) Ideal practice environment and arrangement
   b. *Education: list academic accomplishments*
   c. *Previous positions: brief description of roles and responsibilities*
   d. *Previous teaching experience, publications, awards*

  e. Professional and community organization involvement

C. Contract negotiation

 1. **Compensation**
  a. Salary
  b. Bonus and incentives
  c. Retirement plans
 2. **Benefits**
  a. Vacation
  b. Holidays
  c. Sick leave
 3. **Insurance**
  a. Malpractice
   1) Occurrence
   2) Claims made
  b. Health insurance
  c. Life and disability insurance
 4. **Continuing education benefit**
 5. **Job description**
  a. Lists responsibilities
  b. Defines standards of performance
  c. Reporting mechanism
  d. Pay grade
 6. **Schedule**
 7. **Practice agreements**
  a. Employee agreement: creates an employee-employer relationship governed by labor and employment laws
  b. Collaborative practice agreement: defines how an APRN and physician will work collaboratively

D. Institutional credentialing, privileges

 1. **Rationale**
  a. Defines scope of practice
  b. Delineates role and function
 2. **Process for obtaining credentialing**
  a. Who confers
  b. How to petition

II. APRN EVALUATION

A. Process evaluation

 1. **Job satisfaction**
 2. **Performance**

B. Outcome evaluation

 1. **Quality issues**
 2. **Cost issues**

C. Types of evaluation

1. **Peer review**
   a. *Review by a peer in the same job description*
   b. *Goals: increase professionalism, responsibility, and accountability*
2. **Self-evaluation**
   a. *Rate self against established performance criteria*
   b. *Set goals for next year*
3. **Group evaluation**
   a. *Evaluation done by other staff*
   b. *Use of a standardized instrument*
4. **Administration evaluation**
   a. *Evaluated by administrators*

III. ORGANIZATIONAL DEVELOPMENT

A. Affiliations

1. **National nursing organizations**
2. **State nursing organizations**
3. **Regional organizations**

B. Legislative issues

1. **Licensure**
2. **Prescriptive authority**
3. **State and federal law**
   a. *Scope of practice*
   b. *Credentialing*
   c. *Reimbursement*

IV. ORGANIZATIONAL SCOPE OF PRACTICE

A. ENA definition of APRN
B. Position statement on advance practice in emergency nursing
C. American College of Emergency Physicians (ACEP) policy statement guidelines on the role of nurse practitioners in emergency departments

BIBLIOGRAPHY

Emergency Nurses Association. (1996). Position statement: Advanced practice in emergency nursing. *ENA Position Statements*. Park Ridge, IL: Author.

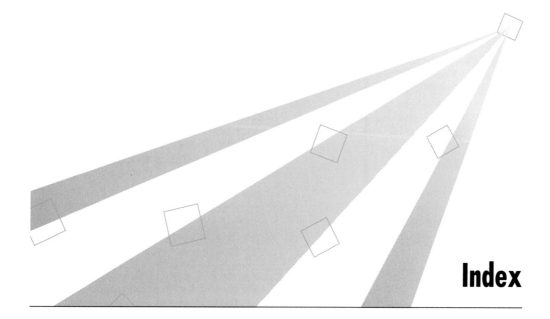

Index

Note: Page numbers in *italics* refer to illustrations; page numbers followed by (t) refer to tables.